Spermatozoa and Sperm Differentiation: Clinical Reproductive Medicine

Spermatozoa and Sperm Differentiation: Clinical Reproductive Medicine

Editor: Orion Solano

AMERICAN
MEDICAL PUBLISHERS
www.americanmedicalpublishers.com

AMERICAN
MEDICAL PUBLISHERS
www.americanmedicalpublishers.com

Cataloging-in-Publication Data

Spermatozoa and sperm differentiation : clinical reproductive medicine / edited by Orion Solano.
p. cm.
Includes bibliographical references and index.
ISBN 979-8-88740-464-6
1. Reproductive health. 2. Spermatozoa--Physiology. 3. Spermatogenesis. 4. Human reproduction.
5. Fertility, Human. 6. Embryology, Human. I. Solano, Orion.
RG133 .S64 2023
613.9--dc23

American Medical Publishers,
41 Flatbush Avenue,
1st Floor, New York,
NY 11217, USA

ISBN 979-8-88740-464-6 (Hardback)

Contents

Preface

The purpose of the book is to provide a glimpse into the dynamics and to present opinions and studies of some of the scientists engaged in the development of new ideas in the field from very different standpoints. This book will prove useful to students and researchers owing to its high content quality.

A spermatozoon or spermatozoa (plural) refers to a motile sperm cell which is the male gamete. It is also called sperm cell. Sperm differentiation is a complicated series of morphological changes that occur in the seminiferous epithelium. Throughout this process, haploid round spermatids undergo significant structural and functional changes that result in highly polarized sperm. Development of new organelles, chromatin condensation and nuclear shaping, removal of residual cytoplasm, and assembly of the sperm flagella are significant changes that take place during the differentiation process. These events need the presence of a cytoskeleton, microtubules, actin filaments, and related motor and non-motor proteins, all of which deliver the vesicular and non-vesicular cargos to the proper intracellular locations. Spermatids have distinct protein trafficking systems that coordinate together to produce these changes. This book aims to shed light on some of the unexplored aspects of sperm differentiation mechanisms. It is a compilation of chapters that discuss the most vital concepts and emerging trends in this area of study. For all those who are interested in clinical reproductive medicine, this book can prove to be an essential guide.

At the end, I would like to appreciate all the efforts made by the authors in completing their chapters professionally. I express my deepest gratitude to all of them for contributing to this book by sharing their valuable works. A special thanks to my family and friends for their constant support in this journey.

Editor

1

Paternal Contributions to Offspring's Health: Role of Sperm Small RNAs in Intergenerational Transmission of Epigenetic Information

*Upasna Sharma**

Department of Molecular, Cell and Developmental Biology, University of California, Santa Cruz, Santa Cruz, CA, United States

Correspondence:
Upasna Sharma
upsharma@ucsc.edu

The most fundamental process for the perpetuation of a species is the transfer of information from parent to offspring. Although genomic DNA contributes to the majority of the inheritance, it is now clear that epigenetic information –information beyond the underlying DNA sequence – is also passed on to future generations. However, the mechanism and extent of such inheritance are not well-understood. Here, I review some of the concepts, evidence, and mechanisms of intergenerational epigenetic inheritance via sperm small RNAs. Recent studies provide evidence that mature sperm are highly abundant in small non-coding RNAs. These RNAs are modulated by paternal environmental conditions and potentially delivered to the zygote at fertilization, where they can regulate early embryonic development. Intriguingly, sperm small RNA payload undergoes dramatic changes during testicular and post-testicular maturation, making the mature sperm epigenome highly unique and distinct from testicular germ cells. I explore the mechanism of sperm small RNA remodeling during post-testicular maturation in the epididymis, and the potential role of this reprograming in intergenerational epigenetic inheritance.

Keywords: sperm, RNA, epigenetic, inheritance, embryo development, exosomes, extracellular vesicles, transgeneration effects

INTRODUCTION

The possibility that our life experiences can influence phenotypes in our descendants has tremendous implications for basic biology and public health and policy (Jirtle and Skinner, 2007). Indeed, there is mounting evidence from worms to mammals, including humans, that parental environment can influence phenotypes in future generations (Rando, 2012; Heard and Martienssen, 2014; Rando and Simmons, 2015). However, the mechanism of such transgenerational inheritance —sometimes referred to as inheritance of acquired traits, or Lamarckian Inheritance— remains mysterious. The inheritance of acquired traits was previously refuted, as there was no known mechanism for the environment to alter the genetic material (DNA) transmitted from parents to offspring. With advances in the field of epigenetics, the inheritance that is not based on DNA sequence but how the DNA sequence is utilized, there is a renewed interest in transgenerational inheritance. Epigenetic information carriers (unlike DNA) are highly dynamic and are often modulated by environmental conditions (Sharma and Rando, 2017), suggesting that the environment experienced by parents may influence the phenotype of offspring via alterations to the gametic "epigenome." However, demonstrating intergenerational inheritance has been challenging in mammals, as such inheritance is a mechanistically complex process that would require epigenetic information to be maintained throughout the disruptive process of epigenetic reprograming during gametogenesis, carried in gametes, delivered to embryos at fertilization, and then influence embryonic development. Furthermore, the inheritance of acquired traits has been discredited by many, because of the so-called "Weismann barrier" that prevents transmission of information from somatic cells to germ cells (and thus to offspring). Paternal contributions to intergenerational epigenetic inheritance have been considered especially unlikely, because of the sheer difference in size between sperm and oocytes.

Challenging these preexisting notions about inheritance, many recent studies in mammals provide evidence that paternal exposure to different environmental stressors, such as diet, psychological stress, toxicants, etc., can influence offspring phenotypes, and sperm epigenome plays a pivotal role in the transmission of such phenotypes. Here, I review recent studies on intergenerational inheritance via male germline, discuss the potential role of small RNAs as epigenetic information carriers in sperm, and explore the mechanisms of such inheritance. Intergenerational inheritance involves transmission of parental environmental effects via exposure of the developing embryo and/or germ cells to the environmental insult (transmission from parent to offspring or grandoffspring). For instance, if a female (F0) pregnant with male offspring is exposed, both its embryo (F1) and germ cells of the embryo (F2) are directly exposed. On the other hand, transgenerational inheritance affects generations that were not directly exposed to the environmental insult (F3 and onwards) (Heard and Martienssen, 2014). I primarily discuss examples of intergenerational inheritance as it is more widely studied in mammals and few examples of transgenerational inheritance are discussed. In addition, I mainly focus on rodent studies, the readers are directed to some excellent recent reviews on transgenerational inheritance in various model organisms (Rando, 2012; Heard and Martienssen, 2014; Rechavi and Lev, 2017; Boskovic and Rando, 2018; Perez and Lehner, 2019). Understanding the mechanism of intergenerational inheritance has important implications for the etiology of human diseases. Many common metabolic disorders, such as diabetes, have both genetic components and contributions from a patient's lifestyle and environment. Only a fraction of the heritability of such diseases can be explained by genetic variation; instead, it is now increasingly appreciated that epigenetic inheritance likely contributes to such conditions (Rando and Simmons, 2015).

INTERGENERATIONAL TRANSMISSION OF PATERNAL ENVIRONMENTAL EFFECTS

Multiple studies in mammals over the past decade have demonstrated that parents pass on information about their environment to their children. In humans, undernutrition in parents has been linked to metabolic diseases in children, with epidemiological studies of the Dutch Hunger Winter of 1944–1945 (Lumey et al., 2007) providing evidence for effects of maternal starvation during pregnancy on the metabolic health of children. In case of the male germline, studies on three generations of family members in Overkalix, Sweden, demonstrated a correlation between food availability to grandfathers and health and mortality rates in their grandchildren (Kaati et al., 2002; Pembrey et al., 2006). Due to the long term interaction of the mother and the developing fetus in the womb, maternal contributions to offspring phenotypes seem plausible. Indeed, alcohol consumption during pregnancy can lead to fetal alcohol syndrome in humans (Jones and Smith, 1973). However, except for a few studies (Huypens et al., 2016), in most of the studies on maternal exposure, it is difficult to separate environmentally induced molecular changes in the oocyte from the direct effect of the environment on the developing fetus (Rando and Simmons, 2015). On the other hand, as fathers mostly contribute just sperm to the developing offspring, mechanistic investigations of paternal effects are more straightforward, and are of great interest (Rando, 2012).

A large number of laboratory studies in rodents have linked paternal treatment regimes with changes in offspring phenotype, such as dietary alterations (Anderson et al., 2006; Carone et al., 2010; Ng et al., 2010; Fullston et al., 2013; Lambrot et al., 2013; Grandjean et al., 2015; Chen et al., 2016; Huypens et al., 2016; Sharma et al., 2016), psychological stress (Dietz et al., 2011; Rodgers et al., 2013; Gapp et al., 2014; Rodgers et al., 2015; Wu et al., 2016), odor fear conditioning (Dias and Ressler, 2014), exposure to endocrine disruptor vinclozolin (Anway et al., 2005) and ethanol exposure (Rompala et al., 2018). In general, to study intergenerational inheritance of paternal phenotypes, male mice are exposed to different environmental conditions (diet, stress, etc.) and mated with control females. The timing and length of exposure vary in different studies and mostly involves either exposure from weaning to sexual maturity or during fetal development. Next, offspring phenotypic changes are monitored, such as altered glucose metabolism in response to a high-fat diet or depressive-like behavior in response to paternal chronic stress.

In rats, paternal consumption of high-fat diet leads to glucose intolerance in F1 female offspring (Ng et al., 2010). Similarly, male mice fed a low protein diet (10 vs. 19% protein, by mass) were found to sire offspring with altered hepatic cholesterol biosynthesis, relative to control offspring (Carone et al., 2010). Additional studies in mice have used interventions ranging from preconception fasting to fetal undernutrition to link paternal nutrition to glucose metabolism in offspring (Anderson et al., 2006; Jimenez-Chillaron et al., 2009). Moreover, multiple studies have investigated the effects of parental psychological stress, such as social defeat stress, early life trauma and chronic variable stress on offspring phenotypes (Dietz et al., 2011; Rodgers et al., 2013; Gapp et al., 2014). These studies report that paternal exposure to psychological stress usually leads to reduced stress sensitivity in offspring, and altered cortisol levels and glucose metabolism often accompany such phenotypes. The earliest studies in transgenerational inheritance examined the effects of exposure of pregnant female rats to endocrine disruptor Vinclozolin. F1 male offspring of vinclozolin exposed mothers displayed infertility, and this defect was transmitted to males until F4 generation (Anway et al., 2005), suggesting that paternal environmental conditions can influence the health of offspring across multiple generations. In recent years, exposure to other toxicants such as carbon tetrachloride, and drugs such as nicotine and cocaine have also been reported to influence offspring phenotypes (Zeybel et al., 2012; Vassoler et al., 2013; Vallaster et al., 2017).

It is still not clear how paternal exposure is linked to phenotypes observed in offspring, and whether those effects are adaptive. In fact, as discussed above, in most cases transmission of paternal environmental effect increases disease susceptibility in offspring. One explanation for such phenotypes comes from the "thrifty phenotype" hypothesis (Hales and Barker, 2001), wherein a compromised *in utero* environment programs offspring for a similar environment after birth, and thus, links poor fetal and infant growth with increased risk of metabolic diseases in adults born in an unmatched *ex utero* environment (Miska and Ferguson-Smith, 2016). For instance, poor nutrient availability during early development programs offspring to withstand a similar environment, leading to diabetes and obesity in subsequent generations in the absence of nutrient deprivation. Furthermore, an adaptive response might only be revealed when offspring are challenged with a specific environmental insult. It was reported that paternal preconception exposure to nicotine induced a higher metabolic tolerance for nicotine as well as other xenobiotics such as cocaine (Vallaster et al., 2017). The offspring showed higher hepatic expression of various genes involved in xenobiotic clearance, suggesting that in the case of paternal exposure to nicotine, the phenotypes observed in offspring are not specific to nicotine but broadly affects offspring tolerance to additional xenobiotics. Interestingly, this protective response was only revealed in offspring that were pre-exposed to nicotine, suggesting that the phenotypes observed in offspring of exposed fathers are influenced by the interaction of paternal environment with the environment of the offspring (Vallaster et al., 2017).

TRANSMISSION OF EPIGENETIC INFORMATION VIA SPERM

Despite the wealth of knowledge that paternal environment can influence offspring health, the mechanism of this inheritance is not well-understood in most cases. The likeliest scenario is that epigenetic information is delivered to the zygote by sperm, although alternative information carriers such as seminal fluid, microbiome, and female's judgment of male quality can also play a role (Dietz et al., 2011; Rando, 2012). Use of assisted reproduction methods such as *in vitro fertilization* (IVF) and foster mothers, where the only contribution from parents is their gametes, allows a direct test of whether paternal environmental information is passed via sperm. A few recent studies reported the effects of paternal exposure (such as diet, stress, etc.) on offspring generated via IVF, similar to those seen in offspring produced using natural mating, suggesting that paternal environmental information is indeed transmitted by sperm (Dias and Ressler, 2014; Chen et al., 2016; Huypens et al., 2016; Sharma et al., 2016). Overall, these studies suggest that paternal environment can influence the health of offspring and this information is transmitted via sperm epigenome, and raise the crucial questions: (1) which epigenetic information molecules in sperm carry environmental information? (2) how does the environment influence those epigenetic signaling molecules, and (3) how do those signals influence offspring gene expression and development? Recent studies provide key insights into these mechanistic questions about the process of intergenerational epigenetic inheritance, as discussed below.

EPIGENETIC INFORMATION CARRIERS IN SPERM

Epigenetic inheritance, the inheritance of phenotypic changes in the absence of changes in DNA sequence, is essential for the maintenance of cell states through cell division. In addition to epigenetic inheritance of cell states during organismal development, there is a growing body of evidence that epigenetic information can be transmitted from one generation to the next, with famous examples including RNA interference in *C. elegans* and paramutation in maize (Fire et al., 1998; Alleman et al., 2006; Heard and Martienssen, 2014; Holoch and Moazed, 2015). Studies of cell-state and transgenerational epigenetic inheritance have identified chromatin structure, DNA modifications, small RNAs, and prions as the main molecular carriers of epigenetic information (Sharma and Rando, 2017). The three most well-characterized epigenetic marks in sperm include histone occupancy and histone modifications, cytosine methylation of DNA, and small non-coding RNAs. Here, I focus on the role of small RNAs in intergenerational inheritance, and briefly review the current understanding of the role of chromatin and DNA methylation in such inheritance [for in depth reviews on epigenetic inheritance via chromatin and DNA methylation, please refer to Heard and Martienssen (2014), Miska and Ferguson-Smith (2016), Boskovic and Rando (2018)].

Chromatin

In eukaryotes, the genomic DNA is wrapped around a core of histone proteins to form a nucleoprotein complex known as chromatin (Kornberg and Lorch, 1999). This wrapping of DNA around the histone core regulates gene expression by modulating the accessibility of the underlying DNA sequence. Furthermore, post-translational modifications of histone proteins add another layer of regulation by recruiting various chromatin modifying enzymes (activators and repressors) to regulate gene expression. Inheritance of chromatin states from one generation to the next in multicellular organisms is complicated by the fact that chromatin undergoes dramatic changes during gametogenesis, fertilization, and early development (Yadav et al., 2018; Hao et al., 2019). In mammals, during the process of spermatogenesis, the majority of canonical histones are replaced with transition proteins, which in turn are replaced with smaller basic proteins known as protamines (Balhorn, 2007). Importantly, a small fraction of the genome escapes this remodeling. The specific regions that maintain histone occupancy during spermatogenesis is unclear, some studies show that a subset of developmentally important gene promoters retain histones (Hammoud et al., 2009, 2014; Brykczynska et al., 2010), while other recent studies report histone retention at repeat-rich regions of the genome (Carone et al., 2014; Yamaguchi et al., 2018). These conflicting results are potentially due to differences in the histone retention assays used in these studies and suggest that potentially multiple populations of nucleosomes exist in mature sperm, and depending on the protocol used, different populations are detected (Rando, 2016). It is unclear whether persisting histones in mature sperm play a role in intergenerational inheritance. A study reported that histone retention did not change in obese and lean men (Donkin et al., 2016). On the other hand, a role for histone modifications in such inheritance is suggested —carbon tetrachloride exposure lead to altered histone acetylation at specific promoters in mouse sperm (Zeybel et al., 2012). Importantly, studies from model organisms and rodents demonstrate that paternal mutations in genes coding for chromatin regulators cause altered phenotypes in offspring that do not inherit the mutation *per se* (Chong et al., 2007; Siklenka et al., 2015). For instance, overexpression of a histone lysine 4 demethylase KDMA1(LSD1) during spermatogenesis lead to impaired development of offspring for three generations, even in offspring lacking KDM1A overexpression (Siklenka et al., 2015). These studies suggest that correct histone modifications and chromatin structure during spermatogenesis is crucial for proper offspring development, and chromatin potentially plays a role in transmission of paternal environmental effects and motivate future studies to elucidate the mechanisms of such inheritance (Rando, 2016).

DNA Methylation

Methylation on the fifth carbon of cytosine results in the formation of 5-methylcytosine (5mC), which is one of the most well-characterized epigenetic information carriers. For instance, cytosine methylation is required for germline epigenetic inheritance of imprinted genes — genes that are expressed from only the maternal or paternal alleles and thus, retain the "memory" of the gender of germline they developed from Bartolomei and Ferguson-Smith (2011). As with chromatin, DNA methylation is also globally erased and reset during two rounds of reprograming, one in primordial germ cells during gametogenesis and the other in preimplantation embryos shortly after fertilization (Hackett and Surani, 2013). Certain regions of the genome escape this global erasure, including the imprinting control regions and transposons (Messerschmidt et al., 2014), suggesting that 5mC in sperm could potentially act as a carrier of paternal environmental information in offspring. Indeed, studies have examined the effects of paternal high-fat or low protein diet (Carone et al., 2010; Wei et al., 2014; Shea et al., 2015; de Castro Barbosa et al., 2016; Donkin et al., 2016), paternal folate deficient diet (Lambrot et al., 2013; Ly et al., 2017), and undernutrition (Radford et al., 2014; Holland et al., 2016) on sperm DNA methylation. Although in most of these studies, only a fraction of the differentially methylated regions are maintained in the next generation, these studies provide a strong premise to further investigate the role of DNA methylation in intergenerational inheritance.

Small Non-coding RNAs

Small RNAs play key roles in multiple, well-established epigenetic inheritance paradigms in model organisms, such as RNA interference in *C. elegans* (Fire et al., 1998) and paramutation in maize (Alleman et al., 2006). Since the discovery of micro RNAs in 1993 (Lee et al., 1993), a multitude of different classes of small RNAs (<40 nts) have been discovered which play critical regulatory roles in biology. The well-studied classes of small RNAs include micro RNAs (miRNAs), endogenous silencing RNAs (endo-siRNAs), and the germ-line enriched piwi-interacting RNAs (piRNAs). In addition, recent advances in RNA-sequencing technology has uncovered additional classes of small RNAs derived from the cleavage of tRNAs known as tRNA-derived small RNAs or tRNA fragments (tRFs). Fragmentation products of ribosomal RNAs are also detected in some biological contexts (Lambert et al., 2019); whether they are functional remains to be determined. Small RNAs primarily function in gene regulation by binding to Argonaute (Ago) family proteins, and this Ago-small RNA complex can regulate gene silencing at different levels, such as (1) transcriptional regulation by targeting DNA methylation and repressive chromatin formation at target gene (Volpe et al., 2002; Chan et al., 2004), (2) post-transcriptional regulation by degradation or deadenylation of target RNA, and (3) translational repression (Bartel, 2009). It is important to note that a subset of tRNA-fragments (mainly tRNA-halves, see below) do not work through the Ago-dependent pathways, and are involved in translational repression by directly interacting with translation machinery, polyribosomes, stress granules, etc. (Ivanov et al., 2011, 2014; Goodarzi et al., 2015; Gebetsberger et al., 2017; Keam et al., 2017; Kim et al., 2017; Dou et al., 2019).

Small RNAs can be distinguished based on their biogenesis and biological function, which in turn is often determined by their size and specific sequence characteristics (Ghildiyal and Zamore, 2009; Czech and Hannon, 2011). miRNAs are ~22 nt small non-coding RNAs processed from precursor RNA molecules. The precursor RNAs are transcribed from either intergenic regions or introns of protein-coding or non-coding RNA genes. miRNAs can also be transcribed as a long transcript from two or more miRNA genes placed adjacent to each other, called clusters, which have similar seed sequence and thus belong to the same family (Ha and Kim, 2014). The precursor transcripts are processed by Ribonuclease III enzyme Drosha to form pre-miRNAs (Lee et al., 2003). Pre-miRNAs are exported to the cytoplasm by Exportin 5 where they are further processed into mature miRNAs by an RNase III endonuclease Dicer and are loaded onto Argonaute (Ago2) to form the miRNA silencing complex (miRISC) (Hutvagner et al., 2001; Lee et al., 2003). miRISC is then recruited to the target mRNAs (mostly at the 3′ UTR in mammals) through partial base-complementarity and represses gene expression by inhibiting translation (Ha and Kim, 2014).

Piwi-interacting RNAs or piRNAs, so called because of their association with PIWI (P-element induced wimpy testis) clade of Argonaute proteins (Aravin et al., 2006; Girard et al., 2006; Grivna et al., 2006; Lau et al., 2006; Watanabe et al., 2006), are highly expressed in germ cells and are required for male fertility —male mice lacking Piwi proteins are sterile (Carmell et al., 2007). In mammals, two major classes of piRNAs have been reported based on their timing of expression and precursor transcripts: (1) pre-pachytene piRNAs: expressed in fetal and newborn mice and are homologous to various retroelements such as LINE elements, and repress transposon expression to maintain germline genomic integrity (Aravin et al., 2007), (2) pachytene piRNAs: derived from intergenic regions, lack repeat sequences, and are proposed to target spermatogenesis-related mRNAs (Li et al., 2013). In flies and vertebrates, piRNAs have preference for 5′ Uracil and 3′ 2′-*O* methylation (Vagin et al., 2006; Kirino and Mourelatos, 2007). Importantly, primary piRNAs can be amplified by producing secondary piRNAs via the so-called ping-pong cycle of amplification (Iwasaki et al., 2015). Mechanistically, piRNAs repress gene expression at both transcriptional level, by promoting *de novo* DNA methylation (Aravin et al., 2008), and post-transcriptionally by cleaving target transposon mRNAs (Reuter et al., 2011).

tRNA-fragments (tRFs) have only recently been studied in depth (Lee and Collins, 2005; Sobala and Hutvagner, 2011; Anderson and Ivanov, 2014; Kumar et al., 2016), and are therefore relatively not well-characterized. tRNAs are well-known for their role in translation as an adaptor molecule for converting information encoded in RNA molecules to peptide chains by delivering amino acids (Hoagland et al., 1958). Small RNAs derived from tRNAs include a diverse variety of RNA species, such as fragments generated by cleavage in anticodon loop known as tRNA halves, or smaller 18–22 nts fragments produced by cleavage in the D or T loops (Keam and Hutvagner, 2015). In addition, tRFs can be derived from 5′ end, 3′ ends, or middle of pre-tRNAs or mature tRNAs (Lee et al., 2009). tRFs were initially thought to be random degradation products of tRNAs. With the advent of sophisticated deep sequencing methods, recent studies revealed that tRFs are generated in a remarkably site-specific manner and are derived from a subset of tRNA isotypes in a given cell type, suggesting that their biogenesis is a highly regulated process (Keam and Hutvagner, 2015). tRNA cleavage has been characterized in several biological contexts, where it is typically induced in response to stress conditions. In budding yeast and *Tetrahymena thermophila*, RNase T2 family endonucleases process tRNAs (Andersen and Collins, 2012), whereas in mammalian cells exposed to stress, the RNase A family member Angiogenin (encoded by *RNase5*) cleaves tRNAs (Fu et al., 2009). tRFs are found in many cell types but are uniquely highly abundant in the germ cells (Peng et al., 2012; Chen et al., 2016; Sharma et al., 2016). For instance, ~70% of small RNAs in mature mammalian sperm are composed of tRFs (Peng et al., 2012; Sharma et al., 2016). Treatment of sperm small RNAs with T4 polynucleotide kinase (PNK) in the absence of ATP, which removes cyclic phosphates from the 3′ ends of RNA molecules and, thus, allows cloning of such RNAs for sequencing, revealed additional tRFs and suggested that RNaseA and/or RNase T2 family endonucleases are involved in the biogenesis of tRFs in the male reproductive tract (Sharma et al., 2018). Functions of tRFs are not well-understood, mostly due to their very recent discovery. Different tRFs might act through distinct effector pathways, as evidenced by the fact that tRFs have been reported to regulate gene expression at the transcriptional, post-transcriptional, and translational level. Proposed functions for tRFs include RNA metabolism, global (Sobala and Hutvagner, 2013) and transcript-specific translation inhibition (Ivanov et al., 2011; Goodarzi et al., 2015), ribosome biogenesis (Kim et al., 2017), targeted cleavage of 3′ UTRs (Elbarbary et al., 2009), regulation of apoptosis (Saikia et al., 2014), and regulation of retroviral elements (Sharma et al., 2016; Schorn et al., 2017).

Since mammalian sperm shed most of their cytoplasm, including RNAs, during development, they were long believed not to carry functional RNAs. However, studies in human sperm reported that sperm carry various RNA species (Ostermeier et al., 2002) and a subset of these RNAs (such as, sperm specific transcripts of Protamine-2 and Clusterin) are delivered to the oocyte (Ostermeier et al., 2004), suggesting their retention in internal structures of sperm head. With recent advances in RNA sequencing it is clear that sperm carry both long (>200 nts) and small RNAs (<200 nts). The long RNAs include mRNAs, long non-coding RNAs, and circular RNAs, and miRNAs, piRNAs, and fragmentation products of tRNAs and rRNAs constitute the major classes of small RNAs in mature mammalian sperm (Godia et al., 2018). A comprehensive database for sperm RNAs has been generated as SpermBase which curates both long and small RNAs in sperm of various species (Schuster et al., 2016b). By utilizing *in situ* hybridization, quantitative real-time PCR, microarrays, and RNA high-throughput sequencing, studies report that sperm RNAs are localized in specific compartments. Small RNAs such as miRNAs and tRFs have been sequenced in detergent-treated-sperm heads (Yan et al., 2008; Peng et al., 2012), suggesting their presence in sperm nucleus. Some miRNAs and tRFs are also present in sperm tail, and piRNAs are relatively more enriched in sperm tail compared to sperm head (Sharma et al., 2018). piRNA enrichment in tail is consistent with the localization of remnants of chromatoid body, which is involved in piRNA biogenesis, in sperm midpiece during maturation (Meikar et al., 2011; de Mateo and Sassone-Corsi, 2014). On the other hand, majority of long (>200 nt, including mRNAs) RNAs are enriched in the outer membrane of sperm and about one-third of sperm long RNAs are estimated to be present within the nuclear/peri-nuclear theca (Johnson et al., 2015). Moreover, a subset of sperm RNAs are potentially deeply embedded in the nuclear matrix of sperm nucleus, in complex with the nuclear DNA, which might be difficult to isolate during RNA extraction (Lalancette et al., 2008). Together, these studies demonstrate that a subset of sperm RNAs are embedded in the nucleus and can be delivered to the oocyte at fertilization.

The first evidence that sperm RNAs can influence offspring phenotypes comes from paramutation studies in mice, wherein, microinjection of purified sperm RNAs from mutant mice into fertilized wild type oocytes lead to transmission of mutant phenotypes to offspring (Rassoulzadegan et al., 2006; Wagner et al., 2008; Grandjean et al., 2009). While these studies focused on sperm total RNAs, more recent studies are focused on small non-coding RNAs in sperm which have the potential to regulate gene expression in early embryos. Mature mammalian sperm have a distinct payload of small RNAs, comprising chiefly of tRFs (~70%), followed by miRNAs as the second most abundant small RNAs and low levels of piRNAs (Peng et al., 2012; Sharma et al., 2016; Hutcheon et al., 2017). Interestingly, abundant tRFs have been reported in sperm of humans, mouse, rat, and bull (Schuster et al., 2016b), suggesting sperm-specific abundance of tRFs is a widespread phenomenon. In addition, fragmentation products of ribosomal RNAs are also present in substantial amount in mature sperm (Chu et al., 2017; Sharma et al., 2018). Some studies have also identified endo-siRNAs and mitochondrial genome enriched small RNAs (mitosRNAs) in mammalian germ cells (Song et al., 2011; Schuster et al., 2016b).

Recent studies provide strong evidence that small RNAs are the environmentally-responsive epigenetic marks in sperm (Fullston et al., 2013; Grandjean et al., 2015; Chen et al., 2016; de Castro Barbosa et al., 2016; Sharma et al., 2016; Zhang et al., 2019). Mice consuming a low protein or high-fat diet have altered levels of small RNAs in mature sperm. A low protein diet leads to upregulation of 5′ fragment of multiple isoacceptors of tRNA-Glycine (tRF-GlyGCC, tRF-GlyTCC, and tRF-GlyCCC), tRNA-LysCTT and tRNA-HisGTT and down-regulation of a miRNA Let7c (Sharma et al., 2016), while a high-fat diet results in an overall increase in the levels of tRFs (~11%) (Chen et al., 2016). In rats, high fat diet consumption also showed changes in specific small RNAs including, piRNAs (piR-025883, piR-015935, piR-036085), miRNAs (Let7c, miR293, miR880) and tRFs (GluCTC) (de Castro Barbosa et al., 2016). tRFs and Let7 miRNA thus seem to be common small RNAs modulated by diet. Mice fed a western diet (high fat and high sugar) also have altered levels of specific miRNAs in their sperm (Grandjean et al., 2015). Moreover, exposure to toxicants, such as vinclozolin and chronic ethanol exposure, affected tRF and miRNA levels (Schuster et al., 2016a; Rompala et al., 2018). Similarly, exposure to psychological stress, such as early life trauma or chronic stress, lead to changes in levels of specific miRNAs (Gapp et al., 2014; Rodgers et al., 2015).

The implication of sperm small RNAs in intergenerational inheritance of paternal environmental conditions was demonstrated by studies using direct microinjections of small RNAs purified from the sperm of exposed males into control zygotes. In one of the first such studies, mice were exposed to maternal separation coupled with unpredictable maternal stress (MSUS) to induce early life stress. The MSUS mice showed depressive-life behavior, and such behavior was transmitted to their offspring. Injection of RNAs purified from sperm of MSUS mice into one-cell control embryos lead to the transmission of a subset of the behavioral and metabolic trait of MSUS mice to their offspring. This study provided the first direct evidence that paternal environmental information is transmitted by sperm RNAs, and identified a specific set of miRNAs that change in MSUS sperm in response to stress (Gapp et al., 2014). Another study examined intergenerational inheritance of paternal chronic stress and identified nine specific miRNAs that were significantly up-regulated in sperm of exposed mice (Rodgers et al., 2013). Injection of these nine miRNAs (in combination) in control zygotes lead to the transmission of paternal behavioral traits to the offspring (Rodgers et al., 2015). Similarly, in the case of high-fat diet paradigm, microinjection of purified tRFs (30–40 nt size RNAs) into control zygotes reproduced metabolic phenotypes in offspring (as seen by natural mating), suggesting that tRFs potentially act as epigenetic information carriers of paternal dietary information (Chen et al., 2016).

Overall, multiple recent studies suggest that various environmental exposures direct distinct small RNA changes in sperm —diet mainly affects tRFs, while psychological stress influences miRNAs. Whether such differences arise from variation in the methods used for sperm small RNA profiling by different groups or distinct environmental insults are signaled to different classes of small RNAs is not clear. Irrespective, these studies provide strong evidence that small RNAs are environmentally-responsive epigenetic molecules in sperm. Moreover, a recent study reported that both small and long RNAs influence paternal exposure phenotypes of early life trauma in offspring, with long and small RNAs regulating different behavioral traits (Gapp et al., 2018). Although the identity of the specific long and small RNAs involved in such inheritance and their mechanism of regulating offspring phenotype remains unknown, these studies suggest that both small and long RNAs potentially play a role in transmitting complex paternal phenotypes to offspring.

Whether one epigenetic mark is more potent at responding to a certain environmental insult is still not clear. Depending on the type of environmental exposure and the developmental timing of exposure, one epigenetic mark might be more responsive compared to the other. For instance, sperm of mice fed a low protein diet from birth to weaning displayed changes in DNA methylation at ribosomal DNA (rDNA) (Holland et al., 2016), however, if mice are challenged with a low protein diet starting at weaning, levels of specific small RNAs change while rDNA methylation remains unaltered (Shea et al., 2015; Sharma et al., 2016). Although sperm epigenome could be modulated by the environment throughout the life of an organism, it is likely more vulnerable during early development, including embryogenesis and primordial germ cell (PGC) development, when rapid cell division and global reprograming take place. Finally, there could be a cross-talk between different epigenetic marks to relay paternal environmental information to offspring.

ROLE OF SOMA-GERMLINE COMMUNICATION IN SHAPING SPERM RNA PAYLOAD

The ability of environmental conditions, such as diet, to influence phenotypes in future generations requires that environmental exposure induces changes in the epigenome of gametes. The nature and mechanism of shaping and altering the epigenome of mammalian gametes are not well-understood. One possibility is that somatic cells communicate information to the gametes and, thus, to progeny. Although the Weismann barrier has long been thought to be a problem for such communication (Liu, 2011), over the past decade, an increasing number of studies have suggested soma-to-germline shipment of RNAs in various model organisms (Bourc'his and Voinnet, 2010). Studies in model organisms (e.g., ciliates, flies, and plants), suggest that during gametogenesis RNAs produced in somatic support cells are transferred into developing germ cells where they regulate genomic integrity (Bourc'his and Voinnet, 2010; Martinez et al., 2016). In mammals, there is no direct contact between the somatic support cells and mature gametes, as found in some of the organisms mentioned above —germline and vegetative nuclei are present in the same cytoplasm in ciliates and plants— making soma-germline communication challenging in mammals. Nonetheless, recent studies provide evidence of RNA-mediated soma-germline communication in mammals (Sharma et al., 2016, 2018; Morgan et al., 2019; Trigg et al., 2019).

Post-testicular sperm maturation takes place in the epididymis, a long, convoluted tubular organ where sperm enter after exiting the testis. Intriguingly, recent studies report that sperm small RNA payload undergoes dramatic changes during epididymal transit. Deep sequencing of small RNAs from sperm at various stages of development revealed that while testicular sperm populations such as spermatocytes, round spermatids, and mature testicular spermatozoa are highly enriched in piRNAs (Kuramochi-Miyagawa et al., 2004; Aravin et al., 2006, 2007; Li et al., 2013; Sharma et al., 2018), mature sperm from the distal cauda epididymis are chiefly comprised of tRFs (Peng et al., 2012; Sharma et al., 2016, 2018). Moreover, even the proximal caput epididymis sperm are highly abundant in tRFs (Sharma et al., 2016), suggesting that tRFs are specifically gained upon entry in the epididymis. Interestingly, miRNAs also undergo dynamic changes during epididymal transit, wherein miRNAs such as miRNA 17–92 cluster, are present in testicular spermatozoa, lost in proximal caput epididymis sperm and then reappear in mature cauda sperm (Nixon et al., 2015; Sharma et al., 2018). These studies provide evidence of a novel RNA reprograming event during post-testicular maturation in the epididymis, and raise the question of how small RNAs are gained/lost during epididymal transit.

During the process of spermatogenesis, spermatozoa shed most of their cytoplasm as residual body (Sprando and Russell, 1987) and in the cytoplasmic droplet (Bloom and Nicander, 1961), a subset of small RNAs are potentially lost through this mechanism (Sharma et al., 2018). More puzzling is the gain of small RNAs in transcriptionally silent mature sperm, and suggest that small RNA increase during epididymal maturation is likely not mediated by intrinsic pathways. Indeed, recent studies report astonishing observations that small RNAs in mature sperm are shipped from surrounding somatic epididymis epithelial cells (Sharma et al., 2016, 2018). Epididymis epithelium is highly abundant in sperm-specific small RNAs (tRFs and miRNAs) (Sharma et al., 2016), and by spatiotemporal metabolic labeling of RNAs (Gay et al., 2013), it was demonstrated that mature sperm carry RNAs initially synthesized in the somatic epididymis tissue (Sharma et al., 2018). Together, these studies provide the first evidence of RNA-mediated soma-germline communication in mammals and suggest that post-testicular maturation in the epididymis shapes the small RNA payload of mature mammalian sperm. Intriguingly, sperm DNA methylation is also modulated during epididymal maturation —specific genes were unmethylated in the mature testicular spermatozoa, but remethylated during epididymal maturation (Ariel et al., 1994). Whether such changes in DNA methylation occur genome-wide and have functional consequences during early development remains unknown. In addition to epididymis, other somatic accessory cells of the male reproductive tract, such as, Leydig cells and Sertoli cells, which are in close proximity to the developing germ cells and serve important roles in spermatogenesis (Sharpe et al., 1990; Rebourcet et al., 2014), may also play a role in shaping the epigenome of developing germ cells.

What is the mechanism of this soma-germline communication? Sperm acquire a multitude of lipids and proteins during epididymal transit (Gervasi and Visconti, 2017). A subset of these proteins and lipids are delivered from epididymis to sperm via extracellular vesicles (EVs) secreted from epididymis epithelium, known as epididymosomes (Rejraji et al., 2006; Sullivan et al., 2007; Koch et al., 2015; Sullivan, 2015, 2016). Recent studies revealed that epididymosomes are highly abundant in small RNAs and have a similar RNA payload to that of mature sperm. Moreover, *in vitro* reconstitution studies revealed that epididymosomes can deliver small RNAs to relatively "immature" testicular spermatozoa (Reilly et al., 2016; Sharma et al., 2016), suggesting that epididymosome-mediated delivery of small RNAs is one mechanism of RNA-mediated communication between somatic epididymis cells and sperm.

Deep sequencing of small RNA profiles of epididymis and epididymosomes revealed that only a subset of small RNAs present in the epididymal epithelium are present in epididymosomes (Belleannee et al., 2013; Reilly et al., 2016; Schuster et al., 2016b), suggesting that instead of being passively released by epididymal epithelial cells, subpopulations of epididymal small RNAs are selectively packaged into epididymosomes. The mechanistic basis of selective sorting of small RNAs into epididymosomes remains unknown. Mechanistic studies on RNA sorting into EVs secreted from activated T-lymphocytes revealed that these EVs have a specific miRNA profile which differs from parent cells, with sumoylated hnRNP2AB1 protein being responsible for sorting miRNAs containing a specific tetranucleotide motif into EVs (Villarroya-Beltri et al., 2013). Potentially, similar mechanisms involving specific sequence motifs and/or RNA binding proteins facilitate selective sorting of small RNAs into epididymosomes. Moreover, recent studies in exosomes (a class of 100–150 nm EVs) secreted from HEK293T cells revealed an exosome-specific post-transcriptional modification in tRNAs (Shurtleff et al., 2017), suggesting an additional mechanism of selective sorting of RNAs into epididymosomes. Importantly, recent studies provide insights in the process of delivery of epididymosomal protein cargo to sperm (Zhou et al., 2019). Sperm plasma membrane has unusually high abundance of polyunsaturated phospholipids which compartmentalize its proteins and lipids into specific domains known as lipid rafts (Kawano et al., 2011). Studies suggest a role of these lipid rafts in coordination of initial epididymosome-sperm interaction (Girouard et al., 2009). Since epididymosomal membrane-bound proteins are not detected on sperm (Gatti et al., 2005), it is speculated that epididymosomes adhere transiently to sperm by tethering to receptors at the post-acrosomal domain of the sperm head, which is followed by formation of a fusion pore (Nixon et al., 2019; Trigg et al., 2019; Zhou et al., 2019).

Intriguingly, epididymosomes are a heterogeneous mix of EVs that can be classified into subcategories based on their size and biogenesis (Sullivan, 2015). The various subpopulations of epididymosomes potentially target different cell types. For instance, a subset of epididymosomes may communicate with maturing sperm (Reilly et al., 2016; Sharma et al., 2016, 2018), another subset between different regions of the epididymis (e.g., lumicrine signaling) (Belleannee et al., 2013), and a third subset between the epididymis and the oviduct following delivery to the female reproductive tract via the seminal fluid. Moreover, epididymosome-mediated small RNA delivery to sperm could potentially be regulated at various levels, for example, by regulating the ability of different EVs to interact with sperm and, possibly, by regulating the subset of sperm that receive cargo from specific classes of EVs.

Other mechanisms of RNA-mediated soma-germline communication potentially involve direct shipment of RNAs to sperm in a complex with RNA binding proteins (RBPs), as has been seen in other mammalian cells (Wang et al., 2010; Arroyo et al., 2011; Sarkies and Miska, 2014). Finally, since ejaculated sperm still has a substantial distance to travel before fertilizing the oocyte in the female reproductive tract, EVs secreted from prostate gland (prostasomes; Sullivan and Saez, 2013) or the female reproductive tract (Al-Dossary et al., 2013), potentially further alter the small RNA payload of fertilization-competent sperm.

The functional significance of epididymis specific small RNA remodeling during post-testicular maturation is not well-understood. Recent studies report that small RNA shipment from the epididymis to sperm is essential for embryo implantation (Conine et al., 2018). Embryos generated using intracytoplasmic sperm injections (ICSIs) of immature sperm from the proximal caput epididymis exhibited misregulation of multiple regulatory genes throughout preimplantation development and eventually failed soon after implantation (Conine et al., 2018). Remarkably, microinjections of small RNAs (18–40 nt) purified from cauda epididymosomes completely rescued the post-implantation embryonic lethality phenotype, suggesting an essential role of epididymosomal RNAs in early embryonic development (Conine et al., 2018). However, these studies contradict prior studies in mice reporting successful generation of offspring from ICSI using caput sperm (Suganuma et al., 2005). As discussed in Conine et al. (2018), these discrepancies could arise from differences in the mouse strain background, age of the male, the timing of embryo implantation and the procedure used for the preparation of sperm heads for ICSI. The latter is of particular importance, since prior studies have documented that epididymosomes interact with sperm in a site specific manner (Griffiths et al., 2008; Zhou et al., 2019), and therefore, inclusion/exclusion of certain parts of the sperm could result in different RNA payload being delivered to the oocyte. Future studies, using mice defective in one or more pathways of epididymosome biogenesis and delivery, will shed more light on the functional consequences of shipment of RNA from the epididymis to sperm and its influence on offspring phenotypes.

ENVIRONMENTAL SIGNALING TO SPERM RNAs

An understanding of how environmental conditions influence epigenetic marks in the gametes is essential to elucidate how paternal environment affects phenotypes in offspring. As discussed above, numerous studies provide evidence that paternal environmental conditions, such as altered diet or stress, influence small RNA levels in sperm, however, the mechanistic understanding of how any of the environmental exposures noted above cause specific changes in sperm small RNA levels is largely lacking. Broadly, paternal environment can affect sperm small RNA levels by (1) regulating the transcription of small RNA precursors, (2) regulating small RNA processing, (3) modulating small RNA decay/stability, (4) influencing sorting of small RNAs into epididymosomes, and (5) affecting delivery of epididymosomal cargo to sperm.

RNA post-transcriptional modifications provide the most compelling potential mechanism of environmental signaling to small RNA levels. RNA modifications can affect RNA base-pairing, the secondary structure of the RNA, and RNA–protein interactions and, thus, add a new layer of transcriptional regulation (Roundtree et al., 2017). Indeed, sperm small RNAs from mice consuming a high-fat diet showed increased levels of 5-methylcytosine (m5C) and *N*-2-methylguanosine (m2G) (Chen et al., 2016) and mice exposed to ethanol were reported to have higher levels of 5′-methylaminomethyl-2-thiouridine (mnm^5s^2U) and formylcytidine (f^5C) (Rompala et al., 2018). Not only do these modifications provide stability to tRFs (Chen et al., 2016), they potentially play a role in intergenerational inheritance of paternal environmental conditions —deletion of a tRNA methyltransferase, Dnmt2, which adds m5C to specific tRNAs, prevents transmission of paternal high-fat phenotype to offspring (Zhang et al., 2018). The modified tRFs potentially remain stable in the oocyte at the time of fertilization and thus allow transmission of paternal epigenetic information. However, in the studies noted above, 30–40 nt small RNA fraction (comprising chiefly of tRFs) were examined to identify modified nucleotides by liquid chromatography with tandem mass spectrometry (LC-MS/MS). It is crucial to identify the precise small RNAs that are modified and the specific location of the modified residue, to better understand the mechanistic basis and functional significance of altered post-transcriptional modifications in response to various environmental stimuli. A combination of mass spectrometry, RNA-sequencing, and affinity pull-down approaches will help resolve these issues. How do changes in environmental conditions lead to changes in tRF modifications? As the levels of tRNA modifications have been shown to respond to nutrient availability (Laxman et al., 2013), dietary changes could affect the levels of critical metabolites, such as *S*-adenosyl methionine (SAM), resulting in global changes in levels of specific tRNA modifications and alterations in tRNA processing and/or stability (Schaefer et al., 2010;

Tuorto et al., 2012; Sharma and Rando, 2017). However, how non-metabolism related environmental exposures, such as ethanol, affect tRF modifications remains mysterious.

Communication between somatic cells and germ cells is not only crucial for the maintenance of germ cell integrity, as suggested in model organisms (Bourc'his and Voinnet, 2010; Martinez et al., 2016), it also provides a potential mechanism for transmitting environmental information to gametes and thereby influencing phenotypes in future generations (**Figure 1**). For instance, epididymis may serve as an environment sensing organ and transmit this information (in the form of small RNAs) to the maturing sperm, and hence, to offspring. Consistent with such possibility, paternal low protein consumption affects small RNA levels throughout the male reproductive tract, including the epididymis (Sharma et al., 2016). Moreover, paternal exposure to ethanol resulted in similar changes in tRF levels in epididymosomes and sperm, suggesting that paternal environmental information is signaled from the epididymis to sperm via epididymosomes (Rompala et al., 2018). Mechanistically, the authors reported reduced expression of Nsun2 —a 5′ cytosine methyltransferase known to prevent tRF biogenesis by inhibiting cleavage of specific tRNAs (Tuorto et al., 2012)— in the epididymis of mice exposed to ethanol (Rompala et al., 2018), suggesting that reduced expression of Nsun2 in the epididymis leads to increased levels of tRFs in epididymosomes, which in turn affects levels of tRFs in sperm. Overall, these studies suggest that epididymis-mediated remodeling of sperm small RNA payload is modulated by the environment, potentially leading to the transmission of environmental information to the next generation (**Figure 1**).

FUNCTIONAL CONSEQUENCES OF SPERM SMALL RNA PAYLOAD

How do changes in sperm small RNAs in response to various environmental conditions result in the transmission of paternally acquired phenotypes in offspring? Mature sperm deliver their RNAs to the oocyte at the time of fertilization, and hence, potentially regulate early embryonic gene expression to affect offspring phenotypes. Indeed, recent studies provide evidence that sperm small RNAs play important, and in some cases, essential role during early development. Microinjection of a synthetic 5′ fragment of tRNA-GlyGCC (tRFGlyGCC) or an inhibitor of tRFGlyGCC —among the most abundant small RNAs in sperm, which is up-regulated in low protein sperm— in control zygotes revealed that tRFGlyGCC represses transcription of a specific set of MERVL retroviral element-driven genes in early embryos (Sharma et al., 2016). While tRFGlyGCC was shown to regulate MERVL expression at the transcriptional level (Sharma et al., 2016), the mechanistic basis of tRF-mediated MERVL-driven gene regulation remains unclear. Intriguingly, genes regulated by tRFGlyGCC were previously shown to be activated during zygotic genome activation in two cell embryos and associated with totipotency program of early embryos (Macfarlan et al., 2012). These findings suggest that tRF-mediated gene expression changes in early embryos potentially lead to altered placental function, which in turn can lead to metabolic phenotypes in offspring as a secondary effect of altered preimplantation development (Sharma et al., 2016). Additionally, 3′ tRFs have been shown to inhibit LTR-retrotransposons in preimplantation trophoblast stem cells (Schorn et al., 2017). Northern blot analysis revealed abundant 3′ tRFs (difficult to sequence with standard small RNA sequencing protocols) in the epididymis and mature sperm (Sharma et al., 2018; Zhang et al., 2018), suggesting that sperm 3′ tRFs potentially play roles in regulating LTR-retrotransposons in preimplantation embryos.

While these studies examined the functions of specific tRFs, another group examined the broad functions of 30–40 nts sperm small RNAs (comprising chiefly of tRFs). Microinjection of 30–40 nts small RNAs purified from sperm of mice fed high-fat diet in control zygotes resulted in altered expression of multiple genes involved in metabolic regulation in eight-cell embryos and blastocysts, suggesting that a cascade of gene expression changes in preimplantation embryos potentially leads to metabolic phenotypes in adult pancreatic islet cells (Chen et al., 2016). Importantly, embryos generated using mice harboring deletion of Dicer, an endonuclease required for miRNAs and endo-siRNAs biogenesis (Ha and Kim, 2014), exhibit reduced developmental potential and altered expression of genes involved in zygotic genome activation (Yuan et al., 2016), further demonstrating that sperm delivered small RNAs play important roles during early development. Overall, these studies point to a role of sperm small RNAs in regulating some crucial steps of early developmental (zygotic genome activation, for instance) and the altered phenotypes in offspring being a secondary downstream effect.

Although, sperm small RNAs are a strong candidate for intergenerational inheritance of paternal environmental effects, many mechanistic questions remain unanswered regarding the delivery and functional consequences of sperm RNAs during early embryonic development. *First,* the RNAs that change in response to environmental conditions are not particularly abundant in sperm. For instance, the most abundant tRFs in sperm are estimated to be at ~100–100,000 molecules per sperm (Sharma et al., 2016). *Second,* the amount of RNA microinjected in the above-mentioned studies is larger than the amount of RNA a single sperm could deliver, and sperm deliver very low amount of RNA at fertilization compared to the amount of RNA in an oocyte. That said, the microinjection studies, along with studies using genetic manipulation of small RNA biogenesis pathways, provide evidence that altering RNA levels or integrity has profound effects on early embryonic development and health of offspring. Moreover, although sperm small RNAs are present in lower abundance, they likely possess some unique features that make them highly efficient in regulating gene expression —potentially due to post-transcriptional modifications (as discussed above) or pre-loading in some RNA-protein effector complexes. Furthermore, epididymosomes adhering to the surface of the sperm might play important regulatory roles in delivering additional RNAs to the female reproductive tract or the oocyte (Sharma and Rando, 2017; Conine et al., 2018). *Three,* since mammals do not express a known RNA-dependent RNA polymerase —found in various

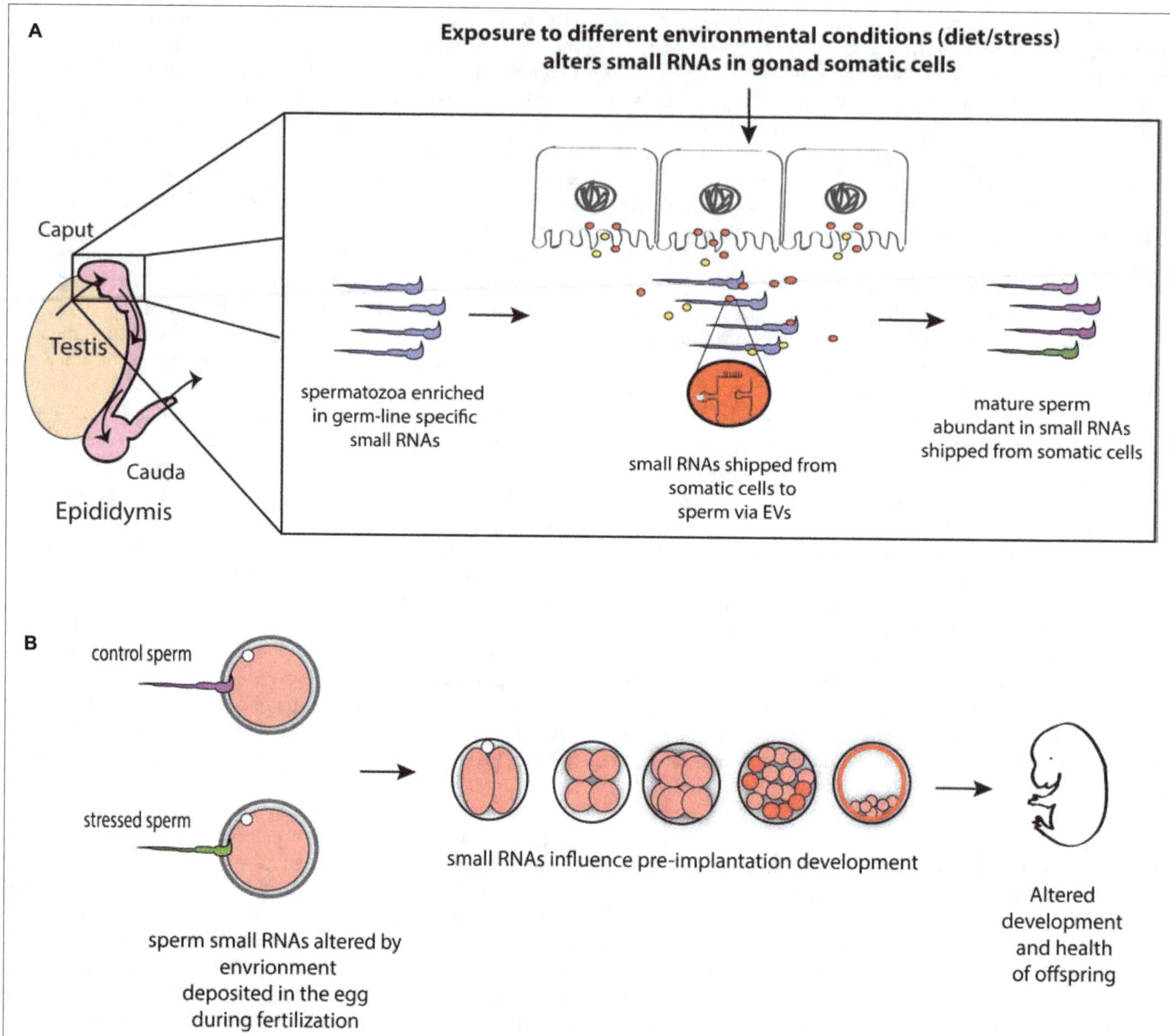

FIGURE 1 | Model for the role of RNA-mediated soma-germline communication in intergenerational inheritance. **(A)** During spermatogenesis and post-testicular maturation, small RNAs generated in the gonad somatic cells (for instance, epididymis) are shipped to sperm via extracellular vesicles (EVs) (and potentially as RNA bound to proteins). The abundance and/or shipment of these small RNAs can be modulated by environmental conditions, leading to an altered small RNA payload of sperm. **(B)** Sperm small RNAs are delivered to the oocyte at fertilization where they potentially affect early embryonic gene expression, resulting in altered early development and health of adult offspring.

model organisms such as plants and worms, where it is involved in amplifying small RNA signals— it is not clear how sperm small RNAs delivered at fertilization will have prolonged effects on phenotypes in adults. Sperm small RNAs likely regulate some crucial developmental events during the first few cell-divisions, which in turn lead to long-lasting effects on offspring phenotypes. Finally, sperm carry multiple additional non-coding RNAs, such as rRNA fragments, piRNAs, snoRNAs, and long non-coding RNAs, future studies should focus on understanding the roles, if any, of these RNAs in shaping offspring phenotypes.

CONCLUSION AND FUTURE PERSPECTIVES

There is a growing body of evidence, from worms to humans, suggesting that parental environment can influence phenotypes in offspring. However, the mechanistic basis of such inheritance is only starting to be understood. Recent advances in our understanding of intergenerational inheritance revealed that paternal environmental information is transmitted to offspring via sperm and that small RNAs are environmentally-responsive epigenetic molecules in sperm. Intriguingly, epididymis-mediated remodeling of sperm small RNA payload may have consequences for early embryonic development and offspring health. As this remodeling can be modulated by paternal environment, it provides a potential mechanism of transmission of environmental information to the next generation. Future studies will focus on elucidating the mechanism of RNA-mediated soma-germline communication and its consequences on offspring health.

These studies have important implications for human reproductive health. For assisted reproduction in humans, in some cases spermatozoa from testicular biopsies are used for fertilizing oocytes. Therefore, elucidating the functional consequences of sperm small RNA remodeling during post-testicular maturation in the epididymis has important implications for assisted reproduction in humans. Moreover, the seminal fluid also contains a high abundance of exosomes enriched in non-coding RNAs (Vojtech et al., 2014) and EVs are found in most of the bodily fluids such as serum and cerebrospinal fluid (Raposo and Stoorvogel, 2013; Colombo et al., 2014). These observations suggest the intriguing possibility that small RNA loaded EVs might play a crucial role in long-range communication at an organismal level and transmit epigenetic information from distant organs to the developing germ cells, and, hence, to the offspring.

Many important questions remain unanswered regarding the role of sperm small RNAs in intergenerational inheritance. For example, how many pieces of information is packaged in sperm — do sperm carry information about the general quality of life or transmit more specific information about various environmental exposures? How does the environment influence the small RNA payload in sperm? How do changes in sperm small RNA levels affect zygote to give rise to altered phenotypes in offspring? Since different paternal exposures, such a high-fat diet or early life trauma, result in a common metabolic phenotypes (for example, glucose intolerance), are some common pathways targeted by distinct classes of small RNAs? Finally, what is the mechanism of transgenerational inheritance? Since mammals lack a known RNA-dependent RNA polymerase, sperm small RNAs potentially influence early embryonic chromatin and/or DNA methylation states to transmit epigenetic information to the future generations. With recent advances in the field of single-cell omics, a more in-depth examination of sperm and embryonic epigenome will help shed light on these and other outstanding questions, and elucidate the mechanism of transgenerational inheritance of acquired traits.

AUTHOR CONTRIBUTIONS

The author confirms being the sole contributor of this work and has approved it for publication.

FUNDING

US was supported by the start-up funds from the University of California, Santa Cruz.

ACKNOWLEDGMENTS

I would like to thank the members of my lab for their helpful discussions on this topic.

REFERENCES

Al-Dossary, A. A., Strehler, E. E., and Martin-Deleon, P. A. (2013). Expression and secretion of plasma membrane Ca2+-ATPase 4a (PMCA4a) during murine estrus: association with oviductal exosomes and uptake in sperm. *PLoS One* 8:e80181. doi: 10.1371/journal.pone.0080181

Alleman, M., Sidorenko, L., McGinnis, K., Seshadri, V., Dorweiler, J. E., White, J., et al. (2006). An RNA-dependent RNA polymerase is required for paramutation in maize. *Nature* 442, 295–298. doi: 10.1038/nature04884

Andersen, K. L., and Collins, K. (2012). Several RNase T2 enzymes function in induced tRNA and rRNA turnover in the ciliate *Tetrahymena*. *Mol. Biol. Cell* 23, 36–44. doi: 10.1091/mbc.E11-08-0689

Anderson, L. M., Riffle, L., Wilson, R., Travlos, G. S., Lubomirski, M. S., and Alvord, W. G. (2006). Preconceptional fasting of fathers alters serum glucose in offspring of mice. *Nutrition* 22, 327–331. doi: 10.1016/j.nut.2005.09.006

Anderson, P., and Ivanov, P. (2014). tRNA fragments in human health and disease. *FEBS Lett.* 588, 4297–4304. doi: 10.1016/j.febslet.2014.09.001

Anway, M. D., Cupp, A. S., Uzumcu, M., and Skinner, M. K. (2005). Epigenetic transgenerational actions of endocrine disruptors and male fertility. *Science* 308, 1466–1469. doi: 10.1126/science.1108190

Aravin, A., Gaidatzis, D., Pfeffer, S., Lagos-Quintana, M., Landgraf, P., Iovino, N., et al. (2006). A novel class of small RNAs bind to MILI protein in mouse testes. *Nature* 442, 203–207. doi: 10.1038/nature04916

Aravin, A. A., Sachidanandam, R., Bourc'his, D., Schaefer, C., Pezic, D., Toth, K. F., et al. (2008). A piRNA pathway primed by individual transposons is linked to de novo DNA methylation in mice. *Mol. Cell* 31, 785–799. doi: 10.1016/j.molcel.2008.09.003

Aravin, A. A., Sachidanandam, R., Girard, A., Fejes-Toth, K., and Hannon, G. J. (2007). Developmentally regulated piRNA clusters implicate MILI in transposon control. *Science* 316, 744–747. doi: 10.1126/science.1142612

Ariel, M., Cedar, H., and Mccarrey, J. (1994). Developmental-changes in methylation of spermatogenesis-specific genes include reprogramming in the epididymis. *Nat. Genetics* 7, 59–63. doi: 10.1038/ng0594-59

Arroyo, J. D., Chevillet, J. R., Kroh, E. M., Ruf, I. K., Pritchard, C. C., Gibson, D. F., et al. (2011). Argonaute2 complexes carry a population of circulating microRNAs independent of vesicles in human plasma. *Proc. Natl. Acad. Sci. U.S.A.* 108, 5003–5008. doi: 10.1073/pnas.1019055108

Balhorn, R. (2007). The protamine family of sperm nuclear proteins. *Genome Biol.* 8, 227. doi: 10.1186/gb-2007-8-9-227

Bartel, D. P. (2009). MicroRNAs: target recognition and regulatory functions. *Cell* 136, 215–233. doi: 10.1016/j.cell.2009.01.002

Bartolomei, M. S., and Ferguson-Smith, A. C. (2011). Mammalian genomic imprinting. *Cold Spring Harb. Perspect. Biol.* 3:a002592. doi: 10.1101/cshperspect.a002592

Belleannee, C., Calvo, E., Caballero, J., and Sullivan, R. (2013). Epididymosomes convey different repertoires of microRNAs throughout the bovine epididymis. *Biol. Reprod.* 89:30. doi: 10.1095/biolreprod.113.110486

Bloom, G., and Nicander, L. (1961). On the ultrastructure and development of the protoplasmic droplet of spermatozoa. *Zeitschrift Fur Zellforschung Und Mikroskopische Anatomie* 55, 833–844. doi: 10.1007/Bf00381652

Boskovic, A., and Rando, O. J. (2018). Transgenerational epigenetic inheritance. *Annu. Rev. Genet.* 52, 21–41. doi: 10.1146/annurev-genet-120417-031404

Bourc'his, D., and Voinnet, O. (2010). A small-RNA perspective on gametogenesis, fertilization, and early zygotic development. *Science* 330, 617–622. doi: 10.1126/science.1194776

Brykczynska, U., Hisano, M., Erkek, S., Ramos, L., Oakeley, E. J., Roloff, T. C., et al. (2010). Repressive and active histone methylation mark distinct promoters in human and mouse spermatozoa. *Nat. Struct. Mol. Biol.* 17, 679–687. doi: 10.1038/nsmb.1821

Carmell, M. A., Girard, A., van de Kant, H. J. G., Bourc'his, D., Bestor, T. H., de Rooij, D. G., et al. (2007). MIWI2 is essential for spermatogenesis and repression of transposons in the mouse male germline. *Dev. Cell* 12, 503–514. doi: 10.1016/j.devcel.2007.03.001

Carone, B. R., Fauquier, L., Habib, N., Shea, J. M., Hart, C. E., Li, R., et al. (2010). Paternally induced transgenerational environmental reprogramming of metabolic gene expression in mammals. *Cell* 143, 1084–1096. doi: 10.1016/j.cell.2010.12.008

Carone, B. R., Hung, J. H., Hainer, S. J., Chou, M. T., Carone, D. M., Weng, Z., et al. (2014). High-resolution mapping of chromatin packaging in mouse embryonic stem cells and sperm. *Dev. Cell* 30, 11–22. doi: 10.1016/j.devcel.2014.05.024

Chan, S. W., Zilberman, D., Xie, Z., Johansen, L. K., Carrington, J. C., and Jacobsen, S. E. (2004). RNA silencing genes control de novo DNA methylation. *Science* 303:1336. doi: 10.1126/science.1095989

Chen, Q., Yan, M., Cao, Z., Li, X., Zhang, Y., Shi, J., et al. (2016). Sperm tsRNAs contribute to intergenerational inheritance of an acquired metabolic disorder. *Science* 351, 397–400. doi: 10.1126/science.aad7977

Chong, S., Vickaryous, N., Ashe, A., Zamudio, N., Youngson, N., Hemley, S., et al. (2007). Modifiers of epigenetic reprogramming show paternal effects in the mouse. *Nat. Genet.* 39, 614–622. doi: 10.1038/ng2031

Chu, C., Yu, L., Wu, B., Ma, L., Gou, L. T., He, M., et al. (2017). A sequence of 28S rRNA-derived small RNAs is enriched in mature sperm and various somatic tissues and possibly associates with inflammation. *J. Mol. Cell Biol.* 9, 256–259. doi: 10.1093/jmcb/mjx016

Colombo, M., Raposo, G., and Thery, C. (2014). biogenesis, secretion, and intercellular interactions of exosomes and other extracellular vesicles. *Annu. Rev. Cell Dev. Biol.* 30, 255–289. doi: 10.1146/annurev-cellbio-101512-122326

Conine, C. C., Sun, F., Song, L., Rivera-Perez, J. A., and Rando, O. J. (2018). Small RNAs gained during epididymal transit of sperm are essential for embryonic development in mice. *Dev. Cell* 46, 470–480.e3. doi: 10.1016/j.devcel.2018.06.024

Czech, B., and Hannon, G. J. (2011). Small RNA sorting: matchmaking for argonautes. *Nat. Rev. Genet.* 12, 19–31. doi: 10.1038/nrg2916

de Castro Barbosa, T., Ingerslev, L. R., Alm, P. S., Versteyhe, S., Massart, J., Rasmussen, M., et al. (2016). High-fat diet reprograms the epigenome of rat spermatozoa and transgenerationally affects metabolism of the offspring. *Mol. Metab.* 5, 184–197. doi: 10.1016/j.molmet.2015.12.002

de Mateo, S., and Sassone-Corsi, P. (2014). Regulation of spermatogenesis by small non-coding RNAs: role of the germ granule. *Semin. Cell Dev. Biol.* 29, 84–92. doi: 10.1016/j.semcdb.2014.04.021

Dias, B. G., and Ressler, K. J. (2014). Parental olfactory experience influences behavior and neural structure in subsequent generations. *Nat. Neurosci.* 17, 89–96. doi: 10.1038/nn.3594

Dietz, D. M., Laplant, Q., Watts, E. L., Hodes, G. E., Russo, S. J., Feng, J., et al. (2011). Paternal transmission of stress-induced pathologies. *Biol. Psychiatry* 70, 408–414. doi: 10.1016/j.biopsych.2011.05.005

Donkin, I., Versteyhe, S., Ingerslev, L. R., Qian, K., Mechta, M., Nordkap, L., et al. (2016). Obesity and bariatric surgery drive epigenetic variation of spermatozoa in humans. *Cell Metab.* 23, 369–378. doi: 10.1016/j.cmet.2015.11.004

Dou, S., Wang, Y., and Lu, J. (2019). Metazoan tsRNAs: biogenesis, evolution and regulatory functions. *Noncoding RNA* 5:E18. doi: 10.3390/ncrna5010018

Elbarbary, R. A., Takaku, H., Uchiumi, N., Tamiya, H., Abe, M., Takahashi, M., et al. (2009). Modulation of gene expression by human cytosolic tRNase Z(L) through 5'-half-tRNA. *PLoS One* 4:e5908. doi: 10.1371/journal.pone.0005908

Fire, A., Xu, S., Montgomery, M. K., Kostas, S. A., Driver, S. E., and Mello, C. C. (1998). Potent and specific genetic interference by double-stranded RNA in Caenorhabditis elegans. *Nature* 391, 806–811. doi: 10.1038/35888

Fu, H., Feng, J., Liu, Q., Sun, F., Tie, Y., Zhu, J., et al. (2009). Stress induces tRNA cleavage by angiogenin in mammalian cells. *FEBS Lett.* 583, 437–442. doi: 10.1016/j.febslet.2008.12.043

Fullston, T., Ohlsson Teague, E. M., Palmer, N. O., DeBlasio, M. J., Mitchell, M., Corbett, M., et al. (2013). Paternal obesity initiates metabolic disturbances in two generations of mice with incomplete penetrance to the F2 generation and alters the transcriptional profile of testis and sperm microRNA content. *FASEB J.* 27, 4226–4243. doi: 10.1096/fj.12-224048

Gapp, K., Jawaid, A., Sarkies, P., Bohacek, J., Pelczar, P., Prados, J., et al. (2014). Implication of sperm RNAs in transgenerational inheritance of the effects of early trauma in mice. *Nat. Neurosci.* 17, 667–669. doi: 10.1038/nn.3695

Gapp, K., van Steenwyk, G., Germain, P. L., Matsushima, W., Rudolph, K. L. M., Manuella, F., et al. (2018). Alterations in sperm long RNA contribute to the epigenetic inheritance of the effects of postnatal trauma. *Mol. Psychiatry* doi: 10.1038/s41380-018-0271-6 [Epub ahead of print].

Gatti, J. L., Metayer, S., Belghazi, M., Dacheux, F., and Dacheux, J. L. (2005). Identification, proteomic profiling, and origin of ram epididymal fluid exosome-like vesicles. *Biol. Reprod.* 72, 1452–1465. doi: 10.1095/biolreprod.104.036426

Gay, L., Miller, M. R., Ventura, P. B., Devasthali, V., Vue, Z., Thompson, H. L., et al. (2013). Mouse TU tagging: a chemical/genetic intersectional method for purifying cell type-specific nascent RNA. *Genes Dev.* 27, 98–115. doi: 10.1101/gad.205278.112

Gebetsberger, J., Wyss, L., Mleczko, A. M., Reuther, J., and Polacek, N. (2017). A tRNA-derived fragment competes with mRNA for ribosome binding and regulates translation during stress. *RNA Biol.* 14, 1364–1373. doi: 10.1080/15476286.2016.1257470

Gervasi, M. G., and Visconti, P. E. (2017). Molecular changes and signaling events occurring in spermatozoa during epididymal maturation. *Andrology* 5, 204–218. doi: 10.1111/andr.12320

Ghildiyal, M., and Zamore, P. D. (2009). Small silencing RNAs: an expanding universe. *Nat. Rev. Genet.* 10, 94–108. doi: 10.1038/nrg2504

Girard, A., Sachidanandam, R., Hannon, G. J., and Carmell, M. A. (2006). A germline-specific class of small RNAs binds mammalian Piwi proteins. *Nature* 442, 199–202. doi: 10.1038/nature04917

Girouard, J., Frenette, G., and Sullivan, R. (2009). Compartmentalization of proteins in epididymosomes coordinates the association of epididymal proteins with the different functional structures of bovine spermatozoa. *Biol. Reprod.* 80, 965–972. doi: 10.1095/biolreprod.108.073551

Godia, M., Swanson, G., and Krawetz, S. A. (2018). A history of why fathers' RNA matters. *Biol. Reprod.* 99, 147–159. doi: 10.1093/biolre/ioy007

Goodarzi, H., Liu, X., Nguyen, H. C., Zhang, S., Fish, L., and Tavazoie, S. F. (2015). Endogenous tRNA-derived fragments suppress breast cancer progression via YBX1 displacement. *Cell* 161, 790–802. doi: 10.1016/j.cell.2015.02.053

Grandjean, V., Fourre, S., De Abreu, D. A., Derieppe, M. A., Remy, J. J., and Rassoulzadegan, M. (2015). RNA-mediated paternal heredity of diet-induced obesity and metabolic disorders. *Sci. Rep.* 5:18193. doi: 10.1038/srep18193

Grandjean, V., Gounon, P., Wagner, N., Martin, L., Wagner, K. D., Bernex, F., et al. (2009). The miR-124-Sox9 paramutation: RNA-mediated epigenetic control of embryonic and adult growth. *Development* 136, 3647–3655. doi: 10.1242/dev.041061

Griffiths, G. S., Galileo, D. S., Reese, K., and Martin-Deleon, P. A. (2008). Investigating the role of murine epididymosomes and uterosomes in GPI-linked protein transfer to sperm using SPAM1 as a model. *Mol. Reprod. Dev.* 75, 1627–1636. doi: 10.1002/mrd.20907

Grivna, S. T., Beyret, E., Wang, Z., and Lin, H. (2006). A novel class of small RNAs in mouse spermatogenic cells. *Genes Dev.* 20, 1709–1714. doi: 10.1101/gad.1434406

Ha, M., and Kim, V. N. (2014). Regulation of microRNA biogenesis. *Nat. Rev. Mol. Cell Biol.* 15, 509–524. doi: 10.1038/nrm3838

Hackett, J. A., and Surani, M. A. (2013). DNA methylation dynamics during the mammalian life cycle. *Philos. Trans. R Soc. Lond. B Biol. Sci.* 368:20110328. doi: 10.1098/rstb.2011.0328

Hales, C. N., and Barker, D. J. (2001). The thrifty phenotype hypothesis. *Br. Med. Bull.* 60, 5–20. doi: 10.1093/bmb/60.1.5

Hammoud, S. S., Low, D. H., Yi, C., Carrell, D. T., Guccione, E., and Cairns, B. R. (2014). Chromatin and transcription transitions of mammalian adult germline stem cells and spermatogenesis. *Cell Stem Cell* 15, 239–253. doi: 10.1016/j.stem.2014.04.006

Hammoud, S. S., Nix, D. A., Zhang, H., Purwar, J., Carrell, D. T., and Cairns, B. R. (2009). Distinctive chromatin in human sperm packages genes for embryo development. *Nature* 460, 473–478. doi: 10.1038/nature08162

Hao, S. L., Ni, F. D., and Yang, W. X. (2019). The dynamics and regulation of chromatin remodeling during spermiogenesis. *Gene* 706, 201–210. doi: 10.1016/j.gene.2019.05.027

Heard, E., and Martienssen, R. A. (2014). Transgenerational epigenetic inheritance: myths and mechanisms. *Cell* 157, 95–109. doi: 10.1016/j.cell.2014.02.045

Hoagland, M. B., Stephenson, M. L., Scott, J. F., Hecht, L. I., and Zamecnik, P. C. (1958). A soluble ribonucleic acid intermediate in protein synthesis. *J. Biol. Chem.* 231, 241–257.

Holland, M. L., Lowe, R., Caton, P. W., Gemma, C., Carbajosa, G., Danson, A. F., et al. (2016). Early-life nutrition modulates the epigenetic state of specific rDNA genetic variants in mice. *Science* 353, 495–498. doi: 10.1126/science.aaf7040

Holoch, D., and Moazed, D. (2015). RNA-mediated epigenetic regulation of gene expression. *Nat. Rev. Genet.* 16, 71–84. doi: 10.1038/nrg3863

Hutcheon, K., McLaughlin, E. A., Stanger, S. J., Bernstein, I. R., Dun, M. D., Eamens, A. L., et al. (2017). Analysis of the small non-protein-coding RNA profile of mouse spermatozoa reveals specific enrichment of piRNAs within mature spermatozoa. *RNA Biol.* 14, 1776–1790. doi: 10.1080/15476286.2017.1356569

Hutvagner, G., McLachlan, J., Pasquinelli, A. E., Balint, E., Tuschl, T., and Zamore, P. D. (2001). A cellular function for the RNA-interference enzyme Dicer in the maturation of the let-7 small temporal RNA. *Science* 293, 834–838. doi: 10.1126/science.1062961

Huypens, P., Sass, S., Wu, M., Dyckhoff, D., Tschop, M., Theis, F., et al. (2016). Epigenetic germline inheritance of diet-induced obesity and insulin resistance. *Nat. Genet.* 48, 497–499. doi: 10.1038/ng.3527

Ivanov, P., Emara, M. M., Villen, J., Gygi, S. P., and Anderson, P. (2011). Angiogenin-induced tRNA fragments inhibit translation initiation. *Mol. Cell* 43, 613–623. doi: 10.1016/j.molcel.2011.06.022

Ivanov, P., O'Day, E., Emara, M. M., Wagner, G., Lieberman, J., and Anderson, P. (2014). G-quadruplex structures contribute to the neuroprotective effects of angiogenin-induced tRNA fragments. *Proc. Natl. Acad. Sci. U.S.A.* 111, 18201–18206. doi: 10.1073/pnas.1407361111

Iwasaki, Y. W., Siomi, M. C., and Siomi, H. (2015). PIWI-Interacting RNA: its biogenesis and functions. *Annu. Rev. Biochem.* 84, 405–433. doi: 10.1146/annurev-biochem-060614-034258

Jimenez-Chillaron, J. C., Isganaitis, E., Charalambous, M., Gesta, S., Pentinat-Pelegrin, T., Faucette, R. R., et al. (2009). Intergenerational transmission of glucose intolerance and obesity by in utero undernutrition in mice. *Diabetes* 58, 460–468. doi: 10.2337/db08-0490

Jirtle, R. L., and Skinner, M. K. (2007). Environmental epigenomics and disease susceptibility. *Nat. Rev. Genet.* 8, 253–262. doi: 10.1038/nrg2045

Johnson, G. D., Mackie, P., Jodar, M., Moskovtsev, S., and Krawetz, S. A. (2015). Chromatin and extracellular vesicle associated sperm RNAs. *Nucleic Acids Res.* 43, 6847–6859. doi: 10.1093/nar/gkv591

Jones, K. L., and Smith, D. W. (1973). Recognition of the fetal alcohol syndrome in early infancy. *Lancet* 302, 999–1001. doi: 10.1016/s0140-6736(73)91092-1

Kaati, G., Bygren, L. O., and Edvinsson, S. (2002). Cardiovascular and diabetes mortality determined by nutrition during parents' and grandparents' slow growth period. *Eur. J. Hum. Genet.* 10, 682–688. doi: 10.1038/sj.ejhg.5200859

Kawano, N., Yoshida, K., Miyado, K., and Yoshida, M. (2011). Lipid rafts: keys to sperm maturation, fertilization, and early embryogenesis. *J. Lipids* 2011:264706. doi: 10.1155/2011/264706

Keam, S. P., and Hutvagner, G. (2015). tRNA-derived fragments (tRFs): emerging new roles for an ancient RNA in the regulation of gene expression. *Life* 5, 1638–1651. doi: 10.3390/life5041638

Keam, S. P., Sobala, A., Ten Have, S., and Hutvagner, G. (2017). tRNA-Derived RNA fragments associate with human multisynthetase complex (MSC) and modulate ribosomal protein translation. *J. Proteome Res.* 16, 413–420. doi: 10.1021/acs.jproteome.6b00267

Kim, H. K., Fuchs, G., Wang, S., Wei, W., Zhang, Y., Park, H., et al. (2017). A transfer-RNA-derived small RNA regulates ribosome biogenesis. *Nature* 552, 57–62. doi: 10.1038/nature25005

Kirino, Y., and Mourelatos, Z. (2007). Mouse Piwi-interacting RNAs are 2'-O-methylated at their 3' termini. *Nat. Struct. Mol. Biol.* 14, 347–348. doi: 10.1038/nsmb1218

Koch, S., Acebron, S. P., Herbst, J., Hatiboglu, G., and Niehrs, C. (2015). Post-transcriptional Wnt signaling governs epididymal sperm maturation. *Cell* 163, 1225–1236. doi: 10.1016/j.cell.2015.10.029

Kornberg, R. D., and Lorch, Y. (1999). Twenty-five years of the nucleosome, fundamental particle of the eukaryote chromosome. *Cell.* 98, 285–294. doi: 10.1016/s0092-8674(00)81958-3

Kumar, P., Kuscu, C., and Dutta, A. (2016). Biogenesis and function of transfer RNA-related fragments (tRFs). *Trends Biochem. Sci.* 41, 679–689. doi: 10.1016/j.tibs.2016.05.004

Kuramochi-Miyagawa, S., Kimura, T., Ijiri, T. W., Isobe, T., Asada, N., Fujita, Y., et al. (2004). Mili, a mammalian member of piwi family gene, is essential for spermatogenesis. *Development* 131, 839–849. doi: 10.1242/dev.00973

Lalancette, C., Miller, D., Li, Y., and Krawetz, S. A. (2008). Paternal contributions: new functional insights for spermatozoal RNA. *J. Cell. Biochem.* 104, 1570–1579. doi: 10.1002/jcb.21756

Lambert, M., Benmoussa, A., and Provost, P. (2019). Small non-coding RNAs derived from eukaryotic ribosomal RNA. *Noncoding RNA* 5:E16. doi: 10.3390/ncrna5010016

Lambrot, R., Xu, C., Saint-Phar, S., Chountalos, G., Cohen, T., Paquet, M., et al. (2013). Low paternal dietary folate alters the mouse sperm epigenome and is associated with negative pregnancy outcomes. *Nat. Commun.* 4:2889. doi: 10.1038/ncomms3889

Lau, N. C., Seto, A. G., Kim, J., Kuramochi-Miyagawa, S., Nakano, T., Bartel, D. P., et al. (2006). Characterization of the piRNA complex from rat testes. *Science* 313, 363–367. doi: 10.1126/science.1130164

Laxman, S., Sutter, B. M., Wu, X., Kumar, S., Guo, X., Trudgian, D. C., et al. (2013). Sulfur amino acids regulate translational capacity and metabolic homeostasis through modulation of tRNA thiolation. *Cell* 154, 416–429. doi: 10.1016/j.cell.2013.06.043

Lee, R. C., Feinbaum, R. L., and Ambros, V. (1993). The C. *elegans heterochronic gene lin*-4 encodes small RNAs with antisense complementarity to lin-14. *Cell* 75, 843–854. doi: 10.1016/0092-8674(93)90529-y

Lee, S. R., and Collins, K. (2005). Starvation-induced cleavage of the tRNA anticodon loop in *Tetrahymena* thermophila. *J. Biol. Chem.* 280, 42744–42749. doi: 10.1074/jbc.M510356200

Lee, Y., Ahn, C., Han, J., Choi, H., Kim, J., Yim, J., et al. (2003). The nuclear RNase III Drosha initiates microRNA processing. *Nature* 425, 415–419. doi: 10.1038/nature01957

Lee, Y. S., Shibata, Y., Malhotra, A., and Dutta, A. (2009). A novel class of small RNAs: tRNA-derived RNA fragments (tRFs). *Genes Dev.* 23, 2639–2649. doi: 10.1101/gad.1837609

Li, X. Z., Roy, C. K., Dong, X., Bolcun-Filas, E., Wang, J., Han, B. W., et al. (2013). An ancient transcription factor initiates the burst of piRNA production during early meiosis in mouse testes. *Mol. Cell* 50, 67–81. doi: 10.1016/j.molcel.2013.02.016

Liu, Y. S. (2011). Inheritance of acquired characters in animals: a historical overview, further evidence and mechanistic explanations. *Italian J. Zool.* 78, 410–417. doi: 10.1080/11250003.2011.562554

Lumey, L. H., Stein, A. D., Kahn, H. S., van der Pal-de Bruin, K. M., Blauw, G. J., Zybert, P. A., et al. (2007). Cohort profile: the Dutch hunger winter families study. *Int. J. Epidemiol.* 36, 1196–1204. doi: 10.1093/ije/drn126

Ly, L., Chan, D., Aarabi, M., Landry, M., Behan, N. A., MacFarlane, A. J., et al. (2017). Intergenerational impact of paternal lifetime exposures to both folic acid deficiency and supplementation on reproductive outcomes and imprinted gene methylation. *Mol. Hum. Reprod.* 23, 461–477. doi: 10.1093/molehr/gax029

Macfarlan, T. S., Gifford, W. D., Driscoll, S., Lettieri, K., Rowe, H. M., Bonanomi, D., et al. (2012). Embryonic stem cell potency fluctuates with endogenous retrovirus activity. *Nature* 487, 57–63. doi: 10.1038/nature11244

Martinez, G., Panda, K., Kohler, C., and Slotkin, R. K. (2016). Silencing in sperm cells is directed by RNA movement from the surrounding nurse cell. *Nat. Plants* 2:16030. doi: 10.1038/nplants.2016.30

Meikar, O., Da Ros, M., Korhonen, H., and Kotaja, N. (2011). Chromatoid body and small RNAs in male germ cells. *Reproduction* 142, 195–209. doi: 10.1530/Rep-11-0057

Messerschmidt, D. M., Knowles, B. B., and Solter, D. (2014). DNA methylation dynamics during epigenetic reprogramming in the germline and preimplantation embryos. *Genes Dev.* 28, 812–828. doi: 10.1101/gad.234294.113

Miska, E. A., and Ferguson-Smith, A. C. (2016). Transgenerational inheritance: models and mechanisms of non-DNA sequence-based inheritance. *Science* 354, 59–63. doi: 10.1126/science.aaf4945

Morgan, C. P., Chan, J. C., and Bale, T. L. (2019). Driving the next generation: paternal lifetime experiences transmitted via extracellular vesicles and their small RNA cargo. *Biol. Psychiatry* 85, 164–171. doi: 10.1016/j.biopsych.2018.09.007

Ng, S. F., Lin, R. C., Laybutt, D. R., Barres, R., Owens, J. A., and Morris, M. J. (2010). Chronic high-fat diet in fathers programs beta-cell dysfunction in female rat offspring. *Nature* 467, 963–966. doi: 10.1038/nature09491

Nixon, B., De Iuliis, G. N., Hart, H. M., Zhou, W., Mathe, A., Bernstein, I. R., et al. (2019). Proteomic profiling of mouse epididymosomes reveals their contributions to post-testicular sperm maturation. *Mol. Cell. Proteomics* 18(Suppl. 1), S91–S108. doi: 10.1074/mcp.RA118.000946

Nixon, B., Stanger, S. J., Mihalas, B. P., Reilly, J. N., Anderson, A. L., Tyagi, S., et al. (2015). The microRNA signature of mouse spermatozoa is substantially modified during epididymal maturation. *Biol. Reprod.* 93:91. doi: 10.1095/biolreprod.115.132209

Ostermeier, G. C., Dix, D. J., Miller, D., Khatri, P., and Krawetz, S. A. (2002). Spermatozoal RNA profiles of normal fertile men. *Lancet* 360, 772–777. doi: 10.1016/S0140-6736(02)09899-9

Ostermeier, G. C., Miller, D., Huntriss, J. D., Diamond, M. P., and Krawetz, S. A. (2004). Reproductive biology: delivering spermatozoan RNA to the oocyte. *Nature* 429:154. doi: 10.1038/429154a

Pembrey, M. E., Bygren, L. O., Kaati, G., Edvinsson, S., Northstone, K., Sjostrom, M., et al. (2006). Sex-specific, male-line transgenerational responses in humans. *Eur. J. Hum. Genet.* 14, 159–166. doi: 10.1038/sj.ejhg.5201538

Peng, H., Shi, J., Zhang, Y., Zhang, H., Liao, S., Li, W., et al. (2012). A novel class of tRNA-derived small RNAs extremely enriched in mature mouse sperm. *Cell Res.* 22, 1609–1612. doi: 10.1038/cr.2012.141

Perez, M. F., and Lehner, B. (2019). Intergenerational and transgenerational epigenetic inheritance in animals. *Nat. Cell. Biol.* 21, 143–151. doi: 10.1038/s41556-018-0242-9

Radford, E. J., Ito, M., Shi, H., Corish, J. A., Yamazawa, K., Isganaitis, E., et al. (2014). In utero undernourishment perturbs the adult sperm methylome and intergenerational metabolism. *Science* 345:1255903. doi: 10.1126/science.1255903

Rando, O. J. (2012). Daddy issues: paternal effects on phenotype. *Cell* 151, 702–708. doi: 10.1016/j.cell.2012.10.020

Rando, O. J. (2016). Intergenerational transfer of epigenetic information in sperm. *Cold Spring Harb. Perspect. Med.* 6:a022988. doi: 10.1101/cshperspect.a022988

Rando, O. J., and Simmons, R. A. (2015). I'm eating for two: parental dietary effects on offspring metabolism. *Cell* 161, 93–105. doi: 10.1016/j.cell.2015.02.021

Raposo, G., and Stoorvogel, W. (2013). Extracellular vesicles: exosomes, microvesicles, and friends. *J. Cell Biol.* 200, 373–383. doi: 10.1083/jcb.201211138

Rassoulzadegan, M., Grandjean, V., Gounon, P., Vincent, S., Gillot, I., and Cuzin, F. (2006). RNA-mediated non-mendelian inheritance of an epigenetic change in the mouse. *Nature* 441, 469–474. doi: 10.1038/nature04674

Rebourcet, D., O'Shaughnessy, P. J., Pitetti, J. L., Monteiro, A., O'Hara, L., Milne, L., et al. (2014). Sertoli cells control peritubular myoid cell fate and support adult Leydig cell development in the prepubertal testis. *Development* 141, 2139–2149. doi: 10.1242/dev.107029

Rechavi, O., and Lev, I. (2017). Principles of transgenerational small RNA inheritance in *Caenorhabditis* elegans. *Curr. Biol.* 27, R720–R730. doi: 10.1016/j.cub.2017.05.043

Reilly, J. N., McLaughlin, E. A., Stanger, S. J., Anderson, A. L., Hutcheon, K., Church, K., et al. (2016). Characterisation of mouse epididymosomes reveals a complex profile of microRNAs and a potential mechanism for modification of the sperm epigenome. *Sci. Rep.* 6:31794. doi: 10.1038/srep31794

Rejraji, H., Sion, B., Prensier, G., Carreras, M., Motta, C., Frenoux, J. M., et al. (2006). Lipid remodeling of murine epididymosomes and spermatozoa during epididymal maturation. *Biol. Reprod.* 74, 1104–1113. doi: 10.1095/biolreprod.105.049304

Reuter, M., Berninger, P., Chuma, S., Shah, H., Hosokawa, M., Funaya, C., et al. (2011). Miwi catalysis is required for piRNA amplification-independent LINE1 transposon silencing. *Nature* 480, 264–267. doi: 10.1038/nature10672

Rodgers, A. B., Morgan, C. P., Bronson, S. L., Revello, S., and Bale, T. L. (2013). Paternal stress exposure alters sperm microRNA content and reprograms offspring HPA stress axis regulation. *J. Neurosci.* 33, 9003–9012. doi: 10.1523/JNEUROSCI.0914-13.2013

Rodgers, A. B., Morgan, C. P., Leu, N. A., and Bale, T. L. (2015). Transgenerational epigenetic programming via sperm microRNA recapitulates effects of paternal stress. *Proc. Natl. Acad. Sci. U.S.A.* 112, 13699–13704. doi: 10.1073/pnas.1508347112

Rompala, G. R., Simons, A., Kihle, B., and Homanics, G. E. (2018). Paternal preconception chronic variable stress confers attenuated ethanol drinking behavior selectively to male offspring in a pre-stress environment dependent manner. *Front. Behav. Neurosci.* 12:257. doi: 10.3389/fnbeh.2018.00257

Roundtree, I. A., Evans, M. E., Pan, T., and He, C. (2017). Dynamic RNA modifications in gene expression regulation. *Cell* 169, 1187–1200. doi: 10.1016/j.cell.2017.05.045

Saikia, M., Jobava, R., Parisien, M., Putnam, A., Krokowski, D., Gao, X. H., et al. (2014). Angiogenin-cleaved tRNA halves interact with cytochrome c, protecting cells from apoptosis during osmotic stress. *Mol. Cell. Biol.* 34, 2450–2463. doi: 10.1128/MCB.00136-14

Sarkies, P., and Miska, E. A. (2014). Small RNAs break out: the molecular cell biology of mobile small RNAs. *Nat. Rev. Mol. Cell Biol.* 15, 525–535. doi: 10.1038/nrm3840

Schaefer, M., Pollex, T., Hanna, K., Tuorto, F., Meusburger, M., Helm, M., et al. (2010). RNA methylation by Dnmt2 protects transfer RNAs against stress-induced cleavage. *Genes Dev.* 24, 1590–1595. doi: 10.1101/gad.586710

Schorn, A. J., Gutbrod, M. J., LeBlanc, C., and Martienssen, R. (2017). LTR-retrotransposon control by tRNA-Derived small RNAs. *Cell* 170, 61–71e.11. doi: 10.1016/j.cell.2017.06.013

Schuster, A., Skinner, M. K., and Yan, W. (2016a). Ancestral vinclozolin exposure alters the epigenetic transgenerational inheritance of sperm small noncoding RNAs. *Environ. Epigenet.* 2:dvw001. doi: 10.1093/eep/dvw001

Schuster, A., Tang, C., Xie, Y., Ortogero, N., Yuan, S., and Yan, W. (2016b). SpermBase: a database for sperm-borne RNA contents. *Biol. Reprod.* 95:99. doi: 10.1095/biolreprod.116.142190

Sharma, U., Conine, C. C., Shea, J. M., Boskovic, A., Derr, A. G., Bing, X. Y., et al. (2016). Biogenesis and function of tRNA fragments during sperm maturation and fertilization in mammals. *Science* 351, 391–396. doi: 10.1126/science.aad6780

Sharma, U., and Rando, O. J. (2017). Metabolic inputs into the epigenome. *Cell Metab.* 25, 544–558. doi: 10.1016/j.cmet.2017.02.003

Sharma, U., Sun, F., Conine, C. C., Reichholf, B., Kukreja, S., Herzog, V. A., et al. (2018). Small RNAs are trafficked from the epididymis to developing mammalian sperm. *Dev. Cell* 46, 481–494.e6. doi: 10.1016/j.devcel.2018.06.023

Sharpe, R. M., Maddocks, S., and Kerr, J. B. (1990). Cell-cell interactions in the control of spermatogenesis as studied using leydig-cell destruction and testosterone replacement. *Am. J. Anat.* 188, 3–20. doi: 10.1002/aja.1001880103

Shea, J. M., Serra, R. W., Carone, B. R., Shulha, H. P., Kucukural, A., Ziller, M. J., et al. (2015). Genetic and epigenetic variation, but not diet, shape the sperm methylome. *Dev. Cell* 35, 750–758. doi: 10.1016/j.devcel.2015.11.024

Shurtleff, M. J., Yao, J., Qin, Y., Nottingham, R. M., Temoche-Diaz, M. M., Schekman, R., et al. (2017). Broad role for YBX1 in defining the small noncoding RNA composition of exosomes. *Proc. Natl. Acad. Sci. U.S.A.* 114, E8987–E8995. doi: 10.1073/pnas.1712108114

Siklenka, K., Erkek, S., Godmann, M., Lambrot, R., McGraw, S., Lafleur, C., et al. (2015). Disruption of histone methylation in developing sperm impairs offspring health transgenerationally. *Science* 350:aab2006. doi: 10.1126/science.aab2006

Sobala, A., and Hutvagner, G. (2011). Transfer RNA-derived fragments: origins, processing, and functions. *Wiley Interdiscip Rev. RNA* 2, 853–862. doi: 10.1002/wrna.96

Sobala, A., and Hutvagner, G. (2013). Small RNAs derived from the 5 end of tRNA can inhibit protein translation in human cells. *RNA Biol.* 10, 553–563. doi: 10.4161/rna.24285

Song, R., Hennig, G. W., Wu, Q., Jose, C., Zheng, H., and Yan, W. (2011). Male germ cells express abundant endogenous siRNAs. *Proc. Natl. Acad. Sci. U.S.A.* 108, 13159–13164. doi: 10.1073/pnas.1108567108

Sprando, R. L., and Russell, L. D. (1987). Comparative study of cytoplasmic elimination in spermatids of selected mammalian species. *Am. J. Anat.* 178, 72–80. doi: 10.1002/aja.1001780109

Suganuma, R., Yanagimachi, R., and Meistrich, M. L. (2005). Decline in fertility of mouse sperm with abnormal chromatin during epididymal passage as revealed by ICSI. *Hum. Reprod.* 20, 3101–3108. doi: 10.1093/humrep/dei169

Sullivan, R. (2015). Epididymosomes: a heterogeneous population of microvesicles with multiple functions in sperm maturation and storage. *Asian J. Androl.* 17, 726–729. doi: 10.4103/1008-682X.155255

Sullivan, R. (2016). Epididymosomes: role of extracellular microvesicles in sperm maturation. *Front. Biosci.* 8, 106–114. doi: 10.2741/s450

Sullivan, R., Frenette, G., and Girouard, J. (2007). Epididymosomes are involved in the acquisition of new sperm proteins during epididymal transit. *Asian J. Androl.* 9, 483–491. doi: 10.1111/j.1745-7262.2007.00281.x

Sullivan, R., and Saez, F. (2013). Epididymosomes, prostasomes, and liposomes: their roles in mammalian male reproductive physiology. *Reproduction* 146, R21–R35. doi: 10.1530/Rep-13-0058

Trigg, N. A., Eamens, A. L., and Nixon, B. (2019). The contribution of epididymosomes to the sperm small RNA profile. *Reproduction* doi: 10.1530/REP-18-0480 [Epub ahead of print].

Tuorto, F., Liebers, R., Musch, T., Schaefer, M., Hofmann, S., Kellner, S., et al. (2012). RNA cytosine methylation by Dnmt2 and NSun2 promotes tRNA stability and protein synthesis. *Nat. Struct. Mol. Biol.* 19, 900–905. doi: 10.1038/nsmb.2357

Vagin, V. V., Sigova, A., Li, C., Seitz, H., Gvozdev, V., and Zamore, P. D. (2006). A distinct small RNA pathway silences selfish genetic elements in the germline. *Science* 313, 320–324. doi: 10.1126/science.1129333

Vallaster, M. P., Kukreja, S., Bing, X. Y., Ngolab, J., Zhao-Shea, R., Gardner, P. D., et al. (2017). Paternal nicotine exposure alters hepatic xenobiotic metabolism in offspring. *eLife* 6:e24771. doi: 10.7554/eLife.24771

Vassoler, F. M., White, S. L., Schmidt, H. D., Sadri-Vakili, G., and Pierce, R. C. (2013). Epigenetic inheritance of a cocaine-resistance phenotype. *Nat. Neurosci.* 16, 42–47. doi: 10.1038/nn.3280

Villarroya-Beltri, C., Gutierrez-Vazquez, C., Sanchez-Cabo, F., Perez-Hernandez, D., Vazquez, J., Martin-Cofreces, N., et al. (2013). Sumoylated hnRNPA2B1 controls the sorting of miRNAs into exosomes through binding to specific motifs. *Nat. Commun.* 4:2980. doi: 10.1038/ncomms3980

Vojtech, L., Woo, S., Hughes, S., Levy, C., Ballweber, L., Sauteraud, R. P., et al. (2014). Exosomes in human semen carry a distinctive repertoire of small non-coding RNAs with potential regulatory functions. *Nucleic Acids Res.* 42, 7290–7304. doi: 10.1093/nar/gku347

Volpe, T. A., Kidner, C., Hall, I. M., Teng, G., Grewal, S. I., and Martienssen, R. A. (2002). Regulation of heterochromatic silencing and histone H3 lysine-9 methylation by RNAi. *Science* 297, 1833–1837. doi: 10.1126/science.1074973

Wagner, K. D., Wagner, N., Ghanbarian, H., Grandjean, V., Gounon, P., Cuzin, F., et al. (2008). RNA induction and inheritance of epigenetic cardiac hypertrophy in the mouse. *Dev. Cell* 14, 962–969. doi: 10.1016/j.devcel.2008.03.009

Wang, K., Zhang, S., Weber, J., Baxter, D., and Galas, D. J. (2010). Export of microRNAs and microRNA-protective protein by mammalian cells. *Nucleic Acids Res.* 38, 7248–7259. doi: 10.1093/nar/gkq601

Watanabe, T., Takeda, A., Tsukiyama, T., Mise, K., Okuno, T., Sasaki, H., et al. (2006). Identification and characterization of two novel classes of small RNAs in the mouse germline: retrotransposon-derived siRNAs in oocytes and germline small RNAs in testes. *Genes Dev.* 20, 1732–1743. doi: 10.1101/gad.1425706

Wei, Y., Yang, C. R., Wei, Y. P., Zhao, Z. A., Hou, Y., Schatten, H., et al. (2014). Paternally induced transgenerational inheritance of susceptibility to diabetes in mammals. *Proc. Natl. Acad. Sci. U.S.A.* 111, 1873–1878. doi: 10.1073/pnas.1321195111

Wu, L., Lu, Y., Jiao, Y., Liu, B., Li, S., Li, Y., et al. (2016). Paternal psychological stress reprograms hepatic gluconeogenesis in offspring. *Cell Metab.* 23, 735–743. doi: 10.1016/j.cmet.2016.01.014

Yadav, T., Quivy, J. P., and Almouzni, G. (2018). Chromatin plasticity: a versatile landscape that underlies cell fate and identity. *Science* 361, 1332–1336. doi: 10.1126/science.aat8950

Yamaguchi, K., Hada, M., Fukuda, Y., Inoue, E., Makino, Y., Katou, Y., et al. (2018). Re-evaluating the localization of sperm-retained histones revealed the modification-dependent accumulation in specific genome regions. *Cell Rep.* 23, 3920–3932. doi: 10.1016/j.celrep.2018.05.094

Yan, W., Morozumi, K., Zhang, J., Ro, S., Park, C., and Yanagimachi, R. (2008). Birth of mice after intracytoplasmic injection of single purified sperm nuclei and detection of messenger RNAs and MicroRNAs in the sperm nuclei. *Biol. Reprod.* 78, 896–902. doi: 10.1095/biolreprod.107.067033

Yuan, S., Schuster, A., Tang, C., Yu, T., Ortogero, N., Bao, J., et al. (2016). Sperm-borne miRNAs and endo-siRNAs are important for fertilization and preimplantation embryonic development. *Development* 143, 635–647. doi: 10.1242/dev.131755

Zeybel, M., Hardy, T., Wong, Y. K., Mathers, J. C., Fox, C. R., Gackowska, A., et al. (2012). Multigenerational epigenetic adaptation of the hepatic wound-healing response. *Nat. Med.* 18, 1369–1377. doi: 10.1038/nm.2893

Zhang, Y., Shi, J., Rassoulzadegan, M., Tuorto, F., and Chen, Q. (2019). Sperm RNA code programmes the metabolic health of offspring. *Nat. Rev. Endocrinol.* 15, 489–498. doi: 10.1038/s41574-019-0226-2

Zhang, Y., Zhang, X., Shi, J., Tuorto, F., Li, X., Liu, Y., et al. (2018). Dnmt2 mediates intergenerational transmission of paternally acquired metabolic disorders through sperm small non-coding RNAs. *Nat. Cell Biol.* 20, 535–540. doi: 10.1038/s41556-018-0087-2

Zhou, W., Stanger, S. J., Anderson, A. L., Bernstein, I. R., De Iuliis, G. N., McCluskey, A., et al. (2019). Mechanisms of tethering and cargo transfer during epididymosome-sperm interactions. *BMC Biol.* 17:35. doi: 10.1186/s12915-019-0653-5

2

Signaling Enzymes Required for Sperm Maturation and Fertilization in Mammals

*Souvik Dey, Cameron Brothag and Srinivasan Vijayaraghavan**

Department of Biological Sciences, Kent State University, Kent, OH, United States

Correspondence:
Srinivasan Vijayaraghavan
svijayar@kent.edu

In mammals, motility and fertilizing ability of spermatozoa develop during their passage through the epididymis. After ejaculation, sperm undergo capacitation and hyperactivation in the female reproductive tract – a motility transition that is required for sperm penetration of the egg. Both epididymal initiation of sperm motility and hyperactivation are essential for male fertility. Motility initiation in the epididymis and sperm hyperactivation involve changes in metabolism, cAMP (cyclic adenosine monophosphate), calcium and pH acting through protein kinases and phosphatases. Despite this knowledge, we still do not understand, in biochemical terms, how sperm acquire motility in the epididymis and how motility is altered in the female reproductive tract. Recent data show that the sperm specific protein phosphatase PP1γ2, glycogen synthase kinase 3 (GSK3), and the calcium regulated phosphatase calcineurin (PP2B), are involved in epididymal sperm maturation. The protein phosphatase PP1γ2 is present only in testis and sperm in mammals. PP1γ2 has a isoform-specific requirement for normal function of mammalian sperm. Sperm PP1γ2 is regulated by three proteins – inhibitor 2, inhibitor 3 and SDS22. Changes in phosphorylation of these three inhibitors and their binding to PP1γ2 are involved in initiation and activation of sperm motility. The inhibitors are phosphorylated by protein kinases, one of which is GSK3. The isoform GSK3α is essential for epididymal sperm maturation and fertility. Calcium levels dramatically decrease during sperm maturation and initiation of motility suggesting that the calcium activated sperm phosphatase (PP2B) activity also decreases. Loss of PP2B results in male infertility due to impaired sperm maturation in the epididymis. Thus the three signaling enzymes PP1γ2, GSK3, and PP2B along with the documented PKA (protein kinase A) have key roles in sperm maturation and hyperactivation. Significantly, all these four signaling enzymes are present as specific isoforms only in placental mammals, a testimony to their essential roles in the unique aspects of sperm function in mammals. These findings should lead to a better biochemical understanding of the basis of male infertility and should lead to novel approaches to a male contraception and managed reproduction.

Keywords: hyperactivation, fertility, PP1γ2, GSK3α, epididymal sperm maturation, PP2B, PKA, contraception

INTRODUCTION

Testicular spermatozoa in mammals are immotile and lack the ability to fertilize eggs. Motility initiation and fertilizing ability develop during their passage through the epididymis (Cooper, 1986; Bedford and Hoskins, 1990). Epididymal maturation is an absolute necessity to produce fertile spermatozoa. Sperm undergo hyperactivation in the female reproductive tract before penetration of the egg. Motile sperm failing to undergo hyperactivation cannot fertilize (Marquez and Suarez, 2008). Understanding the biochemical basis for how motility is attained and modified prior to fertilization is essential for understanding male fertility and infertility.

Sperm flagellar activity and also ciliary motility of somatic cells are known to be regulated by the intracellular mediators cAMP, calcium and pH. Capacitation is operationaly defined as functional modifications that enable sperm to fertilize eggs. Sperm undergo various changes during capacitation: (a) removal of membrane cholesterol followed leading to a decrease in cholesterol to phospholipid ratio (b) membrane hyperpolarization, rise in intra-sperm pH and cAMP levels, (c) increase in calcium uptake, and (d) an increase in protein tyrosine phosphorylation possibily due to increased protein kinase A (PKA) activity (Arcelay et al., 2008; Bailey, 2010; Alvau et al., 2016; Jin and Yang, 2017; Molina et al., 2018). It is generally accepted that these changes during capacitation lead to: (a) the ability of the sperm to bind the oocyte's extracellular matrix, the zona pellucida (ZP) (Si and Olds-Clarke, 1999; Topper et al., 1999) and subsequently undergo the acrosome reaction, (b) hyperactivation, a whiplash flagellar motion required to penetrate the egg (Ho and Suarez, 2001), and (c) the capacity to fuse with the oocyte (Evans and Florman, 2002). Hyperactivation, however, is regulated by similar yet distinct signaling events that distinguish it from capacitation (Marquez and Suarez, 2004).

Considerable progress has been made in understanding changes in sperm cAMP, calcium, and pH during sperm activation and hyperactivation. The proteins responsible for the generation of cAMP, calcium influx and changes in pHi (intracellular pH) have been identified and their functions elucidated by biochemical and genetic approaches. Despite this information, we still do not understand, in biochemical terms, how these second messengers enable sperm to acquire motility in the epididymis and how motility is altered in the female reproductive tract. Our understanding is incomplete because other signaling enzymes can profoundly alter the action and effects of second messengers in sperm. These signaling enzymes, protein phosphatase 1 (PP1), glycogen synthase kinase 3 (GSK3) and the calcium activated phosphatase (PP2B), affect sperm function in the epididymis and in the female reproductive tract. Several reviews detail the roles of sperm cAMP-PKA and calcium metabolism (Visconti et al., 2002; Burton and McKnight, 2007; Buffone et al., 2014; Stival et al., 2016; Freitas et al., 2017; Balbach et al., 2018; Leemans et al., 2019; Stewart and Davis, 2019). Following a brief summary of the actions of cAMP-PKA, calcium and pH, the remainder of the review will be focused largely devoted to examination of the key roles of PP1, GSK3, and calcium activated protein phosphatase, PP2B (PPP3R2/CC) in mediating the actions of the second messengers during sperm maturation and fertilization.

ROLES OF cAMP AND PROTEIN KINASE A IN SPERM FUNCTION

Motility can be induced in demembranated testicular and caput epididymal sperm in the presence of ATP and cAMP, as well as appropriate calcium levels and pH (Lindemann, 1978; Mohri and Yanagimachi, 1980; Yeung, 1984; Lindemann et al., 1987; Bedford and Hoskins, 1990; Lesich et al., 2008). Early studies on the motility effects of phosphodiesterase inhibitors (such as caffeine, theophylline, and IBMX), on intact sperm led to the discovery of the role of cAMP in sperm motility regulation (Dougherty et al., 1976; Jiang et al., 1984). Phosphodiesterase inhibitors or cell permeable cAMP analogs can initiate motility in immotile spermatozoa and stimulate increased motility in motile sperm. Motility activation of demembranated sperm is abrogated in the presence of protein phosphatases in the reactivation medium, suggesting that cAMP mediates its motility effect through protein phosphorylation (Takahashi et al., 1985; Murofushi et al., 1986). An elevation of intra-sperm cAMP is also thought to be involved in motility initiation in the epididymis (Hoskins et al., 1974; Amann et al., 1982; Vijayaraghavan et al., 1985). A unique, hormone insensitive but bicarbonate sensitive, soluble adenylyl cyclase (sAC) is responsible for the synthesis of cAMP in sperm. Sperm cAMP levels should also be regulated by phosphodiesterases (PDEs) enzymes that degrade cAMP. Of the eleven PDEs, PDE1, PDE4, PDE8, PDE10, and PDE11 are present in testis and sperm (Omori and Kotera, 2007; Keravis and Lugnier, 2012).

It is well known that cAMP acts through a protein kinase (PKA). Knockout of the sperm sAC or PKA leads to infertility due to impaired sperm motility and the inability of sperm to undergo hyperactivation (Hess et al., 2005; Xie et al., 2006). Mature sperm contain PKA which is composed of regulatory subunit RIIα and a sperm specific catalytic subunit Cα2. Targeted knock-out of sperm-specific Cα2 results in male infertility. Spermatogenesis in these mutant mice is normal, while kinetic vigor and beat amplitude of epididymal sperm were markedly reduced. Mutant sperm are unable to undergo bicarbonate induced motility stimulation, and hyperactivation. It is known that PKA in cells owes it specificity and function to its localization through anchoring proteins known as AKAPs (Colledge and Scott, 1999). Sperm contain at least two PKA anchoring proteins AKAP 3 and 4 (also known as AKAP110 and 82, respectively) (Lin et al., 1995; Vijayaraghavan et al., 1999). Targeted deletion of AKAP 3 or 4 results in sperm dysfunction and male infertility (Jackson Labs Mouse Repository) (Miki et al., 2002). AKAP82 has been shown to play significant roles mediating the PKA action in murine and human sperm (Moss et al., 1999; Turner et al., 1999).

One of the downstream effects of PKA has been suggested to involve activation of protein tyrosine kinases (PTKs): proline−rich tyrosine kinase 2 (PYK2), ABL (Abelson murine leukemia viral oncogene homolog 1), SRC, and FER

(Baker et al., 2006, 2009; Alvau et al., 2016; Brukman et al., 2019). However, targeted disruption of these PTKs did not impair male fertility. Thus the exact role, of protein tyrosine phosphorylation in sperm function is still not well understood. PKA has also been suggested to regulate cAMP-phosphodiesterase activity. Phosphorylation by PKA has been shown to increase catalytic activities of PDE4 and PDE11 (Sette and Conti, 1996; Yuasa et al., 2000) suggesting a feedback regulation of sperm cAMP levels. Hyper-activated motility in sperm capacitation may also include phospholipase D-dependent actin polymerization (Itach et al., 2012). Thus while it is known that cAMP and PKA are essential in sperm the exact downstream biochemical actions of PKA are still unknown.

THE ROLES OF pHi, CALCIUM AND CatSper CHANNELS IN SPERM FUNCTION

The role of pH in regulating flagellar motion was first recognized in the mechanism underlying activation of sea urchin sperm in sea water, which occurs due to increased pHi mediated by a sodium – proton exchange (Lee et al., 1983). Several studies have now shown that increasing intracellular pH activates motility of sperm in a number of species (Vijayaraghavan et al., 1985; Hamamah and Gatti, 1998; Carr and Acott, 2005; Nishigaki et al., 2014). A change in pHi is also thought to accompany sperm maturation in the epididymis (Vijayaraghavan et al., 1985). Acidic pH and the high concentration of lactate which acts as a membrane permeable proton carrier render sperm immotile in the luminal fluid of the cauda epididymis (Carr et al., 1985; Vijayaraghavan and Hoskins, 1988). Dilution of the quiescent caudal sperm, during ejaculation or in a buffer *in vitro*, results in initiation of vigorous motility. More recently, elevation of pHi has also been recognized to be a key event required for initiation of calcium influx during sperm hyperactivation. Knockout of channels, Slo3, NHE1 (Slca9c) or SLC26A3, responsible for changes in pH renders sperm infertile (Wang et al., 2007; Chen et al., 2009; Santi et al., 2010; Zeng et al., 2011; Chavez et al., 2014; Toure, 2019). A significant advance in understanding hyperactivation came from the discovery of calcium channels (CatSper) as essential mediators of sperm calcium influx. The calcium channel is composed of several essential subunits (Qi et al., 2007; Chang and Suarez, 2011; Singh and Rajender, 2015; Williams et al., 2015; Sun et al., 2017). Alkalinization of the sperm cytosol followed by activation of calcium channels (CatSper) triggers hyperactivation (Carlson et al., 2003; Qi et al., 2007; Lishko and Kirichok, 2010; Chung et al., 2011; Chavez et al., 2014; Lishko and Mannowetz, 2018; Orta et al., 2018). Prevention of the increase in pHi or loss of CatSper leads to infertility. A recent study shows that CatSper channels also mediate Zn^{2+}-dependent stimulation of sperm hyperactivation (Allouche-Fitoussi et al., 2018). A model for sperm hyperactivation incorporating the functions of cAMP-PKA, calcium, and pHi is shown in **Figure 1**. This model is based on those presented in reviews noted earlier on the mechanisms regulating sperm function. Absent in theses models are the essential functions of the signaling enzymes PP1γ2, GSK3α, and PP2B required for sperm motility initiation and fertility.

PROTEIN PHOSPHATASE ISOFORM, PP1γ2 IN SPERM FUNCTION

The presence of a protein kinase in a cell requires a corresponding protein phosphatase. The phosphorylation status of a protein is the result of the opposing activities of protein kinases and protein phosphatases. Based on the observation that protein phosphatases prevent motility initiation of demembranated spermatozoa and also enzyme activity measurements in sperm extracts (Swarup and Garbers, 1982; Takahashi et al., 1985; Murofushi et al., 1986), it was long suspected that a protein phosphatase regulates flagellar motility. However, the identity of the phosphatase and details of its regulation were not known. Research on protein phosphatases was boosted by the discovery of compounds, calyculin A, okadaic acid, and microcystin, isolated from marine organisms that are potent inhibitors of protein phosphatases (Cohen, 1990; Cohen et al., 1990; Fernandez et al., 2002). The inhibitors display distinct inhibition profiles against the serine/threonine phosphatases PP1, PP2A, and PP2B enabling their identification in cellular extracts (da Cruz e Silva et al., 1995). The protein phosphatase inhibitors, calyculin A and okadaic acid, were among the most potent in initiating and stimulating motility of sperm (Smith et al., 1996, 1999; Vijayaraghavan et al., 1996). The inhibitors initiated and stimulated epididymal sperm motility at nanomolar and micromolar concentrations, respectively. The inhibition profile of enzyme activity in sperm extracts suggested that the predominant phosphatase in sperm was protein phosphatase 1 (PP1) along with measurable levels of PP2A. There are four isoforms of PP1, PP1α, PP1β, PP1γ1, and PP1γ2, encoded by three genes (Okano et al., 1997; Lin et al., 1999). The amino acid sequences of all four proteins are essentially identical except at their C-termini. The two PP1 isoforms, PP1γ1 and PP1γ2, are alternate transcripts from a single gene, *Ppp1c* (**Figure 2A**). Based on enzyme activity profiles and western blot analysis, we found that the predominant serine/threonine protein phosphatase in spermatozoa is PP1γ2. High PP1γ2 activity is associated with low sperm motility, while low PP1γ2 activity is associated with vigorous motility (Smith et al., 1996, 1999; Vijayaraghavan et al., 1996). A decline in PP1γ2 activity occurs during epididymal sperm maturation, due to a decrease in its catalytic activity. Other laboratories have shown that the phosphatase inhibitors also promote hyperactivated sperm motility and acrosome reaction (Furuya et al., 1992a,b; Signorelli et al., 2013; Rotfeld et al., 2014; Matsuura and Yogo, 2015; Tsirulnikov et al., 2019). The enzyme PP1γ2 is present in spermatozoa of a wide range of mammalian species including human and non-human primates (Chakrabarti et al., 2007a; Vijayaraghavan et al., 2007).

In most tissues and cells, the loss of any one of the PP1 isoforms is compensated by one of the other isoforms. In yeast the loss of its endogenous protein phosphatase (GLC7) can be functionally replaced by one of the four mammalian PP1

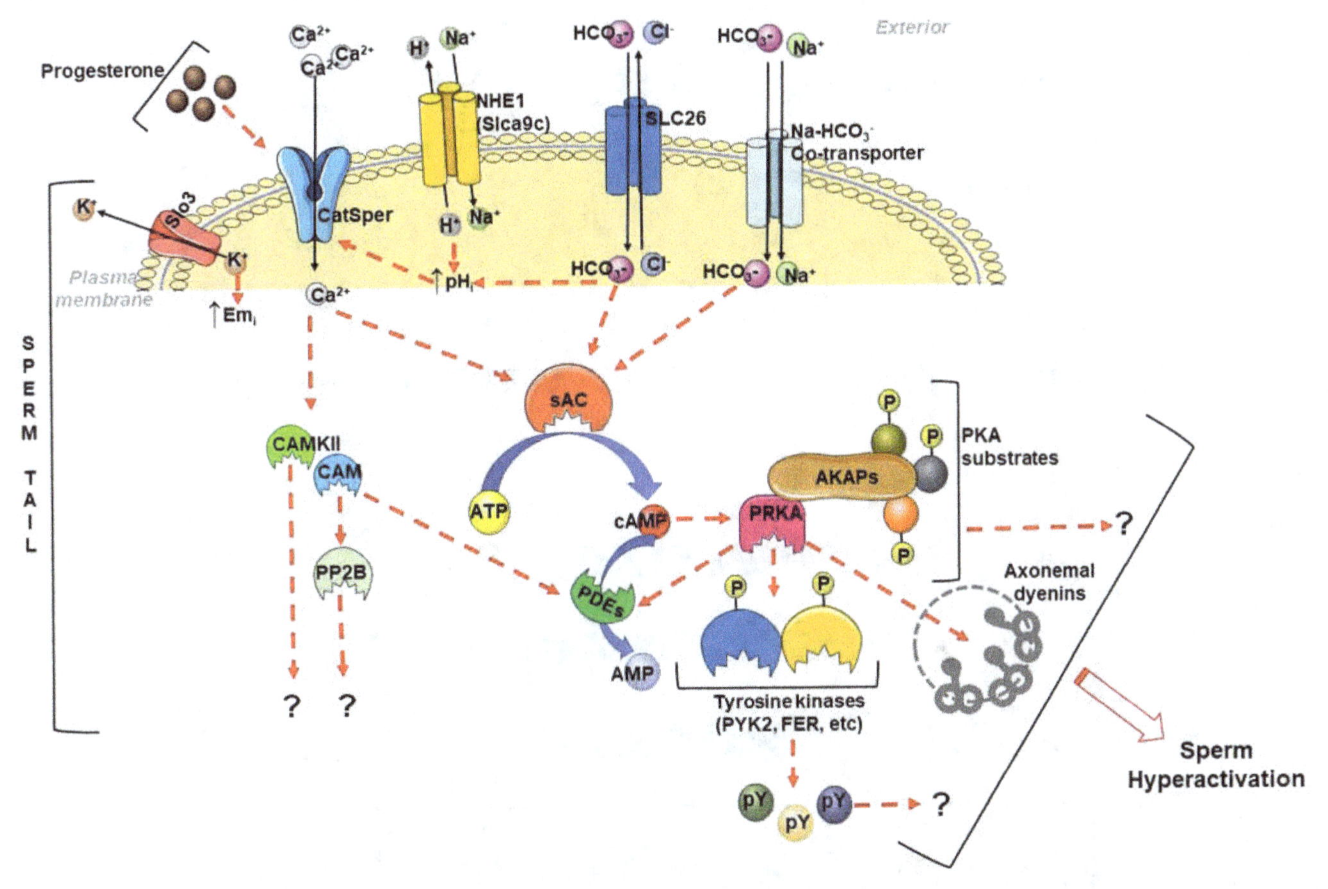

FIGURE 1 | Schematic diagram showing some of the signaling events during sperm hyperactivation. CatSper channels are activated either by progesterone or alkalization of sperm cytosol to permit calcium entry. The Cl^-–HCO_3^- exchanger, SLC26A3 and the Na^+–HCO_3^- co-transporter, and Na^+–H^+ exchanger, NHE1 (Slca9c), aid in alkalization of sperm pHi. Slo3 K^+-channels are activated by alkalization and causes hyperpolarization. Both Ca^{2+} and HCO_3^- stimulate sperm sAC to increase cAMP levels. Cyclic AMP, in turn activates sperm PKA (PRKA), which is expected to phosphorylate several substrates including protein tyrosine kinases (PTKs). Ca^{2+} also activates calmodulin (CAM) and calmodulin dependent phosphatase, calcineurin (PP2B) and a protein kinase CAMKII. The downstream effect and mechanism of action of these enzymes in promoting sperm fertilization is not well understood. Index: dotted arrow indicates activation, upward arrow denotes increase, and question mark (?) indicates unknown mechanism.

isoforms, highlighting their functional equivalence (Gibbons et al., 2007). Because PP1γ2 was implicated in sperm motility it was of interest to see how its loss would affect sperm function. Loss of *Ppp1cc* leads to defects in spermiogenesis and lack of sperm in the epididymis (Varmuza et al., 1999; Chakrabarti et al., 2007b). The enzyme PP1γ2 has a dual role, one, during spermatogenesis and the other in sperm after their exit from the seminiferous tubules. This dual role of PP1γ2 is intriguing because loss of the enzymes of cAMP metabolism and action, sAC or PKA in testis, does not impair sperm morphogenesis or sperm formation. It is likely that other serine/threonine protein kinases along with PP1γ2 are responsible for regulation of protein phosphorylation during spermatogenesis (Kawa et al., 2006; Xu et al., 2007; MacLeod et al., 2014; Cruz et al., 2019). Due to its requirement in spermatogenesis, it is not possible to obtain sperm lacking PP1γ2, which is a limitation for the study of the enzyme in mature sperm.

The only phenotype resulting from the knockout of *Ppp1cc* is male infertility. Females lacking *Ppp1cc* are normal and fertile (**Table 1**). Conditional knockout in post-meiotic developing germ cells also has the same phenotype as the global loss of *Ppp1cc* showing the requirement of *Ppp1cc* only in differentiating germ cells in testis (Sinha et al., 2013). It should be noted that the *Ppp1cc* gene is responsible for expression of both the PP1 isoforms: PP1γ1 and PP1γ2. Since, PP1γ2 is the predominant isoform in testis, it strongly suggests, but does not prove that the reason for male infertility in mice lacking *Ppp1cc* is likely due to the absence of only PP1γ2 in differentiating spermatogenic cells. It was later confirmed that, despite the global absence of PP1γ1, transgenic expression of PP1γ2 driven by the PGK2 promoter in spermatocytes and spermatids of *Ppp1cc* null mice restored spermatogenesis, sperm function, and fertility (Sinha et al., 2012). These data provide compelling evidence that the PP1γ2 isoform expressed only in developing germ cells is sufficient for normal sperm function and fertility.

The phosphatase isoform, PP1γ2, is present only in eutherian mammals. Sperm from non-mammalian species and invertebrates contain one of the three PP1 isoforms – PP1α,

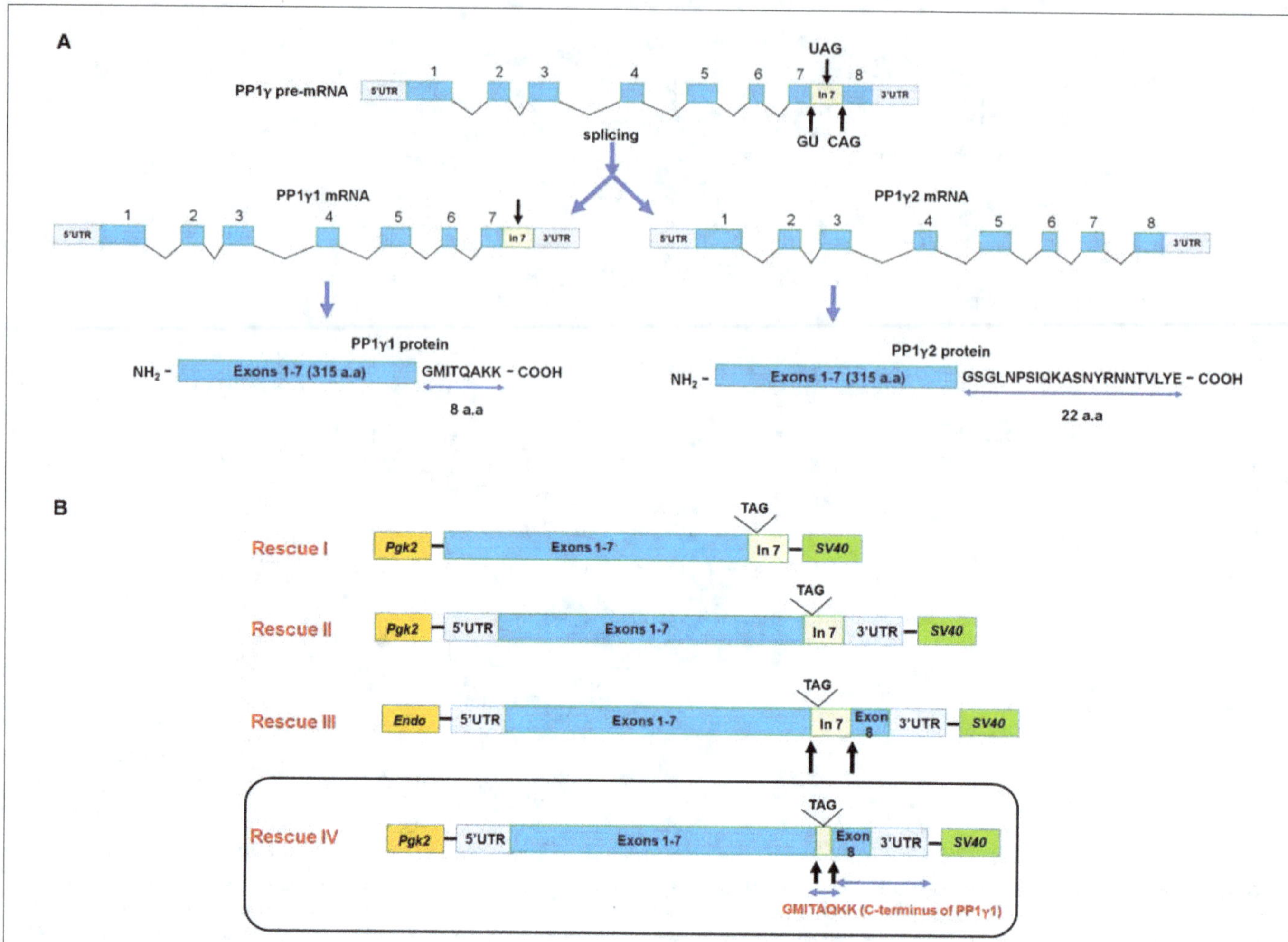

FIGURE 2 | (A) Generation of PP1γ isoforms. The *Ppp1cc* contains 8 exons and 7 introns. The Pp1γ1 mature mRNA (2.3 kb) contains exons 1 through 7. Intron 7 is retained as an extended exon leading to the eight amino acid C-terminus of PP1γ1 (note that "exon 8" is part of its 3′UTR). The PP1γ1 encodes a protein containing 323 amino acids derived from the seven exons along with the 8 amino acid C-terminus from the extended exon 7. In the post-meiotic germ cells in testis the intron 7 is spliced out, thus, producing a shorter Pp1γ2 transcript of approximately 1.7 kb. Exon 8 codes for the 22 amino acid C-terminus in PP1γ2. Thus, the amino acid sequences of PP1γ1 and PP1γ2 are identical in all respects except for their extreme C-termini. **(B)** Constructs for generating transgenic PP1γ1 mice. Rescues I–III constructs contain the entire or a portion of intron 7 which is part of the 3′UTR of the messenger RNA for PP1γ1. There was little or no transgenic expression of PP1γ1 in testis of mice generated from these constructs. The last rescue construct (Rescue IV) lacks the 0.9 kb region of intron 7 following the stop codon in PP1γ1 mRNA. Transcript from this construct will resemble PP1γ2 mRNA except that PP1γ1 protein will be produced. The transgenic mice produced from this construct expressed high testis levels of transgenic PP1γ1 and rescued spermatogenesis but not sperm fertility.

PP1β, or PP1γ1 - which is able to support sperm motility and fertility in these species. The fact that PP1γ2 alone is sufficient for male fertility does not necessarily suggest that the other PP1 isoforms would be unable to functionally replace PP1γ2. Is the requirement for PP1γ2 an evolutionary accident or is there an isoform specific function for it in mammalian sperm? Can expressing the PP1γ1 isoform in testis, restore spermatogenesis and fertility of *Ppp1cc* null mice? Employing the same strategy used in the PP1γ2 transgenic rescue approach, the PGK2 promoter was used to drive transgenic expression of PP1γ1. This approach which was successful for PP1γ2 expression (Sinha et al., 2012), failed to transgenically express PP1γ1 (Dudiki et al., 2019) in testis. The transgene construct in all these failed attempts contained portions of the intron preceding exon 8, which is part of the 3′UTR of the mRNA for PP1γ1 (**Figure 2B**). In the fourth attempt, removal of this entire portion of the 3′UTR in the cDNA in the transgene construct (**Figure 2B**) led to robust expression of PP1γ1 in developing spermatocytes and spermatids (Dudiki et al., 2019). Transgenic expression of PP1γ1 in testis of *Ppp1cc* null mice was able to fully restore spermatogenesis. However, sperm function and fertility were severely compromised in these PP1γ1 rescue mice. Motility of PP1γ1-bearing sperm was diminished and their flagellar beat amplitude was severely dampened (Dudiki et al., 2019). Fertility defects in the rescue mice were most likely due to the inability of sperm bearing PP1γ1 to undergo hyperactivation. Thus PP1γ2 is essential in sperm for its normal function and fertility.

TABLE 1 | Fertility status of knockout mouse lines.

Group	Mouse lines	Fertility status (female)	Fertility status (male)
1	PP1 (*Ppp1cc*) global knockout (Chakrabarti et al., 2007b)	Fertile	Infertile
	PP1γ2 conditional (testis-specific) knockout (Sinha et al., 2013)	Fertile	Infertile
	PP1γ1 rescue (in *Ppp1cc* knockout background) (Dudiki et al., 2019)	Fertile	Sub-fertile
2	GSK3α global knockout (Bhattacharjee et al., 2015)	Fertile	Infertile
	GSK3α conditional (testis-specific) knockout (Bhattacharjee et al., 2018)	Fertile	Infertile
3	GSK3β global knockout (Hoeflich et al., 2000)	Embryonically lethal	
	GSK3β conditional (testis-specific) knockout (Bhattacharjee et al., 2018)	Fertile	Fertile
4	PKACα2 (testis isoform specific) knockout (Nolan et al., 2004)	Fertile	Infertile
5	sAC (*Adcy10*) knockout (Hess et al., 2005; Xie et al., 2006)	Fertile	Infertile
6	PPP3R2 (sperm isoform specific) knockout (Miyata et al., 2015)	Fertile	Infertile
	PPP3CC (sperm isoform specific) knockout (Miyata et al., 2015)	Fertile	Infertile

A specific isoform requirement of a protein is usually thought to arise due to isoform specific binding partners for that protein or due to its unique biochemical activity. An isoform specific function could also be due to the restricted spatio-temporal expression of the protein isoform during cell or tissue development. Despite the knowledge that PP1γ2 is the only PP1 isoform expressed in developing spermatocytes and spermatids (Chakrabarti et al., 2007b). it was anticipated that specific binding proteins for PP1γ2 exist in testis and sperm. However, binding partners of sperm PP1γ2 identified so far are ubiquitous in tissues and organisms and are known to bind to all PP1 isoforms (Goswami et al., 2019). That is, these proteins would bind to any PP1 isoform if present in sperm, just as they do in other cells and tissues. The three protein regulators of PP1γ2 identified are PPP1R2 (inhibitor I2), PPP1R7 (SDS22), and PPP1R11 (inhibitor I3). These three regulators/inhibitors are evolutionarily ancient and conserved across species (Heroes et al., 2013), play key roles in mitosis and other cellular functions (Peggie et al., 2002; Wang et al., 2008; Eiteneuer et al., 2014). Thus, loss of any one them is likely to cause embryonic lethality. It is intriguing that the sperm specific isoform, PP1γ2, is regulated by these ancient, ubiquitous, and essential PP1 binding proteins. The three regulators share localization with PP1γ2 in the head and the principal piece of sperm. The association of inhibitors to PP1γ2 changes during epididymal sperm maturation. In immotile caput epididymal sperm, PPP1R2 and PPP1R7 are not bound to PP1γ2, whereas in motile caudal sperm, all three inhibitors are bound as hetero-dimers or hetero-trimers (Goswami et al., 2019) (**Table 2** and **Figures 3A,B**). In caudal sperm from male mice lacking sAC and GSK3 (see below), where motility and

TABLE 2 | The binding profile of the regulators with PP1γ2 in caput and caudal epididymal sperm is summarized in the table along with data with caudal sperm from Gsk3α knockout, PKA Cα2 knockout and sAC knockout mice where the binding status of sds22 resembles that in wild type caput sperm.

Group	Mouse lines		I2	SDS22	I3
1	Wild type (Goswami et al., 2019)	Caput	Not bound	Not bound	Bound
		Caudal	Bound	Bound	Bound
2	GSK3α global knockout (Goswami et al., 2019)	Caput	Not bound	Not bound	Bound
		Caudal	Bound	Not bound	Bound
3	PKACα2 (testis isoform specific) knockout (Goswami, 2018)	Caput	Not bound	Not bound	Bound
		Caudal	Bound	Not bound	Bound
4	sAC (*Adcy10*) knockout (Goswami et al., 2019)	Caput	Not bound	Not bound	Bound
		Caudal	Bound	Not bound	Bound

Thus, epididymal sperm maturation appears to be altered in these knockout mice.

fertility are impaired, the association of PP1γ2 to the inhibitors resembles immature caput sperm. In sperm containing PP1γ1 the association of these inhibitors are altered resembling that of PP1γ2 in immotile caput epididymal sperm (Goswami et al., 2019) (**Table 2**). It is known that binding of inhibitor 2 to PP1 is regulated by GSK3 (**Figure 3B**). It is likely that binding of the other two inhibitors, PPP1R7 and PPP1R2, to PP1γ2 are also regulated by phosphorylation. Changes in the associations of the regulators with PP1γ2, are likely part of biochemical mechanisms responsible for the development of motility and fertilizing ability of sperm.

A recently identified potential binding protein for PP1γ2 is CCDC181 (Schwarz et al., 2017). It is likely that CCDC181 binds to PP1γ1 and PP1γ2 with differing affinities leading to preferential localization of PP1γ2 to the flagellum. Determination of the protein targets of PP1γ2 in the flagellum and how CCDC181 regulates PP1γ2 is under active investigation.

GLYCOGEN SYNTHASE KINASE 3α, GSK3α, IN SPERM

The enzyme GSK3, a serine/threonine protein kinase, was named GSK-3 because it was discovered after PKA and phosphorylase kinase (GSK-1 and GSK-2). Two other GS kinases, GSK-4 and -5, named based on their relative elution profiles in phospho-cellulose chromatography of muscle extracts, were later renamed as casein kinase 1 and 2, respectively (Parker et al., 1982). The enzyme GSK3, retained its original name even though it was later found to be a key signaling component of a large number of cellular processes (Kaidanovich-Beilin and Woodgett, 2011; Medina and Wandosell, 2011). An array of functions attributed to GSK3 include insulin action, regulation of cell survival, apoptosis, embryonic development, Wnt/β-catenin and hedgehog signaling, and growth factor action. It is also a target for drug development in several clinical disorders including cancer (Jope et al., 2007).

In mammals, GSK3 is ubiquitous and is expressed as two isoforms, GSK3α and GSK3β, encoded by different genes. The catalytic domains of the two isoforms are 98% identical while

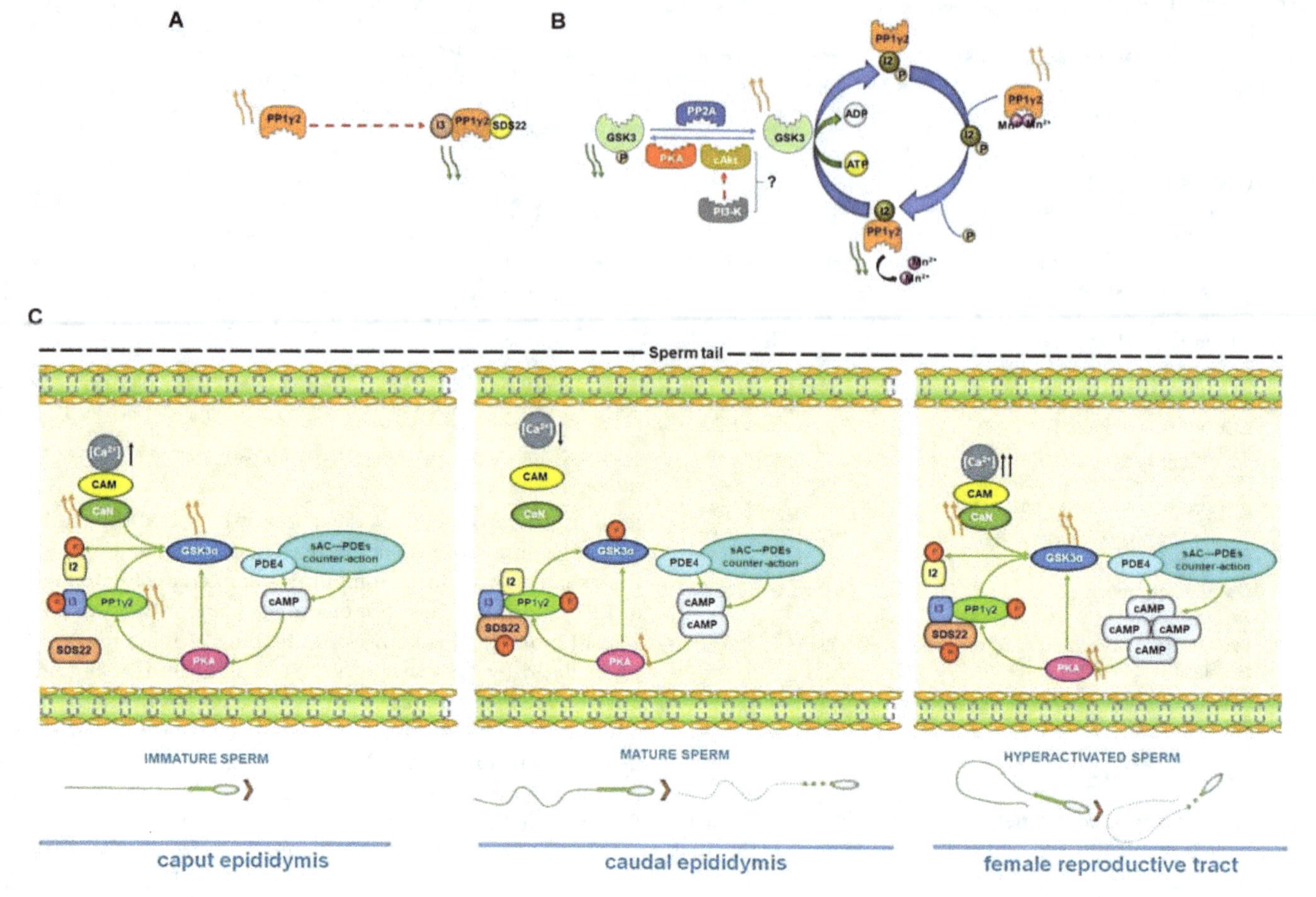

FIGURE 3 | (A–B) Regulation of PP1γ2 activity by I3, SDS22 and I2. **(A)** I3 and SDS bound PP1γ2 is catalytically inactive. Binding of these inhibitors to PP1γ2 is altered in caudal compared to caput sperm and in sperm from infertile transgenic KO mice (see text). **(B)** Inhibitor 2, a regulator of PP1γ2, is known to be phosphorylated by GSK3. In caput but not in caudal epididymal sperm I2 is expected to be phosphorylated due to changes in GSK3 activity. This is one of the ways by which catalytic activity of PP1γ2 is thought to decrease during epididymal sperm maturation. **(C)** Schematic diagram of the proposed interrelationship between GSK3α, PKA Cα2, PP1γ2 and PP2B (PPP3R2/CC) during epididymal sperm maturation and sperm hyperactivation in female reproductive tract. Curved orange arrow(s) indicate relative degree of activities of the enzymes; straight black arrow(s) denote relative level of the ion/protein inside the cell.

their N- and C-termini are distinctive (Woodgett, 1990). While there are reports ascribing distinct roles for each of the isoforms (McNeill and Woodgett, 2010) under most circumstances the two isoforms are redundant and functionally interchangeable. Knockout of *Gsk3β* in mice causes late embryonic lethality (Hoeflich et al., 2000). The inability of GSK3α to substitute for GSK3β in the developing embryo may be due to the non-overlapping expression of the two isoforms. Conditional knockout of the floxed *Gsk3β* alleles on a *Gsk3α* null background show that complete loss of both isoforms impairs signaling and tissue function. However, one allele of *Gsk3β* or *Gsk3α* on a *Gsk3α* or *Gsk3β* null background, respectively, is sufficient to maintain normal Wnt signaling and tissue function (Doble et al., 2007; McNeill and Woodgett, 2010) highlighting the functional redundancy of the two isoforms in most tissues and cell types.

The protein, GSK3 was first discovered as an enzyme responsible for activation of PP1γ2 in bovine sperm (Vijayaraghavan et al., 1996). Both α and β isoforms of GSK3 are present in sperm. Immotile caput sperm contain four-fold higher GSK3 activity than motile caudal epididymal sperm. Both tyrosine phosphorylation (which stimulates catalytic activity) and serine phosphorylation of GSK3 (an inhibitory mechanism) increase significantly in sperm during their passage through the epididymis (Somanath et al., 2004). Incubation of motile or immotile sperm with compounds that activate PKA (e.g., dbcAMP) or inhibit protein phosphatase (e.g., calyculin A) is accompanied by increases in GSK3 serine phosphorylation and motility stimulation. GSK3 tyrosine phosphorylation which is believed to be autoregulatory, remains unchanged during capacitation, while only GSK3α ser21 phosphorylation is altered during this event (Dey et al., 2019a,b).

It was recently shown that *Gsk3α* null mice exhibit male infertility (Bhattacharjee et al., 2015, 2018). Knockout of GSK3α in post-meiotic testicular germ cells, using the Cre-Lox strategy, also results in male infertility. Mice with a testis knockout of GSK3β are normal and fertile. Thus, GSK3α has an isoform specific function in sperm. Analysis of sperm lacking GSK3α showed that adenine nucleotide levels, energy metabolism, and protein phosphatase and kinase activities were affected suggesting impaired sperm maturation in the epididymis. A recent report also documents the role for GSK3 and a non-canonical Wnt signaling during epididymal sperm maturation: loss of Wnt signaling in sperm results in male infertility (Koch et al., 2015). The activity of GSK3α isoform has also been correlated with human sperm motility (Freitas et al., 2019). The inability of GSK3β to replace GSK3α, only in testis and sperm, is surprising given the fact that the two isoforms are functionally interchangeable in most cellular contexts and in tissues. Thus, despite the presence of both GSK3 isoforms, mammalian sperm are unique in their requirement for the GSK3α isoform. Taken together, these studies, support the notion that GSK3α is essential for epididymal sperm maturation, motility, and fertilization.

CALCINEURIN IN SPERM FUNCTION

Calcineurin (also known as PP2B or PPP3C) is a serine/threonine phosphatase regulated by calcium. In response to an elevation of cellular calcium, calmodulin binds to a calmodulin binding region of the catalytic subunit PPP3C. This binding causes an auto-inhibitory arm of calcineurin to move away from the substrate binding site thus activating the enzyme by enabling its access to substrates (Rusnak and Mertz, 2000; Parra and Rothermel, 2017). The catalytic activity of the enzyme is also regulated by calcium binding to a regulatory subunit (PPP3R2). Regulation and function of calcineurin in several cell types has been extensively studied (Rusnak and Mertz, 2000; Parra and Rothermel, 2017). More than two decades ago a role for a calcium regulated protein phosphatase was proposed in the regulation of sperm motility (Tash et al., 1988; Tash and Bracho, 1994). In non-mammalian sperm, calcineurin has been shown to have role in activation of progressive motility and egg activation (Levasseur et al., 2013; Krapf et al., 2014). The catalytic and regulatory subunits of calcineurin are present as testis-specific isoforms, PPP3CC and PPP3R2. It was shown by super resolution microscopy that the catalytic subunit of calcineurin, PPP3CC, is localized near the quadrilateral structures of CatSper in the axoneme (Chung et al., 2014). In CatSper1-deficient spermatozoa, PPP3CC can be seen localized mostly to the axoneme but disappears from the quadrilateral structures. Another report showed that pharmacological inhibition of calmodulin affects protein tyrosine phosphorylation seen during sperm capacitation (Navarrete et al., 2015). In another study, micromolar amounts of FK506 has been demonstrated to prevent sperm acrosomal exocytosis (Castillo Bennett et al., 2010). A recent report now shows that knockout of either *Ppp3CC* or *Ppp3R2* present only in testis and sperm resulted in male infertility (Miyata et al., 2015). Sperm numbers and testis weights in these knockout mice are normal; but sperm motility is impaired with a stiffened mid-piece. The *Ppp3CC* or *Ppp3R2* knockout mice are infertile *in vivo*. Sperm from these knockout mice also cannot fertilize eggs *in vitro*. Surprisingly, wild type sperm treated with the calcineurin inhibitors, FK506 and cyclosporine, did not affect *in vitro* fertilization. Thus, infertility was thought to be due to impaired sperm function in the male reproductive tract. Calcineurin inhibitors injected into mice resulted in reversible male infertility. The investigators concluded that calcineurin was required for epididymal sperm maturation: genetic disruption or pharmacological inhibition *in vivo* affected sperm maturation causing infertility (Miyata et al., 2015).

The questions of how calcineurin may act and how it is activated during epididymal sperm maturation were not addressed. Recent data show that calcineurin and GSK3 are interrelated in their roles in epididymal sperm maturation and absence of calcineurin increases GSK3 phosphorylation resulting in its lower catalytic activity (Dey et al., 2019b). It is suspected that calcineurin regulates mitochondrial energization directly and glycolysis indirectly through its effect on GSK3. It is likely that high calcium levels in immature sperm (Vijayaraghavan and Hoskins, 1989, 1990) activates calcineurin.

INTERRELATIONSHIP BETWEEN PKA, PP1, GSK3α, AND PP2B

As described earlier the requirement and the roles of cAMP and the kinase activated by it, PKA, in sperm are well known. The relationship between PKA and GSK3 in sperm was indicated by the fact that cAMP analogs increased GSK3-α/β phosphorylation, without any isoform specificity. Phosphorylation of both GSK3 α and β isoforms were reduced and its catalytic activity increased in sperm with diminished cAMP (using KH7, a sAC inhibitor), or due to knock out of sAC. That is, GSK3 is a target of PKA phosphorylation. This relationship between GSK3 and PKA was further validated in GSK3α knockout mice. Loss of GSK3α or β by targeted disruption or pharmacological inhibition of the enzyme significantly reduced sperm cAMP levels (Dey et al., 2018). The decrease in cAMP levels was attributed to increased phosphodiesterase activity. Together these data support the possibility that GSK3 and cAMP form an interrelated regulatory loop (Dey et al., 2018).

Inhibition of the predominant sperm protein phosphatase PP1γ2 by calyculin A significantly increased phosphorylation of both GSK3 isoforms (Ser21/9) in caudal epididymal sperm and a concomitant decrease in its catalytic activity. Conversely, increased GSK3 activity is associated with increased PP1γ2 activity. One of the ways by which GSK3 regulates PP1 activity is by its phosphorylation of the inhibitor I2 as discussed earlier. Phosphorylated I2 dissociates from PP1 leading to its activation (**Figure 3B**). The roles of binding and dissociation of PP1γ2 binding proteins due to their reversible phosphorylation is a feature of the regulation of the phosphatase in sperm (Goswami et al., 2019). Sperm PP2A also targets GSK3, without any isoform specificity; however, its role in regulating GSK3 has not been investigated in detail (Dudiki et al., 2015).

New information shows that not only is GSK3 a target of PP1γ2, but it is also regulated by calcineurin. While PP1γ2 acts on both isoforms of GSK3 (Somanath et al., 2004), calcineurin preferentially dephosphorylates only the GSK3α isoform (Dey et al., 2019a,b). Phosphorylation of the GSK3α (Ser21) isoform is elevated in sperm lacking calcineurin (Dey et al., 2019a,b). Following a decrease in their catalytic activities in caudal epididymal sperm during motility initiation, surprisingly the catalytic activities of both GSK3α and calcineurin increase during sperm capacitation and hyperactivation, recapitulating the situation in caput sperm (**Figure 3C**) (Dey et al., 2019a,b). Increased calcineurin activity, presumably following increased sperm Ca^{2+} during hyperactivation is responsible for decreased phosphorylation and increased catalytic activity of GSK3α. Pharmacologic inhibition of calcineurin during capacitation abrogated this decrease in phosphorylation and the increase in GSK3 activity. Increased activities of GSK3α and PP2B appear to be characteristics of not only capacitated sperm, but also, paradoxically, of immature caput epididymal sperm. Thus, phosphatases (PP1γ2 and PP2B) and the kinases (PKA and GSK3) are mechanistically interrelated during epididymal initiation of motility and also during fertilization of the egg (summarized in **Figure 3C**).

THE PROTEINS PP1γ2, GSK3α, PKA Cα2, AND PPP3R2/CC PRESENT ONLY IN SPERM ARE CONSERVED IN MAMMALS

As noted earlier the PP1γ2 isoform in sperm, is present only in mammals. Examination of the available annotated genome databases shows that monotremes and other non-mammalian vertebrates contain the *Ppp1cc* gene but the PP1γ2 isoform cannot form due to the absence of splice sites at exon 7 in the gene. Also absent is a region corresponding to exon 8, which is highly conserved and present in the *Ppp1cc* in all mammals (**Figure 4A**). This PP1γ2 isoform derived from exon 8 has a

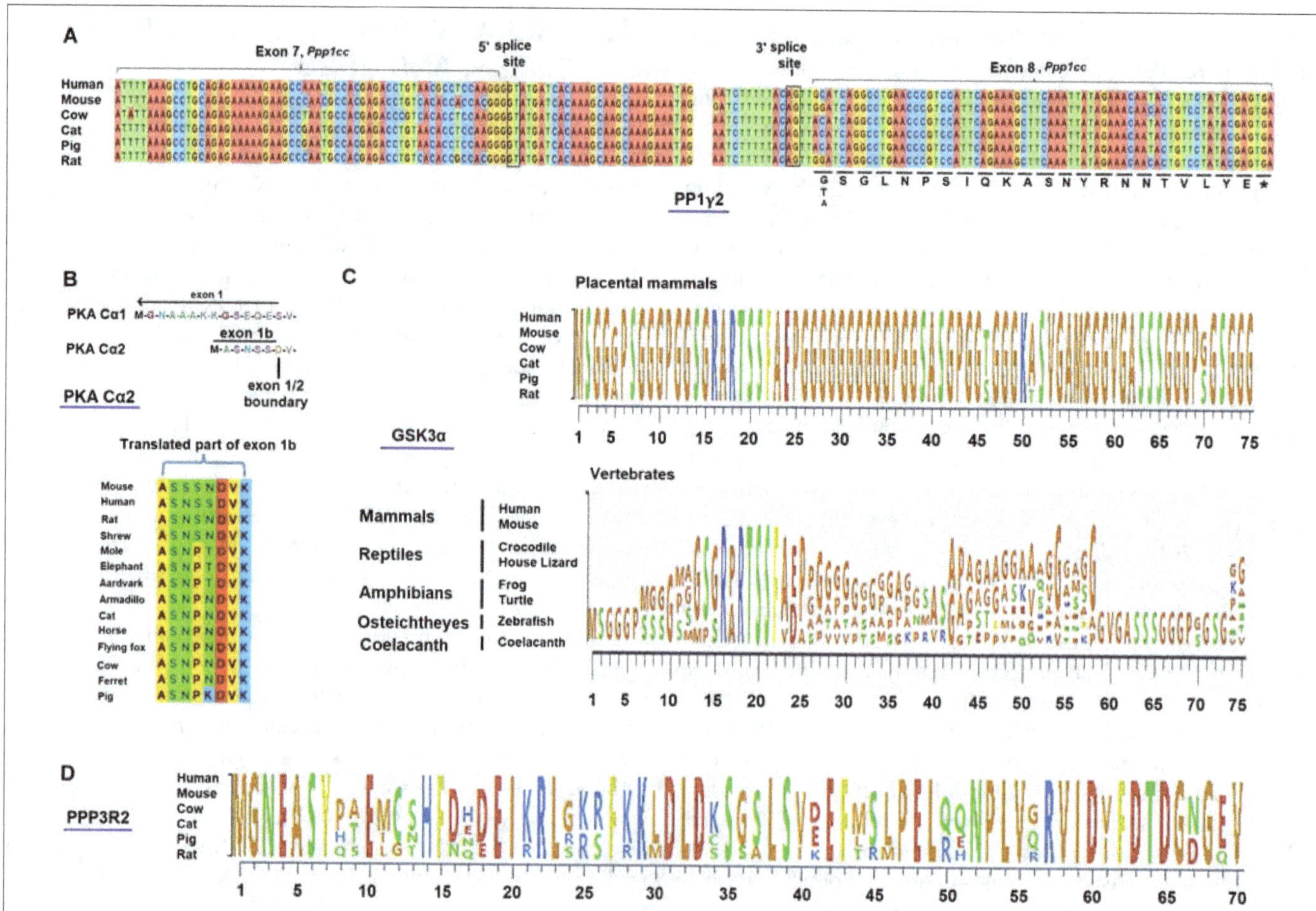

FIGURE 4 | (A) Conservation of C-terminus of PPP1CC2 in mammals. The 5′ and 3′ splice sites for the generation of PP1γ2 in *Ppp1cc* is found only in mammals. These splice sites and a recognizable exon 8 are absent in *Ppp1cc* in the genomes of the duck billed platypus and the non-mammalian vertebrates. The C-terminal 22 amino acid residues (316–337) are virtually identical in all placental mammals for which annotated genomic data bases exist. Sequences from a few of these mammals are shown above. **(B)** PKA catalytic subunit in somatic cells (Cα1) and sperm (Cα2) are derived from alternate exons 1a and 1b. Cα1 is present in somatic cell. Cα2 produced in testis using exon 1b is present only in mammals. Exon 1b is present and conserved in all placental mammals. **(C)** Conservation of GSK3α isoform in mammals. The glycine rich N-terminus of the GSK3 alpha isoform is conserved in placental mammalian species, but not in non-mammalian vertebrates. **(D)** Conservation of testis-specific isoform of PP2B, PPP3R2 (regulatory subunit) across different mammalian species. While the entire PPP3R2 is present and conserved in all mammals only a portion of the N-terminus sequence of PPP3R2 is shown.

unique 22 amino acid C-terminus present and conserved in all mammals (**Figure 4A**). The somatic isoform, PP1γ1 has a six amino acid C-terminus derived from the extended exon 7. Aside from these differences in the C-termini, the rest of 315 amino acid sequences of the both PP1γ1 and PP1γ2 are identical. Why mammalian sperm contain only PP1γ2 is unknown.

It is known that knockout of the enzyme synthesizing cAMP in sperm, sAC, and that of PKA result in male infertility. It is intriguing that the catalytic subunit of PKA is also expressed as a sperm specific isoform (PrkaCA also known as PKA Cα2) with a unique six amino acid N-terminus due to expression of an alternate exon, exon 1b (Agustin et al., 2000; Desseyn et al., 2000; San Agustin and Witman, 2001) (**Figure 4B**). The exon 1a codes for 12 amino acids of the N-terminus of the ubiquitous and the somatic cell version of the catalytic subunit. Aside from this difference in their N-termini the primary sequences of the rest of the catalytic subunits are identical. The reason this different N-terminus is required in testis and sperm remains puzzling because both sperm and somatic cell forms of the PKA catalytic subunits have identical biochemical properties (Vetter et al., 2011). Removal of exon 1b leading to the loss of PKA in sperm, renders males infertile (Nolan et al., 2004). Whether replacement

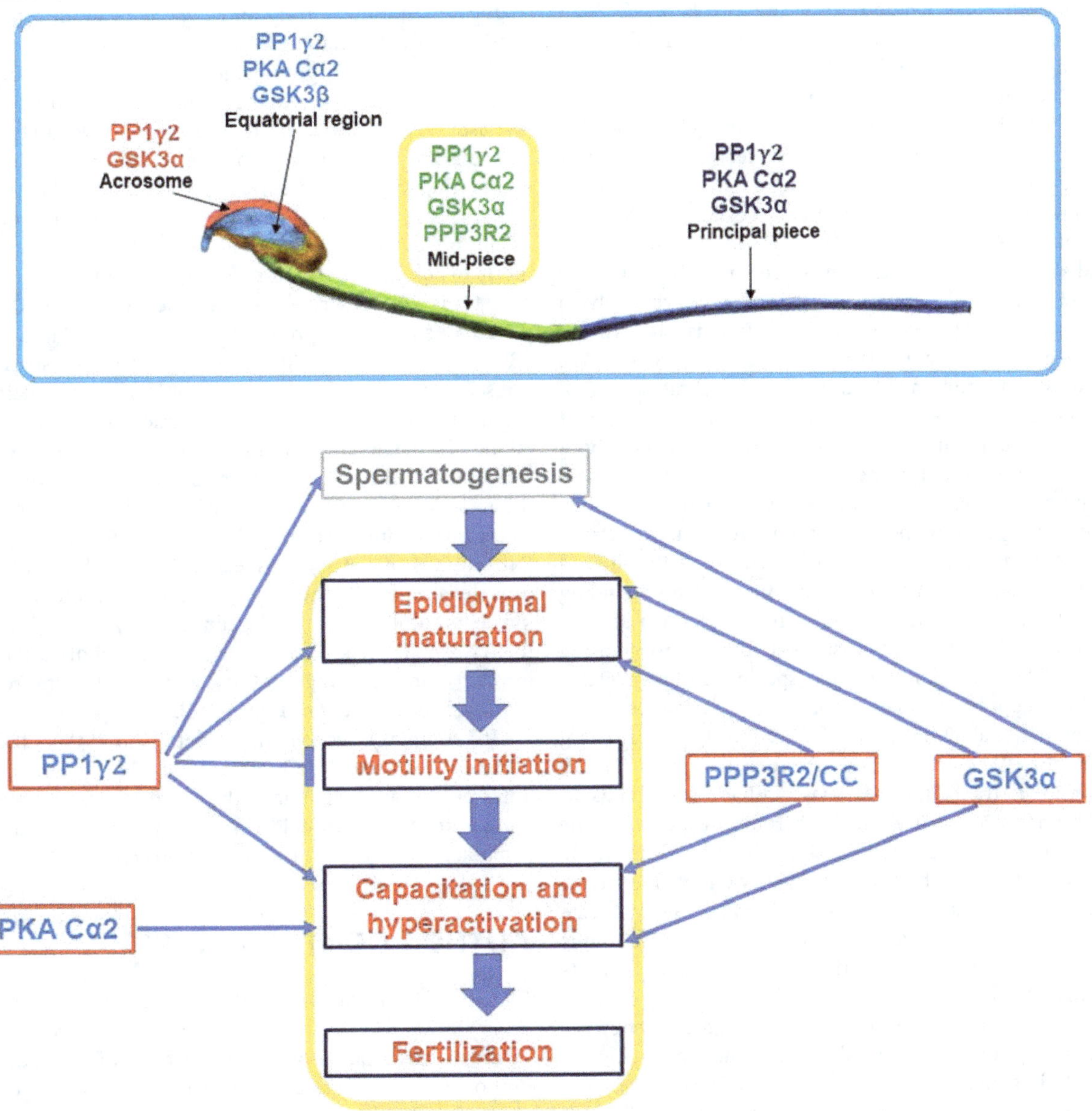

FIGURE 5 | A simplified summary of spatial and temporal organization of GSK3α, PKA Cα2, PP1γ2, and PP2B (PPP3R2/CC). Upper panel image was adopted and modified from Dey et al. (2018, 2019a); it shows localization of these enzymes in different compartments of a sperm cell; all of these four enzyme isoforms co-localizes only in sperm midpiece. Lower panel demonstrates how these enzymes regulate sperm functions starting from its synthesis (i.e., spermatogenesis) till fertilization. (↑) and (T) indicate stimulatory and inhibitory effect, respectively.

of the sperm form of the enzyme with the somatic form of the PKA catalytic subunit would sustain normal sperm function is not known. However, it is intriguing that exon 1b, the sperm specific isoform of PKA, is present only in mammals (Soberg et al., 2017). Non-mammalian species only contain the isoform derived from utilization of exon 1a (**Figure 4B**).

A germ cell–enriched protein, viz. sperm PKA interacting factor (SPIF), was found to be co-expressed and co-regulated with PKACα2 and with t-complex protein (TCP)-11 (Stanger et al., 2016). These three proteins constitute part of a novel trimeric complex in murine spermatozoa. During capacitation, the SPIF undergoes phosphorylation leading to a molecular rearrangement that brings PKACα2 and TCP11 into close proximity of each other. These results could explain how PKA Cα2 functions as a specific isoform complexed with SPIF and TCP11 during capacitation and fertilization.

The GSK3α isoform is essential in mammalian sperm despite the fact both GSK3α and β isoforms are interchangeable in other cells and tissues. GSK3α arose in vertebrates presumably by gene duplication of GSK3β which is the only isoform in invertebrates. Among vertebrates the GSK3α isoform is absent in birds (Alon et al., 2011). Sequence comparison of the extended glycine rich N-terminus present only in GSK3α shows that this sequence segment is highly conserved only in placental mammals. This extended N-terminus is present, but not conserved in non-mammalian vertebrates (**Figure 4C**). We predict that sperm from non-mammalian vertebrates contain only GSK3β and not GSK3α. In fact, we have shown that Xenopus sperm contains only GSK3β despite the fact both GSK3 isoforms are present in the genome of this species. These observations are compatible with the possibility that mammalian sperm contain a GSK3α-specific binding protein. Efforts to identify a isoform-specific binding protein using a two-hybrid approach with testis cDNA yielded a number of GSK3 binding proteins, but these GSK3 interactors were not isoform specific (Freitas et al., 2019). However, a yeast two-hybrid approach using human fetal cDNA yielded four GSK3α-specific binding proteins one of which appears to play a role in regulating circadian rhythm (Zeidner et al., 2011). One of these four GSK3α binding proteins is CENPV which is highly expressed in testis (NCBI, mouse ENCODE transcriptome data). CENPV also binds to tubulin (Honda et al., 2009) and is therefore, expected to be localized along the length of the flagellum. Thus, GSK3α in the flagellum is likely to orchestrate phosphorylation of proteins involved in regulating sperm motility and hyperactivation. The requirement of sperm GSK3α with its conserved of N-terminus suggests a role for it in maturation and fertilization events unique to mammals.

A relatively recent addition to the list of signaling enzymes regulating sperm function is the calcium regulated phosphatase, PP2B. Catalytic activity of PP2B is required in sperm during their passage through the epididymis as is the case with GSK3α. Sperm and testis express specific isoforms of the catalytic and regulatory calcineurin, PPP3CC and PPP3R2, respectively. Examination of the genomic sequences of several species shows that PPP3R2 is present only in eutherian mammalians and its amino acid sequence is remarkably conserved in the 121 mammals for which annotated genomic databases exist (**Figure 4D**).

Several predominantly testis-expressed proteins present in mammalian sperm have been identified as mammal-specific. These include proteins involved in DNA binding, sperm egg binding or those required for required for the unique structural features of mammalian sperm, such as protamine 3, SMCP, and ADAM proteins (Cho, 2012; Luis Villanueva-Canas et al., 2017). However, the observation that the four signaling enzymes suggested to be mechanistically interrelated are mammal specific isoforms is significant, suggesting a unique function in male gametes (**Figure 3C**). The specific isoforms PP1γ2, GSK3, PKA and PP2B play key roles in regulation sperm motility and hyperactivation, a phenomenon unique only to mammals (**Figure 5**). It would appear that their roles in these physiological functions in mammals arise due to their location in the flagellum. **Figure 5** shows the intrasperm localization of these enzymes. It would be interesting to determine if one or more of CatSper complexes located along the flagellum are mammal specific. The two possible binding proteins for PP1γ2 in the flagellum are CCDC181 (Schwarz et al., 2017) and PPP1R32 (Cifuentes et al., 2018), both of which are expressed predominantly or exclusively in the testis. As described above, the GSK3α binding protein CENPV should be present bound to the flagellum because CENPV also binds to tubulin, which in sperm is only present in tail (Honda et al., 2009). Sperm calcineurin has been shown by high resolution microscopy to be localized along the flagellum (Chung et al., 2014). The nature of the binding protein for calcineurin in sperm is not known. Finally, PKA is known to bind AKAP3, which is present along the sperm flagellum (Vijayaraghavan et al., 1999). How the unique N-terminus of the sperm specific PKA catalytic subunit affects this localization is not known. Thus, all the four signaling proteins localized in the flagellum (PP1γ2, GSK3α, PP2B, and PKA) are likely to determine the phosphorylation status of proteins orchestrating motility and metabolism required for normal sperm function (**Figure 3C**).

In summary, considerable data show that the enzymes PP1γ2, GSK3 and PP2B, along with PKA, are mechanistically interrelated in regulating the two physiological processes unique to mammals: epididymal sperm maturation and sperm hyperactivation preceding fertilization (**Figure 5**).

AUTHOR CONTRIBUTIONS

SV and SD contributed to the conception and outline of the review. SD and CB organized the database. SV wrote the first draft of the manuscript. SD wrote the sections of the manuscript. All authors contributed to the manuscript reading and revisions.

FUNDING

This work was funded by the National Institute of Health (SV): R03HD096176 and R21HD086839.

REFERENCES

Agustin, J. T., Wilkerson, C. G., and Witman, G. B. (2000). The unique catalytic subunit of sperm cAMP-dependent protein kinase is the product of an alternative Calpha mRNA expressed specifically in spermatogenic cells. *Mol. Biol. Cell* 11, 3031–3044. doi: 10.1091/mbc.11.9.3031

Allouche-Fitoussi, D., Bakhshi, D., and Breitbart, H. (2018). Signaling pathways involved in human sperm hyperactivated motility stimulated by Zn(2). *Mol. Reprod. Dev.* 85, 543–556.

Alon, L. T., Pietrokovski, S., Barkan, S., Avrahami, L., Kaidanovich-Beilin, O., Woodgett, J. R., et al. (2011). Selective loss of glycogen synthase kinase-3alpha in birds reveals distinct roles for GSK-3 isozymes in tau phosphorylation. *FEBS Lett.* 585, 1158–1162. doi: 10.1016/j.febslet.2011.03.025

Alvau, A., Battistone, M. A., Gervasi, M. G., Navarrete, F. A., Xu, X. R., Sanchez-Cardenas, C., et al. (2016). The tyrosine kinase FER is responsible for the capacitation-associated increase in tyrosine phosphorylation in murine sperm. *Development* 143, 2325–2333. doi: 10.1242/dev.136499

Amann, R. P., Hay, S. R., and Hammerstedt, R. H. (1982). Yield, characteristics, motility and cAMP content of sperm isolated from seven regions of ram epididymis. *Biol. Reprod.* 27, 723–733. doi: 10.1095/biolreprod27.3.723

Arcelay, E., Salicioni, A. M., Wertheimer, E., and Visconti, P. E. (2008). Identification of proteins undergoing tyrosine phosphorylation during mouse sperm capacitation. *Int. J. Dev. Biol.* 52, 463–472. doi: 10.1387/ijdb.072555ea

Bailey, J. L. (2010). Factors regulating sperm capacitation. *Syst. Biol. Reprod. Med.* 56, 334–348. doi: 10.3109/19396368.2010.512377

Baker, M. A., Hetherington, L., and Aitken, R. J. (2006). Identification of SRC as a key PKA-stimulated tyrosine kinase involved in the capacitation-associated hyperactivation of murine spermatozoa. *J. Cell Sci.* 119(Pt 15), 3182–3192. doi: 10.1242/jcs.03055

Baker, M. A., Hetherington, L., Curry, B., and Aitken, R. J. (2009). Phosphorylation and consequent stimulation of the tyrosine kinase c-Abl by PKA in mouse spermatozoa, its implications during capacitation. *Dev. Biol.* 333, 57–66. doi: 10.1016/j.ydbio.2009.06.022

Balbach, M., Beckert, V., Hansen, J. N., and Wachten, D. (2018). Shedding light on the role of cAMP in mammalian sperm physiology. *Mol. Cell. Endocrinol.* 468, 111–120. doi: 10.1016/j.mce.2017.11.008

Bedford, J. M., and Hoskins, D. D. (1990). "The mammalian spermatozoon: morphology, biochemistry and physiology," in *Marshall's Physiology of Reproduction*, ed. G. E. Lamming, (New York, NY: Churchill Livingstone), 379.

Bhattacharjee, R., Goswami, S., Dey, S., Gangoda, M., Brothag, C., Eisa, A., et al. (2018). Isoform-specific requirement for GSK3 alpha in sperm for male fertility. *Biol. Reprod.* 99, 384–394. doi: 10.1093/biolre/ioy020

Bhattacharjee, R., Goswami, S., Dudiki, T., Popkie, A. P., Phiel, C. J., Kline, D., et al. (2015). Targeted disruption of glycogen synthase kinase 3A (GSK3A) in mice affects sperm motility resulting in male infertility. *Biol. Reprod.* 92:65. doi: 10.1095/biolreprod.114.124495

Brukman, N. G., Nunez, S. Y., Puga Molina, L. D. C., Buffone, M. G., Darszon, A., Cuasnicu, P. S., et al. (2019). Tyrosine phosphorylation signaling regulates Ca(2+) entry by affecting intracellular pH during human sperm capacitation. *J. Cell. Physiol.* 234, 5276–5288. doi: 10.1002/jcp.27337

Buffone, M. G., Wertheimer, E. V., Visconti, P. E., and Krapf, D. (2014). Central role of soluble adenylyl cyclase and cAMP in sperm physiology. *Biochim. Biophys. Acta* 1842(12 Pt B), 2610–2620. doi: 10.1016/j.bbadis.2014.07.013

Burton, K. A., and McKnight, G. S. (2007). PKA, germ cells, and fertility. *Physiology* 22, 40–46. doi: 10.1152/physiol.00034.2006

Carlson, A. E., Westenbroek, R. E., Quill, T., Ren, D., Clapham, D. E., Hille, B., et al. (2003). CatSper1 required for evoked Ca2+ entry and control of flagellar function in sperm. *Proc. Natl. Acad. Sci. U.S.A.* 100, 14864–14868. doi: 10.1073/pnas.2536658100

Carr, D. W., and Acott, T. S. (2005). Intracellular pH regulates bovine sperm motility and protein phosphorylation1. *Biol. Reprod.* 41, 907–920. doi: 10.1095/biolreprod41.5.907

Carr, D. W., Usselman, M. C., and Acott, T. S. (1985). Effects of pH, lactate, and viscoelastic drag on sperm motility: a species comparison. *Biol. Reprod.* 33, 588–595. doi: 10.1095/biolreprod33.3.588

Castillo Bennett, J., Roggero, C. M., Mancifesta, F. E., and Mayorga, L. S. (2010). Calcineurin-mediated dephosphorylation of synaptotagmin VI is necessary for acrosomal exocytosis. *J. Biol. Chem.* 285, 26269–26278. doi: 10.1074/jbc.M109.095752

Chakrabarti, R., Cheng, L., Puri, P., Soler, D., and Vijayaraghavan, S. (2007a). Protein phosphatase PP1 gamma 2 in sperm morphogenesis and epididymal initiation of sperm motility. *Asian J. Androl.* 9, 445–452. doi: 10.1111/j.1745-7262.2007.00307.x

Chakrabarti, R., Kline, D., Lu, J., Orth, J., Pilder, S., and Vijayaraghavan, S. (2007b). Analysis of Ppp1cc-null mice suggests a role for PP1gamma2 in sperm morphogenesis. *Biol. Reprod.* 76, 992–1001. doi: 10.1095/biolreprod.106.058610

Chang, H., and Suarez, S. S. (2011). Two distinct Ca(2+) signaling pathways modulate sperm flagellar beating patterns in mice. *Biol. Reprod.* 85, 296–305. doi: 10.1095/biolreprod.110.089789

Chavez, J. C., Ferreira, J. J., Butler, A., De La Vega Beltran, J. L., Trevino, C. L., Darszon, A., et al. (2014). SLO3 K+ channels control calcium entry through CATSPER channels in sperm. *J. Biol. Chem.* 289, 32266–32275. doi: 10.1074/jbc.M114.607556

Chen, W. Y., Xu, W. M., Chen, Z. H., Ni, Y., Yuan, Y. Y., Zhou, S. C., et al. (2009). Cl- is required for HCO3- entry necessary for sperm capacitation in guinea pig: involvement of a Cl-/HCO3- exchanger (SLC26A3) and CFTR. *Biol. Reprod.* 80, 115–123. doi: 10.1095/biolreprod.108.068528

Cho, C. (2012). Testicular and epididymal ADAMs: expression and function during fertilization. *Nat. Rev. Urol.* 9, 550–560. doi: 10.1038/nrurol.2012.167

Chung, J. J., Navarro, B., Krapivinsky, G., Krapivinsky, L., and Clapham, D. E. (2011). A novel gene required for male fertility and functional CATSPER channel formation in spermatozoa. *Nat. Commun.* 2:153.

Chung, J. J., Shim, S. H., Everley, R. A., Gygi, S. P., Zhuang, X., and Clapham, D. E. (2014). Structurally distinct Ca(2+) signaling domains of sperm flagella orchestrate tyrosine phosphorylation and motility. *Cell* 157, 808–822. doi: 10.1016/j.cell.2014.02.056

Cifuentes, M., Baeza, V., Arrabal, P. M., Visser, R., Grondona, J. M., Saldivia, N., et al. (2018). Expression of a novel ciliary protein, IIIG9, during the differentiation and maturation of ependymal cells. *Mol. Neurobiol.* 55, 1652–1664. doi: 10.1007/s12035-017-0434-5

Cohen, P. (1990). The structure and regulation of protein phosphatases. *Adv. Second Messenger Phosphoprotein Res.* 24, 230–235.

Cohen, P., Holmes, C. F., and Tsukitani, Y. (1990). Okadaic acid: a new probe for the study of cellular regulation. *Trends Biochem. Sci.* 15, 98–102. doi: 10.1016/0968-0004(90)90192-e

Colledge, M., and Scott, J. D. (1999). AKAPs: from structure to function. *Trends Cell Biol.* 9, 216–221. doi: 10.1016/s0962-8924(99)01558-5

Cooper, T. G. (1986). *The Epididymis, Sperm Maturation and Fertilization.* Berlin: Springer-Verlag.

Cruz, D. F., Farinha, C. M., and Swiatecka-Urban, A. (2019). Unraveling the Function of lemur tyrosine kinase 2 network. *Front. Pharmacol.* 10:24. doi: 10.3389/fphar.2019.00024

da Cruz e Silva, E. F., Fox, C. A., Ouimet, C. C., Gustafson, E., Watson, S. J., and Greengard, P. (1995). Differential expression of protein phosphatase 1 isoforms in mammalian brain. *J. Neurosci.* 15(5 Pt 1), 3375–3389. doi: 10.1523/jneurosci.15-05-03375.1995

Desseyn, J. L., Burton, K. A., and McKnight, G. S. (2000). Expression of a nonmyristylated variant of the catalytic subunit of protein kinase A during male germ-cell development. *Proc. Natl. Acad. Sci. U.S.A.* 97, 6433–6438. doi: 10.1073/pnas.97.12.6433

Dey, S., Eisa, A., Kline, D., Wagner, F. F., Abeysirigunawardena, S., and Vijayaraghavan, S. (2019a). Roles of glycogen synthase kinase 3 alpha and calcineurin in regulating the ability of sperms to fertilize eggs. *FASEB J.* doi: 10.1096/fj.201902163R

Dey, S., Eisa, A., Opoku, V. W., Kine, D. K., and Vijayaraghavan, S. (2019b). "Mechanistically interrelated roles of calcineurin and GSK3a in regulating the ability of sperm to fertilzie eggs," in *Proceedings of the 44th meeting of the American Society of Andrology*, Chicago, IL, 64.

Dey, S., Goswami, S., Eisa, A., Bhattacharjee, R., Brothag, C., Kline, D., et al. (2018). Cyclic AMP and glycogen synthase kinase 3 form a regulatory loop in spermatozoa. *J. Cell. Physiol.* 233, 7239–7252. doi: 10.1002/jcp.26557

Doble, B. W., Patel, S., Wood, G. A., Kockeritz, L. K., and Woodgett, J. R. (2007). Functional redundancy of GSK-3 alpha and GSK-3 beta in Wnt/beta-catenin signaling shown by using an allelic series of embryonic stem cell lines. *Dev. Cell* 12, 957–971. doi: 10.1016/j.devcel.2007.04.001

Dougherty, K. A., Cockett, A. T., and Urry, R. L. (1976). Caffeine, theophylline, and human sperm motility. *Fertil. Steril.* 27, 541–548.

Dudiki, T., Joudeh, N., Sinha, N., Goswami, S., Eisa, A., Kline, D., et al. (2019). The protein phosphatase isoform PP1gamma1 substitutes for PP1gamma2 to support spermatogenesis but not normal sperm function and fertilitydagger. *Biol. Reprod.* 100, 721–736. doi: 10.1093/biolre/ioy225

Dudiki, T., Kadunganattil, S., Ferrara, J. K., Kline, D. W., and Vijayaraghavan, S. (2015). Changes in carboxy methylation and tyrosine phosphorylation of protein phosphatase PP2A are associated with epididymal sperm maturation and motility. *PLoS One* 10:e0141961. doi: 10.1371/journal.pone.0141961

Eiteneuer, A., Seiler, J., Weith, M., Beullens, M., Lesage, B., Krenn, V., et al. (2014). Inhibitor-3 ensures bipolar mitotic spindle attachment by limiting association of SDS22 with kinetochore-bound protein phosphatase-1. *EMBO J.* 33, 2704–2720. doi: 10.15252/embj.201489054

Evans, J. P., and Florman, H. M. (2002). The state of the union: the cell biology of fertilization. *Nat. Cell Biol.* 4, S57–S63. doi: 10.1038/ncb-nm-fertilityS57

Fernandez, J. J., Candenas, M. L., Souto, M. L., Trujillo, M. M., and Norte, M. (2002). Okadaic acid, useful tool for studying cellular processes. *Curr. Med. Chem.* 9, 229–262. doi: 10.2174/0929867023371247

Freitas, M. J., Silva, J. V., Brothag, C., Regadas-Correia, B., Fardilha, M., and Vijayaraghavan, S. (2019). Isoform-specific GSK3A activity is negatively correlated with human sperm motility. *Mol. Hum. Reprod.* 25, 171–183. doi: 10.1093/molehr/gaz009

Freitas, M. J., Vijayaraghavan, S., and Fardilha, M. (2017). Signaling mechanisms in mammalian sperm motility. *Biol. Reprod.* 96, 2–12. doi: 10.1095/biolreprod.116.144337

Furuya, S., Endo, Y., Oba, M., Matsui, Y., Nozawa, S., and Suzuki, S. (1992a). Protein phosphorylation regulates the mouse sperm acrosome reaction induced by the zona pellucida. *J. Assist. Reprod. Genet.* 9, 384–390. doi: 10.1007/bf01203964

Furuya, S., Endo, Y., Oba, M., Nozawa, S., and Suzuki, S. (1992b). Effects of modulators of protein kinases and phosphatases on mouse sperm capacitation. *J. Assist. Reprod. Genet.* 9, 391–399. doi: 10.1007/bf01203965

Gibbons, J. A., Kozubowski, L., Tatchell, K., and Shenolikar, S. (2007). Expression of human protein phosphatase-1 in *Saccharomyces cerevisiae* highlights the role of phosphatase isoforms in regulating eukaryotic functions. *J. Biol. Chem.* 282, 21838–21847. doi: 10.1074/jbc.M701272200

Goswami, S. (2018). *Identification of Phosphoproteins Involved in Sperm Maturation and Fertility.* Ph.D. dissertation thesis, Kent State University, Kent, OH.

Goswami, S., Korrodi-Gregorio, L., Sinha, N., Bhutada, S., Bhattacharjee, R., Kline, D., et al. (2019). Regulators of the protein phosphatase PP1gamma2, PPP1R2, PPP1R7, and PPP1R11 are involved in epididymal sperm maturation. *J. Cell. Physiol.* 234, 3105–3118. doi: 10.1002/jcp.27130

Hamamah, S., and Gatti, J. L. (1998). Role of the ionic environment and internal pH on sperm activity. *Hum. Reprod.* 13(Suppl. 4), 20–30. doi: 10.1093/humrep/13.suppl_4.20

Heroes, E., Lesage, B., Gornemann, J., Beullens, M., Van Meervelt, L., and Bollen, M. (2013). The PP1 binding code: a molecular-lego strategy that governs specificity. *FEBS J.* 280, 584–595. doi: 10.1111/j.1742-4658.2012.08547.x

Hess, K. C., Jones, B. H., Marquez, B., Chen, Y., Ord, T. S., Kamenetsky, M., et al. (2005). The "soluble" adenylyl cyclase in sperm mediates multiple signaling events required for fertilization. *Dev. Cell* 9, 249–259. doi: 10.1016/j.devcel.2005.06.007

Ho, H. C., and Suarez, S. S. (2001). Hyperactivation of mammalian spermatozoa: function and regulation. *Reproduction* 122, 519–526. doi: 10.1530/rep.0.1220519

Hoeflich, K. P., Luo, J., Rubie, E. A., Tsao, M. S., Jin, O., and Woodgett, J. R. (2000). Requirement for glycogen synthase kinase-3beta in cell survival and NF-kappaB activation. *Nature* 406, 86–90. doi: 10.1038/35017574

Honda, Z., Suzuki, T., and Honda, H. (2009). Identification of CENP-V as a novel microtubule-associating molecule that activates Src family kinases through SH3 domain interaction. *Genes Cells* 14, 1383–1394. doi: 10.1111/j.1365-2443.2009.01355.x

Hoskins, D. D., Stephens, D. T., and Hall, M. L. (1974). Cyclic adenosine 3′:5′-monophosphate and protein kinase levels in developing bovine spermatozoa. *J. Reprod. Fertil.* 37, 131–133. doi: 10.1530/jrf.0.0370131

Itach, S. B., Finklestein, M., Etkovitz, N., and Breitbart, H. (2012). Hyper-activated motility in sperm capacitation is mediated by phospholipase D-dependent actin polymerization. *Dev. Biol.* 362, 154–161. doi: 10.1016/j.ydbio.2011.12.002

Jiang, C. S., Kilfeather, S. A., Pearson, R. M., and Turner, P. (1984). The stimulatory effects of caffeine, theophylline, lysine-theophylline and 3-isobutyl-1-methylxanthine on human sperm motility. *Br. J. Clin. Pharmacol.* 18, 258–262. doi: 10.1111/j.1365-2125.1984.tb02466.x

Jin, S. K., and Yang, W. X. (2017). Factors and pathways involved in capacitation: how are they regulated? *Oncotarget* 8, 3600–3627. doi: 10.18632/oncotarget.12274

Jope, R. S., Yuskaitis, C. J., and Beurel, E. (2007). Glycogen synthase kinase-3 (GSK3): inflammation, diseases, and therapeutics. *Neurochem. Res.* 32, 577–595. doi: 10.1007/s11064-006-9128-5

Kaidanovich-Beilin, O., and Woodgett, J. R. (2011). GSK-3: functional insights from cell biology and animal models. *Front. Mol. Neurosci.* 4:40. doi: 10.3389/fnmol.2011.00040

Kawa, S., Ito, C., Toyama, Y., Maekawa, M., Tezuka, T., Nakamura, T., et al. (2006). Azoospermia in mice with targeted disruption of the Brek/Lmtk2 (brain-enriched kinase/lemur tyrosine kinase 2) gene. *Proc. Natl. Acad. Sci. U.S.A.* 103, 19344–19349. doi: 10.1073/pnas.0603603103

Keravis, T., and Lugnier, C. (2012). Cyclic nucleotide phosphodiesterase (PDE) isozymes as targets of the intracellular signalling network: benefits of PDE inhibitors in various diseases and perspectives for future therapeutic developments. *Br. J. Pharmacol.* 165, 1288–1305. doi: 10.1111/j.1476-5381.2011.01729.x

Koch, S., Acebron, S. P., Herbst, J., Hatiboglu, G., and Niehrs, C. (2015). Post-transcriptional Wnt signaling governs epididymal sperm maturation. *Cell* 163, 1225–1236. doi: 10.1016/j.cell.2015.10.029

Krapf, D., O'Brien, E., Maidagan, P. M., Morales, E. S., Visconti, P. E., and Arranz, S. E. (2014). Calcineurin regulates progressive motility activation of Rhinella (Bufo) arenarum sperm through dephosphorylation of PKC substrates. *J. Cell. Physiol.* 229, 1378–1386. doi: 10.1002/jcp.24571

Lee, H. C., Johnson, C., and Epel, D. (1983). Changes in internal pH associated with initiation of motility and acrosome reaction of sea urchin sperm. *Dev. Biol.* 95, 31–45. doi: 10.1016/0012-1606(83)90004-0

Leemans, B., Stout, T. A. E., De Schauwer, C., Heras, S., Nelis, H., Hoogewijs, M., et al. (2019). Update on mammalian sperm capacitation: how much does the horse differ from other species? *Reproduction* 157, R181–R197. doi: 10.1530/Rep-18-0541

Lesich, K. A., Pelle, D. W., and Lindemann, C. B. (2008). Insights into the mechanism of ADP action on flagellar motility derived from studies on bull sperm. *Biophys. J.* 95, 472–482. doi: 10.1529/biophysj.107.127951

Levasseur, M., Dumollard, R., Chambon, J. P., Hebras, C., Sinclair, M., Whitaker, M., et al. (2013). Release from meiotic arrest in ascidian eggs requires the activity of two phosphatases but not CaMKII. *Development* 140, 4583–4593. doi: 10.1242/dev.096578

Lin, Q., Buckler, E. S. IV, Muse, S. V., and Walker, J. C. (1999). Molecular evolution of type 1 serine/threonine protein phosphatases. *Mol. Phylogenet. Evol.* 12, 57–66. doi: 10.1006/mpev.1998.0560

Lin, R. Y., Moss, S. B., and Rubin, C. S. (1995). Characterization of S-AKAP84, a novel developmentally regulated A kinase anchor protein of male germ cells. *J. Biol. Chem.* 270, 27804–27811. doi: 10.1074/jbc.270.46.27804

Lindemann, C. B. (1978). A cAMP-induced increase in the motility of demembranated bull sperm models. *Cell* 13, 9–18. doi: 10.1016/0092-8674(78)90133-2

Lindemann, C. B., Goltz, J. S., and Kanous, K. S. (1987). Regulation of activation state and flagellar wave form in epididymal rat sperm: evidence for the involvement of both Ca2+ and cAMP. *Cell Motil. Cytoskeleton* 8, 324–332. doi: 10.1002/cm.970080405

Lishko, P. V., and Kirichok, Y. (2010). The role of Hv1 and CatSper channels in sperm activation. *J. Physiol.* 588(Pt 23), 4667–4672. doi: 10.1113/jphysiol.2010.194142

Lishko, P. V., and Mannowetz, N. (2018). CatSper: a unique calcium channel of the sperm flagellum. *Curr. Opin. Physiol.* 2, 109–113. doi: 10.1016/j.cophys.2018.02.004

Luis Villanueva-Canas, J., Ruiz-Orera, J., Agea, M. I., Gallo, M., Andreu, D., and Alba, M. M. (2017). New genes and functional innovation in mammals. *Genome Biol. Evol.* 9, 1886–1900. doi: 10.1093/gbe/evx136

MacLeod, G., Shang, P., Booth, G. T., Mastropaolo, L. A., Manafpoursakha, N., Vogl, A. W., et al. (2014). PPP1CC2 can form a kinase/phosphatase complex with the testis-specific proteins TSSK1 and TSKS in the mouse testis. *Reproduction* 147, 1–12. doi: 10.1530/REP-13-0224

Marquez, B., and Suarez, S. S. (2004). Different signaling pathways in bovine sperm regulate capacitation and hyperactivation. *Biol. Reprod.* 70, 1626–1633. doi: 10.1095/biolreprod.103.026476

Marquez, B., and Suarez, S. S. (2008). Soluble adenylyl cyclase is required for activation of sperm but does not have a direct effect on hyperactivation. *Reprod. Fertil. Dev.* 20, 247–252.

Matsuura, M., and Yogo, K. (2015). TMEM225: a possible protein phosphatase 1 gamma 2 (PP1 gamma 2) regulator localizes to the equatorial segment in mouse spermatozoa. *Mol. Reprod. Dev.* 82, 139–148. doi: 10.1002/mrd.22453

McNeill, H., and Woodgett, J. R. (2010). When pathways collide: collaboration and connivance among signalling proteins in development. *Nat. Rev. Mol. Cell Biol.* 11, 404–413. doi: 10.1038/nrm2902

Medina, M., and Wandosell, F. (2011). Deconstructing GSK-3: the fine regulation of its activity. *Int. J. Alzheimers Dis.* 2011:479249. doi: 10.4061/2011/479249

Miki, K., Willis, W. D., Brown, P. R., Goulding, E. H., Fulcher, K. D., and Eddy, E. M. (2002). Targeted disruption of the Akap4 gene causes defects in sperm flagellum and motility. *Dev. Biol.* 248, 331–342. doi: 10.1006/dbio.2002.0728

Miyata, H., Satouh, Y., Mashiko, D., Muto, M., Nozawa, K., Shiba, K., et al. (2015). Sperm calcineurin inhibition prevents mouse fertility with implications for male contraceptive. *Science* 350, 442–445. doi: 10.1126/science.aad0836

Mohri, H., and Yanagimachi, R. (1980). Characteristics of motor apparatus in testicular, epididymal and ejaculated spermatozoa. *Exp. Cell Res.* 127, 191–196. doi: 10.1016/0014-4827(80)90426-7

Molina, L. C. P., Luque, G. M., Balestrini, P. A., Marin-Briggiler, C. I., Romarowski, A., and Buffone, M. G. (2018). Molecular basis of human sperm capacitation. *Front. Cell Dev. Biol.* 6:72. doi: 10.3389/fcell.2018.00072

Moss, S. B., Turner, R. M. O., Burkert, K. L., Butt, H. V., and Gerton, G. L. (1999). Conservation and function of a bovine sperm A-kinase anchor protein homologous to mouse AKAP82. *Biol. Reprod.* 61, 335–342. doi: 10.1095/biolreprod61.2.335

Murofushi, H., Ishiguro, K., Takahashi, D., Ikeda, J., and Sakai, H. (1986). Regulation of sperm flagellar movement by protein phosphorylation and dephosphorylation. *Cell Motil. Cytoskeleton* 6, 83–88. doi: 10.1002/cm.970060203

Navarrete, F. A., Garcia-Vazquez, F. A., Alvau, A., Escoffier, J., Krapf, D., Sanchez-Cardenas, C., et al. (2015). Biphasic role of calcium in mouse sperm capacitation signaling pathways. *J. Cell. Physiol.* 230, 1758–1769. doi: 10.1002/jcp.24873

Nishigaki, T., José, O., González-Cota, A. L., Romero, F., Treviño, C. L., and Darszon, A. (2014). Intracellular pH in sperm physiology. *Biochem. Biophys. Res. Commun.* 450, 1149–1158. doi: 10.1016/j.bbrc.2014.05.100

Nolan, M. A., Babcock, D. F., Wennemuth, G., Brown, W., Burton, K. A., and McKnight, G. S. (2004). Sperm-specific protein kinase A catalytic subunit Calpha2 orchestrates cAMP signaling for male fertility. *Proc. Natl. Acad. Sci. U.S.A.* 101, 13483–13488. doi: 10.1073/pnas.0405580101

Okano, K., Heng, H., Trevisanato, S., Tyers, M., and Varmuza, S. (1997). Genomic organization and functional analysis of the murine protein phosphatase 1c gamma (Ppp1cc) gene. *Genomics* 45, 211–215. doi: 10.1006/geno.1997.4907

Omori, K., and Kotera, J. (2007). Overview of PDEs and their regulation. *Circ. Res.* 100, 309–327. doi: 10.1161/01.res.0000256354.95791.f1

Orta, G., de la Vega-Beltran, J. L., Martin-Hidalgo, D., Santi, C. M., Visconti, P. E., and Darszon, A. (2018). CatSper channels are regulated by protein kinase A. *J. Biol. Chem.* 293, 16830–16841. doi: 10.1074/jbc.RA117.001566

Parker, P. J., Embi, N., Caudwell, F. B., and Cohen, P. (1982). Glycogen synthase from rabbit skeletal muscle. State of phosphorylation of the seven phosphoserine residues in vivo in the presence and absence of adrenaline. *Eur. J. Biochem.* 124, 47–55. doi: 10.1111/j.1432-1033.1982.tb05904.x

Parra, V., and Rothermel, B. A. (2017). Calcineurin signaling in the heart: the importance of time and place. *J. Mol. Cell. Cardiol.* 103, 121–136. doi: 10.1016/j.yjmcc.2016.12.006

Peggie, M. W., MacKelvie, S. H., Bloecher, A., Knatko, E. V., Tatchell, K., and Stark, M. J. (2002). Essential functions of Sds22p in chromosome stability and nuclear localization of PP1. *J. Cell Sci.* 115(Pt 1), 195–206.

Qi, H., Moran, M. M., Navarro, B., Chong, J. A., Krapivinsky, G., Krapivinsky, L., et al. (2007). All four CatSper ion channel proteins are required for male fertility and sperm cell hyperactivated motility. *Proc. Natl. Acad. Sci. U.S.A.* 104, 1219–1223. doi: 10.1073/pnas.0610286104

Rotfeld, H., Hillman, P., Ickowicz, D., and Breitbart, H. (2014). PKA and CaMKII mediate PI3K activation in bovine sperm by inhibition of the PKC/PP1 cascade. *Reproduction* 147, 347–356. doi: 10.1530/Rep-13-0560

Rusnak, F., and Mertz, P. (2000). Calcineurin: form and function. *Physiol. Rev.* 80, 1483–1521. doi: 10.1152/physrev.2000.80.4.1483

San Agustin, J. T., and Witman, G. B. (2001). Differential expression of the C(s) and Calpha1 isoforms of the catalytic subunit of cyclic 3′,5′-adenosine monophosphate-dependent protein kinase testicular cells. *Biol. Reprod.* 65, 151–164. doi: 10.1095/biolreprod65.1.151

Santi, C. M., Martinez-Lopez, P., de la Vega-Beltran, J. L., Butler, A., Alisio, A., Darszon, A., et al. (2010). The SLO3 sperm-specific potassium channel plays a vital role in male fertility. *FEBS Lett.* 584, 1041–1046. doi: 10.1016/j.febslet.2010.02.005

Schwarz, T., Prieler, B., Schmid, J. A., Grzmil, P., and Neesen, J. (2017). Ccdc181 is a microtubule-binding protein that interacts with Hook1 in haploid male germ cells and localizes to the sperm tail and motile cilia. *Eur. J. Cell Biol.* 96, 276–288. doi: 10.1016/j.ejcb.2017.02.003

Sette, C., and Conti, M. (1996). Phosphorylation and activation of a cAMP-specific phosphodiesterase by the cAMP-dependent protein kinase. Involvement of serine 54 in the enzyme activation. *J. Biol. Chem.* 271, 16526–16534. doi: 10.1074/jbc.271.28.16526

Si, Y. M., and Olds-Clarke, P. (1999). Mice carrying two t haplotypes: sperm populations with reduced zona pellucida binding are deficient in capacitation. *Biol. Reprod.* 61, 305–311. doi: 10.1095/biolreprod61.1.305

Signorelli, J. R., Diaz, E. S., Fara, K., Baron, L., and Morales, P. (2013). Protein phosphatases decrease their activity during capacitation: a new requirement for this event. *PLoS One* 8:e81286. doi: 10.1371/journal.pone.0081286

Singh, A. P., and Rajender, S. (2015). CatSper channel, sperm function and male fertility. *Reprod. Biomed. Online* 30, 28–38. doi: 10.1016/j.rbmo.2014.09.014

Sinha, N., Pilder, S., and Vijayaraghavan, S. (2012). Significant expression levels of transgenic PPP1CC2 in testis and sperm are required to overcome the male infertility phenotype of Ppp1cc null mice. *PLoS One* 7:e47623. doi: 10.1371/journal.pone.0047623

Sinha, N., Puri, P., Nairn, A. C., and Vijayaraghavan, S. (2013). Selective ablation of Ppp1cc gene in testicular germ cells causes oligo-teratozoospermia and infertility in mice. *Biol. Reprod.* 89:128. doi: 10.1095/biolreprod.113.110239

Smith, G. D., Wolf, D. P., Trautman, K. C., da Cruz e Silva, E., Greengard, P., and Vijayaraghavan, S. (1996). Primate sperm contain protein phosphatase 1, a biochemical mediator of motility. *Biol. Reprod.* 54, 719–727. doi: 10.1095/biolreprod54.3.719

Smith, G. D., Wolf, D. P., Trautman, K. C., and Vijayaraghavan, S. (1999). Motility potential of macaque epididymal sperm: the role of protein phosphatase and glycogen synthase kinase-3 activities. *J. Androl.* 20, 47–53.

Soberg, K., Moen, L. V., Skalhegg, B. S., and Laerdahl, J. K. (2017). Evolution of the cAMP-dependent protein kinase (PKA) catalytic subunit isoforms. *PLoS One* 12:e0181091. doi: 10.1371/journal.pone.0181091

Somanath, P. R., Jack, S. L., and Vijayaraghavan, S. (2004). Changes in sperm glycogen synthase kinase-3 serine phosphorylation and activity accompany motility initiation and stimulation. *J. Androl.* 25, 605–617. doi: 10.1002/j.1939-4640.2004.tb02831.x

Stanger, S. J., Law, E. A., Jamsai, D., O'Bryan, M. K., Nixon, B., McLaughlin, E. A., et al. (2016). A novel germ cell protein, SPIF (sperm PKA interacting factor), is essential for the formation of a PKA/TCP11 complex that undergoes conformational and phosphorylation changes upon capacitation. *FASEB J.* 30, 2777–2791. doi: 10.1096/fj.201500136R

Stewart, T. A., and Davis, F. M. (2019). An element for development: calcium signaling in mammalian reproduction and development. *Biochim. Biophys. Acta Mol. Cell Res.* 1866, 1230–1238. doi: 10.1016/j.bbamcr.2019.02.016

Stival, C., Puga Molina Ldel, C., Paudel, B., Buffone, M. G., Visconti, P. E., and Krapf, D. (2016). Sperm capacitation and acrosome reaction in mammalian sperm. *Adv. Anat. Embryol. Cell Biol.* 220, 93–106. doi: 10.1007/978-3-319-30567-7_5

Sun, X. H., Zhu, Y. Y., Wang, L., Liu, H. L., Ling, Y., Li, Z. L., et al. (2017). The Catsper channel and its roles in male fertility: a systematic review. *Reprod. Biol. Endocrinol.* 15:65. doi: 10.1186/s12958-017-0281-2

Swarup, G., and Garbers, D. L. (1982). Phosphoprotein phosphatase activity of sea urchin spermatozoa. *Biol. Reprod.* 26, 953–960. doi: 10.1095/biolreprod26.5.953

Takahashi, D., Murofushi, H., Ishiguro, K., Ikeda, J., and Sakai, H. (1985). Phosphoprotein phosphatase inhibits flagellar movement of Triton models of sea urchin spermatozoa. *Cell Struct. Funct.* 10, 327–337. doi: 10.1247/csf.10.327

Tash, J. S., and Bracho, G. E. (1994). Regulation of sperm motility: emerging evidence for a major role for protein phosphatases. *J. Androl.* 15, 505–509.

Tash, J. S., Krinks, M., Patel, J., Means, R. L., Klee, C. B., and Means, A. R. (1988). Identification, characterization, and functional correlation of calmodulin-dependent protein phosphatase in sperm. *J. Cell Biol.* 106, 1625–1633. doi: 10.1083/jcb.106.5.1625

Topper, E. K., Killian, G. J., Way, A., Engel, B., and Woelders, H. (1999). Influence of capacitation and fluids from the male and female genital tract on the zona binding ability of bull spermatozoa. *J. Reprod. Fertil.* 115, 175–183. doi: 10.1530/jrf.0.1150175

Toure, A. (2019). Importance of SLC26 transmembrane anion exchangers in sperm post-testicular maturation and fertilization potential. *Front. Cell Dev. Biol.* 7:230. doi: 10.3389/fcell.2019.00230

Tsirulnikov, E., Huta, Y., and Breitbart, H. (2019). PKA and PI3K activities during capacitation protect sperm from undergoing spontaneous acrosome reaction. *Theriogenology* 128, 54–61. doi: 10.1016/j.theriogenology.2019.01.036

Turner, R. M. O., Eriksson, R. L. M., Gerton, G. L., and Moss, S. B. (1999). Relationship between sperm motility and the processing and tyrosine phosphorylation of two human sperm fibrous sheath proteins, pro-hAKAP82 and hAKAP82. *Mol. Hum. Reprod.* 5, 816–824. doi: 10.1093/molehr/5.9.816

Varmuza, S., Jurisicova, A., Okano, K., Hudson, J., Boekelheide, K., and Shipp, E. B. (1999). Spermiogenesis is impaired in mice bearing a targeted mutation in the protein phosphatase 1cgamma gene. *Dev. Biol.* 205, 98–110. doi: 10.1006/dbio.1998.9100

Vetter, M. M., Zenn, H. M., Mendez, E., van den Boom, H., Herberg, F. W., and Skalhegg, B. S. (2011). The testis-specific Calpha2 subunit of PKA is kinetically indistinguishable from the common Calpha1 subunit of PKA. *BMC Biochem.* 12:40. doi: 10.1186/1471-2091-12-40

Vijayaraghavan, S., Chakrabarti, R., and Myers, K. (2007). Regulation of sperm function by protein phosphatase PP1gamma2. *Soc. Reprod. Fertil. Suppl.* 63, 111–121.

Vijayaraghavan, S., Critchlow, L. M., and Hoskins, D. D. (1985). Evidence for a role for cellular alkalinization in the cyclic adenosine 3′,5′-monophosphate-mediated initiation of motility in bovine caput spermatozoa. *Biol. Reprod.* 32, 489–500. doi: 10.1095/biolreprod32.3.489

Vijayaraghavan, S., and Hoskins, D. (1989). Quantitation of bovine sperm cytoplasmic calcium with Quin-2 and Fura-2: evidence that external calcium does not have direct access to the sperm cytoplasm. *Cell Calcium* 10, 241–253. doi: 10.1016/0143-4160(89)90007-9

Vijayaraghavan, S., and Hoskins, D. D. (1988). Low molecular weight factor in bovine caudal epididymal fluid that stimulates calcium uptake in caput spermatozoa. *Gamete Res.* 20, 343–352. doi: 10.1002/mrd.1120200309

Vijayaraghavan, S., and Hoskins, D. D. (1990). Changes in the mitochondrial calcium influx and efflux properties are responsible for the decline in sperm calcium during epididymal maturation. *Mol. Reprod. Dev.* 25, 186–194. doi: 10.1002/mrd.1080250212

Vijayaraghavan, S., Liberty, G. A., Mohan, J., Winfrey, V. P., Olson, G. E., and Carr, D. W. (1999). Isolation and molecular characterization of AKAP110, a novel, sperm-specific protein kinase A-anchoring protein. *Mol. Endocrinol.* 13, 705–717. doi: 10.1210/mend.13.5.0278

Vijayaraghavan, S., Stephens, D. T., Trautman, K., Smith, G. D., Khatra, B., da Cruz e Silva, E. F., et al. (1996). Sperm motility development in the epididymis is associated with decreased glycogen synthase kinase-3 and protein phosphatase 1 activity. *Biol. Reprod.* 54, 709–718. doi: 10.1095/biolreprod54.3.709

Visconti, P. E., Westbrook, V. A., Chertihin, O., Demarco, I., Sleight, S., and Diekman, A. B. (2002). Novel signaling pathways involved in sperm acquisition of fertilizing capacity. *J. Reprod. Immunol.* 53, 133–150. doi: 10.1016/s0165-0378(01)00103-6

Wang, D., Hu, J., Bobulescu, I. A., Quill, T. A., McLeroy, P., Moe, O. W., et al. (2007). A sperm-specific Na+/H+ exchanger (sNHE) is critical for expression and in vivo bicarbonate regulation of the soluble adenylyl cyclase (sAC). *Proc. Natl. Acad. Sci. U.S.A.* 104, 9325–9330. doi: 10.1073/pnas.0611296104

Wang, W., Stukenberg, P. T., and Brautigan, D. L. (2008). Phosphatase inhibitor-2 balances protein phosphatase 1 and aurora B kinase for chromosome segregation and cytokinesis in human retinal epithelial cells. *Mol. Biol. Cell* 19, 4852–4862. doi: 10.1091/mbc.E08-05-0460

Williams, H. L., Mansell, S., Alasmari, W., Brown, S. G., Wilson, S. M., Sutton, K. A., et al. (2015). Specific loss of CatSper function is sufficient to compromise fertilizing capacity of human spermatozoa. *Hum. Reprod.* 30, 2737–2746. doi: 10.1093/humrep/dev243

Woodgett, J. R. (1990). Molecular cloning and expression of glycogen synthase kinase-3/factor A. *EMBO J.* 9, 2431–2438. doi: 10.1002/j.1460-2075.1990.tb07419.x

Xie, F., Garcia, M. A., Carlson, A. E., Schuh, S. M., Babcock, D. F., Jaiswal, B. S., et al. (2006). Soluble adenylyl cyclase (sAC) is indispensable for sperm function and fertilization. *Dev. Biol.* 296, 353–362. doi: 10.1016/j.ydbio.2006.05.038

Xu, B., Hao, Z., Jha, K. N., Digilio, L., Urekar, C., Kim, Y. H., et al. (2007). Validation of a testis specific serine/threonine kinase [TSSK] family and the substrate of TSSK1 & 2, TSKS, as contraceptive targets. *Soc. Reprod. Fertil. Suppl.* 63, 87–101.

Yeung, C. H. (1984). Effects of cyclic AMP on the motility of mature and immature hamster epididymal spermatozoa studied by reactivation of the demembranated cells. *Gamete Res.* 9, 99–114. doi: 10.1002/mrd.1120090109

Yuasa, K., Kotera, J., Fujishige, K., Michibata, H., Sasaki, T., and Omori, K. (2000). Isolation and characterization of two novel phosphodiesterase PDE11A variants showing unique structure and tissue-specific expression. *J. Biol. Chem.* 275, 31469–31479. doi: 10.1074/jbc.m003041200

Zeidner, L. C., Buescher, J. L., and Phiel, C. J. (2011). A novel interaction between Glycogen Synthase Kinase-3alpha (GSK-3alpha) and the scaffold protein Receptor for Activated C-Kinase 1 (RACK1) regulates the circadian clock. *Int. J. Biochem. Mol. Biol.* 2, 318–327.

Zeng, X. H., Yang, C., Kim, S. T., Lingle, C. J., and Xia, X. M. (2011). Deletion of the Slo3 gene abolishes alkalization-activated K+ current in mouse spermatozoa. *Proc. Natl. Acad. Sci. U.S.A.* 108, 5879–5884. doi: 10.1073/pnas.1100240108

3

Testicular Structure and Spermatogenesis in the Naked Mole-Rat Is Unique (Degenerate) and Atypical Compared to Other Mammals

Gerhard van der Horst[1]*, Sanet H. Kotzé[2], M. Justin O'Riain[3] and Liana Maree[1]

[1] Department of Medical Biosciences, University of the Western Cape, Bellville, South Africa, [2] Division of Clinical Anatomy, Department of Biomedical Sciences, Stellenbosch University, Stellenbosch, South Africa, [3] Institute for Communities and Wildlife in Africa, Department of Biological Sciences, University of Cape Town, Cape Town, South Africa

***Correspondence:**
Gerhard van der Horst
gvdhorst7@gmail.com

The naked mole-rat (NMR) queen controls reproduction in her eusocial colony by usually selecting one male for reproduction and suppressing gametogenesis in all other males and females. Simplified, polymorphic and slow-swimming spermatozoa in the NMR seem to have been shaped by a low risk of sperm competition. We hypothesize that this unique mammalian social organization has had a dramatic influence on testicular features and spermatogenesis in the NMR. The testicular structure as well as spermatogenic cell types and its organization in breeding, subordinate and disperser males were studied using light microscopy and transmission electron microscopy. Even though the basic testicular design in NMRs is similar to most Afrotheria as well as some rodents with intra-abdominal testes, the Sertoli and spermatogenic cells have many atypical mammalian features. Seminiferous tubules are distended and contain large volumes of fluid while interstitial tissue cover about 50% of the testicular surface area and is mainly composed of Leydig cells. The Sertoli cell cytoplasm contains an extensive network of membranes and a variety of fluid-containing vesicles. Furthermore, Sertoli cells form numerous phagosomes that often appear as extensive accumulations of myelin. Another unusual feature of mature NMR Sertoli cells is mitotic division. While the main types of spermatogonia and spermatocytes are clearly identifiable, these cells are poorly organized and many spermatids without typical intercellular bridges are present. Spermatid heads appear to be malformed with disorganized chromatin, nuclear fragmentation and an ill-defined acrosome formed from star-like Golgi bodies. Rudimentary manchette development corresponds with the occurrence of abnormal sperm morphology. We also hypothesize that NMR testicular organization and spermiation are modified to produce spermatozoa on demand in a short period of time and subsequently use a Sertoli cell "pump" to flush the spermatozoa into short tubuli recti and simplified rete testis. Despite the difficulty in finding cellular associations during spermatogenesis, six spermatogenic stages could be described in the NMR. These numerous atypical and often simplified features of the NMR further supports the notion of degenerative orthogenesis that was selected for due to the absence of sperm competition.

Keywords: spermatogenesis, spermiogenesis, spermiation, staging, Leydig cells, Sertoli cells

INTRODUCTION

Naked mole-rats (NMRs, *Heterocephalus glaber)* represent one of only two eusocial mammals (Jarvis, 1981, 1985; Faulkes et al., 1991; O'Riain et al., 2000) with reproduction typically restricted to a single female (queen) and 1–3 males within large colonies varying from 40 to 90 individuals. Multiple-paternity has been recorded for this species (Faulkes et al., 1997), but usually the queen selects a male for life and most other males and all other females (subordinates) are reproductively suppressed (Faulkes and Abbott, 1991; Faulkes et al., 1991). This restriction of breeding to a small subset of the population presents a low risk for sperm competition and it is assumed to have shaped the sperm structure (simple and low percentage of normal forms) and motility (slow) in this species (van der Horst et al., 2011). It is not evident at what point during spermatogenesis a path is followed which produces the remarkable heterogeneity of morphologically abnormal spermatozoa in the NMR.

Spermatogenesis is a complex but highly coordinated process which is regulated by paracrine, autocrine, juxtacrine, and endocrine pathways (Chocu et al., 2012). Mammalian spermatogenesis is divided into three phases: mitotic divisions of the spermatogonia and differentiation into spermatocytes (spermatocytogenesis); two consecutive meiotic divisions of the spermatocytes to produce spermatids; and differentiation of the spermatids into spermatozoa (spermiogenesis). During spermiogenesis, structural changes occurring in several cellular compartments include repackaging of the chromatin for transport, development of the acrosome, elongating of the tail, formation of the mitochondrial sheath in the midpiece and reduction of cytoplasmic volume. Here after spermatozoa are released into the seminiferous tubule lumen during the process of spermiation. Seasonality, reproductive lifespan, mode of fertilization and sperm competition are all factors that could influence the organization of spermatogenesis within the testis (Ramm et al., 2014).

Although several papers have appeared on spermatogenesis in the NMR since the early 1990s (Faulkes et al., 1991; Yang et al., 2017), these papers covered a general description of spermatogenesis using wax embedding and hematoxylin-eosin stained sections for brightfield microscopy. The emphasis of these studies was to discern the incidence of spermatogenesis, particularly in relation to the presence/absence of spermatozoa. Their general consensus was that spermatogenesis occurs in breeders and non-breeders, particularly if they were kept separate from the queen, providing evidence of her suppressive role in relation to spermatogenesis specifically.

The first study to pursue greater detail of these processes using transmission electron microscopy was by Onyango et al. (1993) focusing exclusively on non-breeders. Despite this shortcoming, they described most of the cell types of spermatogenesis, albeit without any cellular associations, and related their findings to other mammals. While only few late spermatids or spermatozoa were observed in their investigation, van der Horst et al. (2011) and van der Horst and Maree (2014) described the vastly abnormal spermatozoa in NMR breeders, subordinates and dispersers using both stained sperm smears and electron microscopy. The latter two studies concluded that NMR spermatozoa represent a case of degenerative orthogenesis and it was proposed that this was selected for in the absence of sperm competition.

The aim of the current study is to quantify the testicular structure in the NMR, with special reference to spermatogenesis. We hypothesize that due to the lack of sperm competition there will be degenerate testicular features and "relaxed" spermatogenesis. We investigated testicular ultrastructure and spermatogenesis among breeders, subordinates and dispersers and compared our results to other mammals.

MATERIALS AND METHODS

Animal Husbandry

The study population originated from various localities in Kenya, and was comprised of 10 colonies housed in separate artificial burrow systems at the University of Cape Town, South Africa. Husbandry details have been described previously by Jarvis (1991). A total of 26 male NMRs (*Heterocephalus glaber*) were used in this study, including 10 breeders and 10 subordinates from 10 colonies and 6 males that had been isolated from their colonies for a minimum of 2 months. Two of these isolated males had acquired the dispersing male phenotypes (O'Riain et al., 1996). Breeders were adult males confirmed to be in consort with the queen (mutual naso-anal grooming and copulation). Subordinate males were adult males who did not engage in either naso-anal grooming or copulations with their queens. It should be noted that the "subordinate" NMR males referred to in this study is of the same reproductive status as that of "non-breeding" males used in previous NMR studies.

Ethical clearance for the study was obtained from both the University of Cape Town (2005/V7/JOR), the University of the Western Cape (ScR1RC2007/3/30) and Stellenbosch University (P07/09/019). Animals were removed from their custom made burrow systems and anesthetized with halothane by putting a mask over the head. Surgical anesthesia was attained within 5 min and longer exposure to halothane was used to euthanize animals. The entire reproductive system was dissected out and put into

Ham's F10 medium (Invitrogen, Cape Town, South Africa) at 28°C (NMR body temperature) (van der Horst et al., 2011).

Immediately upon removal of the reproductive systems, small sections of representative parts of the testes were fixed in 2.5% phosphate buffered glutaraldehyde (4°C) and were subsequently routinely processed for transmission electron microscopy (TEM). During TEM processing, 1 μm epoxy sections were cut for viewing and final trimming using an ultra-microtome. The 1 μm epoxy sections have been used to great effect in this investigation to provide high quality brightfield light microscopy images at low magnifications for measurement of different parts of the testes (see later). The ultrathin sections have been used for TEM.

Capturing of Images for Light Microscopy, Measurement, and TEM

For brightfield microscopy, a Nikon E50i microscope was used and images were captured using an Ace ACA 1300-200uc Basler camera and the Morphology Module of the Sperm Class Analyzer (SCA, version 6.4.0.64) computer-aided sperm analysis software (Microptic S.L., Barcelona, Spain). The sections investigated for this purpose represented 1 μm epoxy sections stained with toluidine blue. The measurement tool of the SCA system was used to measure the seminiferous tubule diameters and to calculate surface areas for both the interstitial tissue and the seminiferous tubules. For TEM, a Jeol JEM 1011 transmission electron microscope (Advanced Laboratory Solutions, Johannesburg, South Africa) at 80 kV was used to capture micrographs of different testicular cells and compartments for subsequent description. More than 1000 micrographs from all 26 males were studied for description of spermatogenic cell types, cellular associations, and staging (see below).

Statistical Analysis

MedCalc, Version 14 (Mariakerke, Belgium) was used for statistical analyses. Descriptive statistics was used for calculation of averages and standard deviations (SD). Comparisons of testicular morphometry parameters were performed using either ANOVA or Kruskal-Wallis among the different groups and $P < 0.05$ was considered significant.

RESULTS

Testicular Compartments

The interstitial component of the testis in the NMR is large and composed mainly of Leydig cells, blood vessels and lymphatics, representing about 50% of the testicular surface area (**Figure 1A**). Analyses of breeders, subordinates and dispersers of the same body weight and stage of testicular development show that seminiferous tubules occupy about 45 to 55% of the testicular surface area. In NMRs the average diameter of the seminiferous tubules varies from 152 to 240 μm and there are no significant differences ($P = 0.18$) among the three male groups (**Table 1**).

The Leydig cells are arranged in groups (islands) of three or more cells per island and each island is contained within a layer(s) of loose connective tissue (**Figures 1B,C**). The Leydig cells have a spherical or slightly oval nucleus and contain

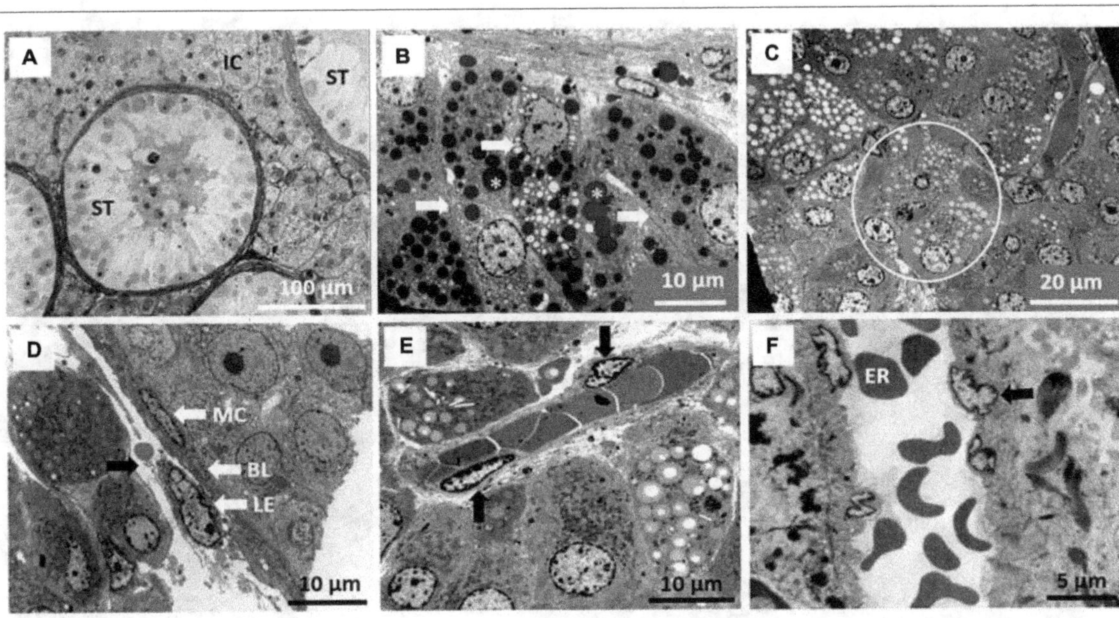

FIGURE 1 | Testicular compartments of the naked mole-rat (NMR). **(A)** Seminiferous tubules (ST) and large interstitial compartment (IC) of the testis. **(B)** Detail of Leydig cells (arrows) arranged in groups of three to four in islands. Lipid droplets (asterisk) are contrasted by osmium tetroxide, appearing black. **(C)** Interstitial compartment containing numerous Leydig cell islands (circle) with lipid content possibly washed out of vesicles during processing. **(D)** Wall of the seminiferous tubules, the lamina propria, consisting of three layers, namely a myoid epithelium (MC), a lymphoid epithelium (LE) and a basal lamina (BL) and arrow indicating lymphatic space. **(E)** Oblique section of arteriole in close association with Leydig cell islands. **(F)** Enhanced view of arteriole in longitudinal section showing endothelial cells (arrow) and erythrocytes (ER).

TABLE 1 | Comparison of seminiferous tubule diameter among three groups of naked mole-rat males (n = 3 for each group and n = 9 in total).

	Average (μm)	±SD (μm)	Range (μm)
Breeders	192.3	20.5	158–240
Subordinates	200.1	18.7	170–234
Dispersers	184.8	20.4	152–219

At least 10 seminiferous tubules were measured per group (100 seminiferous tubules in total).

mainly euchromatin (genetically active). The cytoplasm of the Leydig cell contains numerous mitochondria as well as vesicles with apparently two types of lipid. One type of vesicle appears transluscent/light or containing no lipid or lipid in a particular form. In the second type of vesicle, the lipid appears dark/blue at light microsope level and as electron dense (black) in TEM. These lipid vesicles originate from an extensive network of smooth endoplasmic reticulum. The lymphatic component is clearly defined as sinusoids containing lymph (**Figure 1D**, black arrow). Arterioles are evident (**Figure 1E**) in the interstitial compartment with three to four endothelial cells observed in transverse sections. These blood vessels appear in close association with several islands of interstitial tissue (**Figure 1E**). **Figure 1F** provides an enlarged view of the endothelial wall of an arteriole.

The wall (lamina propria) of the seminiferous tubules consists of three typical layers, namely an inside basal lamina, a myoid epithelial layer and an outer lymphatic endothelium (**Figure 1D**). A detailed description of all the cells contained within the seminiferous tubules (spermatogenic and non-spermatogenic), as well as their cellular associations and accordingly staging of spermatogenesis follows below. These cellular features and organization were noticed in males from all three reproductive groups.

Cell Types of the Seminiferous Epithelium

Sertoli cells in the NMR contain many structural differences compared to other mammals. Their nuclei are usually irregular to ovoid with a prominent nucleolus surrounded by a ring of peri-nucleolar chromatin. In almost all testicular sections of most NMR males, we observed Sertoli cells in division and these cells have an extensive cytoplasm filled with numerous membrane-limited vesicles apparently containing fluid (**Figures 2A,B**). Smaller vesicles seem to coalesce to form large fluid-filled vesicles that might be important in the release of spermatids (see below). The Sertoli cell cytoplasm also often contains many other peculiarities including phagosomes that are described in a separate section below.

Dark and light, large A type spermatogonia as well as B type spermatogonia with prominent nucleoli could be identified (**Figure 2C**). All primary spermatocyte types (pre-leptotene, leptotene, zygotene and pachytene) are present in the NMR testis (**Figures 2D–F**). Dividing primary spermatocytes are clearly designated and some contain intercellular bridges (**Figure 3A**). However, subsequent divisions of these cells do

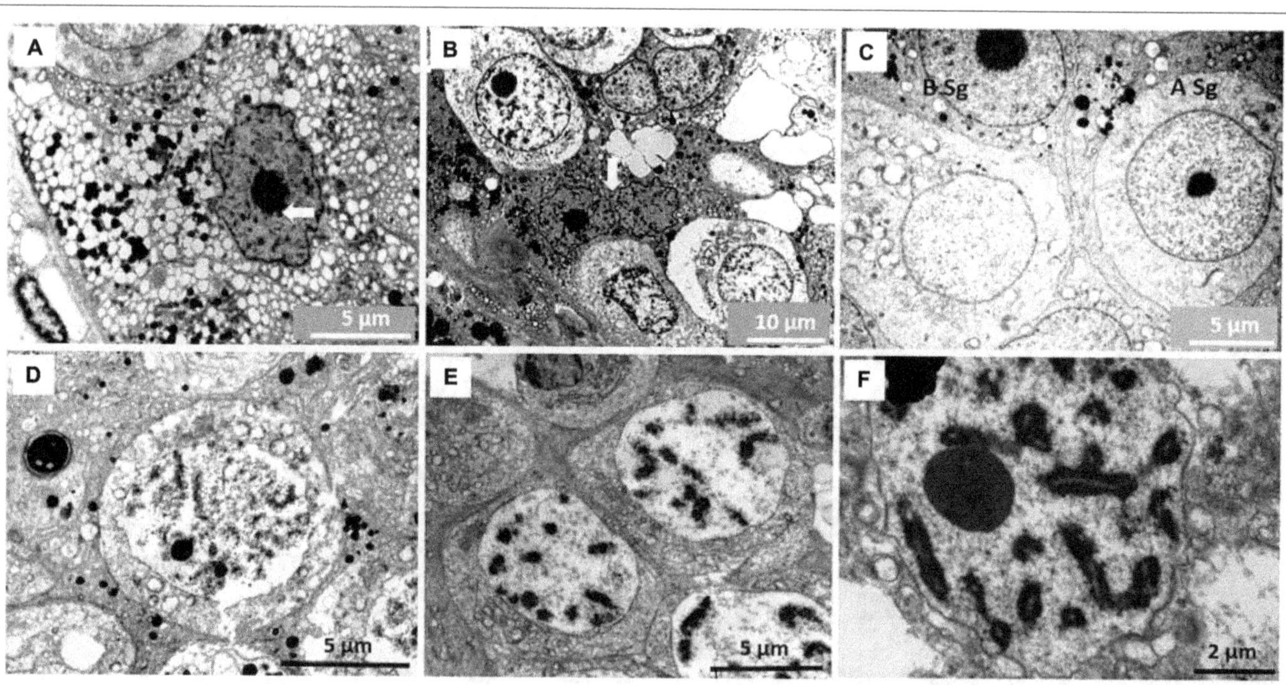

FIGURE 2 | **(A)** Sertoli cell with vast number of fluid-filled vesicles in its cytoplasm. Nucleolus of Sertoli cell is surrounded by peri-nucleolar chromatin (arrow). **(B)** Dividing Sertoli cells (arrow) between two spermatogonia. Similar dividing Sertoli cells are common in all males studied. **(C)** A type spermatogonium (A Sg) and B type spermatogonium (B Sg). **(D)**Leptotene primary spermatocyte. **(E)** Early pachytene primary spematocyte. **(F)** Mid-pachytene primary spermatocyte showing paired chromosomes.

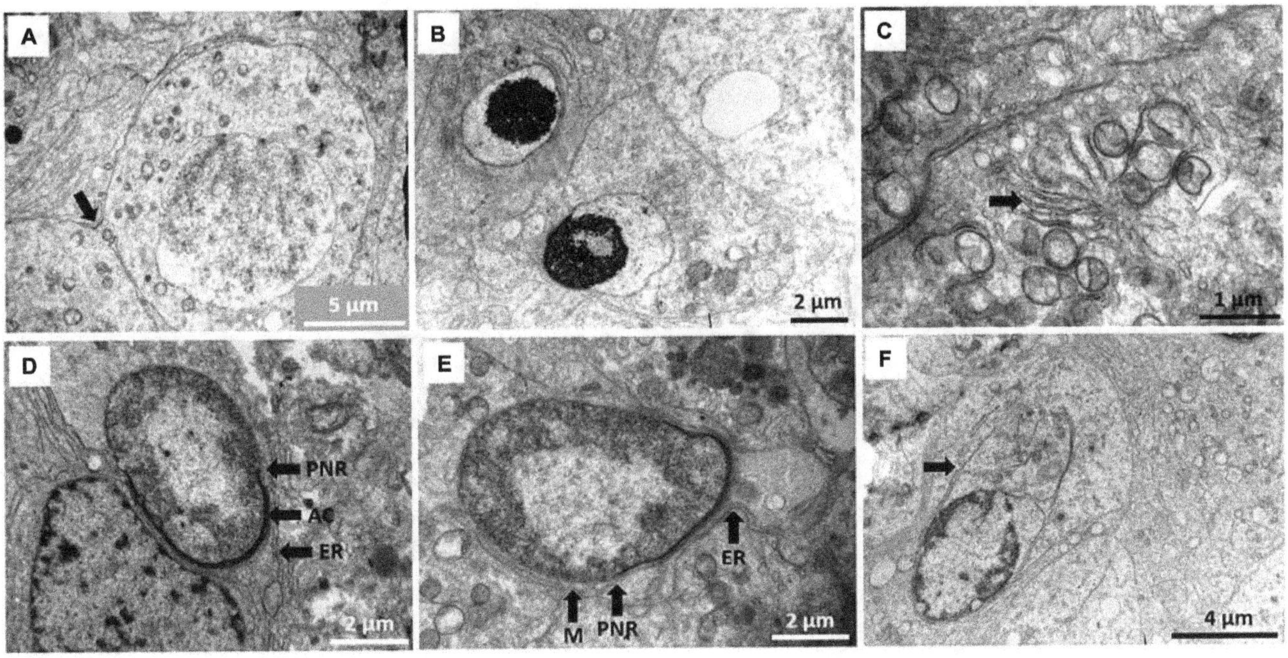

FIGURE 3 | (A) Pre-leptotene primary spermatocyte showing inter-cellular bridge (arrow). **(B)** Early round spermatids showing some nuclear condensation just prior to the cap phase of acrosome formation. **(C)** Star-like Golgi figures (arrow) as part of acrosome formation. Location of Golgi apparatus in Sertoli cell indicated with asterisk in **Figure 4D**. **(D)** Cap phase of spermiogenesis showing acrosome formation (AC) and associated endoplasmic reticulum (ER) as well as the peri-nuclear ring (PNR). **(E)** Start of manchette (M) formation behind peri-nuclear ring (PNR). Endoplasmic reticulum (ER) is associated with the acrosome. **(F)** Caudal tube (arrow) as end phase of manchette.

not appear to have intercellular bridges (see later on number of spermatids released).

The four main developmental phases of spermatids could be designated in the NMR. Early round spermatids (Golgi phase, **Figure 3B**; also see later **Figures 5A,B** for description of spermatid types) are often associated with a large, star-like arrangement of the Golgi apparatus (**Figure 3C**) that eventually appear to contribute to construction of the acrosome. Round to oval spermatids are showing acrosome formation (cap phase, **Figure 3D**; also see later **Figure 5B**) and the peri-nucleolar ring is also formed. Many microtubules are associated with the Golgi phase and also associate with the acrosome.

During the phase of spermatid elongation, a simple/rudimentary manchette of microtubules is formed below the perinuclear ring (**Figure 3E**). This structure is first observed at the acrosome formation stage as a single row of microtubules and in longitudinal sections it appears as a chain of connected microtubules. Several cisternae of endoplasmic reticulum also appear at this stage in the Sertoli cell cytoplasm (usually associated with cell adhesions) and are arranged in the area of the spermatid acrosomal cap (**Figures 3D,E**). In late spermatids with elongated heads, a clear caudal tube (posterior segment of manchette) emerges (**Figure 3F**) at the posterior part of the head and seems to unwind in a snake-like fashion (**Figure 4A**). Elongated spermatids are also depicted in **Figures 5C,D** in the description of spermatid types. It furthermore seems that microtubules at the posterior part of the sperm head break up into small groups of six to eight microtubules and associate with smaller Sertoli cell vesicles (**Figures 4B,C**).

Finally, the release of mature spermatids/spermatozoa from the Sertoli cells appear to be assisted by this microtubule mechanism of forming larger vesicles and accompanied by vast Sertoli cell fluid formation (**Figures 2A, 4B–D**). **Figures 4B–D** typically show residual bodies with two vacuoles presumably form which two spermatids that have been released. We refer to this "excessive" fluid formation (compared to any other mammalian species) as the Sertoli cell pump – a novel adaptation in mammals and unique to the NMR, as will be discussed.

Many spermatid morphological abnormalities are evident during spermiogenesis. The major atypical aspects are the heterogeneity of head morphology and the large number of spermatid and sperm heads showing fragmentation (**Figure 4E**). Many residual bodies seem to contain the remains of the vesicles that released the spermatozoa, many of which are presumably phagocytosed by the Sertoli cells forming phagosomes (**Figures 4E,F**). These phagosomes typically exhibit formation of myelin figures which may be partly related to end products of the phagocytosed material (see section below). A further novel and surprising finding in NMR is the presence of phagocytes (unusual) as part of the seminiferous epithelium (**Figure 4F**).

Staging of Spermatogenesis

Staging of spermatogenesis has only been performed in sections of seminiferous tubules presenting with most spermatogonia,

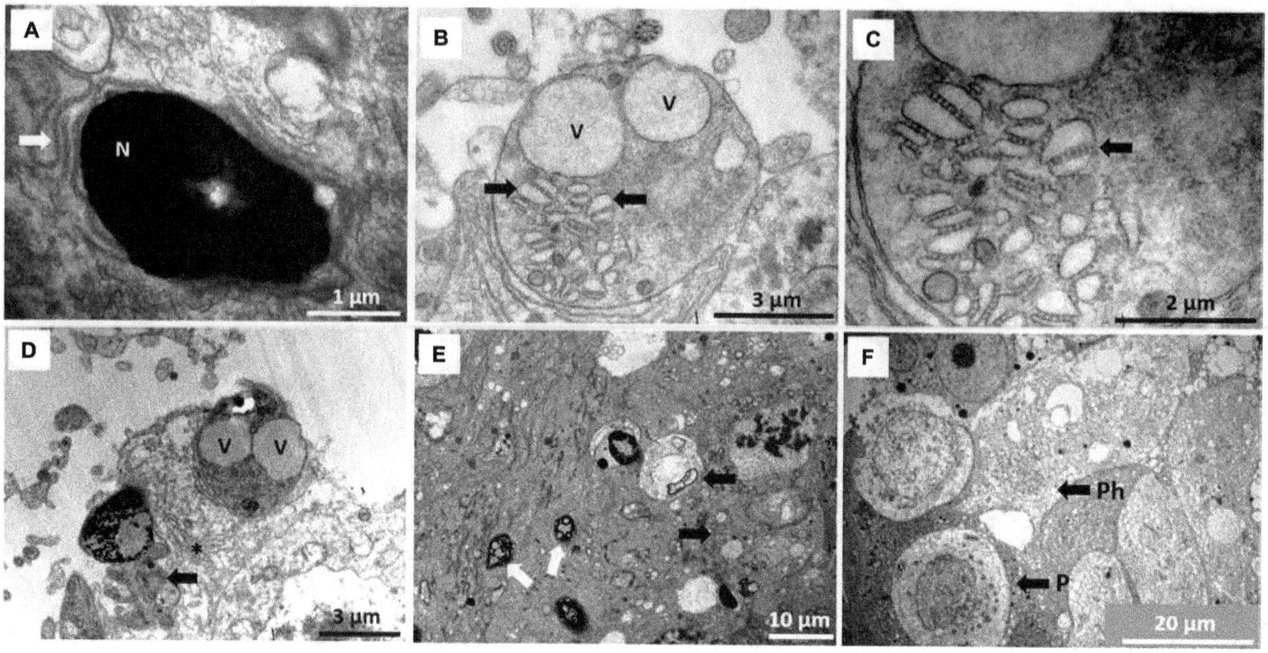

FIGURE 4 | (A) Redundant microtubules presumably of manchette origin forming snake-like arrangement (arrow) posterior to spermatid nucleus (N). **(B)** Microtubules form associations with vesicles (arrows) and seem to be involved in spermiation and vacuoles (V) represent crypts after release of late spermatids/spermatozoa. **(C)** Larger magnification of **(B)** showing the microtubules (arrow) in groups of four to eight apparently involved in movement of vesicles to combine and assist in final stage of spermiation. **(D)** Typical cytoplasmic droplet components are shed before sperm release in seminiferous tubule lumen. Arrow indicates part of process where redundant cytoplasm is eliminated before sperm release from vesicle (V). Asterisk indicates center of a remnant star-like Golgi body. **(E)** Different morphological forms of spermatid heads already showing fragmentation (white arrows) as part of spermiogenesis and phagosomes (black arrows). **(F)** Unusual, typical phagocyte (P) in seminiferous epithelium and phagosomes inside Sertoli cell (Ph).

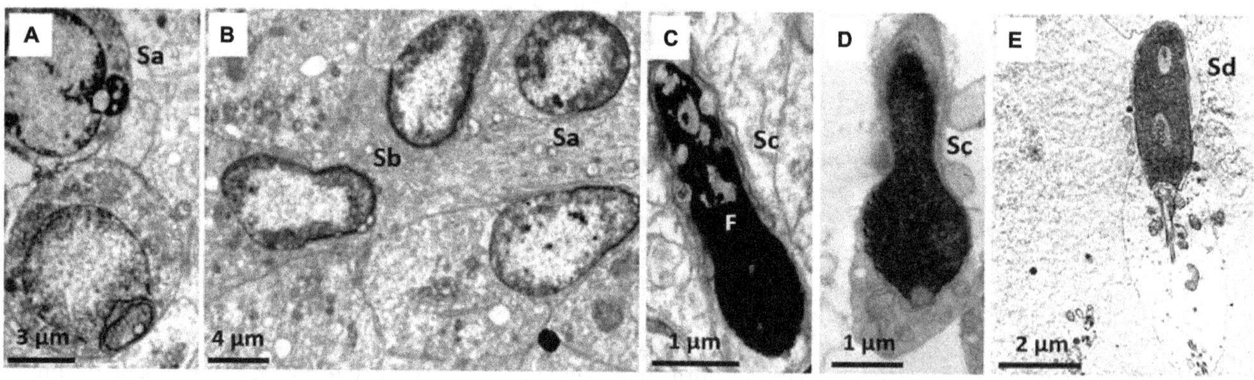

FIGURE 5 | (A–E) Morphological details of the four developmental stages of the spermatids. **(A)** Sa, round spermatid also showing acrosomal granule and part of Golgi phase. **(B)** Sb, spermatid with acrosome formation and slight elongation. **(C)** Sc, elongated spermatid showing fragmentation (F). **(D)** Sc, lobe-shaped elongated spermatid. **(E)** Sd, elongated mature spermatid/sperm.

spermatocytes, spermatids, and spermatozoa and was more distinct in males sacrificed close to estrous of the queen. Spermatogenesis in the NMR appears to be helical, similar to humans, and more than one stage (spermatogenic cellular association) can be designated in a transverse section of the seminiferous tubules. However, defining these cellular associations in NMRs is complicated due to the heterogeneity in spermatid morphology. It was accordingly important to first distinguish the four spermatid developmental stages (**Figure 5**), namely: Sa, representing round spermatids in Golgi phase (**Figures 3B, 5A**); Sb, representing acrosome development, peripheral nuclear condensation and start of elongation (**Figures 3D,E, 5B**); Sc, representing more pronounced elongation and nuclear condensation (**Figures 5C,D**); and Sd, representing mature elongated/mature spermatids (**Figure 5E**).

Despite the limitations posed by spermatid heterogeneity, **Figure 6** illustrates six spermatogenic stages and **Table 2** lists the different cellular associations of spermatogenesis as shown

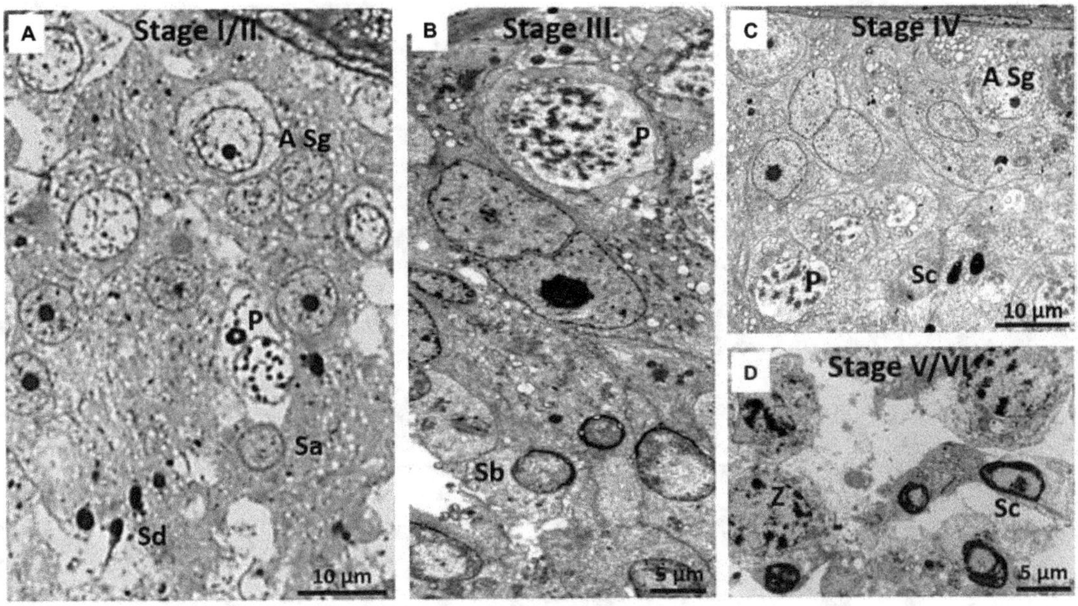

FIGURE 6 | (A–D) Six spermatogenic stages of the NMR. Note that Stages I and II and V and VI show many overlapping features and have been grouped together as Stage I/II and Stage V/VI. Since all stages show A type spermatogonia, they have not been indicated in every stage. **(A)** Stage I/II showing A type spermatogonium (A Sg), pachytene primary spermatocyte (P) and spermatid stages Sa and Sd. **(B)** Stage III, pachytene primary spermatocyte (P), Sb spermatids and Sertoli cell (SC). **(C)** Stage IV, A type spermatogonium (A Sg), pachytene primary spermatocyte (P) and Sc spermatid. **(D)** Stage V/VI with zygotene primary spermatocytes (Z) and Sc spermatids. Only zygotene spermatocytes and Sc spermatids are indicated as this combination distinguishes stage V/VI from the other stages.

TABLE 2 | The cellular associations used in defining the spermatogenic stages of the naked mole-rat.

Stage	Spermatogonia (Sg) and spermatocyte associations	Spermatid types	Depicted
I/II	A type Sg, Leptotene, Pachytene	Sa (round), Sd (elongated)	**Figure 6A**
III	A type Sg, Preleptotene, Pachytene	Sb (acrosome formation)	**Figure 6B**
IV	A type Sg, Leptotene, Pachytene	Sc (condensed/elongated)	**Figure 6C**
V/VI	A type Sg, Zygotene	Sc, Sd (elongated/mature)	**Figure 6D**

Sa, Sb, Sc, Sd = four developmental stages of spermatids.

in these micrographs. Delineation of these six stages was mainly based on an association of spermatogonia, specific primary spermatocytes and the presence of one or two of the four spermatids types. For example, NMR Stage IV contains, as viewed successively from the basal lamina, A type spermatogonia, B type spermatogonia, leptotene and pachytene primary spermatocytes and mainly type Sc spermatids (**Figure 6C**). For the sake of simplicity and difficulty to consistently distinguish between Stages I and II as well as V and VI, they were respectively grouped together as I/II and V/VI (**Table 2**).

Tubuli Recti and the Rete Testis

The transition between a seminiferous tubule and the tubuli recti is shown in **Figure 7A**. The tubuli recti in NMRs are short but have the same basic structure as in other mammals. Their cuboidal type cells contain a very large, irregular nucleus and the cytoplasm forms undulations projecting into the lumen that is packed with glycogen granules (**Figure 7B**). The tubuli recti are confluent with the rete testis which has a large lumen and the cuboidal cells contain short microvilli (**Figure 7C**).

Other Features of the Testis

There are numerous structures/organelles in NMRs not commonly observed in the testis of most mammals. **Figure 8A** shows an example of myelin figures as it occurs in different forms inside the Sertoli cytoplasm and in Leydig cells (**Figure 8B**). These myelin figures present in Sertoli cells seem to form part of phagosomes. Annulate lamellae within the Sertoli cells are indicated in **Figure 8C**. These lamellae form many rows of parallel arranged membranes that seem to constrict at specific points and then expand again. There are many examples of these in NMR testes and they have many different types of arrangement. Rows of parallel-oriented and circular membranes are evident, particularly in the distal parts of Sertoli cells and residual bodies (**Figures 8D–F**). Crystals are present inside the Leydig cells but these do not appear to be a regular feature (**Figure 8G**).

DISCUSSION

It has been well-established in the literature that testicular size is larger in breeders compared to non-breeders in the NMR (Faulkes et al., 1991, 1994; Yang et al., 2017). However, in the

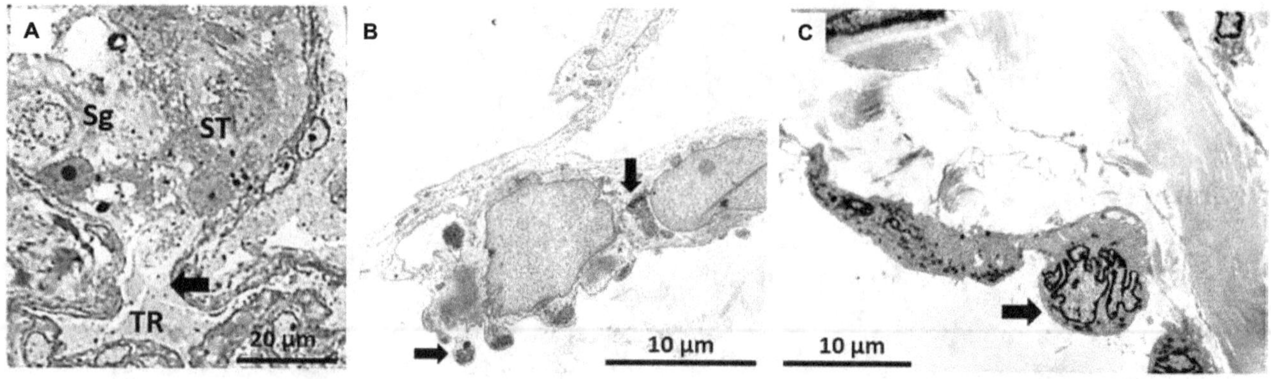

FIGURE 7 | (A) Arrow indicates the transition between seminiferous tubule (ST) [with spermatogonium (Sg) indicated] and tubuli recti (TR). **(B)** Typical epithelium of tubuli recti with glycogen stores, as indicated by two arrows. **(C)** Section of rete testis with polymorph nuclear cells (arrow).

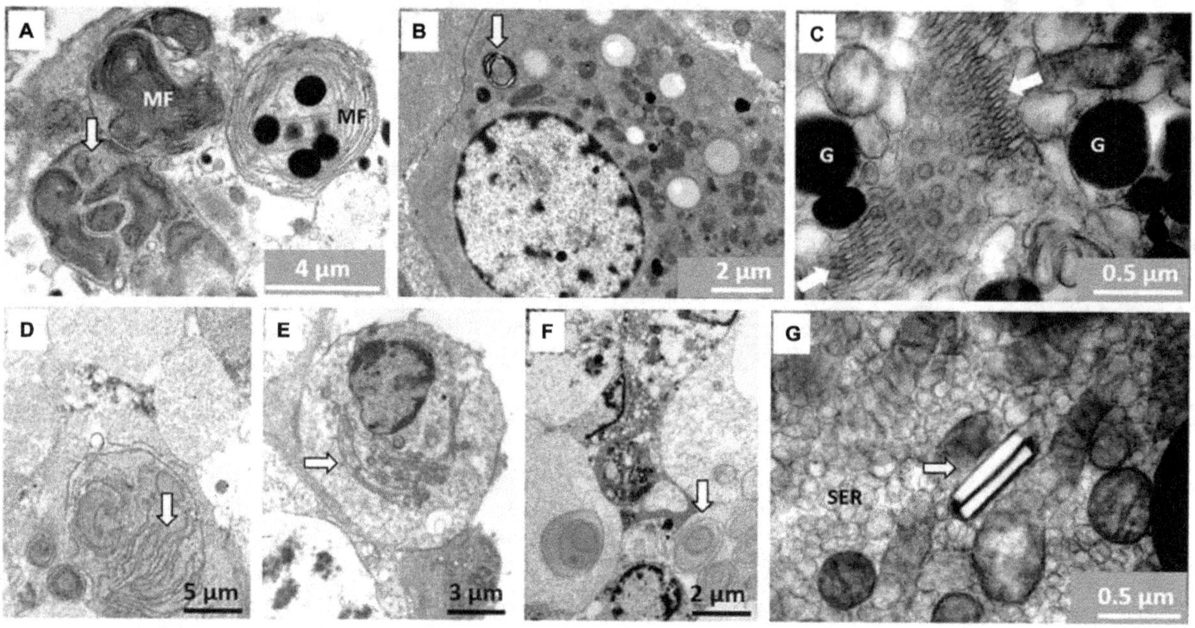

FIGURE 8 | (A–G) Features not commonly seen in the testes of mammals. **(A)** Myelin figures (MF) in the form of concentric layers of presumably lipid composition on right and arrow showing more myelin figures with tighter arranged membranes inside a phagosome. **(B)** Typical myelin figure (arrow) in Leydig cell cytoplasm. **(C)** Annulate lamellae (in between arrows) surrounded by granules (G) in Sertoli cell. **(D–F)** Membranes possibly of agranular endoplasmic reticulum (arrows) in residual body and distal part of Sertoli cell close the seminiferous tubule lumen. **(G)** Two presumably para-crystalline structures arranged in groups of two and surrounded by smooth endoplasmic reticulum (SER).

subsequent discussion we concentrated on the events that occur both in the seminiferous tubules as well as the interstitial cell compartment of breeder, subordinate and disperser NMRs. As we did not find any differences in the cell types among the different groups close to estrous in the queen, the descriptions below will mainly relate to breeders.

Testicular Compartments and Leydig Cells

The NMR has intra-abdominal testes similar to most Afrotheria (e.g., shrews, moles, aardvark, elephant, manatee, and hyrax), also referred to as testiconds in some rodents (van der Horst, 1972). In many of these testiconds the interstitial tissue is considerably expanded during their breeding season compared to most scrotal mammals (Glover and Sale, 1968; Woodall and Skinner, 1989). In the NMRs used in the present study, the interstitial tissue makes up approximately 50% of the testis surface area/volume, which is similar to the 60% reported for NMRs by Fawcett et al. (1973) and confirmed by others (Onyango et al., 1993; Endo et al., 2002). There is no clear reason for this phenomenon and there are exceptions in testiconds with interstitial tissue only comprising about 9% of testicular volume in some shrews (Kisipan et al., 2014).

The volume of interstitial tissue or the area of the testis occupied by seminiferous tubules seem to be linked to levels of sperm competition in some species, with monogamous species or species with limited male intrasexual competition having a smaller testicular area occupied by tubules (delBarco-Trillo et al., 2013; Peirce et al., 2018). An investigation of various murine rodents by Peirce et al. (2018) revealed that in some, but not all, species with a lower relative testis mass (and thus lower sperm competition level), the seminiferous tubules made up 60–70% of the testis area. While no difference between breeders, subordinates and dispersers were found in the current study in terms of the percentage testis area occupied by seminiferous tubules, Mulugeta et al. (2017) indicated a larger interstitial (Leydig) cell content for NMR breeders compared to non-breeders. In another social mole-rat species, Ansell's mole-rat (*Fukomys anselli*), the relative area occupied by Leydig cells and seminiferous tubules was also not significantly different between breeders and non-breeders (Montero et al., 2016).

A special feature of NMR testes is that the seminiferous tubules appear to be filled with fluid and resultantly considerably distended. Despite this observation, the diameter of NMR seminiferous tubules is in the same range as reported for other mole-rats, shrews and murine rodents (Kisipan et al., 2014; Montero et al., 2016; Peirce et al., 2018). Peirce et al. (2018) found a significantly greater mean diameter of the seminiferous tubules in species with a higher compared to those with lower relative testis mass in two of the three murine tribes investigated. Although de Bruin et al. (2012) reported a larger diameter of seminiferous tubules in breeding compared to non-breeding Ansell's mole-rat males, this was not evident in the study by Montero et al. (2016) on the same species or for NMR as reported by Yang et al. (2017) and in the current study.

Another feature that may be unique to NMR is that Leydig cells form islands (three Leydig cells per island) surrounded by regular/loose connective tissue and closely associated with arterioles. We speculate that the two types of vesicles observed in Leydig cells may reflect different stages of steroidogenesis, eventually producing testosterone. The lipid-rich NMR Leydig cell cytoplasm has been reported before (Fawcett et al., 1973; Onyango et al., 1993; Yang et al., 2017), although no mention was made of different types of lipid droplets (translucent vs. dark) encountered. Yang et al. (2017) observed that the Leydig cell area containing lipid droplets, as well as the density of autophagosomes surrounding these droplets, was larger for NMR breeders compared to non-breeders. The latter study linked the lower plasma testosterone levels in non-breeders to a significant decrease in autophagy observed in these males.

Spermatogenesis and Formation of Abnormal Spermatids/Spermatozoa

Spermatogenesis was evident in all males (breeders, subordinates, and dispersers) included in this study, as was reported in numerous previous studies (Faulkes et al., 1991, 1994; Onyango et al., 1993; Mulugeta et al., 2017; Yang et al., 2017). The morphology of the NMR spermatogenic cells, including spermatogonia and spermatocytes, are remarkably similar to that of other mammalian species. Early spermiogenesis in NMR is indeed characterized by the typical main phases such as Golgi phase and cap phase. However, here the similarities end in relation to other mammalian species, with the tail composition and maturation phases being unusual (van der Horst et al., 2011). One exception in the early spermatid phase (Golgi phase) is the formation of bizarre and excessive star-like Golgi bodies which seem to contribute to acrosome formation. These Golgi bodies presumably provide vesicles that will contribute to acrosome formation and its remnants still remain close to spermiation (**Figure 4D**). Furthermore, the elongated spermatids (Sc and Sd) are highly heterogeneous in terms of their head morphology and are often fragmented.

Historically, Fawcett et al. (1971) suggested that manchette formation and function is not related to shaping the form or elongation of the sperm head. Subsequently and recently, several authors have convincingly shown, at both electron microscopic and molecular level, that there are two closely associated developments of cytoskeletal elements linked to protein transport and shaping of the spermatid/sperm head (Lehti and Sironen, 2016; Gunes et al., 2018; Wei and Yang, 2018). The first element is mainly actin-bound (related to ectoplasmic specializations of Sertoli cell) and surrounds both the acrosome area and remainder of the sperm head as part of the acrosome–acroplaxome complex. Secondly, a microtubule-based system that originates below the acrosome and is attached to the peri-nuclear ring is involved in manchette formation and indeed important in elongation of the sperm head as well as determining the morphology of the spermatozoon (Wei and Yang, 2018).

It appears that both the acroplaxome and manchette are temporary structures that, apart from their role in nuclear condensation through elongation, provide an important transport system. The manchette region forms an essential part of intra-microtubule transport (IMT) of a multitude of proteins to the basal body/migrated centrioles in relation to formation of the sperm flagellum. It was suggested that many of these IMT proteins feed into an intra-flagellar transport pathway via several motor proteins (Lehti and Sironen, 2016). Once the sperm tail is formed, the manchette disappears after performing its "zipper" action. This action allows for head elongation due to compression of nuclear proteins that become arginine enriched and converted to smaller protamine molecules and subsequently assist in transport of proteins to the tail (Wei and Yang, 2018). The above authors furthermore provided a large body of evidence that when either manchette formation is faulty/absent or some of the multitude of proteins is lacking, it often results in infertility due to absence of motility.

In the NMR, the manchette appears rudimentary comprising either a single or maximal two layers of microtubules in contrast to other mammals where there are typically multiple layers of microtubules forming a substantial sheath around the posterior part of the sperm head (Fawcett et al., 1971). The high degree of sperm head polymorphisms, fragmentation (ill-condensed chromatin) and short tail lacking a fibrous sheath reported here for late spermatids and previously for spermatozoa (van der Horst et al., 2011) are probably a result of this rudimentary/degenerate manchette. It is thus not surprising that the NMR has many abnormal spermatozoa and poor motility since there is a lack or modification of many key functions in completing spermiogenesis (O'Donnell, 2014).

However, NMR breeders with degenerate spermatozoa are highly successful in impregnating the female, despite van der Horst et al. (2011) and van der Horst and Maree (2014) indicating that mature spermatozoa of NMR breeders are grossly abnormal (only 7% of sperm are morphologically normal) and the percentage motility is less than 14%. These authors explained that in the absence of sperm competition, spermatozoa seem to degenerate and sperm quality decreases dramatically but it is still sufficient to fertilize. Several recent studies on other mammalian and bird species similarly related the presence of a high percentage of abnormal spermatozoa to potentially relaxed sperm competition and a monogamous mating system (Breed et al., 2018; Humann-Guilleminot et al., 2018; Peirce et al., 2018). Dorman et al. (2013) indicated that there seems to be co-evolution of the gametes to aid sperm-zona interactions in the Bandicoot rat (*Bandicota indica*), where a low level of sperm competition is also apparent.

Apart from the correlation between poor NMR sperm morphology/motility and degenerate manchette organization and formation, there are other modifications of the NMR manchette that does not exist or has not been described in other species, which appear to be special adaptations in NMR for sperm release. It is well-known that the manchette essentially disappears in mammals toward the end of spermiogenesis and after flagellar formation. All that remains of the mammalian manchette is its posterior part, namely the caudal tube. In the NMR, the single row of microtubules (caudal tube) seems to remain as a snake-like configuration in relation to the posterior part of the sperm head inside the residual body being formed by the Sertoli cell. Subsequently, the microtubules become re-arranged around small Sertoli cell vesicles, combine to form larger vesicles and these seem to assist to release late spermatids/spermatozoa into the testicular lumen via a Sertoli pressure pump mechanism. Although similar large vesicles in the Sertoli cells are visible or have been reported before in both NMR and Ansell's mole rat, it was referred to as "lesions" or "vacuoles" and its presence was not discussed (Faulkes et al., 1991; Endo et al., 2002; Montero et al., 2016; Yang et al., 2017). Our hypothesis of the pump mechanism shows some similarities to a simplified spermiation process in a species of toad (*Bufo arenarum*) where the endoplasmic reticulum of the Sertoli cell becomes fluid-filled after stimulation by luteinizing hormone and elongated spermatids are pushed out from their crypts in the Sertoli cell (Burgos and Vitale-Calpe, 1967a,b). In the NMR, typically two mature spermatids/sperm are jointly released into the lumen as is evident from the now empty vacuoles of the residual body (**Figure 4**). Spermatozoa are usually released in large groups with still intact intercellular bridges as evident in human (Dym, 1977) and other mammals (Hess and Renato de Franca, 2008). This further supports our notion that there are no intercellular bridges in between spermatids close to being released.

Another NMR sperm feature that has not been observed in other mammals relates to the elimination of the spermatid cytoplasm. In mammals, spermatozoa released from the testis possess a cytoplasmic droplet that is eventually shed in the cauda epididymis or vas deferens. However, NMR spermatozoa released in the seminiferous tubule do not contain a cytoplasmic droplet and it appears that all the redundant organelles have been shed before spermatid/sperm release. This apparent modification in the spermiation process is supported by the fact that Sertoli cells lack typical apical processes that push spermatids into the lumen and stalks of cytoplasm that stay in contact with the spermatids up until final release (Beardsley et al., 2006; O'Donnell, 2014). It is possible that in NMRs an alternative mode of cytoplasmic elimination is used as described for non-mammalian vertebrates (Sprando and Russell, 1988; Russel, 1993) and represents yet another feature potentially related to degenerative orthogenesis and the unique NMR spermiation process.

While the above discussion represents a totally new explanation of the mechanism for the release of spermatozoa from the Sertoli cell it still poses the question of how does this degenerative system relates to fertility, as in all the examples we studied the breeders were proven fathers? In our previous papers we have shown the relationship between sperm degenerate features and fertility and lack of sperm competition (van der Horst et al., 2011; van der Horst and Maree, 2014). Accordingly, it becomes apparent at what stage of spermatogenesis sperm morphology becomes abnormal. The early phases of spermatogenesis seem to be normal in the NMR but then during acrosome formation (cap phase), the manchette dictates development of normal sperm morphology and here it is simplified/degenerate. These observations are in agreement with findings of Mulugeta et al. (2017) on differentially expressed genes in the NMR gonads between breeders and non-breeders which indicated upregulation of genes in breeders that are mainly expressed in the post-meiotic stages of spermatogenesis. A possible explanation for the lower sperm numbers and sperm motility that have been reported in NMR non-breeders compared to breeders (Faulkes et al., 1991, 1994) stems from additional molecular data reported by Mulugeta et al. (2017) which indicated that genes involved in the meiotic cell cycle, male genitalia development, gamete generation, spermatogenesis, and sperm motility are upregulated in breeders.

Staging of Spermatogenesis

Deciphering the spermatogenic stages in the NMR was difficult for two reasons. Firstly, it needs to be emphasized that the well-organized arrangement of groups of specific types of primary spermatocytes or spermatids as in most mammals do not exist in NMRs but rather a more diffuse/disorganized arrangement of these cells. Secondly, there are typically many abnormal spermatids/spermatozoa in the NMR and the basis for staging is to relate a particular association of spermatogonia and spermatocytes to a specific spermatid type. The poorly organized arrangement of the various types of spermatogenic cells, also previously reported by Endo et al. (2002) for non-breeders, is possibly due to the fact that intercellular bridges between closely associated cells are scarce.

In the rat there are 19 different types of spermatids, with each of these spermatids having a specific association with spermatogonia and spermatocyte types, resulting in 14 clear spermatogenic stages (I to XIV). In humans there are only four different spermatid types and accordingly only six spermatogenic stages (I to VI) (Dym, 1977). In the NMR there are also four different types of spermatids that, despite their apparent abnormal and fragmented structure, show some resemblance to those in humans. The spermatid heterogeneity thus posed a challenge to find a coherent system relating to specific spermatid types in defining a specific spermatogenic stage in the NMR. Despite this it was possible to recognize six stages in the NMR that show similarities to human Stages I, II, III, IV, V, and VI. However, in our classification system as indicated in **Table 2** many similarities were evident between Stages I and II as well as V and VI and these stages were respectively grouped together. It may accordingly be then conceived that only four stages are evident in the NMR but due to their closer relationship to human staging (as compared to rodents) we prefer using the human classification rather than delineating a new one for the NMR. We have previously pointed out that in humans whom are largely monogamous there is a low risk of sperm competition (van der Horst and Maree, 2014). Accordingly, it is not surprising to see some similarities between NMR and humans in staging of spermatogenesis. Moreover, complexity in the process of spermatogenesis is in parallel with the evolution of mammals. It appears that the efficiency of spermatogenesis decreased with humans, being less efficient than most mammals such as bulls or rats (Thompson et al., 2018).

While it is accepted that the queen suppresses many aspects of reproduction in the colony, does that mean she suppresses spermatogenesis in all the males all the time? Faulkes et al. (1991) found that while there are differences in testicular weight and size between breeders and non-breeders, all males exhibited spermatogenesis. Our findings agree with Faulkes et al. (1991) and in addition we found that when spermatogenesis is studied at the same period of the estrous cycle in the same colony, breeders, subordinates and dispersers will exhibit similar testicular histology and all may produce and release spermatozoa from the testes. Accordingly, when breeders do not contain spermatozoa in the testis, a non-breeder from the same colony will also not have spermatozoa at that point in time. This observation raises another question: are breeding males also suppressed and do not produce spermatozoa at a certain time in the colony? We have investigated this potential phenomenon which will be deliberated in a separate paper in the near future.

Other Features of the NMR Testis

Myelin figures is considered to be non-specific, concentrically layered, osmiophilic and possibly derived from agranular reticulum. In both the Leydig cells as well as the Sertoli cells there appear areas rich in agranular vesicles and in some parts of the cell they may actually form the concentric layers we observed in these cells in NMR (Neaves, 1973). There is good evidence to suggest that these myelin figures may act as important cholesterol storage centers but are also involved in synthesis of various types of steroids such as testosterone and progesterone (Christensen and Fawcett, 1966). Morita et al. (1999) showed that the myelin figures in testis labeled positively for a family of claudine as in myelinated nerves and are very important in formation of tight junctions. It is accordingly not surprising to find that highly concentrated myelin figures as found in NMR Sertoli and Leydig cells are potentially functional in the testis.

Annulate lamellae within the NMR Sertoli cells form different types of arrangements, one of which rows of parallel-arranged membranes appear to constrict at specific points and then expand again just like the outer nuclear membrane. The bulk of information according to older literature (Wischnitzer, 1970) suggests that these organelles originate from the outer nuclear membrane and are important in messaging between nucleus and cytoplasm. Merisko (1989) attributed that, apart from ATP production and membrane biogenesis, there is macro-molecular trafficking via the pores and regulator of genomic expression. They furthermore seem to associate in many instances with ribosomes and become an active source of protein synthesis. The lamellae in this form can either join rough endoplasmic reticulum or be involved in the formation of endoplasmic reticulum. The most important explanation relating to NMR Sertoli cells is that the vast amount of fluid containing vesicles and membranes as well as the extensive agranular reticulum in Leydig cells may actually also be involved in the formation of annulate lamellae and myelin figures. While we can only speculate, it appears that the rows of parallel or circular membranes in the distal Sertoli cells and residual bodies may be associated with the formation of myelin figures and/or annulate lamellae. Christensen and Fawcett (1966) suggested that these membranes can largely be considered smooth endoplasmic reticulum and accordingly have steroid producing functions as suggested above for myelin figures.

Crystals of Reinke are commonly found in Leydig cells as well as the crystalloid of Charcot-Bottcher in Sertoli cells (Dym, 1977). However, we have found a simple crystal-like structure usually occurring in pairs of two in the Leydig cells of the NMR. These are not products of precipitation of processing material as they are clearly embedded in the cytoplasm. There appear to be many types of so called para-crystalline structures both in Leydig cells as well as in the cytoplasm of Sertoli cells (Sohval et al., 1973). Some are in fact almost tubular like in NMR but none bear a close resemblance. Despite all the speculation about the crystalline structures in Leydig cells there seem to be some association with age. These structures appear in the testes of older men as well as in older animals and do not seem to have a specific function (Sohval et al., 1973).

CONCLUSION

This study used ultrastructural features of the testis to describe both interstitial and testicular components and their associated cell types as well as staging of spermatogenesis in the NMR for the first time. Our results suggest that the main differences in testicular structure and spermiogenesis in NMR compared to other mammals pertains to low levels of sperm competition and supports prior investigations on NMR spermatozoa and investigations on birds and rodents (van der Horst et al., 2011; van der Horst and Maree, 2014). This hypothesis also assists to explain the phenomenon of mature abnormal spermatozoa in

NMR being a function of testicular development/modification, specifically during spermiogenesis.

The testicular compartments of the NMR revealed several aspects that are atypical for a mammalian species and unique for this eusocial species. The NMR interstitial tissue, comprising mostly of Leydig cells, occupies approximately 50% of the surface area/volume of the testis, similar to many other Afrotheria. Seminiferous tubules in NMR show all the typical cell types expected during spermatogenesis with some important exceptions. Mitotic divisions of the Sertoli cells are often found and their cytoplasm is packed with fluid-filled vesicles. These vesicles merge and eventually forms part of our hypothesized Sertoli cell pump which, in addition to other adaptations for a simplified spermiation process, assists to release mature spermatids into the seminiferous tubule lumen. Instead of several spermatids being closely associated not more than two spermatids are found in close vicinity to each other and their release is typically associated with copious amounts of fluid being released in the lumen which appears to assist spermatid release and hence support our Sertoli cell pump hypothesis.

The most prominent feature in which NMR spermiogenesis differs from that of other mammals is in the structure and formation of the manchette which is simplified/degenerate in NMR. Since manchette formation involving many rows of microtubules is associated with producing normal shaped spermatids and normal sperm morphology, it is expected that there will be many diverse and abnormal sperm forms in NMR. Furthermore, the "remnants" of the manchette is modified in NMR and seems to be associated with the release of spermatids from the Sertoli cells. Intercellular bridges are present during early phases of spermatogenesis but then seem to "disappear" and are not present in spermatids. The lack of a cytoplasmic droplet during release of sperm into the seminiferous tubule lumen emphasize further modification/simplification compared to other mammals and relate to degenerative orthogenesis.

ETHICS STATEMENT

The animal study was reviewed and approved by University of Cape Town (2005/V7/JOR), the University of the Western Cape (ScR1RC2007/3/30), and Stellenbosch University (P07/09/019).

AUTHOR CONTRIBUTIONS

GH and LM collated the results and drafted the manuscript. All authors read and approved the final manuscript and designed the study, sampling and analyzed the data.

ACKNOWLEDGMENTS

The authors express their gratitude to Prof. J. U. M. Jarvis for her interest in the study and for initially supplying electron micrographs of NMR spermatozoa and rete testis. Ms. N. Muller, Electron Microscopy Unit, Tygerberg Hospital, South Africa, is thanked for her assistance with the preparation of the TEM samples and the electron micrographs.

REFERENCES

Beardsley, A., Robertson, D. M., and O'Donnell, L. (2006). A complex containing α6β1-integrin and phosphorylated focal adhesion kinase between sertoli cells and elongated spermatids during spermatid release from the seminiferous epithelium. *J. Endocrinol.* 190, 759–770. doi: 10.1677/joe.1.06867

Breed, W. G., Hassan, H., Ganzalez, M., McLennan, H. J., Leigh, C. M., and Heaney, L. R. (2018). Interspecific diversity of testes mass and sperm morphology in the Philippine chrotomyine rodents: implications for differences in breeding systems across the species. *Reprod. Fertil. Dev.* 31, 705–711. doi: 10.1071/RD18278

Burgos, M. H., and Vitale-Calpe, R. (1967a). The fine structure of the sertoli cell-spermatozoon relationship in the toad. *J. Ultrastruct. Res.* 19, 221–237. doi: 10.1016/s0022-5320(67)80217-x

Burgos, M. H., and Vitale-Calpe, R. (1967b). The mechanism of spermiation in the toad. *Am. J. Anat.* 120, 227–252.

Chocu, S., Calvel, P., Rollan, A. D., and Pineau, C. (2012). Spermatogenesis in mammals: proteomic insights. *Syst. Biol. Reprod. Med.* 58, 179–190. doi: 10.3109/19396368.2012.691943

Christensen, A. K., and Fawcett, D. (1966). The fine structure of testicular interstitial cells in mice. *Am. J. Anat.* 118, 551–572. doi: 10.1002/aja.1001180214

de Bruin, P. R., Viljoen, H., Sichilima, A. M., and Bennett, N. C. (2012). Socially induced infertility in Ansell's mole-rat: are there depressed hormone levels in the non-reproductive males and females? *J. Zool.* 286, 15–21. doi: 10.1111/j.1469-7998.2011.00841.x

delBarco-Trillo, J., Tourmente, M., and Roldan, E. R. S. (2013). Metabolic rate limits the effect of sperm competition on mammalian spermatogenesis. *PLoS One* 8:e76510. doi: 10.1371/joural.pone.0076510

Dorman, F., Balsamo, O., Leigh, C., and Breed, W. G. (2013). Co-evolution of gametes of the greater bandicoot rat, bandicota indica – a murine rodent from South-East Asia. *Acta Zool.* 95, 392–396. doi: 10.1111/azo.12036

Dym, M. (1977). "The male reproductive system," in *Histology*, eds L. Weiss, and R. O. Greep, (New York: McGraw-Hill), 979–1038.

Endo, H., Okanoya, K., Park, T. J., Sasaki, M., Tanemura, K., Kimura, J., et al. (2002). Localization of the cytochrome P450 side-chain cleavage enzyme in the inactive testis of the naked mole-rat. *Zool. Sci.* 19, 673–678. doi: 10.2108/zsj.19.673

Faulkes, C. G., and Abbott, D. H. (1991). Social control of reproduction in breeding and non-breeding male naked mole-rats (*Heterocephalus glaber*). *J. Reprod. Fertil.* 93, 427–435. doi: 10.1530/jrf.0.0930427

Faulkes, C. G., Abbott, D. H., and Jarvis, J. U. M. (1991). Social suppression of reproduction in male naked mole-rats, *Heterocephalus glaber*. *J. Reprod. Fertil.* 91, 593–604. doi: 10.1530/jrf.0.0910593

Faulkes, C. G., Abbott, D. H., O'Brien, H. P., Lau, L., Roy, R., Wayne, R. K., et al. (1997). Micro- and macrogeographical genetic structure of colonies of naked mole-rats *Heterocephalus glaber*. *Mol. Ecol.* 6, 615–628. doi: 10.1046/j.1365-294x.1997.00227.x

Faulkes, C. G., Trowell, S. N., Jarvis, J. U. M., and Bennett, N. C. (1994). Investigation of numbers and motility of spermatozoa in reproductively active and socially suppressed males of two eusocial African mole-rats, the naked mole-rat (*Heterocephalus glaber*) and the damaraland mole-rat (*Cryptomys damarensis*). *J. Reprod. Fertil.* 100, 411–416. doi: 10.1530/jrf.0.1000411

Fawcett, D. W., Anderson, W. A., and Phillips, D. M. (1971). Morphogenic factors influencing the shape of the sperm head. *Dev. Biol.* 26, 220–251. doi: 10.1016/0012-1606(71)90124-2

Fawcett, D. W., Neaves, W. B., and Flores, M. N. (1973). Comparitive observations on intertubular lymphatics and the organization of the interstitial tissue of the mammalian testis. *Biol. Reprod.* 9, 500–532. doi: 10.1093/biolreprod/9.5.500

Glover, T. D., and Sale, T. B. (1968). The reproductive system of male rock hyrax *(Procavia* and *Heterohyrax). J. Zool. Lond.* 156, 351–362. doi: 10.1111/j.1469-7998.1968.tb04358.x

Gunes, S., Sengupta, P., Henkel, R., Alguraigari, A., Sinigaglia, M. M., Kayal, M., et al. (2018). Microtubular dysfunction and male infertility. *World J. Mens Health* doi: 10.5534/wjmh.180066 [Epub ahead of print].

Hess, R. A., and Renato de Franca, L. (2008). "Spermatognesis and cycle of the seminiferous epithelium," in *Molecular Mechanisms in Spermatognesis*, ed. C. Y. Cheng, (Berlin: Springer Science+Business Media), 1–15.

Humann-Guilleminot, S., Blévin, P., Azou-Barré, A., Yacouman, A., Gabrielsen, G. W., Chastel, O., et al. (2018). Sperm collection in black-legged kittiwakes and characterization of sperm velocity and morphology. *Avain Res.* 9:24. doi: 10.1186/s40657-018-0117-6

Jarvis, J. U. M. (1981). Eusociality in a mammal: cooperative breeding in naked mole-rat colonies. *Science* 212, 571–573. doi: 10.1126/science.7209555

Jarvis, J. U. M. (1985). Ecological studies on *Heterocephalus glaber*, the naked mole-rat, in Kenya. *Nat. Geogr. Soc. Res. Rep.* 20, 429–437. doi: 10.1111/mec.13358

Jarvis, J. U. M. (1991). "Reproduction of naked mole-rats," in *The Biology of the Naked Mole-Rat*, eds P. W. Sherman, J. U. M. Jarvis, and R. D. Alexander, (Princeton: Princeton University Press), 384–425. doi: 10.1515/9781400887132-016

Kisipan, M. L., Oduor-Okelo, D., Makanya, A. N., and Onyango, D. W. (2014). The structure, morphometry and vascular perfusion of the testis in the rufous sengi (*Elephantulus rufescens*). *J. Morphol. Sci.* 31, 146–155. doi: 10.4322/jms.054613

Lehti, M. S., and Sironen, A. (2016). Formation and function of the manchette and flagellum during spermatogenesis. *Reproduction* 151, R43–R54. doi: 10.1530/REP-15-0310

Merisko, E. M. (1989). Annulate lamellae: an organelle in search of a function. *Tissue Cell* 21, 343–354. doi: 10.1016/0040-8166(89)90049-9

Montero, A. G., Vole, C., Burda, H., Malkemper, E. P., Holtze, S., Morhart, M., et al. (2016). Non-breeding eusocial mole-rats produce viable sperm – spermiogram and functional testicular morphology of *Fukomys anselli*. *PLoS One* 11:e0150112. doi: 10.1371/journal.pone.050112

Morita, K., Sasaki, H., Fujimotot, K., Furuse, M., and Tsukita, S. (1999). Claudin-11OSP-based tight junctions of myelin shetahs in brainand sertoli cells in testis. *J. Cell Biol.* 145, 579–588. doi: 10.1083/jcb.145.3.579

Mulugeta, E., Marion-Poll, L., Gentien, D., Ganswindt, S. B., Ganswindt, A., Bennett, N. C., et al. (2017). *Molecular Insights into the Pathways Underlying Naked Mole-Rat Eusociality. bioRxiv.* [Preprint]. Available at: https://www.biorxiv.org/content /10.1101/209932v1.supplementary-material (accessed May 31, 2019).

Neaves, W. B. (1973). Changes in testicular leydig cells and in plasma testosterone levels among seasonally breeding rock hyrax. *Biol. Reprod.* 8, 451–466. doi: 10.1093/biolreprod/8.4.451

O'Donnell, L. (2014). Mechanisms of spermiogenesis and spermiation and how they are disturbed. *Spermatogenesis* 4:e979623. doi: 10.4161/21565562.2014.979623

Onyango, D. W., Oduor-Okelo, D., and Otiang'a-Owiti, G. E. (1993). Ultrastructural study of the testis on non-breeding naked mole-rat (*Heterocephalus glaber*, Ruppel). *Ann. Anat.* 175, 447–452. doi: 10.1016/s0940-9602(11)80111-1

O'Riain, M. J., Jarvis, J. U. M., Alexander, R., Buffenstein, R., and Peeters, C. (2000). Morphological castes in a vertebrate. *Proc. Natl. Acad. Sci. U.S.A.* 97, 13194–13197. doi: 10.1073/pnas.97.24.13194

O'Riain, M. J., Jarvis, J. U. M., and Faulkes, G. C. (1996). A dispersive morph in the naked mole-rat. *Nature* 380, 619–621. doi: 10.1038/380619a0

Peirce, E. J., McLennan, H. J., Tuke, J., Leigh, C. M., and Breed, W. G. (2018). Evolution of the testis and spermatozoon in mice and rats (Subfamily Murinae) in the absence of sperm competition. *J. Zool.* 306, 56–58. doi: 10.1111/jzo.12573

Ramm, S. A., Schrärer, L., Ehmcke, J., and Wistuba, J. (2014). Sperm competition and the evolution of spermatogenesis. *Mol. Hum. Reprod.* 20, 1169–1179. doi: 10.1093/molehr/gau070

Russel, L. (1993). "Role in spermiation," in *The Sertoli cell*, eds L. D. Russel, and M. D. Griswold, (Clearwater, FL: Cache River Press), 269–302.

Sohval, A. R., Gabrilove, J. L., and Churg, J. (1973). Ultrastructure of Leydig cell paracrystalline inclusions, possibly related to Reinke crystals in the normal human testis. *Z. Zellforsch. Mikrosk. Anat.* 142, 13–26. doi: 10.1007/bf00306701

Sprando, R. L., and Russell, L. D. (1988). Spermiogenesis in the red-ear turtle (*Pseudemys scripta*) and the domestic fowl (*Gallus domesticus*): a study of cytoplasmic events including cell volume changes and cytoplasmic elimination. *J. Morphol.* 198, 95–118. doi: 10.1002/jmor.1051980110

Thompson, S. K., Kutchy, N. A., Kwok, S., Rosyada, Z. N. A., Imumorin, I. G., Purwantara, B., et al. (2018). Sperm: comparative morphology and function related to altered reproductive strategies and fertility in mammals. *Prof. Anim. Sci.* 34, 558–565. doi: 10.15232/pas.2018-1748

van der Horst, G. (1972). Seasonal effects on the anatomy and histology of the reproductive tract of the male rodent mole *Bathyergus suillus suillus* (Schreber). *Zool. Afr.* 7, 491-520.

van der Horst, G., and Maree, L. (2014). Sperm form and function in the absence of sperm competition (Invited review). *Mol. Reprod. Dev.* 81, 204–216. doi: 10.1002/mrd.22277

van der Horst, G., Maree, L., Kotzé, S. H., and O'Riain, M. J. (2011). Sperm structure and motility in the eusocial naked mole-rat, *Heterocephalus glaber*: a case of degenerative orthogenesis in the absence of sperm competition? *BMC Evol. Biol.* 11:351. doi: 10.1186/1471-2148-11-351

Wei, Y.-L., and Yang, W.-X. (2018). The acroframosome-acroplaxome-manchette axis may function in sperm head shaping and male fertility. *Gene* 660, 28–40. doi: 10.1016/j.gene.2018.03.059

Wischnitzer, S. (1970). The annulate lamellae. *Int. Rev. Cytol.* 27, 65–100. doi: 10.1016/S0074-7696(08)61246-2

Woodall, P. F., and Skinner, J. D. (1989). Seasonality of reproduction in male rock elephant shrews *Elephantulus myurus*. *J. Zool. Lond.* 217, 203–212. doi: 10.1111/j.1469-7998.1989.tb02482.x

Yang, W., Li, L., Huang, X., Kan, G., Lin, L., Cheng, J., et al. (2017). Levels of leydig cell autophagy regulate the fertility of male naked-mole rats. *Oncotarget* 8, 98677–98690. doi: 10.18632/oncotarget.22088

4

Essential Role of Sperm-Specific PLC-Zeta in Egg Activation and Male Factor Infertility

Alaaeldin Saleh[1], Junaid Kashir[2,3,4], Angelos Thanassoulas[1], Bared Sa ieh-Garabedian[1], F. Anthony Lai[1,5] and Michail Nomikos[1*]

[1] Member of QU Health, College of Medicine, Qatar University, Doha, Qatar, [2] College of Medicine, Alfaisal University, Riyadh, Saudi Arabia, [3] Department of Comparative Medicine, King Faisal Specialist Hospital and Research Center, Riyadh, Saudi Arabia, [4] School of Biosciences, Cardiff University, Cardiff, United Kingdom, [5] Biomedical Research Center, Qatar University, Doha, Qatar

*Correspondence:
Michail Nomikos
mnomikos@qu.edu.qa;
mixosn@yahoo.com

Sperm-specific phospholipase C zeta (PLCζ) is widely considered to be the physiological stimulus responsible for generating calcium (Ca^{2+}) oscillations that induce egg activation and early embryonic development during mammalian fertilization. In the mammalian testis, PLCζ expression is detected at spermiogenesis following elongated spermatid differentiation. Sperm-delivered PLCζ induces Ca^{2+} release via the inositol 1,4,5-trisphosphate ($InsP_3$) signaling pathway. PLCζ is the smallest known mammalian PLC isoform identified to date, with the simplest domain organization. However, the distinctive biochemical properties of PLCζ compared with other PLC isoforms contribute to its unique potency in stimulating cytosolic Ca^{2+} oscillations within mammalian eggs. Moreover, studies describing PLCζ "knockout" mouse phenotypes confirm the supreme importance of PLCζ at egg activation and monospermic fertilization in mice. Importantly, a number of clinical reports have highlighted the crucial importance of PLCζ in human fertilization by associating PLCζ deficiencies with certain forms of male factor infertility. Herein, we give an update on recent advances that have refined our understanding of how sperm PLCζ triggers Ca^{2+} oscillations and egg activation in mammals, while also discussing the nature of a potential "alternative" sperm factor. We summarise PLCζ localization in mammalian sperm, and the direct links observed between defective PLCζ protein in sperm and documented cases of male infertility. Finally, we postulate how this sperm protein can be used as a potential diagnostic marker, and also as a powerful therapeutic agent for treatment of certain types of male infertility due to egg activation failure or even in more general cases of male subfertility.

Keywords: sperm, phospholipase C zeta, PLC zeta, egg activation, fertilization

SPERM PLCζ IS THE PRIMARY STIMULUS FOR EGG ACTIVATION AND EARLY EMBRYONIC DEVELOPMENT

In mammalian fertilization, the fertilizing spermatozoon stimulates egg activation, a fundamental event that initiates embryonic development (Nomikos et al., 2017a). It is well established that the most crucial event of egg activation is an acute increase in cytosolic free Ca^{2+} concentrations, which in mammals occurs in the form of long-lasting Ca^{2+} oscillations that commence at or directly following gamete fusion, and persist for several hours beyond meiotic completion (Stricker, 1999; Malcuit et al., 2006; Kashir et al., 2013a). This Ca^{2+} signaling paradigm is essential for the completion of the multiple events of egg activation. However, previous archetypes of our understanding regarding the distinct events of egg activation and the events controlling them are continuously being unraveled and questioned, with specifics still being investigated. It is, however, clear that Ca^{2+}-release is an integral component of egg activation in all species studied to date (Cran et al., 1988; Swann and Ozil, 1994; Jones, 1998; Nomikos et al., 2012; Limatola et al., 2019b). Over the last few decades, a number of sperm-derived molecules had been proposed as potential soluble sperm factors responsible for the generation of Ca^{2+} oscillations during mammalian fertilization (for more information see Nomikos et al., 2012, 2013a, 2017a). The fact that sperm-induced Ca^{2+} oscillations are caused by activation of the inositol 1,4,5-trisphosphate ($InsP_3$) signaling pathway (Miyazaki et al., 1992) suggested that the sperm factor might itself be a phospholipase C (PLC) isoform (Jones et al., 1998).

In 2002, a novel testis-specific PLC, termed PLC zeta (PLCζ), was discovered (Saunders et al., 2002) and abundant experimental evidence has accumulated over the years suggesting that PLCζ fulfills all prerequisite criteria of the soluble sperm factor responsible for the generation of Ca^{2+} oscillations at mammalian fertilization (Cox et al., 2002; Saunders et al., 2002, 2007; Knott et al., 2005; Kouchi et al., 2005; Nomikos et al., 2005, 2013b, 2017a; Swann et al., 2006; Yu et al., 2008; Kashir et al., 2012a). Upon sperm-egg fusion, PLCζ is proposed to be delivered by the fertilizing sperm into the ooplasm, triggering the Ca^{2+} oscillations via the $InsP_3$ signaling pathway, through the hydrolysis of its membrane-bound phospholipid substrate, PIP_2 (Saunders et al., 2002; Nomikos, 2015). The importance of this sperm specific protein in mammalian fertilization has been further highlighted by numerous clinical studies directly linking defects or deficiencies in human PLCζ with documented cases of male factor infertility (Yoon et al., 2008; Heytens et al., 2009; Nomikos et al., 2011a, 2017b; Kashir et al., 2012b,c; Escoffier et al., 2016; Torra-Massana et al., 2019).

Intriguingly, two recent independent studies described the phenotype of a PLCζ "knockout" mouse (Hachem et al., 2017; Nozawa et al., 2018). By using multiple transgenic models of PLCζ "knockout" mice generated by CRISPR/Cas methodology, both studies reported that males can produce offspring, albeit with significantly reduced litter numbers (~25%). Interestingly, both studies showed that sperm lacking functional PLCζ protein failed to induce Ca^{2+} release when microinjected into mouse eggs by ICSI. However, *in vitro* fertilisation (IVF) with such sperm, produced atypical and delayed patterns of Ca^{2+} oscillations (lower in number and frequency) with a high degree of polyspermy and activation failure, compared to the robust, physiological pattern triggered by physiological PLCζ-induced egg activation (Nozawa et al., 2018; Satouh and Ikawa, 2018).

Perhaps the atypical and delayed pattern of Ca^{2+} release, observed alongside the low number of embryos and offspring, could be spontaneous activation, unrelated to Ca^{2+} release, which is common in some strains of mice (Cheng et al., 2012), alongside with the introduction of PLCζ knockout sperm. Indeed, eggs that had been fertilized by knockout sperm also displayed multiple pronuclei, consistent with the inability of a sufficient polyspermy block (Nozawa et al., 2018). Critically, however, eggs fertilized with PLCζ knockout sperm exhibited a total of 3–4 oscillations in total, initiating following a 1-h delay. This was in contrast to normal fertilization where 3–4 oscillations were observed per hour over 3–4 h (Nozawa et al., 2018; Satouh and Ikawa, 2018). Such observations perhaps suggest that sperm containing a second molecule with Ca^{2+} releasing activity, albeit weaker than PLCζ (Jones, 2018). From such results, one could potentially posit that perhaps PLCζ is not an absolute requirement for natural fertilization, and that perhaps an alternative "primitive" or "cryptic" sperm factor may also be involved in leading to egg activation (Nozawa et al., 2018; Satouh and Ikawa, 2018).

It is possible that such a factor could be one of the previously proposed unsuccessful candidates for the "sperm factor," including tr-kit (Sette et al., 2002), citrate synthase (Harada et al., 2007), or PAWP (Aarabi et al., 2010), which while not contributing to the majority of Ca^{2+} release at oocyte activation, may have a contributory function, especially, in the absence of PLCζ. However, it is worth noting that none of the aforementioned proteins is able to elicit Ca^{2+} release in the specific manner required for oocyte activation at physiological levels within sperm (Kashir et al., 2014; Nomikos et al., 2014; Satouh et al., 2015), while none of the alternatively proposed sperm factors (apart from PLCζ) has been shown to be directly involved in IP_3-mediated Ca^{2+} release (Kashir et al., 2014). Furthermore, we cannot exclude the possibility that another sperm-associated enzyme, which might be only able to achieve critical levels due to absence of PLCζ in the sperm of PLCζ knockout mice, might play the role of the "cryptic" factor triggering embryogenesis by a distinct mechanism.

Theories regarding RNA involvement are also questionable since the total amount of PLCζ RNA present within sperm may not be enough to elicit any Ca^{2+} release. On the other hand, this may have been altered as part of genetic compensation.

Intriguingly, starfish eggs pre-injected with heparin (which also blocks $InsP_3$ receptor function) to disrupt cytoskeletal arrangement were unable to exhibit a rapid Ca^{2+} wave response upon interaction with sperm, instead exhibiting a much more delayed pattern of release, and failed to prevent polyspermy. Furthermore, the amplitude of subsequent Ca^{2+} peaks were reduced, exhibiting an effect similar to observations made with sperm from PLCζ-null mice. In starfish, it was suggested that heparin- or age-induced hyperpolymerization of the cortical actin disrupted actin cytoskeleton dynamics at fertilization influenced Ca^{2+} release (Puppo et al., 2008; Santella et al., 2015; Limatola et al., 2019a), potentially also impacting upon subsequent events in egg activation such as cortical granule exocytosis. It is thus possible that due to the lack of a sufficient response at fertilization due to deficient/absent PLCζ, a similar effect was observed in the PLCζ-null mice, where similar symptoms of insufficient Ca^{2+} release and increased polyspermy were also observed. Indeed, it may be the case that the low number and frequency

Abbreviations: ART, assisted reproductive technology; Ca^{2+}, calcium; ICSI, intracytoplasmic sperm injection; $InsP_3$, inositol 1,4,5-trisphosphate; PI(3)P, phosphatidylinositol 3-phosphate; PI(5P), phosphatidylinositol 5-phosphate; PIP_2, phosphatidylinositol 4,5-bisphosphate; PLCζ, phospholipase C zeta.

of Ca^{2+} observed could be due to events surrounding actin polymerization or associated $InsP_3$-independent events of Ca^{2+} release (such as influx). However, these mechanisms are poorly understood in mammals, and require further investigation to fully ascertain.

It is clear that both Hachem et al. (2017) and Nozawa et al. (2018) represent keystone studies that support the notion that PLCζ is the primary physiological stimulus that triggers the required specific pattern of Ca^{2+} oscillations, ensuring monospermy and eventually successful egg activation and early embryonic development (Hachem et al., 2017; Nozawa et al., 2018; Swann, 2018). Moreover, the presence of an alternative factor in other species and especially in humans is still questionable, particularly taking into consideration all the documented cases of male factor infertility due to PLCζ deficiencies. However, this is an intriguing area of investigation that ongoing studies are now aiming to address. It would be interesting to examine how the increasing body of invertebrate animal work will direct the mammalian side of the coin in the future, particularly with relation to the early influence exerted by the egg actin cytoskeleton upon patterns of Ca^{2+} release and fertilization as is being unraveled in starfish. Furthermore, integral studies are required in particularly livestock mammalian models to demonstrate whether PLCζ-loss resembles the mouse and/or human scenarios. Perhaps of particular interest should be attempts to generate transgenic knockout models of PLCζ in porcine or bovine systems. While this would of course be considerably harder to perform than in the mouse, such data would undoubtedly assist in ascertaining the validity of "cryptic factor" theories. Further experiments that would be prudent would be to examine the specific timing of the reduced profiles of Ca^{2+} release in relation to PLCζ knockout sperm-egg fusion and fertilization. Are such reduced frequency and amplitude oscillations due to fusion of a single sperm, or the cumulative effect of multiple sperm-egg fusion events? It is necessary that such experiments are performed to ascertain fully the conflicting data generated from knockout studies thus far.

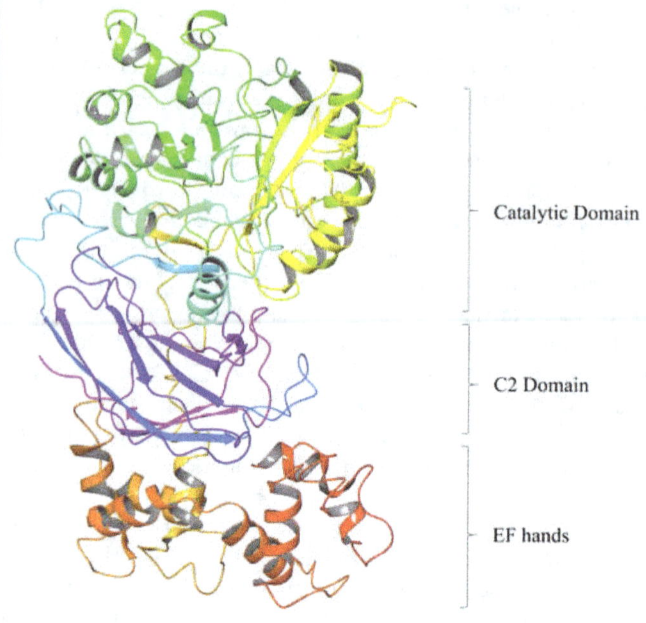

FIGURE 1 | Homology modeling of Human PLCζ (3D ribbon representation) predicted using 1DJI.B PDB entry as template based on a target-template alignment by the Prime homology modeling tool of the Schrödinger Suite (DeLano Scientific LLC, Schrödinger).

SPERM PLCζ STRUCTURE AND DOMAIN ORGANIZATION

Phospholipase C zeta is currently the smallest known mammalian PLC isoform (~70–75 kDa in size) with the most elementary domain organization (Cox et al., 2002; Saunders et al., 2002; Nomikos et al., 2013a, 2017a). Despite this, PLCζ exhibits uniquely supreme potency in triggering Ca^{2+} oscillations within the fertilizing egg compared to other somatic PLCs. This is attributed to its novel biochemical characteristics, arising from the essential role of its domains that contribute to the unique biological function and mode of regulation of this distinctive PLC isozyme (Nomikos, 2015; Nomikos et al., 2017a). PLCζ domain structure consists of four tandem EF hand domains at the N-terminus, the catalytic X and Y domain in the center of the molecule, followed by a single C2 domain at the C-terminus (**Figure 1**; Nomikos et al., 2017a). All these domains are common to other PLC isoforms. The X and Y catalytic domains are separated by a short segment, the XY-linker, which through its net positive charge plays an important role in targeting PLCζ to intracellular membranes by direct electrostatic interactions with its negatively charged substrate, PIP_2 (Nomikos et al., 2007, 2011b). The XY-linker region differs considerably between PLC isozymes (Nomikos et al., 2013a). By contrast, the XY catalytic domain between PLC isoforms is the most highly conserved region (Nomikos, 2015).

The XY domain of PLCζ shares ~60% sequence similarity to that of all PLCs and is responsible for PIP_2 hydrolysis (Nomikos et al., 2005). The EF hands are Ca^{2+}-binding motifs and in PLCζ these domains play a vital role in its high Ca^{2+} sensitivity compared with the other somatic PLCs, allowing PLCζ to be active at resting Ca^{2+} levels within the egg cytosol, when PLCζ enters after sperm-egg fusion (Nomikos et al., 2005). Additionally, we have demonstrated that the first EF-hand domain of PLCζ, which contains a cluster of basic amino acid residues, plays an essential role together with the XY-linker region, in the interaction of PLCζ with the PIP_2-containing membranes (Nomikos et al., 2015b). The C-terminal C2 domain of PLCζ, comprising ~120 amino acid residues is essential for PLCζ function, as targeted deletion or replacement of this domain by the corresponding domain from PLCδ1 abolishes the Ca^{2+}-oscillation-inducing activity of PLCζ in eggs, without altering its enzymatic activity or Ca^{2+} sensitivity (Nomikos et al., 2005; Theodoridou et al., 2013). We have provided biochemical evidence that this domain directly interacts with the membrane phospholipids, PI(3)P, and PI(5)P and have suggested that C2 association with these phospholipids may facilitate in the membrane targeting of PLCζ (Theodoridou et al., 2013; Nomikos, 2015).

PLCζ IN MAMMALIAN SPERM

Phospholipase C zeta mRNA has been identified during both early and late stages of spermatogenesis in mice and pigs (Yoneda et al., 2006; Young et al., 2009; Bedford-Guaus et al., 2011; Kaewmala et al., 2012). Specific localization patterns, however, remain elusive in the literature throughout the various spermatogenic cells within the testes (Kashir et al., 2018). Aarabi et al. (2012) indicated that PLCζ is integrated as part of the acrosome during the Golgi phase of human and mouse spermiogenesis (Aarabi et al., 2012), suggesting that observable PLCζ levels are diminished gradually throughout spermatid elongation (Kashir et al., 2018). PLCζ was originally identified in mouse sperm extract fractions that were able to induce Ca^{2+} release. Subsequent immunofluorescence analysis indicated a post-acrosomal localization for PLCζ; a component of the post-acrosomal sheath (Saunders et al., 2002; Fujimoto et al., 2004; Young et al., 2009). Nevertheless, PLCζ has been identified in the sperm of various mammalian species, and usually tends to be found within the sperm head in distinct subcellular regions, postulating differential functional roles for each population (Amdani et al., 2013; Kashir et al., 2014, 2018).

While in mouse and porcine sperm, PLCζ has been observed mainly at acrosomal and post-acrosomal regions (Fujimoto et al., 2004; Young et al., 2009; Nakai et al., 2011; Kaewmala et al., 2012), in equine sperm, PLCζ was recorded at the acrosome, equatorial segment, and head mid-piece, as well as the principle piece of the flagellum (Bedford-Guaus et al., 2011; Kashir et al., 2018). Several PLCζ populations were observed in humans in multiple studies including the acrosomal, equatorial and post-acrosomal regions of the sperm head, with a potential tail localization (Grasa et al., 2008; Yoon et al., 2008; Young et al., 2009; Kashir et al., 2013b, 2018; Escoffier et al., 2015; Yelumalai et al., 2015; Yeste et al., 2016). While there is consensus regarding PLCζ localization in mouse sperm, the veracity of the multiple populations identified in other mammalian sperm (particularly in humans) remains debated (Nomikos et al., 2017a; Kashir et al., 2018). In human sperm, this variation in PLCζ localization is not only limited to observations between different studies but substantial variability in the PLCζ localization pattern was found even within the same study (Kashir et al., 2013b).

Despite numerous efforts to examine PLCζ localization within mammalian sperm, significant concern surrounds the specificity of the majority of antibodies used to date. More specifically, most antibodies used in the literature are unable to demonstrate a consistent motif of recognizing a single band following immunoblotting of human sperm, often detecting multiple protein bands other than, or in addition to, that of the expected size for native PLCζ protein. Compounded by this non-specificity, multiple groups have identified varying populations between mouse and human sperm, even using the same antibodies, suggesting that varying protocols and the use of different antibodies are the main source of inconsistent results between studies (Grasa et al., 2008; Yoon et al., 2008; Heytens et al., 2009; Kashir et al., 2011a,b, 2013b; Aarabi et al., 2012).

Addressing such concerns, we recently generated highly epitope-specific PLCζ polyclonal antibodies against human, mouse, and porcine PLCζ, that exhibit high consistency throughout numerous studies for both recombinant and native PLCζ (Nomikos et al., 2013b, 2014, 2015a; Theodoridou et al., 2013). Furthermore, we have also developed specific antigen unmasking/retrieval protocols, which we previously demonstrated are essential to enhance the visualization efficacy of PLCζ in mammalian sperm (Kashir et al., 2017). Using these enhanced protocols and materials, we have identified PLCζ in the acrosomal and post-acrosomal, acrosomal and equatorial, and post-acrosomal and equatorial compartments of mouse, human, and porcine sperm, respectively. Furthermore, we have also consistently observed potential tail localization in all species (Kashir et al., 2017). **Figure 2** demonstrates the expression and distribution of PLCζ in mouse sperm using our specific polyclonal antibodies and our recently developed and reported protocols (Kashir et al., 2017). It is now imperative that these specific antibodies and protocols are applied in a systematic manner to examine whether particular localization patterns or profiles of PLCζ exhibit any relationships between male fertility parameters, or indeed between fertility treatment outcomes.

Another intriguing question is how PLCζ, despite its high Ca^{2+}-sensitivity and its potent enzymatic activity, is kept in an inactive state within the sperm, especially when it is likely to be present in much higher concentrations in a single spermatozoon than within the fertilizing egg. Indeed, our previous work where it was shown that PLCζ is inactive in somatic cells even at levels over 1000 times that at which it is active in eggs (Phillips et al., 2011), suggests that either PLCζ has an essential binding-partner within the egg, or that other factors within sperm and somatic cells may inhibit its catalytic activity.

REDUCED EXPRESSION LEVELS AND ABNORMAL FORMS OF SPERM PLCζ LEAD TO MALE INFERTILITY

Infertility is estimated to affect ~15% of couples, with male infertility affecting ~7% of men worldwide (Kashir et al., 2010). While genetic causes of male infertility are estimated to underlie ~30% of such cases (Harton and Tempest, 2012; Jungwirth et al., 2012; Hotaling, 2014), ~50% of cases of male infertility remain unexplained (Kashir et al., 2018). While most forms of infertility can now be treated via a collection of laboratory techniques collectively termed ART, a number of conditions such as severe male infertility (19–57% of cases) cannot yet been treated (Botezatu et al., 2014). Despite the fact that powerful ART methods such as IVF or ICSI can successfully treat some infertility cases, it is concerning that this is achieved only after several fertility treatment cycles. A significant causative factor may be recurrent implantation failure, which even after fertility treatment leads to infertility (Polanski et al., 2014; Kashir et al., 2018).

Considering the indispensable contribution of PLCζ to fertilization, defects in either egg activation, or in PLCζ

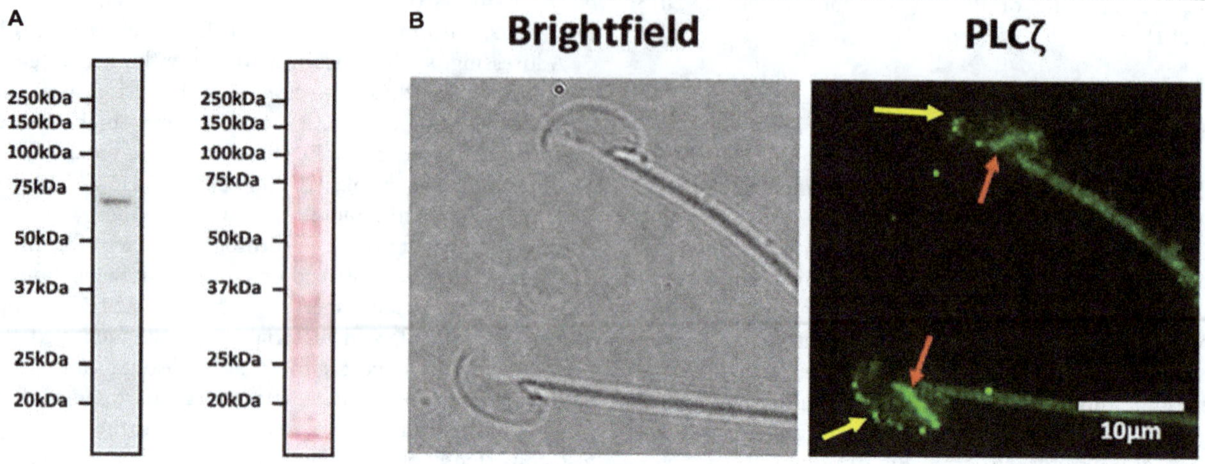

FIGURE 2 | (A) Representative immunoblot image obtained using a highly specific anti-PLCζ polyclonal antibody identifying a single protein band corresponding to the molecular weight of native mouse PLCζ (~74 kDa). Left image indicates immunoblot specificity, while the right image shows ponceau-stained membranes. 1×10^6 mouse sperm were loaded per lane. **(B)** Representative immunofluorescence image illustrating representative localization of native PLCζ in mouse sperm. Image was captured at 100X, and brightfield (left panel) and green fluorescence (right panel; PLCζ) images were obtained. Yellow arrows indicate acrosomal populations, while red arrows indicate post-acrosomal localization of PLCζ in mouse sperm, Scale bar indicates 10 μm.

protein itself, may underlie conditions of male infertility where fertilization failure occurs. The first evidence came from studies that reported sperm of infertile men, which consistently failed to fertilize eggs following routine IVF or ICSI, and were either unable to induce Ca^{2+} release upon microinjection into mouse eggs, or produced highly abnormal Ca^{2+} transients which were reduced in frequency and amplitude (Yoon et al., 2008; Heytens et al., 2009). Furthermore, such sperm also exhibited reduced or absent levels, as well as abnormal localization patterns, of PLCζ within the sperm head (Heytens et al., 2009; Kashir et al., 2011a,b, 2013b), suggesting that deficiencies in PLCζ protein may underlie currently unknown cases of male factor infertility. In a clinical scenario, in contrast to other causes, complete fertilization failure is attributed to egg activation failure in a species-specific manner (Kashir et al., 2010, 2018).

Moreover, PLCζ gene abrogation in patients diagnosed with egg activation deficiency is now increasingly being reported within the scientific literature. The first two PLCζ mutations were identified in the gene of an infertile male, whose sperm was unable to trigger the normal pattern of Ca^{2+} oscillations, leading to egg activation failure and potentially to his infertility (Heytens et al., 2009; Kashir et al., 2011b, 2012b,c). Both mutations were reported within the active catalytic site domains of PLCζ (X and Y), disrupting local protein structural folding to cause reduction of enzymatic activity, subsequently leading to highly abnormal Ca^{2+} transients unable to initiate egg activation (Kashir et al., 2011b). Both mutations were reported to be heterozygous, with one mutation being inherited from the patient's father and the other from the patient's mother, indicating for the first time that such maternally inherited loss-of-activity mutations can lead to male infertility (Kashir et al., 2012b,c; Nomikos et al., 2017a). Subsequently, a further mutation in homozygosis was later reported by Escoffier et al. (2016) from two infertile brothers. This mutation is located within the C2 domain of PLCζ (Escoffier et al., 2016). Intriguingly, this PLCζ mutant displayed similar enzymatic activity to wild type PLCζ, but displayed a dramatically reduced relative binding-affinity to PI(3)P and PI(5)P-containing liposomes (Nomikos et al., 2017a). More importantly, this genetic report by Escoffier et al. (2016) and the identification of this novel missense homozygous PLCζ mutation in these infertile brothers after whole exomic sequencing, strongly indicates that absence or defects in PLCζ protein alone is sufficient to prevent human egg activation by the sperm, suggesting that PLCζ is essential for human egg activation and thus human fertilization.

Furthermore, single nucleotide polymorphisms (SNPs) have also been reported by Yoon et al. (2008) and more recently by Ferrer-Vaquer et al. (2016), either within the PLCζ coding sequence or its associated bi-directional promoter in human patients (Nomikos et al., 2017a).

Interestingly, Torra-Massana et al. (2019) very recently reported six new PLCζ mutations after screening an egg activation deficiency group, one of which was previously described (Kashir et al., 2012b,c), in addition to four novel single-nucleotide missense mutations, located in the EF-hands, the X catalytic and C2 domains; while the sixth mutation identified was a frameshift variant, which was predicted to generate a truncated protein at the X-Y linker region (Torra-Massana et al., 2019). While further analysis indicated a potential deleterious effect of some of these mutations upon PLCζ activity within eggs, further biochemical analysis is required to ascertain whether such variants of PLCζ are deleterious as claimed at physiological levels, needing their accurate quantification in sperm and eggs. However, it is now clear that deleterious mutations in PLCζ may be more widespread than previously thought, appearing not only in the catalytic active site, but also in other vital regulatory regions of this essential sperm protein, afflicting its membrane and/or substrate binding, its Ca^{2+} sensitivity, as well as its enzymatic activity.

Despite the relatively high success rate of ICSI in overcoming cases of failed fertilization after IVF, ~30% of such cases still repeatedly fail ICSI (Flaherty et al., 1998; van der Westerlaken et al., 2005). Low global pregnancy success rates following ART have been attributed to poor embryogenesis following fertility treatment (Fauque et al., 2007; Pelinck et al., 2010). Importantly, such poor embryonic competency can be directly linked to PLCζ and competency of egg activation (Nomikos et al., 2017a; Kashir et al., 2018). Injection of increasing levels of PLCζ in human eggs results in increasing frequencies and amplitudes of Ca^{2+} oscillations (Yamaguchi et al., 2017), which in turn affects subsequent gene expression (Ducibella et al., 2002, 2006). Furthermore, the frequency and amplitude of Ca^{2+} oscillations has been shown to play an important role in compaction, and blastocyst formation (Swann and Ozil, 1994; Miyazaki and Ito, 2006). Finally, taking into consideration that the rate of progression to the 2- and 4-cell stages of human eggs following fertilization has been suggested as an indicator of normal embryogenesis (Wong et al., 2010), PLCζ-driven Ca^{2+} oscillations may not only be required for egg activation, but can also be equally important for subsequent embryogenesis. Thus, abnormalities in sperm PLCζ levels may underlie not only infertility through fertilization failure, but also cases of male subfertility, whereby enough PLCζ may be delivered into the eggs to trigger activation, but prove insufficient for embryonic competence.

CLINICAL APPLICATIONS OF PLCζ AND FUTURE DIRECTIONS

Currently, cases of defective egg activation are clinically resolved using assisted egg activation (AOA), involving artificially mediated Ca^{2+} release (Santella and Dale, 2015; Kashir et al., 2018). Ca^{2+} ionophores like ionomycin, calcimycin are currently used to overcome unexplained fertilization failure in couples, who repeatedly fail ICSI cycles (Fawzy et al., 2018; Norozi-Hafshejani et al., 2018). Recently, a meta-analysis indicated that use of Ca^{2+} ionophores significantly improved fertilization and implantation rates in ICSI (Murugesu et al., 2017). However, Ca^{2+} ionophores induce a single Ca^{2+} transient, unlike the endogenous specific physiological pattern of Ca^{2+} oscillations observed during normal fertilization (Rinaudo et al., 1997). In fact, microinjection of human recombinant PLCζ yielded higher blastocyst development rates than Ca^{2+} ionophore treatment (Sanusi et al., 2015). Thus, PLCζ has long represented a physiologically endogenous alternative method to clinically treat cases of egg activation failure/deficiency, which would involve the *in vitro* production of active, purified versions of human recombinant PLCζ protein. Indeed, following initial difficulties, multiple studies made advancements in the production of such a desired product (Kashir et al., 2011b; Yoon et al., 2012), culminating in efforts by Nomikos et al. (2013b) who made a significant breakthrough by generating purified, highly active recombinant PLCζ, capable of inducing physiological patterns of Ca^{2+} oscillations following microinjection into mouse and human eggs (Nomikos et al., 2013b). More importantly, recombinant PLCζ was able to effectively rescue failed egg activation in a prototype of male infertility (Nomikos et al., 2013b). Further attempts to develop the use of recombinant PLCζ protein as a therapeutic agent in a clinical setting are currently in progress, in order to eliminate any potential cytotoxic effects during embryonic development and confirm the overall safety of exogenous PLCζ on the subsequent offspring.

Finally, PLCζ not only represents a promising clinical therapeutic agent, but also a potentially powerful diagnostic biomarker, which may help in determining the criteria and requirements of the fertility treatment of male patients, significantly decreasing the number of cycles needed for a successful pregnancy to occur. Taking into consideration that PLCζ analysis might be beneficial to identify not only cases of ICSI-failure but also cases of male subfertility, a simple immunocytological approach to routinely examine PLCζ protein in sperm is currently widely regarded as a cost-effective approach, which could be easily applied by the majority of IVF clinics worldwide. However, it is essential that studies focus on the reliable investigation of PLCζ parameters in relation to sperm health, using robust protocols and ultra-specific antibodies, before such clinical promise can be achieved. Indeed, significant issues remain regarding such analyses, particularly in humans, where PLCζ antibodies used recognize multiple protein bands in addition to the full-length PLCζ protein. The same antibodies have also been used to identify different immunoblotting profiles (for detailed review see Kashir et al., 2018). Predictably, such shortcomings have led to conflicting results between the association of specific PLCζ localization patterns and quantification levels.

ETHICS STATEMENT

Use of mouse sperm cells was carried out in accordance with the principles of the Basel Declaration and recommendations of the Animal Care and Use Committee (ACUC) at the Office of Research Affairs (ORA) at the King Faisal Specialist Hospital and Research Center, Riyadh, Saudi Arabia. The protocols utilized for the relevant study (RAC-216004) were approved by the ACUC.

AUTHOR CONTRIBUTIONS

AS, JK, AT, and MN prepared the first draft of the manuscript, which was revised and approved by all authors.

FUNDING

This work was supported by the Qatar University student grant to AS and FL (QUST-1-CMED-2020-3). JK was supported by a Healthcare Research Fellowship Award (HF-14-16) made by Health and Care Research Wales (HCRW), alongside a National Science, Technology, and Innovation plan (NSTIP) project grant (15-MED4186-20) awarded by the King Abdulaziz City for Science and Technology (KACST).

REFERENCES

Aarabi, M., Qin, Z., Xu, W., Mewburn, J., and Oko, R. (2010). Sperm-borne protein, PAWP, initiates zygotic development in Xenopus laevis by eliciting intracellular calcium release. *Mol. Reprod. Dev.* 77, 249–256. doi: 10.1002/mrd.21140

Aarabi, M., Yu, Y., Xu, W., Tse, M. Y., Pang, S. C., Yi, Y. J., et al. (2012). The testicular and epididymal expression profile of PLCzeta in mouse and human does not support its role as a sperm-borne oocyte activating factor. *PLoS One* 7:e33496. doi: 10.1371/journal.pone.0033496

Amdani, S. N., Jones, C., and Coward, K. (2013). Phospholipase C zeta (PLCzeta): oocyte activation and clinical links to male factor infertility. *Adv. Biol. Regul.* 53, 292–308. doi: 10.1016/j.jbior.2013.07.005

Bedford-Guaus, S. J., McPartlin, L. A., Xie, J., Westmiller, S. L., Buffone, M. G., and Roberson, M. S. (2011). Molecular cloning and characterization of phospholipase C zeta in equine sperm and testis reveals species-specific differences in expression of catalytically active protein. *Biol. Reprod.* 85, 78–88. doi: 10.1095/biolreprod.110.089466

Botezatu, A., Socolov, R., Socolov, D., Iancu, I. V., and Anton, G. (2014). Methylation pattern of methylene tetrahydrofolate reductase and small nuclear ribonucleoprotein polypeptide N promoters in oligoasthenospermia: a case-control study. *Reprod. Biomed Online* 28, 225–231. doi: 10.1016/j.rbmo.2013.10.010

Cheng, Y., Zhong, Z., and Latham, K. E. (2012). Strain-specific spontaneous activation during mouse oocyte maturation. *Fertil. Steril.* 98, 200–206. doi: 10.1016/j.fertnstert.2012.03.060

Cox, L. J., Larman, M. G., Saunders, C. M., Hashimoto, K., Swann, K., and Lai, F. A. (2002). Sperm phospholipase Czeta from humans and cynomolgus monkeys triggers Ca2+ oscillations, activation and development of mouse oocytes. *Reproduction* 124, 611–623. doi: 10.1530/rep.0.1240611

Cran, D. G., Moor, R. M., and Irvine, R. F. (1988). Initiation of the cortical reaction in hamster and sheep oocytes in response to inositol trisphosphate. *J. Cell Sci.* 91(Pt 1), 139–144.

Ducibella, T., Huneau, D., Angelichio, E., Xu, Z., Schultz, R. M., Kopf, G. S., et al. (2002). Egg-to-embryo transition is driven by differential responses to Ca(2+) oscillation number. *Dev. Biol.* 250, 280–291. doi: 10.1006/dbio.2002.0788

Ducibella, T., Schultz, R. M., and Ozil, J. P. (2006). Role of calcium signals in early development. *Semin. Cell Dev. Biol.* 17, 324–332. doi: 10.1016/j.semcdb.2006.02.010

Escoffier, J., Lee, H. C., Yassine, S., Zouari, R., Martinez, G., Karaouzene, T., et al. (2016). Homozygous mutation of PLCZ1 leads to defective human oocyte activation and infertility that is not rescued by the WW-binding protein PAWP. *Hum. Mol. Genet.* 25, 878–891. doi: 10.1093/hmg/ddv617

Escoffier, J., Yassine, S., Lee, H. C., Martinez, G., Delaroche, J., Coutton, C., et al. (2015). Subcellular localization of phospholipase Czeta in human sperm and its absence in DPY19L2-deficient sperm are consistent with its role in oocyte activation. *Mol. Hum. Reprod.* 21, 157–168. doi: 10.1093/molehr/gau098

Fauque, P., Leandri, R., Merlet, F., Juillard, J. C., Epelboin, S., Guibert, J., et al. (2007). Pregnancy outcome and live birth after IVF and ICSI according to embryo quality. *J. Assist. Reprod. Genet.* 24, 159–165. doi: 10.1007/s10815-007-9115-z

Fawzy, M., Emad, M., Mahran, A., Sabry, M., Fetih, A. N., Abdelghafar, H., et al. (2018). Artificial oocyte activation with SrCl2 or calcimycin after ICSI improves clinical and embryological outcomes compared with ICSI alone: results of a randomized clinical trial. *Hum. Reprod.* 33, 1636–1644. doi: 10.1093/humrep/dey258

Ferrer-Vaquer, A., Barragan, M., Freour, T., Vernaeve, V., and Vassena, R. (2016). PLCzeta sequence, protein levels, and distribution in human sperm do not correlate with semen characteristics and fertilization rates after ICSI. *J. Assist. Reprod. Genet.* 33, 747–756. doi: 10.1007/s10815-016-0718-0

Flaherty, S. P., Payne, D., and Matthews, C. D. (1998). Fertilization failures and abnormal fertilization after intracytoplasmic sperm injection. *Hum. Reprod.* 13(Suppl. 1), 155–164. doi: 10.1093/humrep/13.suppl_1.155

Fujimoto, S., Yoshida, N., Fukui, T., Amanai, M., Isobe, T., Itagaki, C., et al. (2004). Mammalian phospholipase Czeta induces oocyte activation from the sperm perinuclear matrix. *Dev. Biol.* 274, 370–383. doi: 10.1016/j.ydbio.2004.07.025

Grasa, P., Coward, K., Young, C., and Parrington, J. (2008). The pattern of localization of the putative oocyte activation factor, phospholipase Czeta, in uncapacitated, capacitated, and ionophore-treated human spermatozoa. *Hum. Reprod.* 23, 2513–2522. doi: 10.1093/humrep/den280

Hachem, A., Godwin, J., Ruas, M., Lee, H. C., Ferrer Buitrago, M., Ardestani, G., et al. (2017). PLCzeta is the physiological trigger of the Ca(2+) oscillations that induce embryogenesis in mammals but conception can occur in its absence. *Development* 144, 2914–2924. doi: 10.1242/dev.150227

Harada, Y., Matsumoto, T., Hirahara, S., Nakashima, A., Ueno, S., Oda, S., et al. (2007). Characterization of a sperm factor for egg activation at fertilization of the newt Cynops pyrrhogaster. *Dev. Biol.* 306, 797–808. doi: 10.1016/j.ydbio.2007.04.019

Harton, G. L., and Tempest, H. G. (2012). Chromosomal disorders and male infertility. *Asian. J. Androl.* 14, 32–39. doi: 10.1038/aja.2011.66

Heytens, E., Parrington, J., Coward, K., Young, C., Lambrecht, S., Yoon, S. Y., et al. (2009). Reduced amounts and abnormal forms of phospholipase C zeta (PLCzeta) in spermatozoa from infertile men. *Hum. Reprod.* 24, 2417–2428. doi: 10.1093/humrep/dep207

Hotaling, J. M. (2014). Genetics of male infertility. *Urol. Clin. North Am.* 41, 1–17. doi: 10.1016/j.ucl.2013.08.009

Jones, K. T. (1998). Ca2+ oscillations in the activation of the egg and development of the embryo in mammals. *Int. J. Dev. Biol.* 42, 1–10.

Jones, K. T. (2018). Mammalian sperm contain two factors for calcium release and egg activation: phospholipase C zeta and a cryptic activating factor. *Mol. Hum. Reprod.* 24, 465–468. doi: 10.1093/molehr/gay038

Jones, K. T., Cruttwell, C., Parrington, J., and Swann, K. (1998). A mammalian sperm cytosolic phospholipase C activity generates inositol trisphosphate and causes Ca2+ release in sea urchin egg homogenates. *FEBS Lett.* 437, 297–300. doi: 10.1016/s0014-5793(98)01254-x

Jungwirth, A., Giwercman, A., Tournaye, H., Diemer, T., Kopa, Z., Dohle, G., et al. (2012). European association of urology guidelines on male infertility: the 2012 update. *Eur. Urol.* 62, 324–332. doi: 10.1016/j.eururo.2012.04.048

Kaewmala, K., Uddin, M. J., Cinar, M. U., Grosse-Brinkhaus, C., Jonas, E., Tesfaye, D., et al. (2012). Investigation into association and expression of PLCz and COX-2 as candidate genes for boar sperm quality and fertility. *Reprod. Domest. Anim.* 47, 213–223. doi: 10.1111/j.1439-0531.2011.01831.x

Kashir, J., Buntwal, L., Nomikos, M., Calver, B. L., Stamatiadis, P., Ashley, P., et al. (2017). Antigen unmasking enhances visualization efficacy of the oocyte activation factor, phospholipase C zeta, in mammalian sperm. *Mol. Hum. Reprod.* 23, 54–67. doi: 10.1093/molehr/gaw073

Kashir, J., Deguchi, R., Jones, C., Coward, K., and Stricker, S. A. (2013a). Comparative biology of sperm factors and fertilization-induced calcium signals across the animal kingdom. *Mol. Reprod. Dev.* 80, 787–815. doi: 10.1002/mrd.22222

Kashir, J., Heindryckx, B., Jones, C., De Sutter, P., Parrington, J., and Coward, K. (2010). Oocyte activation, phospholipase C zeta and human infertility. *Hum. Reprod. Update* 16, 690–703. doi: 10.1093/humupd/dmq018

Kashir, J., Heynen, A., Jones, C., Durrans, C., Craig, J., Gadea, J., et al. (2011a). Effects of cryopreservation and density-gradient washing on phospholipase C zeta concentrations in human spermatozoa. *Reprod. Biomed Online* 23, 263–267. doi: 10.1016/j.rbmo.2011.04.006

Kashir, J., Jones, C., and Coward, K. (2012a). Calcium oscillations, oocyte activation, and phospholipase C zeta. *Adv. Exp. Med. Biol.* 740, 1095–1121. doi: 10.1007/978-94-007-2888-2_50

Kashir, J., Jones, C., Lee, H. C., Rietdorf, K., Nikiforaki, D., Durrans, C., et al. (2011b). Loss of activity mutations in phospholipase C zeta (PLCzeta) abolishes calcium oscillatory ability of human recombinant protein in mouse oocytes. *Hum. Reprod.* 26, 3372–3387. doi: 10.1093/humrep/der336

Kashir, J., Jones, C., Mounce, G., Ramadan, W. M., Lemmon, B., Heindryckx, B., et al. (2013b). Variance in total levels of phospholipase C zeta (PLC-zeta) in human sperm may limit the applicability of quantitative immunofluorescent analysis as a diagnostic indicator of oocyte activation capability. *Fertil. Steril.* 99, 107–117. doi: 10.1016/j.fertnstert.2012.09.001

Kashir, J., Konstantinidis, M., Jones, C., Heindryckx, B., De Sutter, P., Parrington, J., et al. (2012b). Characterization of two heterozygous mutations of the oocyte activation factor phospholipase C zeta (PLCzeta) from an infertile man by use of minisequencing of individual sperm and expression in somatic cells. *Fertil. Steril.* 98, 423–431. doi: 10.1016/j.fertnstert.2012.05.002

Kashir, J., Konstantinidis, M., Jones, C., Lemmon, B., Lee, H. C., Hamer, R., et al. (2012c). A maternally inherited autosomal point mutation in human phospholipase C zeta (PLCzeta) leads to male infertility. *Hum. Reprod.* 27, 222–231. doi: 10.1093/humrep/der384

Kashir, J., Nomikos, M., and Lai, F. A. (2018). Phospholipase C zeta and calcium oscillations at fertilisation: the evidence, applications, and further questions. *Adv. Biol. Regul.* 67, 148–162. doi: 10.1016/j.jbior.2017.10.012

Kashir, J., Nomikos, M., Lai, F. A., and Swann, K. (2014). Sperm-induced Ca2+ release during egg activation in mammals. *Biochem. Biophys. Res. Commun.* 450, 1204–1211. doi: 10.1016/j.bbrc.2014.04.078

Knott, J. G., Kurokawa, M., Fissore, R. A., Schultz, R. M., and Williams, C. J. (2005). Transgenic RNA interference reveals role for mouse sperm phospholipase Czeta in triggering Ca2+ oscillations during fertilization. *Biol. Reprod.* 72, 992–996. doi: 10.1095/biolreprod.104.036244

Kouchi, Z., Shikano, T., Nakamura, Y., Shirakawa, H., Fukami, K., and Miyazaki, S. (2005). The role of EF-hand domains and C2 domain in regulation of enzymatic activity of phospholipase Czeta. *J. Biol. Chem.* 280, 21015–21021. doi: 10.1074/jbc.M412123200

Limatola, N., Vasilev, F., Chun, J. T., and Santella, L. (2019a). Altered actin cytoskeleton in ageing eggs of starfish affects fertilization process. *Exp. Cell Res.* 381, 179–190. doi: 10.1016/j.yexcr.2019.05.007

Limatola, N., Vasilev, F., Chun, J. T., and Santella, L. (2019b). Sodium-mediated fast electrical depolarization does not prevent polyspermic fertilization in *Paracentrotus lividus* eggs. *Zygote* 27, 241–249. doi: 10.1017/S0967199419000364

Malcuit, C., Kurokawa, M., and Fissore, R. A. (2006). Calcium oscillations and mammalian egg activation. *J. Cell Physiol.* 206, 565–573. doi: 10.1002/jcp.20471

Miyazaki, S., and Ito, M. (2006). Calcium signals for egg activation in mammals. *J. Pharmacol. Sci.* 100, 545–552. doi: 10.1254/jphs.cpj06003x

Miyazaki, S., Yuzaki, M., Nakada, K., Shirakawa, H., Nakanishi, S., Nakade, S., et al. (1992). Block of Ca2+ wave and Ca2+ oscillation by antibody to the inositol 1,4,5-trisphosphate receptor in fertilized hamster eggs. *Science* 257, 251–255. doi: 10.1126/science.1321497

Murugesu, S., Saso, S., Jones, B. P., Bracewell-Milnes, T., Athanasiou, T., Mania, A., et al. (2017). Does the use of calcium ionophore during artificial oocyte activation demonstrate an effect on pregnancy rate? A meta-analysis. *Fertil. Steril.* 108, 468– 462. doi: 10.1016/j.fertnstert.2017.06.029

Nakai, M., Ito, J., Sato, K., Noguchi, J., Kaneko, H., Kashiwazaki, N., et al. (2011). Pre-treatment of sperm reduces success of ICSI in the pig. *Reproduction* 142, 285–293. doi: 10.1530/rep-11-0073

Nomikos, M. (2015). Novel signalling mechanism and clinical applications of sperm-specific PLCzeta. *Biochem. Soc,. Trans.* 43, 371–376. doi: 10.1042/BST20140291

Nomikos, M., Blayney, L. M., Larman, M. G., Campbell, K., Rossbach, A., Saunders, C. M., et al. (2005). Role of phospholipase C-zeta domains in Ca2+-dependent phosphatidylinositol 4,5-bisphosphate hydrolysis and cytoplasmic Ca2+ oscillations. *J. Biol. Chem.* 280, 31011–31018. doi: 10.1074/jbc.M500629200

Nomikos, M., Elgmati, K., Theodoridou, M., Calver, B. L., Cumbes, B., Nounesis, G., et al. (2011a). Male infertility-linked point mutation disrupts the Ca2+ oscillation-inducing and PIP(2) hydrolysis activity of sperm PLCzeta. *Biochem. J.* 434, 211–217. doi: 10.1042/BJ20101772

Nomikos, M., Elgmati, K., Theodoridou, M., Calver, B. L., Nounesis, G., Swann, K., et al. (2011b). Phospholipase Czeta binding to PtdIns(4,5)P2 requires the XY-linker region. *J. Cell Sci.* 124(Pt 15), 2582–2590. doi: 10.1242/jcs.083485

Nomikos, M., Kashir, J., and Lai, F. A. (2017a). The role and mechanism of action of sperm PLC-zeta in mammalian fertilisation. *Biochem. J.* 474, 3659–3673. doi: 10.1042/BCJ20160521

Nomikos, M., Kashir, J., Swann, K., and Lai, F. A. (2013a). Sperm PLCzeta: from structure to Ca2+ oscillations, egg activation and therapeutic potential. *FEBS Lett.* 587, 3609–3616. doi: 10.1016/j.febslet.2013.10.008

Nomikos, M., Mulgrew-Nesbitt, A., Pallavi, P., Mihalyne, G., Zaitseva, I., Swann, K., et al. (2007). Binding of phosphoinositide-specific phospholipase C-zeta (PLC-zeta) to phospholipid membranes: potential role of an unstructured cluster of basic residues. *J. Biol. Chem.* 282, 16644–16653. doi: 10.1074/jbc.M701072200

Nomikos, M., Stamatiadis, P., Sanders, J. R., Beck, K., Calver, B. L., Buntwal, L., et al. (2017b). Male infertility-linked point mutation reveals a vital binding role for the C2 domain of sperm PLCzeta. *Biochem. J.* 474, 1003–1016. doi: 10.1042/BCJ20161057

Nomikos, M., Yu, Y., Elgmati, K., Theodoridou, M., Campbell, K., Vassilakopoulou, V., et al. (2013b). Phospholipase Czeta rescues failed oocyte activation in a prototype of male factor infertility. *Fertil. Steril.* 99, 76–85. doi: 10.1016/j.fertnstert.2012.08.035

Nomikos, M., Sanders, J. R., Kashir, J., Sanusi, R., Buntwal, L., Love, D., et al. (2015a). Functional disparity between human PAWP and PLCzeta in the generation of Ca2+ oscillations for oocyte activation. *Mol. Hum. Reprod.* 21, 702–710. doi: 10.1093/molehr/gav034

Nomikos, M., Sanders, J. R., Parthimos, D., Buntwal, L., Calver, B. L., Stamatiadis, P., et al. (2015b). Essential role of the EF-hand domain in targeting sperm phospholipase czeta to membrane phosphatidylinositol 4,5-Bisphosphate (PIP2). *J. Biol. Chem.* 290, 29519–29530. doi: 10.1074/jbc.M115.658443

Nomikos, M., Sanders, J. R., Theodoridou, M., Kashir, J., Matthews, E., Nounesis, G., et al. (2014). Sperm-specific post-acrosomal WW-domain binding protein (PAWP) does not cause Ca2+ release in mouse oocytes. *Mol. Hum. Reprod.* 20, 938–947. doi: 10.1093/molehr/gau056

Nomikos, M., Swann, K., and Lai, F. A. (2012). Starting a new life: sperm PLC-zeta mobilizes the Ca2+ signal that induces egg activation and embryo development: an essential phospholipase C with implications for male infertility. *Bioessays* 34, 126–134. doi: 10.1002/bies.201100127

Norozi-Hafshejani, M., Tavalaee, M., Azadi, L., Bahadorani, M., and Nasr-Esfahani, M. H. (2018). Effects of assisted oocyte activation with calcium- ionophore and strontium chloride on in vitro ICSI outcomes. *Iran. J. Basic Med. Sci.* 21, 1109–1117. doi: 10.22038/IJBMS.2018.30422.7331

Nozawa, K., Satouh, Y., Fujimoto, T., Oji, A., and Ikawa, M. (2018). Sperm-borne phospholipase C zeta-1 ensures monospermic fertilization in mice. *Sci. Rep.* 8, 1315.

Pelinck, M. J., Hoek, A., Simons, A. H., Heineman, M. J., van Echten-Arends, J., and Arts, E. G. (2010). Embryo quality and impact of specific embryo characteristics on ongoing implantation in unselected embryos derived from modified natural cycle in vitro fertilization. *Fertil. Steril.* 94, 527–534. doi: 10.1016/j.fertnstert.2009.03.076

Phillips, S. V., Yu, Y., Rossbach, A., Nomikos, M., Vassilakopoulou, V., Livaniou, E., et al. (2011). Divergent effect of mammalian PLCzeta in generating Ca(2)(+) oscillations in somatic cells compared with eggs. *Biochem. J.* 438, 545–553. doi: 10.1042/BJ20101581

Polanski, L. T., Baumgarten, M. N., Quenby, S., Brosens, J., Campbell, B. K., and Raine-Fenning, N. J. (2014). What exactly do we mean by 'recurrent implantation failure'? A systematic review and opinion. *Reprod. Biomed Online* 28, 409–423. doi: 10.1016/j.rbmo.2013.12.006

Puppo, A., Chun, J. T., Gragnaniello, G., Garante, E., and Santella, L. (2008). Alteration of the cortical actin cytoskeleton deregulates Ca2+ signaling, monospermic fertilization, and sperm entry. *PLoS One* 3:e3588. doi: 10.1371/journal.pone.0003588

Rinaudo, P., Pepperell, J. R., Buradgunta, S., Massobrio, M., and Keefe, D. L. (1997). Dissociation between intracellular calcium elevation and development of human oocytes treated with calcium ionophore. *Fertil. Steril.* 68, 1086–1092. doi: 10.1016/s0015-0282(97)00406-8

Santella, L., and Dale, B. (2015). Assisted yes, but where do we draw the line? *Reprod. Biomed Online* 31, 476–478. doi: 10.1016/j.rbmo.2015.06.013

Santella, L., Limatola, N., and Chun, J. T. (2015). Calcium and actin in the saga of awakening oocytes. *Biochem. Biophys. Res. Commun.* 460, 104–113. doi: 10.1016/j.bbrc.2015.03.028

Sanusi, R., Yu, Y., Nomikos, M., Lai, F. A., and Swann, K. (2015). Rescue of failed oocyte activation after ICSI in a mouse model of male factor infertility by recombinant phospholipase Czeta. *Mol. Hum. Reprod.* 21, 783–791. doi: 10.1093/molehr/gav042

Satouh, Y., and Ikawa, M. (2018). New insights into the molecular events of mammalian fertilization. *Trends Biochem. Sci.* 43, 818–828. doi: 10.1016/j.tibs.2018.08.006

Satouh, Y., Nozawa, K., and Ikawa, M. (2015). Sperm postacrosomal WW domain-binding protein is not required for mouse egg activation. *Biol. Reprod.* 93, 94. doi: 10.1095/biolreprod.115.131441

Saunders, C. M., Larman, M. G., Parrington, J., Cox, L. J., Royse, J., Blayney, L. M., et al. (2002). PLC zeta: a sperm-specific trigger of Ca(2+) oscillations in eggs and embryo development. *Development* 129, 3533–3544.

Saunders, C. M., Swann, K., and Lai, F. A. (2007). PLCzeta, a sperm-specific PLC and its potential role in fertilization. *Biochem. Soc. Symp.* 23-36. doi: 10.1042/BSS0740023

Sette, C., Paronetto, M. P., Barchi, M., Bevilacqua, A., Geremia, R., and Rossi, P. (2002). Tr-kit-induced resumption of the cell cycle in mouse eggs requires activation of a Src-like kinase. *EMBO J.* 21, 5386–5395. doi: 10.1093/emboj/cdf553

Stricker, S. A. (1999). Comparative biology of calcium signaling during fertilization and egg activation in animals. *Dev. Biol.* 211, 157–176. doi: 10.1006/dbio.1999.9340

Swann, K. (2018). The role of Ca(2+) in oocyte activation during in vitro fertilization: insights into potential therapies for rescuing failed fertilization. *Biochim. Biophys. Acta Mol. Cell Res.* 1865(11 Pt B), 1830–1837. doi: 10.1016/j.bbamcr.2018.05.003

Swann, K., and Ozil, J. P. (1994). Dynamics of the calcium signal that triggers mammalian egg activation. *Int. Rev. Cytol.* 152, 183–222. doi: 10.1016/s0074-7696(08)62557-7

Swann, K., Saunders, C. M., Rogers, N. T., and Lai, F. A. (2006). PLCzeta(zeta): a sperm protein that triggers Ca2+ oscillations and egg activation in mammals. *Semin. Cell Dev. Biol.* 17, 264–273. doi: 10.1016/j.semcdb.2006.03.009

Theodoridou, M., Nomikos, M., Parthimos, D., Gonzalez-Garcia, J. R., Elgmati, K., Calver, B. L., et al. (2013). Chimeras of sperm PLCzeta reveal disparate protein domain functions in the generation of intracellular Ca2+ oscillations in mammalian eggs at fertilization. *Mol. Hum. Reprod.* 19, 852–864. doi: 10.1093/molehr/gat070

Torra-Massana, M., Cornet-Bartolome, D., Barragan, M., Durban, M., Ferrer-Vaquer, A., Zambelli, F., et al. (2019). Novel phospholipase C zeta 1 mutations associated with fertilization failures after ICSI. *Hum. Reprod.* 34, 1494–1504. doi: 10.1093/humrep/dez094

van der Westerlaken, L., Helmerhorst, F., Dieben, S., and Naaktgeboren, N. (2005). Intracytoplasmic sperm injection as a treatment for unexplained total fertilization failure or low fertilization after conventional in vitro fertilization. *Fertil. Steril.* 83, 612–617. doi: 10.1016/j.fertnstert.2004.08.029

Wong, C. C., Loewke, K. E., Bossert, N. L., Behr, B., De Jonge, C. J., Baer, T. M., et al. (2010). Non-invasive imaging of human embryos before embryonic genome activation predicts development to the blastocyst stage. *Nat. Biotechnol.* 28, 1115–1121. doi: 10.1038/nbt.1686

Yamaguchi, T., Ito, M., Kuroda, K., Takeda, S., and Tanaka, A. (2017). The establishment of appropriate methods for egg-activation by human PLCZ1 RNA injection into human oocyte. *Cell Calcium.* 65, 22–30. doi: 10.1016/j.ceca.2017.03.002

Yelumalai, S., Yeste, M., Jones, C., Amdani, S. N., Kashir, J., Mounce, G., et al. (2015). Total levels, localization patterns, and proportions of sperm exhibiting phospholipase C zeta are significantly correlated with fertilization rates after intracytoplasmic sperm injection. *Fertil. Steril.* 104, 561.e4, 567.e4. doi: 10.1016/j.fertnstert.2015.05.018

Yeste, M., Jones, C., Amdani, S. N., Yelumalai, S., Mounce, G., da Silva, S. J., et al. (2016). Does advancing male age influence the expression levels and localisation patterns of phospholipase C zeta (PLCzeta) in human sperm? *Sci. Rep.* 6:27543. doi: 10.1038/srep27543

Yoneda, A., Kashima, M., Yoshida, S., Terada, K., Nakagawa, S., Sakamoto, A., et al. (2006). Molecular cloning, testicular postnatal expression, and oocyte-activating potential of porcine phospholipase Czeta. *Reproduction* 132, 393–401. doi: 10.1530/rep.1.01018

Yoon, S. Y., Eum, J. H., Lee, J. E., Lee, H. C., Kim, Y. S., Han, J. E., et al. (2012). Recombinant human phospholipase C zeta 1 induces intracellular calcium oscillations and oocyte activation in mouse and human oocytes. *Hum. Reprod.* 27, 1768–1780. doi: 10.1093/humrep/des092

Yoon, S. Y., Jellerette, T., Salicioni, A. M., Lee, H. C., Yoo, M. S., Coward, K., et al. (2008). Human sperm devoid of PLC, zeta 1 fail to induce Ca(2+) release and are unable to initiate the first step of embryo development. *J. Clin. Invest.* 118, 3671–3681. doi: 10.1172/JCI36942

Young, C., Grasa, P., Coward, K., Davis, L. C., and Parrington, J. (2009). Phospholipase C zeta undergoes dynamic changes in its pattern of localization in sperm during capacitation and the acrosome reaction. *Fertil. Steril.* 91 (5 Suppl.), 2230–2242. doi: 10.1016/j.fertnstert.2008.05.021

Yu, Y., Saunders, C. M., Lai, F. A., and Swann, K. (2008). Preimplantation development of mouse oocytes activated by different levels of human phospholipase C zeta. *Hum. Reprod.* 23, 365–373. doi: 10.1093/humrep/dem350

5

Determination of a Robust Assay for Human Sperm Membrane Potential Analysis

*Carolina Baro Graf[1,2], Carla Ritagliati[1], Cintia Stival[1], Paula A. Balestrini[3], Mariano G. Buffone[3] and Darío Krapf[1,2]**

[1] CONICET-UNR, Laboratoty of Cell Signal Transduction Networks, Instituto de Biología Molecular y Celular de Rosario, Rosario, Argentina, [2] UNR, Laboratorio de Medicina Reproductiva, Facultad de Ciencias Bioquímicas y Farmacéuticas, Rosario, Argentina, [3] Consejo Nacional de Investigaciones Científicas y Tecnológicas, Instituto de Biología y Medicina Experimental, Buenos Aires, Argentina

Correspondence:
Darío Krapf
krapf@ibr-conicet.gov.ar

Mammalian sperm must undergo a complex process called capacitation in order to fertilize the egg. During this process, hyperpolarization of the sperm plasma membrane has been mostly studied in mouse, and associated to its importance in the preparation to undergo the acrosome reaction (AR). However, despite the increasing evidence of membrane hyperpolarization in human sperm capacitation, no reliable techniques have been set up for its determination. In this report we describe human sperm membrane potential (*Em*) measurements by a fluorimetric population assay, establishing optimal conditions for *Em* determination. In addition, we have conducted parallel measurements of the same human sperm samples by flow cytometry and population fluorimetry, before and after capacitation, to conclusively address their reliability. This integrative analysis sets the basis for the study of *Em* in human sperm allowing future work aiming to understand its role in human sperm capacitation.

Keywords: membrane potential, population fluorimetry, sperm capacitation, human sperm, carbocyanine dye, diSC3(5)

INTRODUCTION

During fertilization, the sperm cell has a simple and fundamental goal: to merge with the oocyte and deliver its genetic material. However, mammalian sperm are not able to fertilize an oocyte shortly after ejaculation. To gain fertilizing competence, they must go through a process called sperm capacitation. Capacitation includes a complex series of molecular events that normally take place in the female genital tract but can be mimicked *in vitro* in defined media. This process prepares sperm to acquire hyperactivated motility (HA) and to undergo the acrosome reaction (AR) upon stimulation (Chang, 1951; Austin, 1952).

At the molecular level, sperm capacitation is associated with increased membrane fluidity, changes in intracellular ion concentrations (Visconti et al., 2011), hyperpolarization of the sperm plasma membrane (Zeng et al., 1995; Hernández-González et al., 2006), increased activity of protein kinase A (PKA) (Krapf et al., 2010), and protein tyrosine phosphorylation (Arcelay et al., 2008). Data regarding capacitation has been acquired in different mammalian species. Moreover, due to the complexity of the capacitation process, each of these events has been studied independently.

Thus, knowledge regarding how these events interconnect to regulate capacitation is mostly unavailable.

One important molecular process leading to the capacitated state is hyperpolarization of the sperm plasma potential, which has been mostly studied in mouse (Zeng et al., 1995; Hernández-González et al., 2006; De La Vega-Beltran et al., 2012). In this species, *Em* hyperpolarization has been shown to be both necessary and sufficient for sperm to undergo stimulated AR (De La Vega-Beltran et al., 2012). The mechanisms that drive *Em* hyperpolarization in mouse sperm involve the opening of the potassium channel Slo3 (Chávez et al., 2013), since sperm from Slo3 KO mice fail to hyperpolarize during capacitation. Most importantly, these sperm do not undergo acrosomal reaction upon stimulation (Santi et al., 2010; Yang et al., 2011), and, as expected from these data, Slo3 KO male mice are sterile. Despite the clear importance of membrane hyperpolarization during mouse sperm capacitation, this *Em* change has not been studied in detail in human sperm. A few reports have independently analyzed *Em* of sperm samples: while Linares-Hernández et al. (1998) reported an *Em* for non-capacitated sperm of around −40 mV, Patrat et al. (2005) reported that capacitated sperm exhibit an *Em* of about −58 mV. Both studies used fluorimetric population assays using the carbocyanine $DiSC_3(5)$. In addition, a qualitative study suggested by flow cytometry that human sperm undergo hyperpolarization during capacitation (Brewis et al., 2000). It is worth noticing that the consortium of Drs. Treviño and Darszon, further substantiated these qualitative findings, showing by flow cytometry that a subpopulation of human sperm hyperpolarizes during capacitation (López-González et al., 2014). However, these studies did not measure *Em* changes quantitatively on the same sample, i.e., during capacitation, which is crucial for proper human sperm analysis considering the biological variabilities found in these cells.

Despite the clear importance of hyperpolarization in mouse sperm cells, data regarding human sperm is scarce. Our manuscript presents an integrative study, since the same samples have been evaluated through flow cytometry analysis and population *Em* measurements, both before and after capacitation. We have established a solid reproducible methodology. Moreover, our data show that hyperpolarization is observed in human sperm along incubation in capacitating conditions, although alternative behaviors are also reported here. Finally, the methodology and implications of *Em* hyperpolarization in human sperm are herein discussed.

MATERIALS AND METHODS

Reagents

Chemicals were obtained from the following sources: bovine serum albumin (BSA) and HEPES were purchased from Sigma (St. Louis, MO, United States). Propidium iodide (PI) from Santa Cruz (Santa Cruz, CA, United States), 3,3-dipropylthiadicarbocyanine iodide [$DiSC_3(5)$] from Invitrogen (Carlsbad, United States). All other chemicals were of analytical grade.

Ethical Statement

The study protocol was approved by the Bioethics Committee of the Instituto de Biología y Medicina Experimental (CONICET). All subjects gave written informed consent in accordance with the Declaration of Helsinki.

Culture Media

HEPES-buffered human tubal fluid (HTF) was used throughout the study, containing (in mM) 4.7 KCl, 0.3 KH_2PO_2, 90.7 NaCl, 41.2 $MgSO_4$, 2.8 Glucose, 1.6 $CaCl_2$, 3.4 Sodium Piruvate, 60 Sodium Lactate, 23.8 HEPES, and was termed non-capacitating media. For capacitating media, 15 mM $NaHCO_3$, and 0.5% w/v BSA were added. In all cases, pH was adjusted to 7.4 with NaOH.

Human Sperm Preparation

Semen samples were obtained by masturbation from 10 healthy donors after 3–5 days of abstinence and analyzed following WHO recommendations (World Health Organization, 2010). All samples fulfilled semen parameters (total fluid volume, sperm concentration, motility, viability, and morphology) according to WHO normality criteria. Samples were allowed to liquefy for 1 h at 37°C in water bath. Then, sperm ejaculates were allowed to swim-up in non-capacitating HTF media (see above) at 37°C for 1 h. Motile selected spermatozoa were washed 5 min 400 × *g*. Conditions were performed in 400 μl of non-capacitating or capacitating media to a final cell concentration of 7×10^6 cells/ml for fluorimetric population assays and 1.25×10^6 cells/ml for flow cytometry measurements. Sperm were capacitated for 3 h at 37°C.

Determination of Membrane Potential by Flow Cytometry

Sperm plasma membrane potential (*Em*) was assessed using different concentrations of $DiSC_3(5)$ for 10 min, for proper determination of dye concentration. Unless specified, dye concentration was then of 50 nM. In addition, 2 μM of PI was added 30 s before collecting data to monitor viability. Data were recorded as individual cellular events using a BD FACSAria™ II cell sorter flow cytometer (BD Biosciences). Forward scatter (FSC) and side scatter (SSC) fluorescence data were collected from 20,000 events per sample. Debris and cell aggregates were excluded from analysis by gating side vs. FSC cytogram. Negative stain for PI was selected for living cells and positive cells for $DiSC_3(5)$ were detected using the filter for allophycocyanine (APC) (660/20). Normalization was performed by adding 1 μM valinomycin and 39.6 mM KCl. Data were analyzed using FACS Diva and FlowJo software (Tree Star 10.0.7r2).

Determination of Membrane Potential by Fluorimetric Population Assay

After incubation in each condition, human sperm, at a concentration of 3×10^6 sperm in 1.7 ml, were loaded with $DiSC_3(5)$ at different concentrations to determine the ideal dye concentration. Unless specified, dye concentration was determined at 1 μM (dissolved in DMSO at 5 mM). Sperm were transferred to a gently stirred cuvette at 37°C, and the fluorescence was monitored with a Varian Cary

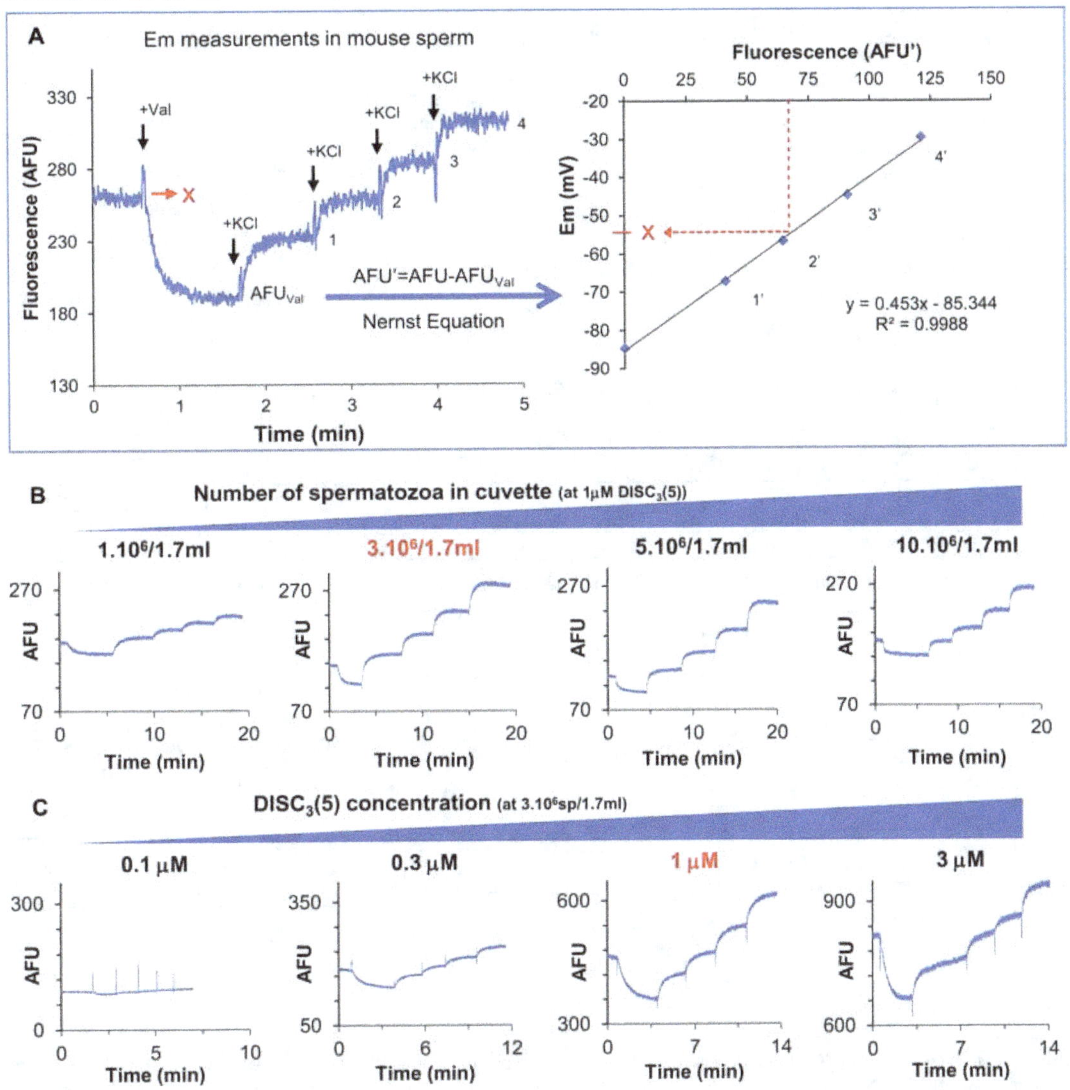

FIGURE 1 | Optimization of a population fluorimetry assay to determine human sperm membrane potential (*Em*). **(A)** *Em* measurement in mouse sperm. Left panel shows a representative trace, indicating valinomycin, and KCl additions. Right panel corresponds to the resulting calibration curve obtained after calculating *Em* for each fluorescence value using the Nernst equation. The initial fluorescence value is then interpolated to reach the resting membrane potential value. **(B)** Representative fluorescence traces using different human sperm concentrations at 1 μM $DiSC_3(5)$. Optimal number of sperm is indicated in red. **(C)** Representative fluorescence traces using different dye concentrations, at constant sperm number (3×10^6/1.7 ml). Optimal dye concentration is indicated in red.

Eclipse fluorescence spectrophotometer at 620/670 nm excitation/emission wavelengths. Recordings were initiated when steady-state fluorescence was reached (approximately 10 min). Calibration was performed by adding 1 μM valinomycin and sequential additions of KCl (in μL): 4, 4, 7, and 15 for calibration curve 1; 8, 13.34, 13.1, and 13.3 for calibration curve 2; 1.67, 3.4, 5.95, and 10.2 for calibration curve 3. Unless specified, calibration curve 1 was used. Final sperm membrane potentials were obtained by linearly interpolating the theoretical *Em* values against arbitrary fluorescence units of each trace. The theoretical *Em* values were obtained using Nernst equation, considering 120 mM the internal K^+ concentration in sperm. This internal calibration for each determination compensates for variables that influence the absolute fluorescence values.

Statistical Analysis

One-way repeated measures analysis of variance was used to compare between *Em* values obtained with different calibration curves. Statistical significances are indicated in the figure legends.

RESULTS

Em Measurement in Human Sperm

Em measurements were performed with a positively charged carbocyanine probe, $DiSC_3(5)$. This dye partitions into sperm cells according to their membrane potential but independently on the nature of ionic fluxes, rendering it suitable for potential measurements of the plasma membrane. The technique has

A

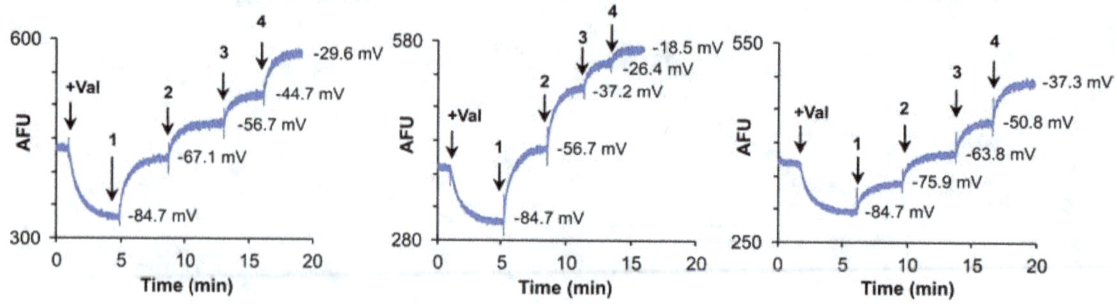

↓	KCl 2M (µL)	External K⁺ (mM)	Em (mV)
Val	0	5.04	-84.7
1	4	9.72	-67.1
2	4	14.38	-56.7
3	7	22.49	-44.7
4	15	39.63	-29.6

Obtained value: -63.5 mV

↓	KCl 2M (µL)	External K⁺ (mM)	Em (mV)
Val	0	5.04	-84.7
1	8.00	14.38	-56.7
2	13.34	29.77	-37.2
3	13.10	44.66	-26.4
4	13.30	59.95	-18.5

Obtained value: -64.5 mV

↓	KCl 2M (µL)	External K⁺ (mM)	Em (mV)
Val	0	5.04	-84.7
1	1.67	7.01	-75.9
2	3.40	10.99	-63.8
3	5.95	17.90	-50.8
4	10.20	29.65	-37.3

Obtained value: -66.9 mV

B

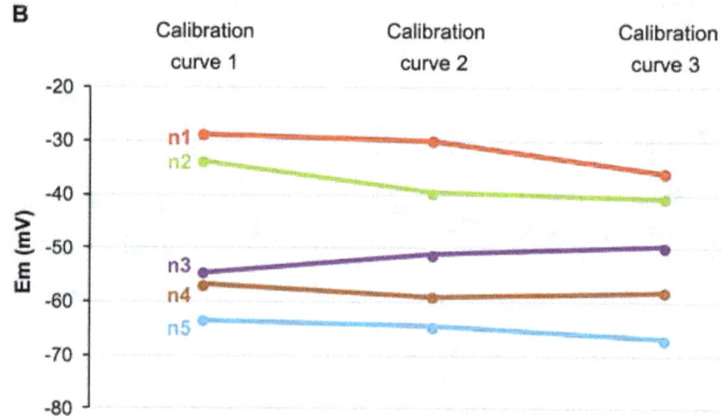

Obtained values (mV)

Curve 1	Curve 2	Curve 3
-28.9	-30.1	-35.9
-33.8	-39.6	-40.7
-54.5	-51.2	-49.7
-56.9	-59.1	-58.1
-63.5	-64.5	-66.9

FIGURE 2 | Calibration of *Em* measurements. **(A)** Upper panels show fluorescence traces for each calibration curve tested (1–3), indicating *Em* values after sequential KCl additions. Lower panels show KCl volume added, external K^+ concentration and *Em* obtained for each addition. Finally, the resting membrane potential of each measurement is indicated. **(B)** Membrane potential values obtained after testing the described calibration curves in five different samples. No significant differences were observed, $p > 0.05$.

long been used in mouse sperm, in a robust and reproducible way, as shown in **Figure 1A** (Chou et al., 1989; Zeng et al., 1995; Demarco et al., 2003). The dye is added to the sperm suspension, where it partitions into the cells originating a decrease in fluorescence due to accumulation of the dye in the lipid bilayer of the cells, in a less-fluorescent form (Plášek and Hrouda, 1991). *Em* hyperpolarization favors the influx of more dye to the cell, resulting in decreased extracellular fluorescence. Once the dye gives a stable signal, reached after a 10 min incubation in the sperm suspension, calibration starts by adding valinomycin (a K^+ ionophore) followed by sequential additions of KCl, increasing extracellular K^+ concentration to different known values. The original resting potential can be obtained following the Nernst equation, provided that the membrane behaves as a K^+ electrode where the internal K^+ concentration is 120 mM (Darszon et al., 1999; **Figures 1A,B**).

At appropriate concentrations of sperm and probe, this method provides a highly reproducible value of plasma membrane potential. In order to analyze optimal conditions for human sperm, both sperm and probe concentrations were assayed. When the probe was fixed at 1 µM, shifting sperm cell number from 1×10^6 to 1×10^7 (in a cuvette containing 1.7 ml) gave different responses. The best dynamic range was observed when 3×10^6 sperm were used (1.76×10^6 sperm/ml) (**Figure 1C**). Once the optimal sperm number was determined, different $DiSC_3(5)$ concentrations were tested. As seen in **Figure 1C**, no other concentration improved signal to noise ratio when compared to 1 µM $DiSC_3(5)$. Accordingly, 1 µM dye and 3×10^6 sperm/1.7 ml where taken as optimal conditions for the subsequent analysis of human sperm *Em*. Even though $DiSC_3(5)$ bears a short alkyl group that renders it poorly hydrophobic, migration to the mitochondria cannot be totally

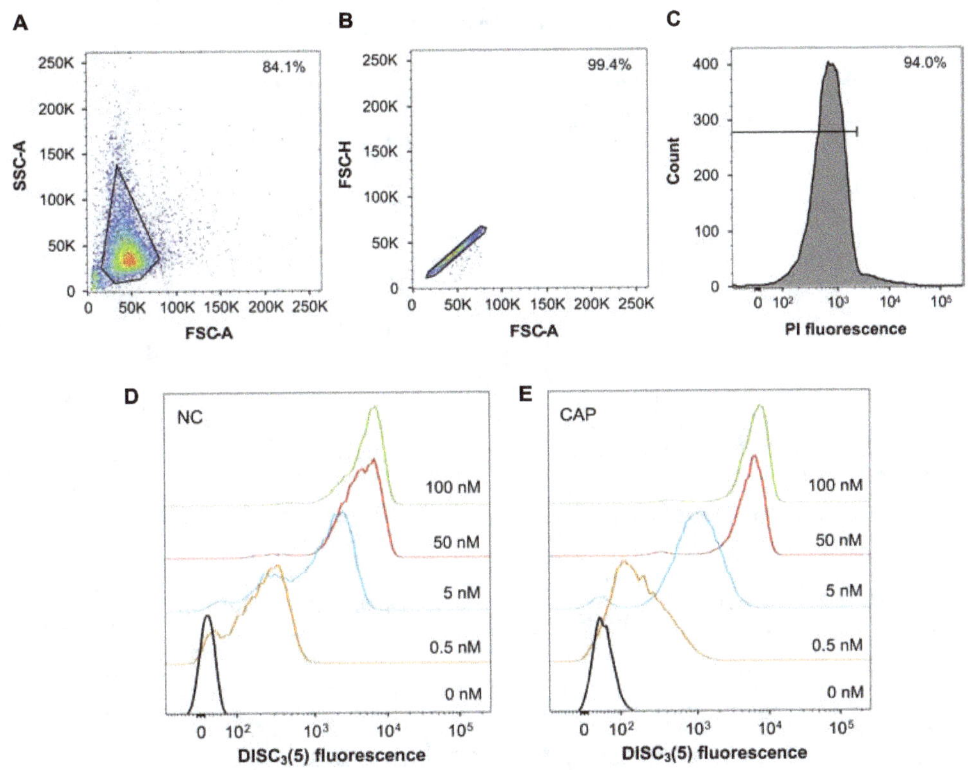

FIGURE 3 | Optimization of a flow cytometry assay to determine human sperm membrane potential. **(A)** Dot plot of side (SSC-A) vs. forward (FSC-A) scatter for each sample. Region of interest to eliminate cellular debris is shown. **(B)** The forward scatter height (FSC-H) vs. forward scatter area (FSC-A) profile was used to exclude cell aggregates and large cells from the analysis. **(C)** Histogram of PI fluorescence where live cells (low stain) were selected. **(D)** Human sperm were incubated with different dye concentrations in non-capacitating (left panel) and **(E)** capacitating conditions (right panel) by flow cytometry to determine optimal loading conditions.

excluded, which would originate minor contributions to the observed *Em*. However, as showed in **Supplementary Figure 1**, the mitochondrial electron transport inhibitor rotenone did not affect DiSC$_3$(5) signal. Thus, *Em* measurements of both non capacitated and capacitated sperm were unaffected by mitochondrial dysfunction, further substatntiating that mitochondrial contribution is negligible.

Calibration of *Em* Measurements

In order to avoid errors due to dye loading or sperm concentration differences, every measurement carries an internal calibration curve after fluorescence stabilization (Ritagliati et al., 2018). As shown in **Figure 2A**, calibration was performed by adding 1 μM valinomycin and sequential additions of KCl. Initial potassium concentration equals 5.04 mM KCl; then, additions of a 2 M KCl solution, sequentially rose KCl concentration to 9.72, 14.38, 22.49, and 39.63 mM, corresponding to *Em* of −84.7, −67.1, −56.7, −44.7, and −29.6 mV, respectively. With the aim of assessing the strength of this method applied to human sperm samples, three different calibration curves were performed (**Figure 2A**, curves 1-3), varying the concentration of KCl added. In the examples shown in **Figure 2A**, the resting membrane potentials were of −63.5, −64.5, and −66.9 mV for calibration curves 1-3, respectively. This procedure was performed on 5 different sperm samples. As shown in **Figure 2B**, the technique showed no significant variations among different calibration curves, supporting the strength of the methodology.

Comparative Analysis Between Flow Cytometry and Fluorometric Population Assays

Up to now, the few studies that have reported *Em* measurements in human sperm have mostly used flow cytometry, while only a couple of them have used the fluorescent population assay, in either capacitated or non-capacitated sperm. However, quantitative measurements of *Em* during capacitation is clearly missing. Thus, we decided to analyze human sperm *Em* during capacitation, using both flow cytometry and population fluorimetry approaches.

Firstly, in order to establish appropriate working conditions, sperm were loaded with 50 nM DiSC$_3$(5) and run on a flow cytometer. A plot of cell complexity (SSC-A) vs. cell size (FSC-A) is shown in **Figure 3A**, detailing the gating used to eliminate cell debris and aggregates. The selection of individual cells was confirmed using the FSC-H vs. FSC-A plot (**Figure 3B**). Live cells were selected after co-staining sperm with PI, normally obtaining a cellular viability >90% (**Figure 3C**). This representative set up was performed after loading cells with

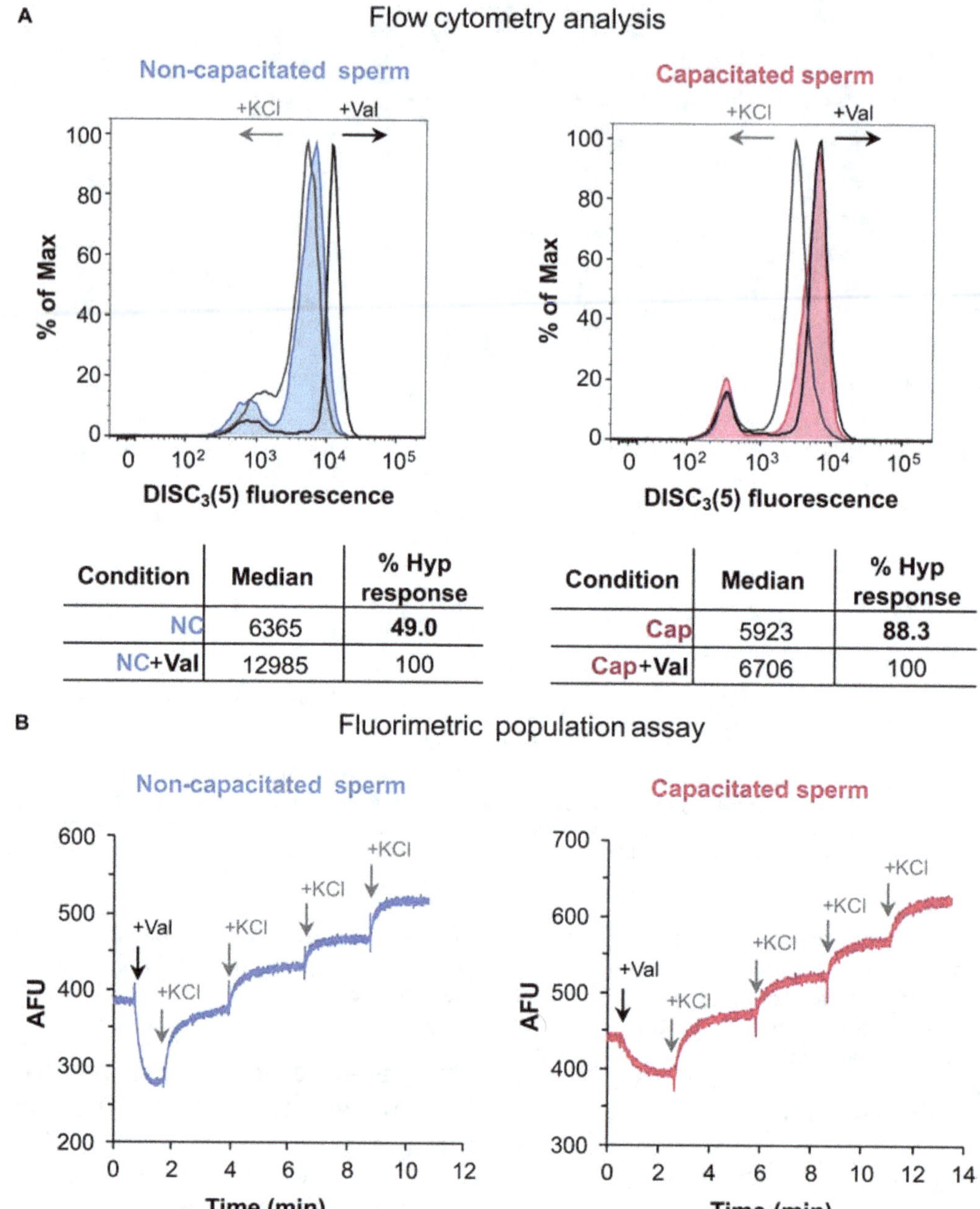

Condition	Median	% Hyp response
NC	6365	**49.0**
NC+**Val**	12985	100

Condition	Median	% Hyp response
Cap	5923	**88.3**
Cap+**Val**	6706	100

Condition	AFU	Em (mV)
NC	385.8	**-63.1**
NC+**Val**	278.8	-84.7

Condition	AFU	Em (mV)
Cap	398.2	**-74.5**
Cap+**Val**	471.6	-84.7

FIGURE 4 | Human sperm membrane potential determination by flow cytometry and population fluorimetry. **(A)** Flow cytometry analysis of human sperm in non-capacitating (left panel) and capacitating conditions (right panel). Valinomycin addition causes an increase of fluorescence, in accordance to a hyperpolarized state; KCl addition causes a decrease of fluorescence, as expected for a depolarized state. Each histogram plots percentage of maximum (% of Max) vs. DiSC3(5) fluorescence, obtained by normalizing to the peak height at the mode of the distribution – so the maximum *Y*-axis value in the absolute-count histogram becomes 100% of total. Lower panel shows median values obtained before and after valinomycin addition. Hyperpolarization response is normalized against valinomycin addition. **(B)** Population fluorimetric assay of human sperm in non-capacitating (left panel) and capacitating conditions (right panel). In this case valinomycin addition causes a decrease in fluorescence, as expected for a hyperpolarized state; KCl sequential additions increase extracellular fluorescence, depolarizing the sample. Lower panel shows fluorescence values for initial and hyperpolarized states, with their corresponding membrane potential value (in mV). These results are representative of one experiment (*n* = 5).

different $DiSC_3(5)$ concentrations (0.5–100 nM), for both non-capacitated (**Figure 3D**) and capacitated sperm (**Figure 3E**). From these data, 50 nM $DiSC_3(5)$ resulted the concentration of choice, being the lowest concentration tested with highest intracellular fluorescence. Final cell concentration was fixed to 1.25×10^6 sperm/ml.

Secondly, these conditions were used to analyze *Em* by flow cytometry, as shown in **Figure 4A**. In flow cytometry using $DiSC_3(5)$ (a cationic dye), increased fluorescence correlates to *Em* hyperpolarization since more dye enters the cell. Addition of valinomycin further increases fluorescence, as the sperm cells hyperpolarize (**Figure 4A**). Subsequent addition of KCl caused the expected depolarization of the sperm cells, rendering lower values of fluorescence. When a capacitated sperm sample was analyzed, valinomycin only caused a slight increase in fluorescence (**Figure 4A**). However, KCl highly depolarized these hyperpolarized cells. Thus, it could be inferred from these data, that this sample suffered hyperpolarization during capacitation.

In order to compare *Em* measurements of two samples by flow cytometry, the median fluorescence was obtained after valinomycin addition, corresponding to the maximum hyperpolarization state. The median value from the initial state (before valinomycin addition) of each sample can then be used to calculate a normalized degree of hyperpolarization (**Figure 4A**). Accordingly, in non-capacitating conditions the hyperpolarization degree was 49% shifting to 88.3% in capacitating conditions. This normalization is necessary not only for a semi-quantitative analysis, but also when performing a qualitative comparison between conditions (i.e., NC and CAP), since dye concentrations could differ among them.

When the same sperm sample incubated under either non-capacitating or capacitating conditions were analyzed by fluorimetry, values of −63.1 and −74.5 mV were obtained, supporting the data obtained by flow cytometry (**Figure 4B**). It is worth noticing that occasionally, approximately 10% of samples, exhibited unexpected behaviors when analyzed by flow cytometry: upon addition of valinomycin, instead of causing hyperpolarization, a shift to a depolarized state was observed (**Supplementary Figure 2**). When these samples were analyzed by fluorimetry, it was observed that, as expected, valinomycin caused an initial hyperpolarization that is, however, immediately followed by a sustained depolarization (**Supplementary Figure 2**). This result indicates that what was observed as a valinomycin-triggered depolarization, was in fact a later compensation by still unknown ion fluxes, and further supporting the strength of fluorimetric measurements.

DISCUSSION

In mouse sperm, changes in the sperm plasma membrane potential (*Em*) associated with sperm capacitation have been studied for more than 20 years (Zeng et al., 1995). Cauda epidydimal mouse sperm have a depolarized *Em* of ∼ −40 mV, which hyperpolarizes to ∼ −60 mV when capacitation takes place reviewed by Stival et al. (2016). These values of mouse sperm *Em* have been conducted using fluorimetric measurements and constitute an average value of a population known to be far from homogenous. Thus, when other techniques as single cell microscopy (Arnoult et al., 1999) or flow cytometry (López-González et al., 2014; Escoffier et al., 2015) were used, two clear sperm sub-populations displaying different *Em* were observed. One of these sub-populations remains at a depolarized state, while the other shifts to a relatively hyperpolarized value of *Em* (∼ −80 mV) (Arnoult et al., 1999). These findings are consistent with the observation that only a fraction of the sperm cells are capable to undergo the AR (Salicioni et al., 2007).

In human sperm, it has been recently proposed that certain *Em* shift is associated with normal sperm function, as assessed by electrophysiology and IVF outcome (Brown et al., 2016). However, this study involved laborious techniques that hampered the analysis of many cells per patient. Other studies involved the qualitative analysis of *Em* in human sperm by flow cytometry (Brewis et al., 2000) and analysis of either non-capacitated or capacitated sperm by fluorimetry (Linares-Hernández et al., 1998; Patrat et al., 2005). Considering the importance of the study of *Em* in human sperm using straightforward techniques, we aimed to standardize a reliable method for the analysis of *Em* during human sperm capacitation.

We have satisfactorily established the optimal conditions to quantitatively measure human sperm *Em* using the carbocyanine $DiSC_3(5)$ with a fluorimeter in a population assay. But most importantly, we have compared two different methods, i.e., flow cytometry and population fluorimetry, by using the same sperm sample. Our data indicate that *Em* analysis by flow cytometry is a robust and reproducible methodology, when proper normalization for loading control is performed. However, it is important to highlight results that, although very reproducible, are to date difficult to understand. After addition of valinomycin, some samples experience an initial hyperpolarization that is followed by a depolarization. These behaviors are easily followed by fluorimetry, and can then be analyzed accordingly. However, when cytometry is used, due to technical time limitations, depolarization is observed instead of the expected valinomycin driven hyperpolarization. Thus, even though both techniques give the same end point result, cytometry might omit this particular behavior, and give a confusing result.

The mechanisms that regulate the hyperpolarization of human sperm plasma membrane during capacitation are poorly understood. Plasma membrane permeability to the ionic media at any given time defines the cell *Em*. Thus, *Em* changes during capacitation reflect changes of ion permeability. The most relevant ions are Na^+, K^+, and Cl^-, which have an equilibrium potential of +40, −80, and −40 mV, respectively. Considering these ion's equilibrium, closure of Na^+ transport as well as opening of a K^+ channel could drive hyperpolarization. In mouse, the current knowledge points toward a high contribution of K^+ to this phenomenon. However, the situation is far from clear in human sperm. Re-depolarization might in turn be associated to opening of Na^+ channels and/or Cl^- channels, shifting the equilibrium to more positive values. The methodology herein described is ideal for standardizing a technique that could aid in the study of human *Em* physiology.

ETHICS STATEMENT

The study protocol was approved by the Bioethics Committee of the Instituto de Biologa y Medicina Experimental (CONICET). All subjects gave written informed consent in accordance with the Declaration of Helsinki.

AUTHOR CONTRIBUTIONS

CBG, CR, CS, and PB conducted the experiments. All authors analyzed the data and revised final version of the manuscript. CBG, CR, MGB, and DK conceived the study. CBG, CR, and DK wrote the manuscript.

FUNDING

This work was supported by grants from the Agencia Nacional de Promoción Científica y Tecnológica de Argentina, PICT 2015-2294 (awarded to MGB), and PICT 2015-3164 and PICT 2017-3217 (awarded to DK). CBG is recipient of a scholarship from the National Research Council of Argentina.

REFERENCES

Arcelay, E., Salicioni, A. M., Wertheimer, E., and Visconti, P. E. (2008). Identification of proteins undergoing tyrosine phosphorylation during mouse sperm capacitation. *Int. J. Dev. Biol.* 52, 463–472. doi: 10.1387/ijdb.072555ea

Arnoult, C., Kazam, I. G., Visconti, P. E., Kopf, G. S., Villaz, M., and Florman, H. M. (1999). Control of the low voltage-activated calcium channel of mouse sperm by egg ZP3 and by membrane hyperpolarization during capacitation. *Proc. Natl. Acad. Sci. U.S.A.* 96, 6757–6762. doi: 10.1073/pnas.96.12.6757

Austin, C. R. (1952). The capacitation of the mammalian sperm. *Nature* 170:326. doi: 10.1038/170326a0

Brewis, I. A., Morton, I. E., Mohammad, S. N., Browes, C. E., and Moore, H. D. (2000). Measurement of intracellular calcium concentration and plasma membrane potential in human spermatozoa using flow cytometry. *J. Androl.* 21, 238–249. doi: 10.1002/j.1939-4640.2000.tb02101.x

Brown, S. G., Publicover, S. J., Mansell, S. A., Lishko, P. V., Williams, H. L., Ramalingam, M., et al. (2016). Depolarization of sperm membrane potential is a common feature of men with subfertility and is associated with low fertilization rate at IVF. *Hum. Reprod.* 31, 1147–1157. doi: 10.1093/humrep/dew056

Chang, M. (1951). Fertilizing capacity of spermatozoa deposited into the fallopian tubes. *Nat. Rev. Mol. Cell Biol.* 168, 697–698. doi: 10.1038/168697b0

Chávez, J. C., de la Vega-Beltrán, J. L., Escoffier, J., Visconti, P. E., Treviño, C. L., Darszon, A., et al. (2013). Ion permeabilities in mouse sperm reveal an external trigger for SLO3-Dependent hyperpolarization. *PLoS One* 8:e60578. doi: 10.1371/journal.pone.0060578

Chou, K., Chen, J., Yuan, S., and Haug, A. (1989). The membrane potential changes polarity during capacitation of murine epididymal sperm. *Biochem. Biophys. Res. Commun.* 165, 58–64. doi: 10.1016/0006-291X(89)91033-4

Darszon, A., Labarca, P., Nishigaki, T., and Espinosa, F. (1999). Ion channels in sperm physiology. *Physiol. Rev.* 79, 481–510. doi: 10.1111/j.1469-7998.2006.00165.x

De La Vega-Beltran, J. L., Sánchez-Cárdenas, C., Krapf, D., Hernandez-González, E. O., Wertheimer, E., Treviño, C. L., et al. (2012). Mouse sperm membrane potential hyperpolarization is necessary and sufficient to prepare sperm for the acrosome reaction. *J. Biol. Chem.* 287, 44384–44393. doi: 10.1074/jbc.M112.393488

Demarco, I. A., Espinosa, F., Edwards, J., Sosnik, J., De la Vega-Beltrán, L., Hockensmith, J. W., et al. (2003). Involvement of a Na+/HCO3- cotransporter in mouse sperm capacitation. *J. Biol. Chem.* 278, 7001–7009. doi: 10.1074/jbc.M206284200

Escoffier, J., Navarrete, F., Haddad, D., Santi, C. M., Darszon, A., and Visconti, P. E. (2015). Flow cytometry analysis reveals that only a subpopulation of mouse sperm undergoes hyperpolarization during capacitation. *Biol. Reprod.* 92:121. doi: 10.1095/biolreprod.114.127266

Hernández-González, E. O., Sosnik, J., Edwards, J., Acevedo, J. J., Mendoza-Lujambio, I., López-González, I., et al. (2006). Sodium and epithelial sodium channels participate in the regulation of the capacitation-associated hyperpolarization in mouse sperm. *J. Biol. Chem.* 281, 5623–5633. doi: 10.1074/jbc.M508172200

Krapf, D., Arcelay, E., Wertheimer, E. V., Sanjay, A., Pilder, S. H., Salicioni, A. M., et al. (2010). Inhibition of ser/Thr phosphatases induces capacitation-associated signaling in the presence of Src kinase inhibitors. *J. Biol. Chem.* 285, 7977–7985. doi: 10.1074/jbc.M109.085845

Linares-Hernández, L., Guzmán-Grenfell, A. M., Hicks-Gomez, J. J., and González-Martínez, M. T. (1998). Voltage-dependent calcium influx in human sperm assessed by simultaneous optical detection of intracellular calcium and membrane potential. *Biochim. Biophys. Acta* 372, 1–12. doi: 10.1016/S0005-2736(98)00035-2

López-González, I., Torres-Rodríguez, P., Sánchez-Carranza, O., Solís-López, A., Santi, C. M., Darszon, A., et al. (2014). Membrane hyperpolarization during human sperm capacitation. *Mol. Hum. Reprod.* 20, 619–629. doi: 10.1093/molehr/gau029

Patrat, C., Serres, C., and Jouannet, P. (2005). Progesterone induces hyperpolarization after a transient depolarization phase in human spermatozoa1. *Biol. Reprod.* 66, 1775–1780. doi: 10.1095/biolreprod66.6.1775

Plášek, J., and Hrouda, V. (1991). Assessment of membrane potential changes using the carbocyanine dye, diS-C3-(5): synchronous excitation spectroscopy studies. *Eur. Biophys. J.* 19, 183–188. doi: 10.1007/BF00196344

Ritagliati, C., Baro Graf, C., Stival, C., and Krapf, D. (2018). Regulation mechanisms and implications of sperm membrane hyperpolarization. *Mech. Dev.* 154, 33–43. doi: 10.1016/j.mod.2018.04.004

Salicioni, A. M., Platt, M. D., Wertheimer, E. V., Arcelay, E., Allaire, A., Sosnik, J., et al. (2007). Signalling pathways involved in sperm capacitation. *Soc. Reprod. Fertil. Suppl.* 65, 245–259.

Santi, C. M., Martínez-López, P., de la Vega-Beltrán, J. L., Butler, A., Alisio, A., Darszon, A., et al. (2010). The SLO3 sperm-specific potassium channel plays a vital role in male fertility. *FEBS Lett.* 584, 1041–1046. doi: 10.1016/j.febslet.2010.02.005

Stival, C., Puga Molina, L. D. C., Paudel, B., Buffone, M. G., Visconti, P. E., and Krapf, D. (2016). Sperm capacitation and acrosome reaction in mammalian sperm. *Adv. Anat. Embryol. Cell Biol.* 220, 93–106. doi: 10.1007/978-3-319-30567-7-5

Visconti, P. E., Krapf, D., de la Vega-Beltrán, J. L., Acevedo, J. J., and Darszon, A. (2011). Ion channels, phosphorylation and mammalian sperm capacitation. *Asian J. Androl.* 13, 395–405. doi: 10.1038/aja.2010.69

World Health Organization (2010). *WHO Laboratory Manual for The Examination and Processing Of Human Semen.* Geneva: World Health Organisation.

Yang, C., Zeng, X.-H., Kim, S. T., Lingle, C. J., and Xia, X.-M. (2011). Deletion of the Slo3 gene abolishes alkalization-activated K+ current in mouse spermatozoa. *Proc. Natl. Acad. Sci. U.S.A.* 108, 5879–5884. doi: 10.1073/pnas.1100240108

Zeng, Y., Clark, E. N., and Florman, H. M. (1995). Sperm membrane potential: hyperpolarization during capacitation regulates zona pellucida-dependent acrosomal secretion. *Dev. Biol.* 171, 554–563. doi: 10.1006/dbio.1995.1304

6

Mechanism of Acrosome Biogenesis in Mammals

Muhammad Babar Khawar[1,2], *Hui Gao*[1] *and Wei Li*[1,2*]

[1] *State Key Laboratory of Stem Cell and Reproductive Biology, Institute of Zoology, Chinese Academy of Sciences, Beijing, China,*

[2] *University of Chinese Academy of Sciences, Beijing, China*

***Correspondence:**
Wei Li
leways@ioz.ac.cn

During sexual reproduction, two haploid gametes fuse to form the zygote, and the acrosome is essential to this fusion process (fertilization) in animals. The acrosome is a special kind of organelle with a cap-like structure that covers the anterior portion of the head of the spermatozoon. The acrosome is derived from the Golgi apparatus and contains digestive enzymes. With the progress of our understanding of acrosome biogenesis, a number of models have been proposed to address the origin of the acrosome. The acrosome has been regarded as a lysosome-related organelle, and it has been proposed to have originated from the lysosome or the autolysosome. Our review will provide a brief historical overview and highlight recent findings on acrosome biogenesis in mammals.

Keywords: acrosome biogenesis, autolysosome, lysosomes, globozoospermia, spermiogenesis

INTRODUCTION

Sexual reproduction requires the fusion of two gametes in a critical multistep process termed fertilization. To ensure the success of fertilization, each step needs to proceed in a very precise manner. One of the key steps that ensures successful fertilization is acrosome reaction (AR). Sperm-egg fusion is a carbohydrate-dependent event that takes place via interaction between several glycan-binding molecules (receptors) present on the sperm plasma membrane with their corresponding glycans (ligands) localized to the zona pellucida (oocyte) (Yanagimachi, 1994; Tulsiani et al., 1997; Shur, 1998; Töpfer-Petersen, 1999; Wassarman, 1999). This irreversible interaction of the gametes leads to a calcium-mediated signal transduction cascade of events that results in the release of the acrosomal contents via exocytosis, which is termed AR. Several hydrolytic and proteolytic acrosomal enzymes are released in order to facilitate sperm fusion with the oocyte (Ikawa et al., 2010). Any structural or functional acrosomal abnormality could impair sperm fusion, and ultimately result in infertility. Moreover, studies have shown that intra-cytoplasmic insemination with sperm containing acrosomal abnormalities did not lead to successful fertilization, even in the absence of fertilization barriers, because the oocyte was unable to be efficiently activated (Nasr-Esfahani et al., 2008, 2010a,b). Only intracytoplasmic sperm injection (ICSI) followed by assisted oocyte activation with calcium ionophore was found to achieve high live birth-rates (Shang et al., 2019). Thus, the acrosome is indispensable for fertilization.

Acrosome biogenesis in mammals is accompanied with spermatid differentiation during spermiogenesis, which is characterized by the transformation of a spermatid into a spermatozoon. The process continues throughout the reproductive lifespan of the male. Although the acrosome morphology varies from species to species, two basic parts make up the acrosome in all mammals: (1) a large anterior part that varies in shape (paddle, hook, and spatula-like) and in size (Bedford, 2014) and (2) an equatorial segment (ES), which is the smaller and thinner part of the acrosome found in the middle of the sperm head. The acrosomal contents are enclosed in a single membrane that is generally divided into an outer acrosomal membrane (OAM) and an inner acrosomal membrane (IAM). The OAM lies immediately beneath the plasma membrane of the spermatid and both of these membranes fuse at the time of AR (Yanagimachi, 2011). The IAM lies above the nuclear envelope as a cap and does not fuse during AR. The luminal contents are heterogeneous and are usually categorized as soluble and particulate material. The soluble material is comprised of hydrolytic enzymes that take part in AR and help to disperse the oocyte coverings. The particulate material is the acrosomal matrix that facilitates the sperm-oocyte interaction during fertilization by providing a stable protein scaffold (Buffone et al., 2004; Suryavathi et al., 2015).

Researchers have characterized the process of spermiogenesis in mice, and they have identified 16 steps, with acrosome biogenesis being a key event. Acrosome biogenesis is classically divided into four major phases: Golgi (1–3 steps), cap (4–7 steps), acrosome (elongation) (8–12 steps), and maturation (final) phases (13–16 steps) (**Figure 1**). This four-phase division of acrosome biogenesis was proposed more than half-a-century ago, based mainly on light microscopic analysis of testicular sections stained with periodic acid–Schiff (PAS) (Clermont and Leblond, 1955).

The 1st phase is called the Golgi phase because the Golgi apparatus is an essential organelle that supports early spermiogenesis (Leblond and Clermont, 1952; Hess, 1990; Russell et al., 1993). During the 1st phase, the Golgi apparatus is very active in producing several glycoproteins, and the trans-Golgi network gives rise to several small proacrosomal vesicles that are required for the formation of a mature acrosome. These proacrosomal granules fuse to form a large solitary acrosomal granule near the concave region of the nuclear surface. The central part of the acrosomal granule is bound to the nuclear envelope while the peripheral part is associated with the perinuclear theca (**BOX 1**; **Figure 2**). In the 2nd (Cap) phase, the acrosomal granule becomes enlarged with glycoprotein-rich contents. Moreover, it begins to flatten upon touching the nuclear envelope, and spreads over the nucleus to form a cap. At the same time, the Golgi complex moves to the nascent neck region located in the distal end. The acrosomal granule gradually covers 1/3 of the nuclear surface and spreads, transforming into a very thin layer (**Figure 1**). Near the distal end of the developing acrosome, the "acroplaxome" can be found, which is an important structure that supports spermiogenesis. It consists of a marginal ring, which consists of an acrosomal plate that is made up of keratin and F-actin (**BOX 1**; **Figure 2**). At the time of elongation of the spermatid head, the marginal ring is associated with the growing edge of the acrosome and the nuclear surface (nuclear plate). Thus, acroplaxome not only binds the acrosome with the nucleus but also ensures the developing acrosomal cap remains anchored to the nuclear envelope undergoing elongation (Kierszenbaum et al., 2003). In the 3rd (acrosomal) phase, the acrosomal system begins to migrate over the ventral surface of the elongating spermatid nucleus and this migration ends in step 14 spermatid (**BOX 1**; **Figure 1**; Hess and de Franca, 2008). At this stage, the acrosome undergoes condensation and attaches itself to the IAM, while chromatin also undergoes intense condensation. Several cytoskeletal proteins including calmodulin (Camatini et al., 1992), actin (Talbot and Kleve, 1978), and α-spectrin-like antigens (Virtanen et al., 1984), play very important roles in the acrosomal organization. The elongating spermatids show initiation of manchette microtubule formation near the nuclear ring region (perinuclear ring), thinning of the cytoplasm and a gradual orientation of the acrosome toward the overlying plasma membrane (**BOX 1**; **Figure 2**). The 4th (maturation) phase involves a few changes in nuclear morphology and acrosomal migration. Condensation of the nucleus continues and acrosomal granule spreads over the entire acrosomal membrane and the acrosome differentiates into anterior and posterior regions. The anterior portion becomes the acrosome apex, while the rest of the acrosome covers nearly all the nuclear surface, except the part attached to the sperm tail (Russell et al., 1993). Moreover, excess cytoplasm, cytoplasmic components (lipids) and multiple unwanted organelles including mitochondria, vesicles, and ribosomes are disposed of in the form of cytoplasmic droplets prior to spermiation (**Figure 1**; Hess et al., 1993; Russell et al., 1993; De Franca et al., 1995). The resulting residual bodies released from spermatids are taken up and digested by Sertoli cells. Although, the morphogenetic process of the acrosome is well studied, the precise molecular mechanism of sperm acrosome biogenesis is not yet fully understood. Here, we describe the most recent progress that has been made in understanding the molecular mechanism underlying acrosome biogenesis.

THE MOLECULAR MECHANISM UNDERLYING ACROSOME BIOGENESIS

Several ER and Golgi-associated proteins actively participate in acrosome biogenesis. The endoplasmic reticulum (ER) is the main site of protein synthesis and folding (Vitale et al., 1993), while the Golgi apparatus directs glycosylation, processing, and sorting of newly synthesized proteins by the ER. The biosynthesis of some acrosome-specific proteins, such as acrosin, starts during the meiotic pachytene stage and continues as round spermatids enter the elongation stage (Anakwe and Gerton, 1990; Kashiwabara et al., 1990; Escalier et al., 1991). These proteins then enter the exocytic route and are transported to their respective targeted area in the form of proacrosomal granules that originate from the Golgi apparatus. The presence of these proacrosomal granules in the pachytene stage has been confirmed by numerous studies (Nicander and Ploen, 1969; Fawcett, 1975; Anakwe and Gerton, 1990; Suarezquian et al., 1991; Ramalho-Santos et al., 2002). Moreover, the presence of several ER-associated proteins such as protein O-mannosyltransferase 1 (POMT1) (Prados et al., 2007), POMT2 (Willer et al., 2002) and Calreticulin (Nakamura et al., 1993), have also been detected in the acrosome. Another ER-associated protein that has been detected in mouse testes is HSP90B1 (gp96/Grp94; glucose-related protein 94) (Asquith et al., 2005; Yang and Li, 2005). Germ cell-specific *Hsp90b1* knockout resulted in spermatozoa characterized by globular/abnormal heads, similar to those in

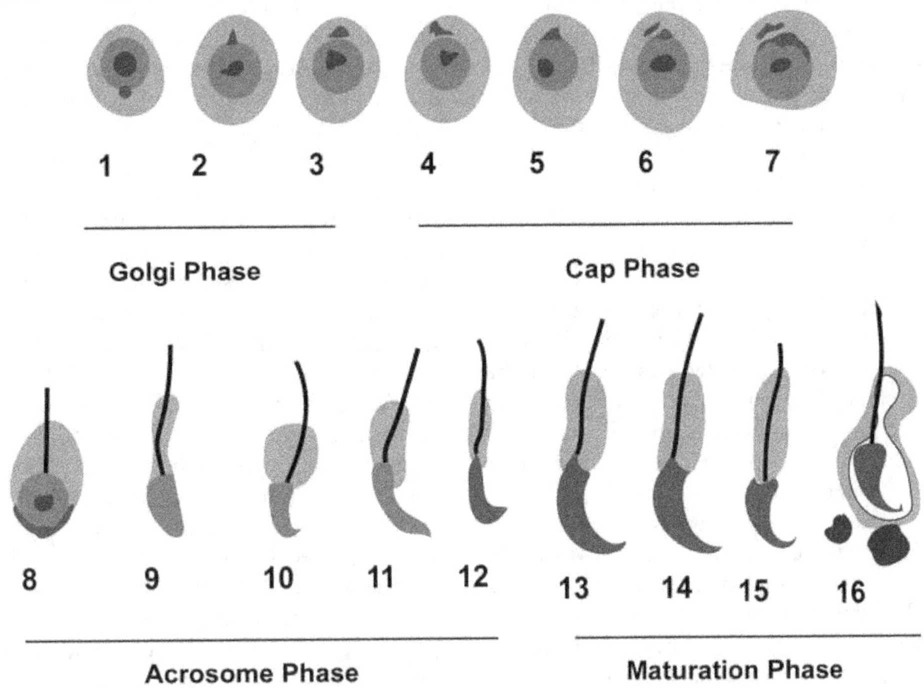

FIGURE 1 | Schematic representation of the phases of acrosome biogenesis in mouse. Round spermatids are transformed into mature spermatozoa in four different phases: Golgi (1–3), Cap (4–7), Acrosome (8–12), and maturation phase (13–16). The whole process of spermiogenesis is comprised of 16 steps in mouse.

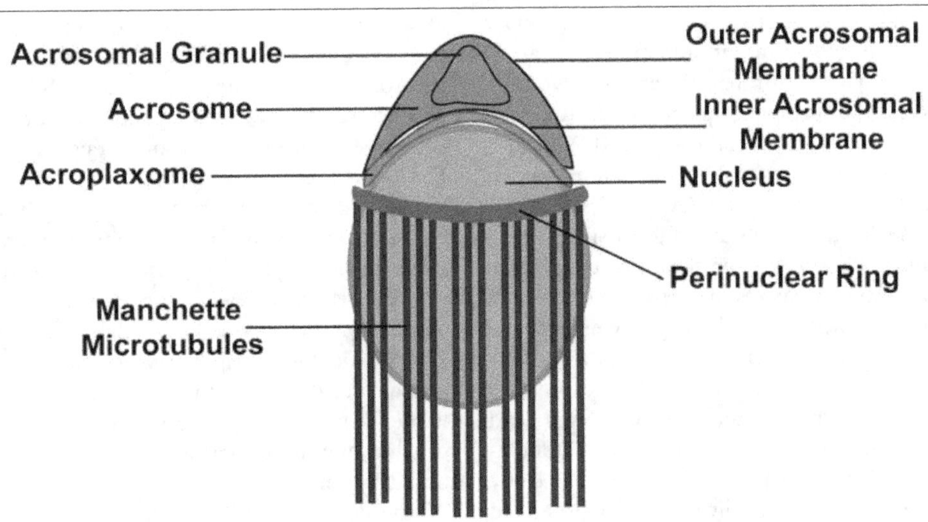

FIGURE 2 | Schematic illustration of a developing spermatid. Developing spermatid has an elongating nucleus surrounded by a perinuclear ring and manchette microtubules. The acrosome lies above the nucleus and is attached to the nucleus with assistance from the acroplaxome.

globozoospermia syndrome (Audouard and Christians, 2011). Therefore, HSP90B1 has been suggested to be a testis-specific chaperone and to be required for the proper folding of acrosomal proteins. The impairment of protein folding during HSP90B1 deficiency suggests an important role of ER protein folding in acrosome biogenesis. β-Glucosidase 2 (GBA2) is another ER-associated protein, and is involved in the metabolism of bile acid–glucose conjugates (Matern et al., 1997). GBA2 disruption results in the formation of abnormal spermatozoa characterized by enlarged heads and the absence of acrosome (Yildiz et al., 2006). In short, these proteins are indispensable for acrosome biogenesis.

In addition, the highly dynamic trafficking of the Golgi-derived vesicles is also involved in acrosome biogenesis. For instance, several Golgi proteins, including Golgin-95/GM130, Golgin-97, Giantin, and β-COP have been found in acrosomal associated membranes (Moreno and Schatten, 2000; Moreno et al., 2000; Ramalho-Santos et al., 2001; Hermo et al., 2010). Among these proteins, β-COP and Clathrin have been described to participate in anterograde and retrograde transport of vesicles during acrosome formation (Martínez-Menárguez et al., 1996b; Moreno et al., 2000; Ramalho-Santos et al., 2001). Golgi-derived vesicle trafficking during acrosome biogenesis can generally be divided into three steps: vesicle formation, trafficking, and fusion. Some of the important proteins that contribute to these three events are described below.

Vesicle formation and trafficking are key events of acrosome biogenesis. Stromal membrane-associated protein 2 (SMAP2) regulates the production of clathrin-coated vesicles from the trans-Golgi network (TGN) by interacting with CALM (Clathrin and the Clathrin assembly protein) and Syntaxin 2 (a component of SNARE complex that helps in membrane fusion), contributing to acrosome biogenesis (Funaki et al., 2013). GOPC (Golgi-associated PDZ- and coiled-coil motif-containing protein) was identified as a frizzled-interacting protein that is involved in vesicular trafficking from the Golgi apparatus (Yao et al., 2001). GOPC is predominantly localized in the trans-Golgi region in round spermatids and plays an important role in the transport and fusion of the proacrosomal vesicles with the growing acrosome (Yao et al., 2002). Golgin subfamily A member 3 (GOLGA3) is another Golgi-associated protein that is highly expressed during the round spermatid stage and is believed to contribute to acrosome biogenesis by interacting with GOPC (Banu et al., 2002; Hicks and Machamer, 2005; Bentson et al., 2013). Another important protein that is involved in protein transport is protein interacting with C kinase 1 (PICK1), which is primarily localized around the Golgi apparatus in spermatids (Arvan and Castle, 2013). PICK1 regulates vesicle trafficking from the Golgi apparatus to the developing acrosome by interacting with GOPC (Xiao et al., 2009). Hence, Golgi-associated proteins are of great significance in vesicle formation and trafficking during acrosome biogenesis. Autophagic machinery also participates in acrosome biogenesis by regulating vesicular trafficking. Autophagy refers to the intracellular catabolic pathway which is responsible for the degradation and recycling of organelles and cytosolic proteins via autophagosomes (double-membrane vesicle) (Yang and Klionsky, 2009; Mizushima and Levine, 2010). Microtubule-associated protein 1A/1B-light chain 3 (LC3) activated by autophagy related protein 7 (ATG7) is delivered to Golgi-derived vacuoles either directly or indirectly (via phagophores) where the activated protein either facilitates the fusion of vesicles or guides them toward the nucleus (Wang et al., 2014). These investigations suggest that the autophagic pathway might be involved in acrosome biogenesis.

Proacrosomal granules undergo fusion with each other to form a single large acrosomal granule at the nuclear surface. Vesicle fusion requires SNARE complexes that help in the fusion of opposing membranes (Rizo and Südhof, 2002; Ungermann and Langosch, 2005; Zhao and Brunger, 2016). Moreover, the disruption of fatty acid desaturase 2 (FADS2) results in Syntaxin 2 scattering, which eventually impairs acrosome formation (Roqueta-Rivera et al., 2011). TATA element Modulatory Factor (TMF/ARA160) is another Golgi-associated protein required for the fusion of vesicles to the targeted membrane (Bel et al., 2012; Miller et al., 2013), and interruption of its expression leads to a complete absence of the acrosomes, suggesting that TMF/ARA160 probably supports the transport and docking of proacrosomal vesicles to the nucleus (Lerer-Goldshtein et al., 2010). Human Rev-binding (HRB) is another critical protein required for the docking of Golgi-derived proacrosomal vesicles; it binds to the cytosolic side of proacrosomal vesicles and links the Golgi apparatus and the nuclear surface (Kang-Decker et al., 2001). Polypeptide N-acetylgalactosaminyltransferase 3 (GALNT3) is located in the cis-medial region of the Golgi, and its disruption leads to failure of proacrosomal vesicles fusion and transport to nuclear surface suggesting the significance of protein O-glycosylation in acrosome biogenesis (Miyazaki et al., 2013). Besides, many other proteins important for vesicle formation or trafficking such as SMAP2 and GOPC also contribute to the fusion of proacrosomal vesicles (Yao et al., 2002; Funaki et al., 2013).

In addition to the transportation to the concave region of the nuclear surface and fusion to form a single large acrosomal granule, the attachment and spreading of the acrosome over the nucleus is also very important to its function. Sperm acrosome-associated 1 (SPACA1), an acrosomal membrane protein, participates in the process of acrosome attachment to the nucleus and the disruption of SPACA1 leads to the detachment of the acrosome from the nucleus (Fujihara et al., 2012). Zona pellucida-binding protein 1 (ZPBP1) is another important protein localized on the periphery of the acrosomal membrane (Lin et al., 2007; Yu et al., 2009), its absence results in the compaction failure of the acrosome and subsequently leads to acrosome fragmentation (Lin et al., 2007). Fer Testis (FerT) is a member of Fes/Fps (nonreceptor tyrosine kinases family), and it regulates cytoskeletal reorganization, cell adhesion, and vesicular transport (Greer, 2002) by attaching itself to the cytosolic surface of OAM and coexists with phosphorylated cortactin (an F-actin regulator protein) in the acroplaxome (Kierszenbaum, 2006; Kierszenbaum et al., 2008). Developmental pluripotency-associated 19-like 2 (DPY19L2) acts as a bridge between the nucleus and the acroplaxome, and its deficiency leads to a loss of the acrosome due to disruption of the nuclear/acroplaxome junction (Pierre et al., 2012). Similarly, disruption of Lamin A/C (a structural component of the nuclear envelope) (Dittmer and Misteli, 2011) leads to acrosome fragmentation and malformed acrosome (Shen et al., 2014). A vast array of specific proteins is involved in acrosome biogenesis and any defect may result in malformation of the acrosome and eventually lead to infertility (**Table 1**; **Figure 3**).

Although most acrosomal substances are transported to the developing acrosome via the ER-Golgi route (Fawcett and Hollenberg, 1963; Clermont and Tang, 1985), numerous other routes are also suspected to exist for the transfer of acrosomal components to the developing acrosome. Toshimori (1998) has reported the existence of an extra-Golgi tract and a Golgi tract, which includes a Golgi-acrosomal granule tract and a Golgi-head cap tract (Toshimori, 1998).

TABLE 1 | Mouse models related to acrosome biogenesis.

	Protein	Function	Phenotype	References
Vesicle formation and trafficking	Hsp90b1	Folds, degrades, and activates ER proteins	Globozospermia	Audouard and Christians, 2011
	GBA2	Glycolipid hydrolase	Globozospermia Glucosylceramide accumulation Disruption of Sertoli-germ cell communication	Yildiz et al., 2006
	GOPC	Transport of proacrosomal granules from Golgi to the acrosome	Globozoospermia Absence of perinuclear theca Absence of coiled-coiltail	Ito et al., 2004; Suzuki-Toyota et al., 2004
	Hrb	Nucleocytoplasmic trafficking Proacrosomal vesicles fusion Acroplaxome formation	Globozoospermia Weak acrosomal vesicle binding to nucleus	Kang-Decker et al., 2001; Kierszenbaum et al., 2004
	Vps54	Endosomes to the trans-Golgi vesicular trafficking	Lack of acrosome Globozospermia	Paiardi et al., 2011
	Sirt1	Recruits LC3 to Golgi-derived vesicles Recruits GOPC and PICK1 to nucleus-associated acrosomal vesicles	Globozospermia	Liu et al., 2017
	Atg7	Recruits LC3 to Golgi-derived vesicles Recruits GOPC and PICK1 to nucleus-associated acrosomal vesicles	Globozospermia	Wang et al., 2014
	PICK1	Involved in proacrosomal granules trafficking	Globozospermia	Xiao et al., 2009
Vesicular fusion	GM130	Vesicular fusion into a single large acrosome vesicle	Lack of acrosomes Aberrant mitochondrial sheath assembly Globozospermia	Han et al., 2017
	AU040320	Vesicular fusion into a single large acrosome vesicle	Lack of acrosomes Globozospermia	Guidi et al., 2018
Anchor the acrosome to the nucleus	DPY19L2	Anchor the cytoskeleton to the nuclear envelope	Dissociation of acroplaxome Globozospermia	Pierre et al., 2012
	ZPBP1	Acrosomal protein	Globozospermia Acrosomal fragmentation Disassembly of protein matrix	Lin et al., 2007
	SPACA1	Supports sperm-egg interaction	Disrupted acroplaxome Failure of acrosome thinning	Fujihara et al., 2012
	Csnk2a2	Nucleus and acrosome formation	Lack of acrosome Acrosomal detachment from nucleus Acrosomal scrap	Xu et al., 1999
	SPAG4L/4L-2	Involved in nucleo-cytoskeleton complex formation Acrosomal vesicle docking to the nucleus	Globozospermia	Frohnert et al., 2010

POTENTIAL WAYS FOR THE ORIGIN OF ACROSOME

Previously, immunocytochemical investigations of glycoprotein synthesis in the Golgi established the acrosome as a direct Golgi derivate (Friend and Fawcett, 1974; Tang et al., 1982; Aguas and da Silva, 1985; Anakwe and Gerton, 1989; Moreno et al., 2000). Later, the acrosome was proposed to be a specialized lysosome based on an acidic pH, protease activities and the presence of hyaluronidase (Hartree and Srivastava, 1965; Allison and Hartree, 1970). A non-lysosomal origin of the acrosome has also been proposed (Martínez-Menárguez et al., 1996a). Martínez-Menárguez et al. (1996a) reported the absence of two well known lysosomal markers; lysosomal membrane glycoprotein (lgp) 120 and mouse Lamp-1 in acrosomal membranes. Moreover, acrosomal and proacrosomal vesicles both lacked two important endosomal markers, cation-dependent and -independent mannose 6-phosphate receptors suggesting some lysosomal features are absent in the acrosomes (Martínez-Menárguez et al., 1996a). In addition, small GTPases were found to be associated with acrosome development (Ramalho-Santos et al., 2001), leading researchers to postulate that the acrosome is a unique cellular organelle, and could be considered a secretory granule (Moreno, 2003). More recently, the acrosome has been suggested as a novel lysosome-related organelle (LRO) (Berruti et al., 2010; Berruti and Paiardi, 2011, 2015). The details of our understanding about acrosome biogenesis are given below:

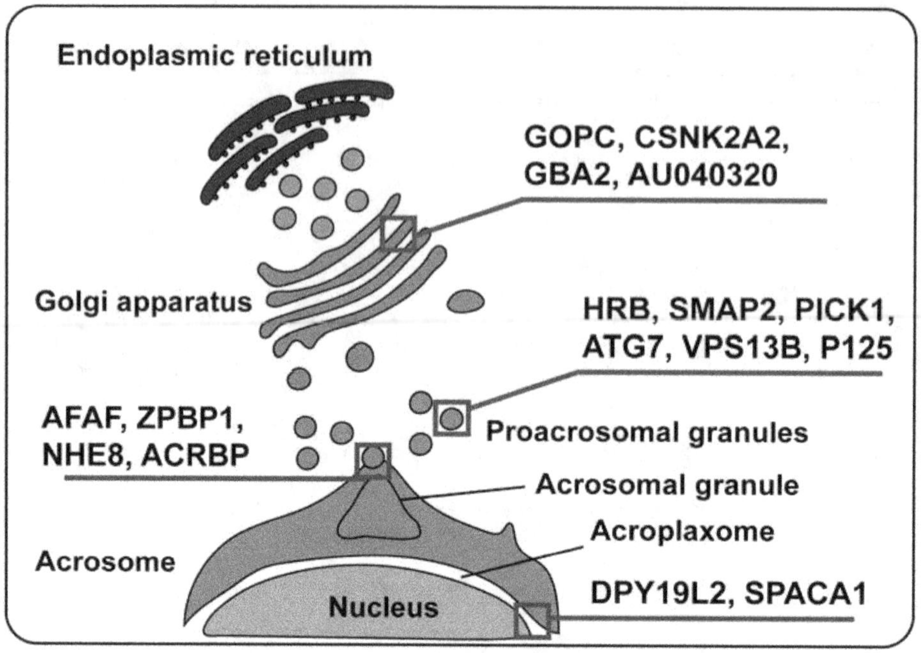

FIGURE 3 | Various proteins are involved in acrosome biogenesis. Several proteins play significant roles in the whole process of acrosome biogenesis, which can be divided into four processes: vesicle formation, vesicular trafficking, vesicular fusion, and acrosome binding to the nucleus. Squares depict the main action of various proteins mentioned in the figure.

Is the Acrosome a Direct Golgi Derivative?

The release of acrosomal contents, during AR, led to concerns and questions about how acrosomal substances are synthesized and stored. To answer these questions, researchers turned their center of investigation toward biosynthetic pathways, especially those of the trans-Golgi network. In line with this, the synthesis, target, and fate of a number of acrosomal proteins in conjunction with lysosomal (Lamp-1, cathepsin D) and Golgi markers (giantin, β-COP, golgin 97) have been precisely examined using immunocytochemical techniques (Aguas and da Silva, 1985; Anakwe and Gerton, 1989; Martínez-Menárguez et al., 1996b; Moreno et al., 2000; Ramalho-Santos et al., 2001). Subsequently, some of these acrosomal-associated proteins were found to be produced in the Golgi complex of spermatocytes (cells that lack an acrosome) and later transported to the acrosome (Anakwe and Gerton, 1989; Escalier et al., 1991). These results were in complete accordance with the previous findings (Fawcett and Bloom, 1986). Therefore, the acrosome was interpreted to be directly derived from the Golgi complex, which acts as a source for membrane and protein contents. In other words, the TGN could be considered the main player during acrosome development, and no lysosome-related characteristics needed to be attributed to the acrosomal vacuole. Meanwhile, more investigations were carried out to identify the origin of acrosomal proteins, their trafficking, and sorting. Consequently, some novel roles of acrosomal proteins were revealed. For instance, acrosin was found to be stored in an inactive state as proacrosin and only activated by the protease acrolysin (McRorie et al., 1976) at the time of AR. Activated acrosin accelerates the release of acrosomal contents by dispersing the acrosomal matrix (Mao and Yang, 2013). Therefore, acrosin is now believed to help in not only the cleavage and subsequent activation of acrosome-specific proteases but also their release via exocytosis (Mao and Yang, 2013). These results were consistent with previous findings (Baba et al., 1994) that showed disruption of acrosin did not affect fecundity but led to a delayed fertilization rate in mice. However, some data exist that are not concordant with the idea that the acrosome is directly derived from Golgi. For instance, the Golgi apparatus detaches from the acrosomal space and moves in the opposite direction during the late capping phase. Furthermore, differentiating spermatids are characterized by the presence of an atypical micro-tubular organization. For example, a cortical microtubule array, despite the absence of centrosome, has been observed in the Golgi phase and tends to disappear during the formation of the manchette, which is a transient structure over the nuclear envelope at the late capping phase (Cherry and Hsu, 1984; Moreno and Schatten, 2000). In fact, this idea is so deep-rooted in the field that a variety of proteins in somatic cells that are involved in endocytosis have also been investigated, and were found to play a role in the biosynthetic/anterograde pathway, supporting acrosome biogenesis in spermatids (Berruti and Paiardi, 2011, 2015). Hence, in spite of contrary reports, a large majority of the reproductive-research community still supports the idea that the acrosome is a direct Golgi derivative.

Is the Acrosome a Secretory Granule?

The notion that the acrosome is a direct Golgi derivative prevailed until the emergence of reports strengthened earlier evidence for the presence of a range of hydrolytic enzymes and a low pH maintained by the activity of V-ATPase (Sun-Wada et al., 2002). These characteristics were found to be common between lysosomes and acrosomes. Moreover, two Rab family members were identified to be involved in endocytosis and acrosome development, such as Rab5 (Simonsen et al., 1998) and Rab7 (Ramalho-Santos et al., 2001), respectively. Although acrosomes and lysosomes share several common characteristics, there are also dissimilarities. As mentioned earlier, the acrosome has been suggested to be a modified secretory granule (Moreno and Alvarado, 2006). For instance, serine proteinases (unique to testis), AM67 (a secretory component protein), acrosin acrogranin (Ohmura et al., 1999; Abou-Haila and Tulsiani, 2000) and exocytotic properties support the idea that the acrosome could be considered analogous to a secretory granule. Secretory granules are known to carry luminal protein contents that are directly delivered by the biosynthetic pathway to the targeted organelle and do not traverse to other parts of the endosomal system (Arvan and Castle, 1998). Secretory lysosomes, however, receive proteins through biosynthetic and endocytic pathways and serve as both degradative and secretory compartments (Blott and Griffiths, 2002). Secretory lysosomes are also mostly found in hematopoietic lineage-derived cells. To solve the mystery of whether the acrosome is really a secretory lysosome, Lamp-1 and Lamp-2 (lysosome specific proteins) were studied in detail during spermiogenesis. Results showed that both Lamp-1 and Lamp-2 were found to link with cytoplasmic vesicles only and not to the growing acrosome (Moreno, 2003). Although AR is usually associated with a somatic cell exocytosis, it still has several exclusive characteristics. For instance, AR is an irreversible "all-or-nothing" event. Moreover, in contrast to a single large vacuole of sperm, there are several secretory vesicles in cells that show exocytosis. In addition, AR takes place only once in each sperm because once the acrosome has reacted, it cannot be replaced by further biogenesis. Similarly, acrosomal membranes are lost and cannot be recycled at the time of AR (Berruti, 2016). In each sperm, only a single secretory granule exists, in contrast to the numerous secretory vesicles found in most other exocytotic cells. A feature that makes the acrosome unique is that the acrosome remains undocked prior to the required exocytosis stimulus, which is in contrast to other granules that are docked even before the application of the relevant stimulus (**Table 2**; Zanetti and Mayorga, 2009; Tsai et al., 2010; Rodríguez et al., 2011, 2012). Another interpretation has also been made in regards to secretory granule/lysosome nature of acrosome. Sperm traversing through the zona pellucida doesn't show any enzymatic lysis in eutherian (Bedford, 1998). A physical thrust, from the sperm head's structure was implicated in vitelline coat invasion (Bedford, 1998; Berruti, 2016). This investigation pointed out the importance of the "exocytotic" release of the acrosomal contents to penetrate the zona pellucida.

TABLE 2 | Similarities and differences between acrosome and secretory granules of other exocytotic cells.

Feature	Sperm (acrosome)	Exocytotic cells (secretory granule)
SIMILARITIES		
Secretory components in common	AM67	AM67
Exocytosis	Present	Present
Enzymes in common	Serine proteinases	Serine proteinases
DIFFERENCES		
No. of secretory granules	Single (one)	Numerous
Granular docking	Undocked	Docked
Exocytosis	Once	Multiple times
Regeneration/replacement	Once reacted, can't be replaced	Can be replaced or reproduced
Membrane recycling	No membrane recycling	Membranes are recycled

Is the Acrosome a Lysosome-Related Organelle?

The acrosome contains a vast array of acidic hydrolytic enzymes that are essential for the AR to take place normally and help the sperm to bind and dissolve the oocyte coverings during the exocytic release at the time of fertilization (Hartree and Srivastava, 1965; Allison and Hartree, 1970; Jin et al., 2011). Initially, researchers identified the lysosomal enzyme, hyaluronidase, and later several other hydrolytic enzymes such as acid phosphatase (another lysosomal enzyme), glycohydrolases, proteases, esterases, and aryl sulfatases in the acrosomes. These findings led to the suggestion that the acrosome is nothing unique, but a specially modified lysosome that has evolved to facilitate the fertilization process (Hartree and Srivastava, 1965; Allison and Hartree, 1970; Zaneveld and De Jonge, 1991; Tulsiani et al., 1998). Further strengthening this hypothesis was the characterization of analogous histochemical properties, the acidic pH of both the organelles (Allison and Hartree, 1970) and pro-acrosomal vesicle biogenesis in the Golgi apparatus (**Table 3**; Burgos and Fawcett, 1955; Dooher and Bennett, 1973). Among all the acrosomal enzymes, acrosin remains the most well-characterized protease (McRorie and Williams, 1974), but its location in the acrosome remains controversial. Is acrosin associated with the IAM, in the vicinity of the acrosomal membrane, or in the acrosomal matrix (Polakoski and Zaneveld, 1976; Shams-Borhan et al., 1979; Berruti and Martegani, 1982, 1984; Castellani-Ceresa et al., 1983)? In contrast, many believed acrosin existed to help sperm progress through the zona pellucida, and was therefore named the zona pellucida proteolytic enzyme/zona-penetrating enzyme (Chang and Hunter, 1975). Previously, a main research focus was to determine the function of different hydrolytic enzymes, especially acrosomal enzymes involved in the swift focal lysis of the outer coverings of the oocyte for fertilization. Researchers believed that the acrosome was a specialized lysosome, and enzymatic lysis would be required for sperm–oocyte fusion. But no consensus existed to unite both of those ideas (Bedford, 2014). The belief that the "acrosome is a specially modified lysosome" was finally shattered with the advent of gene-knockout technology, which revealed that acrosin is not indispensable for fertilization (Baba et al., 1994). In the

TABLE 3 | Similarities between acrosome and lysosome.

Feature	Acrosome	Lysosome
Enzymes in common	Hyaluronidase, proteinases (acrosin), esterases, neuraminidases, acid phosphatases	Hyaluronidase, proteinases, esterases, neuraminidases, acid phosphatases
pH	Acidic	Acidic
Origin	Golgi Apparatus	Golgi Apparatus

BOX 1 | Glossary.

Perinuclear theca: a condensed cytoskeletal structure that encompasses the nucleus of the mammalian spermatozoa, except near the tail implantation region. The structure consists of two distinct regions, a subacrosomal layer/perforatorium, and postacrosomal regions.

Acroplaxome (Greek words akros, topmost; platys, flat; soma, body): a structure located in the sub-acrosomal space that holds the developing acrosome to the spermatid nucleus.

Manchette: is a temporary structure that persists only during elongation and encompasses the elongating spermatid head. The structure lies below the marginal ring of the acroplaxome and consists of a perinuclear ring and inserted microtubular mantle.

Step 14 Spermatid: Spermiogenesis occurs in 16 steps (1-16) in mice. Step 14 spermatids are characterized by chromatin condensation, nucleus elongation, and transformation of the head in sickle a shape.

past few years, the acrosome was suggested to be a lysosome-related organelle (LRO) based on findings that acrosome biogenesis involves both the biosynthetic and endocytic pathways (Berruti et al., 2010; Berruti and Paiardi, 2011).

LROs are special membrane-bound organelles that received cargo from early endosomal intermediates and link biosynthetic and endosomal systems (Delevoye et al., 2009). LROs show a unique morphology, composition, and physiology and represent the resident cell. It has been suggested that the acrosome is an LRO, and it receives diverse protein cargos from more non-redundant pathways that contribute to acrosome biogenesis. It could therefore be construed that the lytic contents are primarily delivered from the ER-Golgi-TGN route while the acrosomal matrix scaffold and membranous constituents are contributed by the early endosome–endosome intermediates-TGN route. In addition, the complexity of the structure and physiology of the mature LRO is supported by the involvement of several routes. In line with this, several acrosomal features such as high spatial regulation of acrosome biogenesis, highly polarized location, and "modular" organization of its ingredients are consistent with the proposed nature of the acrosome as an LRO (Marks et al., 2013). Proteomic analysis data (Guyonnet et al., 2012) also uncovered unique analogies of biogenesis and protein contents between acrosomes and LROs. For instance, melanosome biogenesis follows four developmental stages (Seiji et al., 1963) that are similar to acrosome biogenesis. Furthermore, both the melanosome matrix and the acrosomal matrix can self-aggregate. Theses matrices both possess a core made up of a firm amyloidogenic structure that is later transformed into a functional matrix by successive attachment of several proteins (Delevoye et al., 2009; Guyonnet et al., 2012). Recently, we found that germ cell-specific *atg7*-knockout mice produce a globozoospermia-like phenotype due to a malformed acrosome, and autophagy was found to mediate the proacrosomal vesicle transport or fusion in the acrosome (Wang et al., 2014). Thus, the acrosome is proposed to have originated from an autolysosome rather than a lysosome alone. In support of this hypothesis, Sirt1 (sirtuin 1) and Tbc1d20 (TBC1 domain family, member 20) have been found to be involved in acrosome biogenesis and regulate autophagic flux (Sidjanin et al., 2016; Liu et al., 2017).

PERSPECTIVE AND CONCLUDING REMARKS

Although the origin and the first appearance of acrosomes are yet to be determined, it could have originated from the simplest eukaryotes, such as yeast. A prerequisite for yeast mating is the formation of shmoo tips/ projections (Merlini et al., 2013), which show several features similar to the typical acrosome, such as the presence of degradative enzymes and the trafficking of some vesicles. Therefore, the primary form of the acrosome could have developed very early in the evolutionary history. Nevertheless, the existence of a true acrosome can be traced back to the evolution of heterogamy, heterozygosity, and cross-fertilization. Initially, all organisms were homogametic, and most were self-fertilizing. Later, some organisms evolved cross-fertilization. To better adapt the ever-changing circumstances of the earth (Shields, 1982; Schmidt-Rhaesa, 2007; Stearns, 2013), protective coverings around eggs developed to ensure gamete integrity, and sperms needed to arm with a powerful weapon in its arsenal, the acrosome, to evade these protective gamete vestments (Schmidt-Rhaesa, 2007). This review provides a brief historical overview and highlights new break-through on acrosome biogenesis. The acrosome might be generated from a combination of many membrane trafficking systems during gametes fusion, and it might have evolved during the arms race between sperm and ovum. A collective effort to uncover unidentified components, their interactions, and their regulatory mechanism(s) is urgently needed to elucidate a more complete picture of this highly complicated secretory vesicle. Our current era definitely will be a time of deep understanding of acrosome biogenesis.

AUTHOR CONTRIBUTIONS

MK collected the data, drew the figures, and wrote the manuscript. HG revised the figures and the manuscript. WL proposed the idea and revised the manuscript.

FUNDING

This work was funded by the Strategic Priority Research Program of the Chinese Academy of Sciences (Grant No. XDA16020701), the National Key R&D Program of China (Grant No. 2016YFA0500901), and the National Natural Science Foundation of China (Grant No. 91649202).

REFERENCES

Abou-Haila, A., and Tulsiani, D. R. (2000). Mammalian sperm acrosome: formation, contents, and function. *Arch. Biochem. Biophys.* 379, 173–182. doi: 10.1006/abbi.2000.1880

Aguas, A. P., and da Silva, P. P. (1985). The acrosomal membrane of boar sperm: a Golgi-derived membrane poor in glycoconjugates. *J. Cell Biol.* 100, 528–534. doi: 10.1083/jcb.100.2.528

Allison, A., and Hartree, E. F. (1970). Lysosomal enzymes in the acrosome and their possible role in fertilization. *Reproduction* 21, 501–515. doi: 10.1530/jrf.0.0210501

Anakwe, O., and Gerton, G. L. (1989). Acrosome biogenesis begins during meiosis: evidence from the synthesis and distribution of an acrosomal glycoprotein, acrogranin, during guinea pig spermatogenesis. *Biol. Reprod.* 42, 317–328. doi: 10.1095/biolreprod42.2.317

Anakwe, O. O., and Gerton, G. L. (1990). Acrosome biogenesis begins during meiosis - evidence from the synthesis and distribution of an acrosomal glycoprotein, acrogranin, during guinea-pig spermatogenesis. *Biol. Reprod.* 42, 317–328.

Arvan, P., and Castle, D. (1998). Sorting and storage during secretory granule biogenesis: looking backward and looking forward. *Biochem. J.* 332, 593–610. doi: 10.1042/bj3320593

Arvan, P., and Castle, D. (2013). Neuroendocrinology: regulated secretory cells go to the BAR for a bud. *Nat. Rev. Endocrinol.* 9:443. doi: 10.1038/nrendo.2013.121

Asquith, K. L., Harman, A. J., McLaughlin, E. A., Nixon, B., and Aitken, R. J. (2005). Localization and significance of molecular chaperones, heat shock protein 1, and tumor rejection antigen gp96 in the male reproductive tract and during capacitation and acrosome reaction. *Biol. Reprod.* 72, 328–337. doi: 10.1095/biolreprod.104.034470

Audouard, C., and Christians, E. (2011). Hsp90b1 knockout targeted to male germline: a mouse model for globozoospermia. *Fertil. Steril.* 95, 1475–1477. e1474. doi: 10.1016/j.fertnstert.2010.12.006

Baba, T., Azuma, S., Kashiwabara, S.-,i., and Toyoda, Y. (1994). Sperm from mice carrying a targeted mutation of the acrosin gene can penetrate the oocyte zona pellucida and effect fertilization. *J. Biol. Chem.* 269, 31845–31849.

Banu, Y., Matsuda, M., Yoshihara, M., Kondo, M., Sutou, S., and Matsukuma, S. (2002). Golgi matrix protein gene, Golga3/Mea2, rearranged and re-expressed in pachytene spermatocytes restores spermatogenesis in the mouse. *Mol. Reprod. Dev.* 61, 288–301. doi: 10.1002/mrd.10035

Bedford, J. (1998). Mammalian fertilization misread? Sperm penetration of the eutherian zona pellucida is unlikely to be a lytic event. *Biol. Reprod.* 59, 1275–1287. doi: 10.1095/biolreprod59.6.1275

Bedford, J. M. (2014). Singular features of fertilization and their impact on the male reproductive system in eutherian mammals. *Reproduction* 147, R43–R52. doi: 10.1530/REP-13-0436

Bel, S., Elkis, Y., Lerer-Goldstein, T., Nyska, A., Shpungin, S., and Nir, U. (2012). Loss of TMF/ARA160 protein renders colonic mucus refractory to bacterial colonization and diminishes intestinal susceptibility to acute colitis. *J. Biol. Chem.* 287, 25631–25639. doi: 10.1074/jbc.M112.364786

Bentson, L. F., Agbor, V. A., Agbor, L. N., Lopez, A. C., Nfonsam, L. E., Bornstein, S. S., et al. (2013). New point mutation in Golga3 causes multiple defects in spermatogenesis. *Andrology* 1, 440–450. doi: 10.1111/j.2047-2927.2013.00070.x

Berruti, G. (2016). Towards defining an 'origin'—the case for the mammalian acrosome. *Semin. Cell Dev. Biol.* 59, 46–53. doi: 10.1016/j.semcdb.2016.01.013

Berruti, G., and Martegani, E. (1982). Cytochemical demonstration that acrosin is unavailable in intact ejaculated boar and bull spermatozoa. *J. Exp. Zool.* 222, 149–154. doi: 10.1002/jez.1402220206

Berruti, G., and Martegani, E. (1984). Dansylalanyllysylchloromethyl ketone as a fluorescent probe for localization of acrosin activity in boar and human spermatozoa. *J. Histochem. Cytochem.* 32, 526–530. doi: 10.1177/32.5.6371133

Berruti, G., and Paiardi, C. (2011). Acrosome biogenesis: revisiting old questions to yield new insights. *Spermatogenesis* 1, 95–98. doi: 10.4161/spmg.1.2.16820

Berruti, G., and Paiardi, C. (2015). USP8/UBPy-regulated sorting and the development of sperm acrosome: the recruitment of MET. *Reproduction* 149, 633–644. doi: 10.1530/REP-14-0671

Berruti, G., Ripolone, M., and Ceriani, M. (2010). USP8, a regulator of endosomal sorting, is involved in mouse acrosome biogenesis through interaction with the spermatid ESCRT-0 complex and microtubules. *Biol. Reprod.* 82, 930–939. doi: 10.1095/biolreprod.109.081679

Blott, E. J., and Griffiths, G. M. (2002). Secretory lysosomes. *Nat. Rev. Mol. Cell Biol.* 3:122. doi: 10.1038/nrm732

Buffone, M. G., Foster, J. A., and Gerton, G. L. (2004). The role of the acrosomal matrix in fertilization. *Int. J. Dev. Biol.* 52, 511–522. doi: 10.1387/ijdb.072532mb

Burgos, M. H., and Fawcett, D. W. (1955). Studies on the fine structure of the mammalian testis: I. Differentiation of the spermatids in the cat (*Felis domestica*). *J. Cell Biol.* 1, 287–300. doi: 10.1083/jcb.1.4.287

Camatini, M., Colombo, A., and Bonfanti, P. (1992). Cytoskeletal elements in mammalian spermiogenesis and spermatozoa. *Microsc. Res. Tech.* 20, 232–250. doi: 10.1002/jemt.1070200303

Castellani-Ceresa, L., Berruti, G., and Colombo, R. (1983). Immunocytochemical localization of acrosin in boar spermatozoa. *J. Exp. Zool.* 227, 297–304. doi: 10.1002/jez.1402270213

Chang, M., and Hunter, R. (1975). "Capacitation of mammalian sperm: biological and experimental aspects," in *Handbook of Physiology*, Vol. 5, ed R. O. Greep (Washington, DC: American Physiology Society), 339–351.

Cherry, L. M., and Hsu, T. (1984). Antitubulin immunofluorescence studies of spermatogenesis in the mouse. *Chromosoma* 90, 265–274. doi: 10.1007/BF00287034

Clermont, Y., and Leblond, C. (1955). Spermiogenesis of man, monkey, ram and other mammals as shown by the "periodic acid-Schiff" technique. *Am. J. Anat.* 96, 229–253. doi: 10.1002/aja.1000960203

Clermont, Y., and Tang, X. (1985). Glycoprotein synthesis in the *Golgi apparatus* of spermatids during spermiogenesis of the rat. *Anat. Rec.* 213, 33–43. doi: 10.1002/ar.1092130106

De Franca, L. R., Ye, S. J., Ying, L., Sandberg, M., and Russell, L. D. (1995). Morphometry of rat germ cells during spermatogenesis. *Anat. Rec.* 241, 181–204. doi: 10.1002/ar.1092410206

Delevoye, C., Hurbain, I., Tenza, D., Sibarita, J.-B., Uzan-Gafsou, S., Ohno, H., et al. (2009). AP-1 and KIF13A coordinate endosomal sorting and positioning during melanosome biogenesis. *J. Cell Biol.* 187, 247–264. doi: 10.1083/jcb.200907122

Dittmer, T. A., and Misteli, T. (2011). The lamin protein family. *Genome Biol.* 12:222. doi: 10.1186/gb-2011-12-5-222

Dooher, G., and Bennett, D. (1973). Fine structural observations on the development of the sperm head in the mouse. *Am. J. Anat.* 136, 339–361. doi: 10.1002/aja.1001360307

Escalier, D., Gallo, J. M., Albert, M., Meduri, G., Bermudez, D., David, G., et al. (1991). Human acrosome biogenesis - immunodetection of proacrosin in primary spermatocytes and of its partitioning pattern during meiosis. *Development* 113, 779–788.

Fawcett, D. W. (1975). Gametogenesis in the male: prospects for its control. *Symp. Soc. Dev. Biol.* 25–53. doi: 10.1016/B978-0-12-612979-3.50009-1

Fawcett, D. W., and Bloom, W. (1986). *A Textbook of Histology*. Philadelphia, PA: WB Saunders Company, 614–628.

Fawcett, D. W., and Hollenberg, R. D. (1963). Changes in the acrosome of guinea pig spermatozoa during passage through the epididymis. *Z. Zellforsch. Mikrosk. Anat.* 60, 276–292. doi: 10.1007/BF00350481

Friend, D. S., and Fawcett, D. W. (1974). Membrane differentiations in freeze-fractured mammalian sperm. *J. Cell Biol.* 63, 641–664. doi: 10.1083/jcb.63.2.641

Frohnert, C., Schweizer, S., and Hoyer-Fender, S. (2010). SPAG4L/SPAG4L-2 are testis-specific SUN domain proteins restricted to the apical nuclear envelope of round spermatids facing the acrosome. *Mol. Hum. Reprod.* 17, 207–218. doi: 10.1093/molehr/gaq099

Fujihara, Y., Satouh, Y., Inoue, N., Isotani, A., Ikawa, M., and Okabe, M. (2012). SPACA1-deficient male mice are infertile with abnormally shaped sperm heads reminiscent of globozoospermia. *Development* 139, 3583–3589. doi: 10.1242/dev.081778

Funaki, T., Kon, S., Tanabe, K., Natsume, W., Sato, S., Shimizu, T., et al. (2013). The Arf GAP SMAP2 is necessary for organized vesicle budding from the trans-Golgi network and subsequent acrosome formation in spermiogenesis. *Mol. Biol. Cell* 24, 2633–2644. doi: 10.1091/mbc.e13-05-0234

Greer, P. (2002). Closing in on the biological functions of Fps/Fes and Fer. *Nat. Rev. Mol. Cell Biol.* 3, 278–289. doi: 10.1038/nrm783

Guidi, L. G., Holloway, Z. G., Arnoult, C., Ray, P. F., Monaco, A. P., Molnár, Z., et al. (2018). AU040320 deficiency leads to disruption of acrosome biogenesis and infertility in homozygous mutant mice. *Sci. Rep.* 8:10379. doi: 10.1038/s41598-018-28666-6

Guyonnet, B., Zabet-Moghaddam, M., SanFrancisco, S., and Cornwall, G. A. (2012). Isolation and proteomic characterization of the mouse sperm acrosomal matrix. *Mol. Cell. Proteomics* 11, 758–774. doi: 10.1074/mcp.M112.020339

Han, F., Liu, C., Zhang, L., Chen, M., Zhou, Y., Qin, Y., et al. (2017). Globozoospermia and lack of acrosome formation in GM130-deficient mice. *Cell Death Dis.* 8:e2532. doi: 10.1038/cddis.2016.414

Hartree, E., and Srivastava, P. (1965). Chemical composition of the acrosomes of ram spermatozoa. *Reproduction* 9, 47–60. doi: 10.1530/jrf.0.0090047

Hermo, L., Pelletier, R. M., Cyr, D. G., and Smith, C. E. (2010). Surfing the wave, cycle, life history, and genes/proteins expressed by testicular germ cells. Part 2: changes in spermatid organelles associated with development of spermatozoa. *Microsc. Res. Tech.* 73, 279–319. doi: 10.1002/jemt.20787

Hess, R. A. (1990). Quantitative and qualitative characteristics of the stages and transitions in the cycle of the rat seminiferous epithelium: light microscopic observations of perfusion-fixed and plastic-embedded testes. *Biol. Reprod.* 43, 525–542. doi: 10.1095/biolreprod43.3.525

Hess, R. A., and de Franca, L. R. (2008). "Spermatogenesis and cycle of the seminiferous epithelium," in *Molecular Mechanisms in Spermatogenesis*, ed C. Y. Cheng (New York, NY: Springer), 1–15.

Hess, R. A., Miller, L. A., Kirby, J. D., Margoliash, E., and Goldberg, E. (1993). Immunoelectron microscopic localization of testicular and somatic cytochromes c in the seminiferous epithelium of the rat. *Biol. Reprod.* 48, 1299–1308. doi: 10.1095/biolreprod48.6.1299

Hicks, S. W., and Machamer, C. E. (2005). Isoform-specific interaction of golgin-160 with the Golgi-associated protein PIST. *J. Biol. Chem.* 280, 28944–28951. doi: 10.1074/jbc.M504937200

Ikawa, M., Inoue, N., Benham, A. M., and Okabe, M. (2010). Fertilization: a sperm's journey to and interaction with the oocyte. *J. Clin. Invest.* 120, 984–994. doi: 10.1172/JCI41585

Ito, C., Suzuki-Toyota, F., Maekawa, M., Toyama, Y., Yao, R., Noda, T., et al. (2004). Failure to assemble the peri-nuclear structures in GOPC deficient spermatids as found in round-headed spermatozoa. *Arch. Histol. Cytol.* 67, 349–360. doi: 10.1679/aohc.67.349

Jin, M., Fujiwara, E., Kakiuchi, Y., Okabe, M., Satouh, Y., Baba, S. A., et al. (2011). Most fertilizing mouse spermatozoa begin their acrosome reaction before contact with the zona pellucida during *in vitro* fertilization. *Proc. Natl. Acad. Sci. U.S.A.* 108, 4892–4896. doi: 10.1073/pnas.1018202108

Kang-Decker, N., Mantchev, G. T., Juneja, S. C., McNiven, M. A., and van Deursen, J. M. (2001). Lack of acrosome formation in Hrb-deficient mice. *Science* 294, 1531–1533. doi: 10.1126/science.1063665

Kashiwabara, S., Arai, Y., Kodaira, K., and Baba, T. (1990). Acrosin biosynthesis in meiotic and postmeiotic spermatogenic cells. *Biochem. Biophys. Res. Commun.* 173, 240–245. doi: 10.1016/S0006-291X(05)81047-2

Kierszenbaum, A. L. (2006). Tyrosine protein kinases and spermatogenesis: truncation matters. *Mol. Reprod. Dev.* 73, 399–403. doi: 10.1002/mrd.20456

Kierszenbaum, A. L., Rivkin, E., and Tres, L. L. (2003). Acroplaxome, an F-actin–keratin-containing plate, anchors the acrosome to the nucleus during shaping of the spermatid head. *Mol. Biol. Cell* 14, 4628–4640. doi: 10.1091/mbc.e03-04-0226

Kierszenbaum, A. L., Rivkin, E., and Tres, L. L. (2008). Expression of Fer testis (FerT) tyrosine kinase transcript variants and distribution sites of FerT during the development of the acrosome-acroplaxome-manchette complex in rat spermatids. *Dev. Dynam.* 237, 3882–3891. doi: 10.1002/dvdy.21789

Kierszenbaum, A. L., Tres, L. L., Rivkin, E., Kang-Decker, N., and Van Deursen, J. M. (2004). The acroplaxome is the docking site of Golgi-derived myosin Va/Rab27a/b-containing proacrosomal vesicles in wild-type and Hrb mutant mouse spermatids. *Biol. Reprod.* 70, 1400–1410. doi: 10.1095/biolreprod.103.025346

Leblond, C., and Clermont, Y. (1952). Spermiogenesis of rat, mouse, hamster and guinea pig as revealed by the "periodic acid-fuchsin sulfurous acid" technique. *Am. J. Anat.* 90, 167–215. doi: 10.1002/aja.1000900202

Lerer-Goldshtein, T., Bel, S., Shpungin, S., Pery, E., Motro, B., Goldstein, R. S., et al. (2010). TMF/ARA160: a key regulator of sperm development. *Dev. Biol.* 348, 12–21. doi: 10.1016/j.ydbio.2010.07.033

Lin, Y.-N., Roy, A., Yan, W., Burns, K. H., and Matzuk, M. M. (2007). Loss of zona pellucida binding proteins in the acrosomal matrix disrupts acrosome biogenesis and sperm morphogenesis. *Mol. Cell. Biol.* 27, 6794–6805. doi: 10.1128/MCB.01029-07

Liu, C., Song, Z., Wang, L., Yu, H., Liu, W., Shang, Y., et al. (2017). Sirt1 regulates acrosome biogenesis by modulating autophagic flux during spermiogenesis in mice. *Development* 144, 441–451. doi: 10.1242/dev.147074

Mao, H.-T., and Yang, W.-X. (2013). Modes of acrosin functioning during fertilization. *Gene* 526, 75–79. doi: 10.1016/j.gene.2013.05.058

Marks, M. S., Heijnen, H. F., and Raposo, G. (2013). Lysosome-related organelles: unusual compartments become mainstream. *Curr. Opin. Cell Biol.* 25, 495–505. doi: 10.1016/j.ceb.2013.04.008

Martínez-Menárguez, J., Geuze, H., and Ballesta, J. (1996b). Identification of two types of beta-COP vesicles in the Golgi complex of rat spermatids. *Eur. J. Cell Biol.* 71, 137–143.

Martínez-Menárguez, J. A., Geuze, H. J., and Ballesta, J. (1996a). Evidence for a nonlysosomal origin of the acrosome. *J. Histochem. Cytochem.* 44, 313–320. doi: 10.1177/44.4.8601690

Matern, H., Heinemann, H., Legler, G., and Matern, S. (1997). Purification and characterization of a microsomal bile acid β-glucosidase from human liver. *J. Biol. Chem.* 272, 11261–11267. doi: 10.1074/jbc.272.17.11261

McRorie, R. A., Turner, R. B., Bradford, M. M., and Williams, W. L. (1976). Acrolysin, the aminoproteinase catalyzing the initial conversion of proacrosin to acrosin in mammalian fertilization. *Biochem. Biophys. Res. Commun.* 71, 492–498. doi: 10.1016/0006-291X(76)90814-7

McRorie, R. A., and Williams, W. L. (1974). Biochemistry of mammalian fertilization. *Annu. Rev. Biochem.* 43, 777–802. doi: 10.1146/annurev.bi.43.070174.004021

Merlini, L., Dudin, O., and Martin, S. G. (2013). Mate and fuse: how yeast cells do it. *Open Biol.* 3:130008. doi: 10.1098/rsob.130008

Miller, V. J., Sharma, P., Kudlyk, T. A., Frost, L., Rofe, A. P., Watson, I. J., et al. (2013). Molecular insights into vesicle tethering at the Golgi by the conserved oligomeric Golgi (COG) complex and the golgin TATA element modulatory factor (TMF). *J. Biol. Chem.* 288, 4229–4240. doi: 10.1074/jbc.M112.426767

Miyazaki, T., Mori, M., Yoshida, C. A., Ito, C., Yamatoya, K., Moriishi, T., et al. (2013). Galnt3 deficiency disrupts acrosome formation and leads to oligoasthenoteratozoospermia. *Histochem. Cell Biol.* 139, 339–354. doi: 10.1007/s00418-012-1031-3

Mizushima, N., and Levine, B. (2010). Autophagy in mammalian development and differentiation. *Nat. Cell Biol.* 12:823. doi: 10.1038/ncb0910-823

Moreno, R. D. (2003). Differential expression of lysosomal associated membrane protein (LAMP-1) during mammalian spermiogenesis. *Mol. Reprod. Dev.* 66, 202–209. doi: 10.1002/mrd.10342

Moreno, R. D., and Alvarado, C. P. (2006). The mammalian acrosome as a secretory lysosome: new and old evidence. *Mol. Reprod. Dev.* 73, 1430–1434. doi: 10.1002/mrd.20581

Moreno, R. D., Ramalho-Santos, J., Sutovsky, P., Chan, E. K., and Schatten, G. (2000). Vesicular traffic and Golgi apparatus dynamics during mammalian spermatogenesis: implications for acrosome architecture. *Biol. Reprod.* 63, 89–98. doi: 10.1095/biolreprod63.1.89

Moreno, R. D., and Schatten, G. (2000). Microtubule configurations and post-translational α-tubulin modifications during mammalian spermatogenesis. *Cell Motil. Cytoskeleton* 46, 235–246. doi: 10.1002/1097-0169(200008)46:4<235::AID-CM1>3.0.CO;2-G

Nakamura, M., Moriya, M., Baba, T., Michikawa, Y., Yamanobe, T., Arai, K., et al. (1993). An endoplasmic-reticulum protein, calreticulin, is transported into the acrosome of rat sperm. *Exp. Cell Res.* 205, 101–110. doi: 10.1006/excr.1993.1063

Nasr-Esfahani, M. H., Deemeh, M. R., and Tavalaee, M. (2010a). Artificial oocyte activation and intracytoplasmic sperm injection. *Fertil. Steril.* 94, 520–526. doi: 10.1016/j.fertnstert.2009.03.061

Nasr-Esfahani, M. H., Razavi, S., Javdan, Z., and Tavalaee, M. (2008). Artificial oocyte activation in severe teratozoospermia undergoing intracytoplasmic sperm injection. *Fertil. Steril.* 90, 2231–2237. doi: 10.1016/j.fertnstert.2007.10.047

Nasr-Esfahani, M. H., Tavalaee, M., Reza Deemeh, M., Arbabian, M., and Parrington, J. (2010b). Can assessment of total acrosin activity help predict failed or low fertilization rate ICSI for implementation of artificial oocyte activation? *Open Androl. J.* 2, 19–26.

Nicander, L., and Ploen, L. (1969). Fine structure of spermatogonia and primary spermatocytes in rabbits. *Z. Zellforsch. Mikrosk. Anat.* 99, 221–234. doi: 10.1007/BF00342223

Ohmura, K., Kohno, N., Kobayashi, Y., Yamagata, K., Sato, S., and Kashiwabara, S.-,i., et al. (1999). A homologue of pancreatic trypsin is localized in the acrosome of mammalian sperm and is released during acrosome reaction. *J. Biol. Chem.* 274, 29426–29432. doi: 10.1074/jbc.274.41.29426

Paiardi, C., Pasini, M. E., Gioria, M., and Berruti, G. (2011). Failure of acrosome formation and globozoospermia in the wobbler mouse, a Vps54 spontaneous recessive mutant. *Spermatogenesis* 1, 52–62. doi: 10.4161/spmg.1.1.14698

Pierre, V., Martinez, G., Coutton, C., Delaroche, J., Yassine, S., Novella, C., et al. (2012). Absence of Dpy19l2, a new inner nuclear membrane protein, causes globozoospermia in mice by preventing the anchoring of the acrosome to the nucleus. *Development* 139, 2955–2965. doi: 10.1242/dev.077982

Polakoski, K. L., and Zaneveld, L. J. D. (1976). "Proacrosin," in *Methods in Enzymology, Vol. LV, Proteolytic Enzymes, Part B*, ed L. Lorand (New York, NY: Academic Press), 325–331.

Prados, B., Pena, A., Cotarelo, R. P., Valero, M. C., and Cruces, J. (2007). Expression of the murine Pomt1 gene in both the developing brain and adult muscle tissues and its relationship with clinical aspects of Walker-Warburg syndrome. *Am. J. Pathol.* 170, 1659–1668. doi: 10.2353/ajpath.2007.061264

Ramalho-Santos, J., Moreno, R. D., Wessel, G. M., Chan, E. K., and Schatten, G. (2001). Membrane trafficking machinery components associated with the mammalian acrosome during spermiogenesis. *Exp. Cell Res.* 267, 45–60. doi: 10.1006/excr.2000.5119

Ramalho-Santos, J., Schatten, G., and Moreno, R. D. (2002). Control of membrane fusion during spermiogenesis and the acrosome reaction. *Biol. Reprod.* 67, 1043–1051. doi: 10.1095/biolreprod67.4.1043

Rizo, J., and Südhof, T. C. (2002). Snares and Munc18 in synaptic vesicle fusion. *Nat. Rev. Neurosci.* 3, 641–653. doi: 10.1038/nrn898

Rodríguez, F., Bustos, M. A., Zanetti, M. N., Ruete, M. C., Mayorga, L. S., and Tomes, C. N. (2011). α-SNAP prevents docking of the acrosome during sperm exocytosis because it sequesters monomeric syntaxin. *PLoS ONE* 6:e21925. doi: 10.1371/journal.pone.0021925

Rodríguez, F., Zanetti, M. N., Mayorga, L. S., and Tomes, C. N. (2012). Munc18-1 controls SNARE protein complex assembly during human sperm acrosomal exocytosis. *J. Biol. Chem.* 287, 43825–43839. doi: 10.1074/jbc.M112.409649

Roqueta-Rivera, M., Abbott, T. L., Sivaguru, M., Hess, R. A., and Nakamura, M. T. (2011). Deficiency in the omega-3 fatty acid pathway results in failure of acrosome biogenesis in mice. *Biol. Reprod.* 85, 721–732. doi: 10.1095/biolreprod.110.089524

Russell, L. D., Ettlin, R. A., Hikim, A. P. S., and Clegg, E. D. (1993). Histological and histopathological evaluation of the testis. *Int. J. Androl.* 16, 83–83. doi: 10.1111/j.1365-2605.1993.tb01156.x

Schmidt-Rhaesa, A. (2007). *The Evolution of Organ Systems*. Oxford: Oxford University Press.

Seiji, M., Fitzpatrick, T. B., and Simpson, R. (1963). Chemical composition and terminology of specialized organelles (melanosomes and melanin granules) in mammalian melanocytes. *Nature* 197:1082. doi: 10.1038/1971082a0

Shams-Borhan, G., Huneau, D., and Fléchon, J. E. (1979). Acrosin does not appear to be bound to the inner acrosomal membrane of bull spermatozoa. *J. Exp. Zool.* 209, 143–149. doi: 10.1002/jez.1402090117

Shang, Y.-L., Zhu, F.-X., Yan, J., Chen, L., Tang, W.-H., Xiao, S., et al. (2019). Novel DPY19L2 variants in globozoospermic patients and the overcoming this male infertility. *Asian J. Androl.* 21, 183–189. doi: 10.4103/aja.aja_79_18

Shen, J., Chen, W., Shao, B., Qi, Y., Xia, Z., Wang, F., et al. (2014). Lamin A/C proteins in the spermatid acroplaxome are essential in mouse spermiogenesis. *Reproduction* 148, 479–487. doi: 10.1530/REP-14-0012

Shields, W. M. (1982). *Philopatry, Inbreeding, and the Evolution of Sex*. State University of New York Press.

Shur, B. D. (1998). Is sperm galactosyltransferase a signaling subunit of a multimeric gamete receptor? *Biochem. Biophys. Res. Commun.* 250, 537–543. doi: 10.1006/bbrc.1998.9274

Sidjanin, D., Park, A. K., Ronchetti, A., Martins, J., and Jackson, W. T. (2016). TBC1D20 mediates autophagy as a key regulator of autophagosome maturation. *Autophagy* 12, 1759–1775. doi: 10.1080/15548627.2016.1199300

Simonsen, A., Lippe, R., Christoforidis, S., Gaullier, J.-M., Brech, A., Callaghan, J., et al. (1998). EEA1 links PI (3) K function to Rab5 regulation of endosome fusion. *Nature* 394, 494–498. doi: 10.1038/28879

Stearns, S. C. (2013). *The Evolution of Sex and Its Consequences*. Basel: Birkhäuser.

Suarezquian, C. A., An, Q., Jelesoff, N., and Dym, M. (1991). The Golgi-apparatus of rat pachytene spermatocytes during spermatogenesis. *Anat. Record* 229, 16–26. doi: 10.1002/ar.1092290104

Sun-Wada, G.-H., Imai-Senga, Y., Yamamoto, A., Murata, Y., Hirata, T., Wada, Y., et al. (2002). A proton pump ATPase with testis-specific E1-subunit isoform required for acrosome acidification. *J. Biol. Chem.* 277, 18098–18105. doi: 10.1074/jbc.M111567200

Suryavathi, V., Panneerdoss, S., Wolkowicz, M. J., Shetty, J., Sherman, N. E., Flickinger, C. J., et al. (2015). Dynamic changes in equatorial segment protein 1 (SPESP1) glycosylation during mouse spermiogenesis. *Biol. Reprod.* 92, 121–116. doi: 10.1095/biolreprod.114.121095

Suzuki-Toyota, F., Ito, C., Toyama, Y., Maekawa, M., Yao, R., Noda, T., et al. (2004). The coiled tail of the round-headed spermatozoa appears during epididymal passage in GOPC-deficient mice. *Arch. Histol. Cytol.* 67, 361–371. doi: 10.1679/aohc.67.361

Talbot, P., and Kleve, M. G. (1978). Hamster sperm cross react with antiactin. *J. Exp. Zool.* 204, 131–136. doi: 10.1002/jez.1402040112

Tang, X., Lalli, M., and Clermont, Y. (1982). A cytochemical study of the Golgi apparatus of the spermatid during spermiogenesis in the rat. *Am. J. Anat.* 163, 283–294. doi: 10.1002/aja.1001630402

Töpfer-Petersen, E. (1999). Carbohydrate-based interactions on the route of a spermatozoon to fertilization. *Hum. Reprod. Update* 5, 314–329. doi: 10.1093/humupd/5.4.314

Toshimori, K. (1998). Maturation of mammalian spermatozoa: modifications of the acrosome and plasma membrane leading to fertilization. *Cell Tissue Res.* 293, 177–187. doi: 10.1007/s004410051110

Tsai, P.-S., Garcia-Gil, N., Van Haeften, T., and Gadella, B. M. (2010). How pig sperm prepares to fertilize: stable acrosome docking to the plasma membrane. *PLoS ONE* 5:e11204. doi: 10.1371/journal.pone.0011204

Tulsiani, D. R., Abou-Haila, A., Loeser, C. R., and Pereira, B. M. (1998). The biological and functional significance of the sperm acrosome and acrosomal enzymes in mammalian fertilization. *Exp. Cell Res.* 240, 151–164. doi: 10.1006/excr.1998.3943

Tulsiani, D. R., Yoshida-Komiya, H., and Araki, Y. (1997). Mammalian fertilization: a carbohydrate-mediated event. *Biol. Reprod.* 57, 487–494. doi: 10.1095/biolreprod57.3.487

Ungermann, C., and Langosch, D. (2005). Functions of SNAREs in intracellular membrane fusion and lipid bilayer mixing. *J. Cell Sci.* 118, 3819–3828. doi: 10.1242/jcs.02561

Virtanen, I., Badley, R., Paasivuo, R., and Lehto, V. (1984). Distinct cytoskeletal domains revealed in sperm cells. *J. Cell Biol.* 99, 1083–1091. doi: 10.1083/jcb.99.3.1083

Vitale, A., Ceriotti, A., and Denecke, J. (1993). The role of the endoplasmic-reticulum in protein-synthesis, modification and intracellular-transport. *J. Exp. Bot.* 44, 1417–1444. doi: 10.1093/jxb/44.9.1417

Wang, H., Wan, H., Li, X., Liu, W., Chen, Q., Wang, Y., et al. (2014). Atg7 is required for acrosome biogenesis during spermatogenesis in mice. *Cell Res.* 24, 852–869. doi: 10.1038/cr.2014.70

Wassarman, P. M. (1999). Mammalian fertilization: molecular aspects of gamete adhesion, exocytosis, and fusion. *Cell* 96, 175–183. doi: 10.1016/S0092-8674(00)80558-9

Willer, T., Amselgruber, W., Deutzmann, R., and Strahl, S. (2002). Characterization of POMT2, a novel member of the PMT protein O-mannosyltransferase family specifically localized to the acrosome of mammalian spermatids. *Glycobiology* 12, 771–783. doi: 10.1093/glycob/cwf086

Xiao, N., Kam, C., Shen, C., Jin, W., Wang, J., Lee, K. M., et al. (2009). PICK1 deficiency causes male infertility in mice by disrupting acrosome formation. *J. Clin. Invest.* 119, 802–812. doi: 10.1172/JCI36230

Xu, X., Toselli, P. A., Russell, L. D., and Seldin, D. C. (1999). Globozoospermia in mice lacking the casein kinase II α′ catalytic subunit. *Nat. Genet.* 23, 118–121. doi: 10.1038/12729

Yanagimachi, R. (1994). "Mammalian fertilization," in *The Physiology of Reproduction*, Vol. 1, eds E. Knobil and J. D. Neill (New York, NY: Raven Press), 189–317.

Yanagimachi, R. (2011). Mammalian sperm acrosome reaction: where does it begin before fertilization? *Biol. Reprod.* 85, 4–5. doi: 10.1095/biolreprod.111.092601

Yang, Y., and Li, Z. (2005). Roles of heat shock protein gp96 in the ER quality control: redundant or unique function? *Mol. Cell.* 20, 173–182.

Yang, Z., and Klionsky, D. J. (2009). "An overview of the molecular mechanism of autophagy," in *Autophagy in Infection and Immunity* (Berlin; Heidelberg: Springer), 1–32.

Yao, R., Ito, C., Natsume, Y., Sugitani, Y., Yamanaka, H., Kuretake, S., et al. (2002). Lack of acrosome formation in mice lacking a Golgi protein, GOPC. *Proc. Natl. Acad. Sci. U.S.A.* 99, 11211–11216. doi: 10.1073/pnas.162027899

Yao, R., Maeda, T., Takada, S., and Noda, T. (2001). Identification of a PDZ domain containing Golgi protein, GOPC, as an interaction partner of frizzled. *Biochem. Biophys. Res. Commun.* 286, 771–778. doi: 10.1006/bbrc.2001.5430

Yildiz, Y., Matern, H., Thompson, B., Allegood, J. C., Warren, R. L., Ramirez, D. M., et al. (2006). Mutation of β-glucosidase 2 causes glycolipid storage disease and impaired male fertility. *J. Clin. Invest.* 116, 2985–2994. doi: 10.1172/JCI29224

Yu, Y., Vanhorne, J., and Oko, R. (2009). The origin and assembly of a zona pellucida binding protein, IAM38, during spermiogenesis. *Microsc. Res. Tech.* 72, 558–565. doi: 10.1002/jemt.20696

Zanetti, N., and Mayorga, L. S. (2009). Acrosomal swelling and membrane docking are required for hybrid vesicle formation during the human sperm acrosome reaction. *Biol. Reprod.* 81, 396–405. doi: 10.1095/biolreprod.109.076166

Zaneveld, L., and De Jonge, C. (1991). "Mammalian sperm acrosomal enzymes and the acrosome reaction," in *A Comparative Overview of Mammalian Fertilization* (Springer), 63–79.

Zhao, M., and Brunger, A. T. (2016). Recent advances in deciphering the structure and molecular mechanism of the AAA+ ATPase N-ethylmaleimide-sensitive factor (NSF). *J. Mol. Biol.* 428, 1912–1926. doi: 10.1016/j.jmb.2015.10.026

7

The Role of Sperm Centrioles in Human Reproduction – The Known and the Unknown

Tomer Avidor-Reiss[1,2], Matthew Mazur[1,2], Emily L. Fishman[1] and Puneet Sindhwani[1,2]*

[1] Department of Biological Sciences, College of Natural Sciences and Mathematics, The University of Toledo, Toledo, OH, United States,
[2] Department of Urology, College of Medicine and Life Sciences, The University of Toledo, Toledo, OH, United States

***Correspondence:**
Tomer Avidor-Reiss
tomer.avidorreiss@utoledo.edu

Each human spermatozoon contains two remodeled centrioles that it contributes to the zygote. There, the centrioles reconstitute a centrosome that assembles the sperm aster and participate in pronuclei migration and cleavage. Thus, centriole abnormalities may be a cause of male factor infertility and failure to carry pregnancy to term. However, the precise mechanisms by which sperm centrioles contribute to embryonic development in humans are still unclear, making the search for a link between centriole abnormalities and impaired male fecundity particularly difficult. Most previous investigations into the role of mammalian centrioles during fertilization have been completed in murine models; however, because mouse sperm and zygotes appear to lack centrioles, these studies provide information that is limited in its applicability to humans. Here, we review studies that examine the role of the sperm centrioles in the early embryo, with particular emphasis on humans. Available literature includes case studies and case-control studies, with a few retrospective studies and no prospective studies reported. This literature has provided some insight into the morphological characteristics of sperm centrioles in the zygote and has allowed identification of some centriole abnormalities in rare cases. Many of these studies suggest centriole involvement in early embryogenesis based on phenotypes of the embryo with only indirect evidence for centriole abnormality. Overall, these studies suggest that centriole abnormalities are present in some cases of sperm with asthenoteratozoospermia and unexplained infertility. Yet, most previously published studies have been restricted by the laborious techniques (like electron microscopy) and the limited availability of centriolar markers, resulting in small-scale studies and the lack of solid causational evidence. With recent progress in sperm centriole biology, such as the identification of the unique composition of sperm centrioles and the discovery of the atypical centriole, it is now possible to begin to fill the gaps in sperm centriole epidemiology and to identify the etiology of sperm centriole dysfunction in humans.

Keywords: centriole, sperm, embrio, cilium, centrosome, infertility, male factor, reproduction

INTRODUCTION

Centrioles are essential for animal development and physiology, as demonstrated by a variety of experiments that have tested the centriole's role directly (Bettencourt-Dias et al., 2011). Most of these experiments have been performed *in vitro*, in human immortalized cells, or in animal models, limiting our knowledge of the centriole's role in human reproduction. In general, the centriole's role is expected to be similarly essential in humans because of its conservation throughout animal evolution (Carvalho-Santos et al., 2011). However, the centrioles of sperm and the early embryo of murine animals are exceptions to this evolutionary conservation (**Figure 1**). While humans and many other mammals have centrioles in their spermatozoa and early embryos, mice, rats, and hamsters (the most common experimental mammals) do not have recognizable centrioles in their spermatozoa and early embryos (Schatten et al., 1986; Sathananthan et al., 1996; Phillips et al., 2014). These major differences in centriole appearance raise the question: *What exactly is the role of the centriole in human fertilization and early embryonic development?*

One extreme and unlikely idea is that sperm centrioles are not needed in humans because they are undetectable in mice sperm and appear to be expendable for murine live birth. However, an alternative hypothesis is that mice have evolved a novel biology of sperm and early embryonic centrioles, and, therefore, studying their role in reproduction is not applicable to their role in human reproduction and their clinical implication. Indeed, all studied non-murine mammals *do* have centrioles in their sperm and early embryo, and, in certain animals, some evidence indicates that these centrioles are necessary. Here, we will explore this evidence and the fact that the sperm of humans and non-murine mammals have two centrioles (one with typical structure and one atypical), not one, as was concluded in the past (Avidor-Reiss and Fishman, 2018). We start with a brief general introduction to centrioles, then progress to discussion of sperm and early embryonic centrioles. Then, we describe clinical studies that implicate the centriole in human reproduction. Finally, we propose future directions to resolve the question of the role of the sperm centriole role in the embryo. This review focuses on the role of the mature sperm (spermatozoon) centrioles in the zygote, and it does not address the role of centrioles in germline (spermatogonia, spermatocyte, and meiosis) development [reviewed in Riparbelli and Callaini (2011)].

MOST DIVIDING ANIMAL CELLS HAVE PRECISELY TWO CENTRIOLES WITH A CONSERVED BARREL SHAPE

Centrioles are evolutionarily conserved cellular components essential for fertilization, cell development, and animal physiology through their function in the cell [reviewed in Nigg and Raff (2009)]. The centriole is a cylinder built from nine triplet microtubules arranged in a ring-like formation to form a barrel structure. In the centrosome, the centrioles are surrounded by pericentriolar material (PCM) (Vorobjev and Chentsov Yu, 1982) [reviewed in Lange and Gull (1996), Mennella et al. (2012)]. In cilia and flagella, the centriole triplets are continuous with the doublet microtubules of the axoneme. Centrioles are composed of more than one hundred proteins (Preble et al., 2000) [reviewed in Winey and O'Toole (2014), Nigg and Holland (2018)], and, while new components of centriolar protein structure continue to be discovered, determining their functionality can be a challenge, both because they often have essential roles in early development [reviewed in Schatten and Sun (2010)], and because their function may vary from one cell type to another [previously reviewed in Loncarek and Bettencourt-Dias (2018)].

Most cells have two centrioles during early interphase. Most centrioles form by "duplication," where each of the two-preexisting centrioles direct the formation of one new procentriole, providing a mechanism to control the number of centrioles formed. Centrioles may infrequently form *de novo*, in the absence of preexisting centrioles or in specialized cell types, but often times, this mechanism results in too many centrioles being formed (Loncarek and Khodjakov, 2009; Shahid and Singh, 2018). Progression from a procentriole to a mature centriole correlates with cell-cycle progression (Lange and Gull, 1996). A pair of centrioles is made of the cell's older mother centriole and a younger daughter centriole. As a result, the number of centrioles in the cell oscillates between two centrioles during early interphase and four centrioles during late interphase and mitosis (Fukasawa, 2007).

Centrioles are integral to the cilia, which confer motility and extra-cellular communication potential to the cell. In most cell types, the cilium is formed by the mature centriole within the cell, which is known as the basal body [reviewed in Avidor-Reiss and Gopalakrishnan (2013)]. However, it was recently proposed that in sperm, the flagellum is formed by the younger daughter centriole, but this proposal requires further support (Garanina et al., 2019). Centrioles are also involved in the cell division process, but their contributions vary in distinct cell types. In general, centrioles recruit PCM to form a centrosome. This centrosome associates with microtubules to assemble an aster that localizes to the spindle poles during mitosis. The asters' main function is to determine the axis of cell division and the number of spindle poles (Bobinnec et al., 1998). Interestingly, some animal cells [oocytes, importantly (Calarco et al., 1972)] and many plant cells (Joshi and Palevitz, 1996) lack centrioles. This implies that centrioles are not necessary in all cell types and that some cells can successfully complete mitosis and cellular organization without centriolar influence. Therefore, the significance of centrioles may vary in the several cell types that normally contain them.

HUMAN MATURE OOCYTES HAVE NO CENTRIOLES

Oocytes contain most of the elements necessary for zygotic development (i.e., Golgi, ER, and proteasomes), including centriolar and PCM proteins, but they lack assembled centrioles. Oocyte centrioles are eliminated, either by extrusion or inactivation, during oogenesis in humans and most studied animals (Hertig and Adams, 1967; Sathananthan et al., 1985; Schatten et al., 1986; Pickering et al., 1988; Crozet, 1990; Navara et al., 1994; Crozet et al., 2000) [reviewed in Sathananthan et al. (2006)]. Limited studies have explored the mechanism of oocyte centriole elimination, but they propose a mechanism reliant on some of the same proteins that are involved in centrosome biology, such as PLK1 (Pimenta-Marques et al., 2016). Centriole elimination by the oocyte necessitates contribution of both

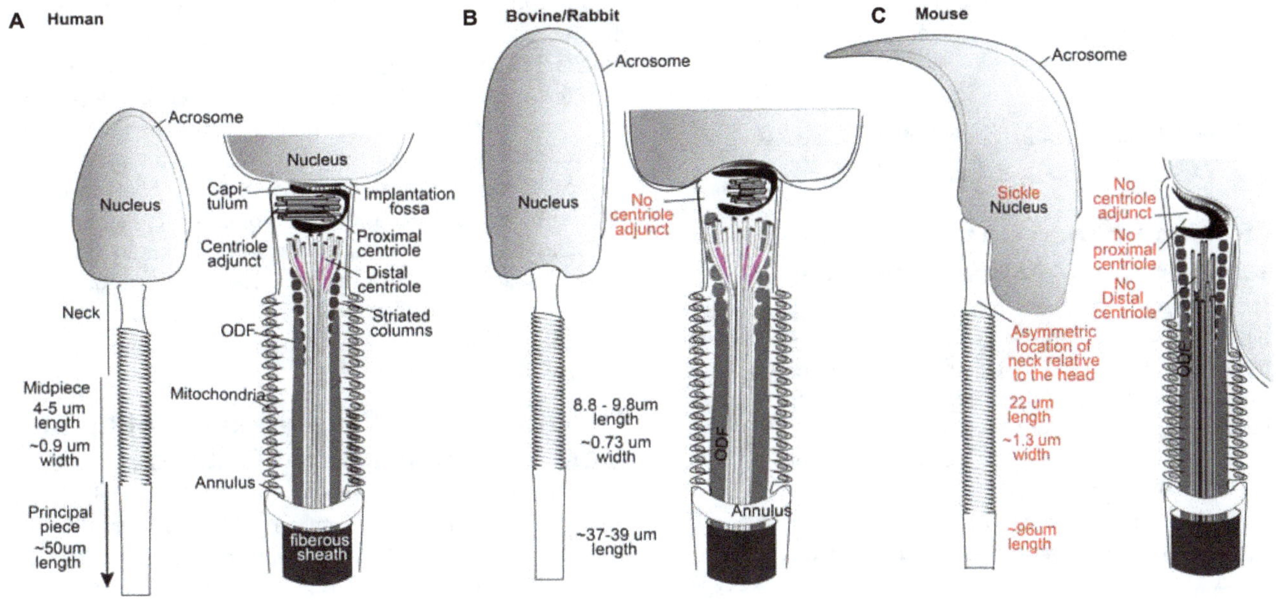

FIGURE 1 | The spermatozoa of human **(A)**, bovine, and rabbit **(B)** share many properties not found in mice **(C)**, including the presence of one typical and one atypical centriole. Drawings are based on electron microscopy of Zamboni and Stefanini (1971), Fawcett (1975), and Ounjai et al. (2012). Mammalian sperm dimensions are from Cummins and Woodall (1985).

spermatozoan centrioles to the zygote to ensure an appropriate number of centrioles in the embryo cell (Connolly et al., 1986; Schatten, 1994; Manandhar et al., 2005; Pimenta-Marques et al., 2016). More information can be found in a recent review on how animal oocytes assemble spindles in the absence of the centriole at Severson et al. (2016).

MOUSE SPERMATOZOON AND ZYGOTE HAVE NO RECOGNIZABLE CENTRIOLES

In mice, centriole inheritance to the embryo diverges from other mammalian models. In mice, centrioles appear to completely degenerate during spermiogenesis (Manandhar et al., 1998), and, as a result, sperm centrioles may not be present within the zygote (Schatten, 1994; Hewitson et al., 1997) (**Figure 1C**). It has been proposed that zygotic centrioles are inherited maternally or form *de novo* (Schatten et al., 1985, 1986, 1991; Gueth-Hallonet et al., 1993; Hewitson et al., 1997). The support for non-paternal inheritance is based on several observations, including: (1) zygotes do not appear to have a dominant sperm aster and, instead, have maternal mini-asters, (2) the sperm axoneme is present in the oocyte but lacks microtubules and shows no association with mitotic poles, (3) centrioles are observed only starting in the 32/64 cell stage of early embryos (Gueth-Hallonet et al., 1993), and (4) intracytoplasmic sperm injection (ICSI) with disassociated sperm nuclei is sufficient for embryo development (Kuretake et al., 1996; Yan et al., 2008). The question of *why* the centrioles of the murine zygote are not inherited from the sperm, as is seen with other mammals, remains unanswered.

PARTHENOGENIC CELLS HAVE AN UNREGULATED NUMBER OF CENTRIOLES

The ability to form a parthenogen (an embryo that is developed from an unfertilized egg that lacks centrioles) and parthenogenic cell lines is often referenced to suggest that sperm centrioles are not essential in mammals. However, it is important to note that mammalian parthenogenesis does not lead to viable offspring (Wininger, 2004). It has been proposed that imprinting defects are the main barrier to viability in mammalian parthenogenesis (Kono, 2006; Miller et al., 2019), but concomitant centriole abnormalities present during mammalian parthenogenesis may also contribute to this barrier.

The importance of sperm centrioles in mammalian parthenogenic embryos is apparent, in that parthenogenic cells have an abnormal number of centrioles, as expected from a *de novo* mechanism of centriole formation (Brevini et al., 2012). In the absence of preexisting centrioles (as would be expected in parthenogenesis), an unregulated number of centrioles is expected to form *de novo* in the activated oocytes or subsequent cell types of the embryo (Hinchcliffe, 2011). The presence of too many or too few centrioles, as is observed in mammalian parthenogenic cell lines, can lead to chromosomal instability and, ultimately, cell death (Sir et al., 2013; Godinho and Pellman, 2014). These centriole abnormalities can partially explain the presence of high levels of chromosomal abnormalities in parthenogenic embryos and their ultimate inability to develop viable offspring (Bhak et al., 2006). Therefore, it is possible that non-murine zygotes need two centrioles to produce a viable embryo, and further study of parthenogenic centrioles is necessary, particularly to determine at what stage they form, how many are formed, and how they function.

MOST MAMMALIAN SPERMATOZOA AND ZYGOTES HAVE CENTRIOLES

The Spermatozoon Neck Has One Typical and One Atypical Centriole

The spermatozoon is a streamlined, motile cell that is made of a head and tail and a neck that contains the two centrioles (**Figure 1**). The head carries half of the genetic material of the embryo, along with proteolytic proteins within the acrosome that help in reaching the oocyte (Cox et al., 2002; Yoon et al., 2008). The tail is a specialized cilium that propels the sperm cell to meet the egg (Basiri et al., 2014; Avidor-Reiss and Leroux, 2015). Spermatozoon morphology is variable across mammals due to evolutionary pressure, making it one of the most diverse cells when compared with the corresponding cell type in other species (Gomendio and Roldan, 2008; Breed et al., 2014). Importantly, a major difference is exhibited between human and mouse spermatozoa. While human sperm, like that of most other mammals, is morphologically broad and flat (spatula-shaped), mouse sperm is curved, long, and narrow (sickle-shaped) (**Figure 1A**). In humans and most other mammals, the tail is attached to the head near its center, but in mice, the attachment is to the side of the head (**Figure 1C**). Also, the tail dimensions are very similar between humans and other mammals, but the mouse tail is about twice the length of that of humans. Mice exhibit substantial evolutionary conservation of many of the critical developmental processes in other mammals and, in general, are a beneficial model. However, the differences described above suggest that some aspects of murine sperm have evolved differently than and away from other mammals, including humans. Therefore, translating information on this topic from mice to humans requires caution.

The human sperm neck contains two centrioles as well as a specialized PCM. The proximal centriole (PC) is found just near the head base, and the distal centriole (DC) is located further from the head, attached to the base of the axoneme (**Figure 1A**). During sperm formation, the PC forms a centriolar adjunct that is thought to organize the development of the neck region and to guide the manchette to form the axis of nuclear flattening (Fawcett and Phillips, 1969; Lehti and Sironen, 2016). At the same time, the DC microtubules extend to form the axonemal microtubules of the tail (Fawcett and Phillips, 1969). The centrioles become embedded in structural material, including the capitulum around the PC, the striated columns filling most of the neck, and the outer dense fibers (ODFs) (**Figure 1A**). The capitulum and the striated columns form a specialized PCM that also contains centrosomal proteins (Fawcett and Phillips, 1969; Fishman et al., 2018).

The mature spermatozoon obtains its unique streamlined morphology and composition during spermiogenesis [reviewed in Avidor-Reiss and Fishman (2018)]. Early spermatids contain both a PC and a DC with typical centriole structure and composition. The fate of the DC and PC during spermatid differentiation into spermatozoa varies according to animal species, but both centrioles are present in mature spermatozoa of humans and most other mammals. The "centriole remodeling" that occurs during differentiation leaves one centriole that maintains a typical structure (the PC) and one that obtains an atypical structure (the DC). This structure consists of splayed microtubules doublets and centrosomal proteins but maintains the ability to function in the zygote (Fishman et al., 2018). What remains unknown is the usefulness, unique function, and fate in the embryo of these remodeled centrioles and specialized PCM.

The Two Sperm Centrioles Function in Most Mammalian Early Embryos

Most dividing cells require two centrioles, each of which localizes to one of the spindle poles that mediate chromatid separation between daughter cells when the cell divides. The same is expected for the first cell of the embryo (the zygote). Also, immediately after sperm-egg fusion, the sperm centrioles form an aster, and, shortly thereafter, the two sperm centrioles undergo "duplication," forming two new daughter centrioles [reviewed in Avidor-Reiss and Fishman (2018)]. Finally, at some point in embryonic development, centrioles are expected to template a primary cilium. While the timing for this is unknown in humans and non-murine animals, in mice, the first primary cilia have been observed in blastocysts with 64–100 cells, only after implantation on epiblast cells (Bangs et al., 2015). Based on these functions, sperm centrioles are widely expected to be essential in the embryo for development.

In many animals, such as worms and fish, centrosome reduction results in the elimination of PCM proteins, with little or no apparent change to centriole structure. In insects, the two centrioles are modified, one slightly and one so dramatically that it was only recently discovered (Gottardo et al., 2015; Khire et al., 2016; Dallai et al., 2017; Fishman et al., 2017). The oocyte contains appropriate PCM material that joins with the spermatozoan centrioles after they are introduced. The necessity of both sperm centrioles and maternal PCM for embryo development has been demonstrated in flies (Blachon et al., 2014), nematodes [reviewed in Leidel and Gonczy (2005)], and fish (Yabe et al., 2007). These publications suggest that in many animals, remodeled sperm centrioles are essential in the embryo, and, therefore, the lack of an integral role for sperm centrioles in mice is an exception.

The paternal inheritance of the PC in the zygote has been well established in several mammalian models. The presence of sperm centrioles in the zygote has been demonstrated in cows (Navara et al., 1994), sheep (Le Guen and Crozet, 1989), primates (Simerly et al., 1995; Wu et al., 1996), and pigs (Kim et al., 1996). However, the essential functions of zygotic centrioles in these models have not been directly demonstrated. Remodeling of zygotic centrioles has been established through ultrastructural and some immunological studies in cows (Long et al., 1993; Navara et al., 1994; Sutovsky et al., 1996; Sutovsky and Schatten, 1997), sheep (Le Guen and Crozet, 1989; Crozet, 1990; Crozet et al., 2000), rabbits (Longo, 1976; Szollosi and Ozil, 1991;

Yllera-Fernandez et al., 1992; Pinto-Correia et al., 1994; Terada et al., 2000), and cats (Comizzoli et al., 2006). More recently, it was shown that cow zygotes also inherit a second atypical centriole (the DC) (Fishman et al., 2018). This inheritance pattern suggests that centrioles *may* play an important role in the developing zygote; however, it is unclear exactly *what* and *how* these centrioles may be contributing.

THE ZYGOTE OF HUMANS INHERITS TWO FUNCTIONAL SPERM CENTRIOLES

Though studies in humans are lacking, two sperm centrioles are likely present in the early zygotes and four during mitosis. The human zygote inherits the PC from sperm, which is well established (Sathananthan et al., 1991). Also, the human zygote is likely to inherit the DC because (1) the spermatozoa have a remodeled DC that is attached to the axoneme (Fishman et al., 2018), and (2) the base of the axoneme is located at one of the spindle poles (Asch et al., 1995; Van Blerkom, 1996; Simerly et al., 1999; Kovacic and Vlaisavljevic, 2000).

Kai et al. (2015) showed the presence of two centrosomes in zygotes with two pronuclei (presumably fertilized by a single sperm) by immunofluorescence staining for centrosomes. Sathananthan et al. (1991) identified centrioles within the centrosomes of zygotes with two pronuclei by electron microscopy following *in vitro* fertilization; two centrosomes with one or two centrioles were observed. Both Kai et al. (2015) and Sathananthan et al. (1991) have observed four centrosomes in early zygotes with three pronuclei, suggesting that dispermic embryos provide extra centrioles that form extra centrosomes. Interestingly, only three and not four spindle poles were observed in these zygotes. The presence of only three poles in dispermic embryos, despite the presence of four centrosomes, raises the question of whether the number of poles is determined by the sperm centrioles or pronuclei. However, these studies are consistent with the idea that human sperm normally contribute two centrioles to the zygote.

After membrane fusion, the centrosome forms one sperm aster near the head, which then enlarges throughout most of the zygote cytoplasm (Van Blerkom, 1996; Simerly et al., 1999). During pronuclear migration, this aster splits into two. Later, each aster localizes to one pole of the forming bipolar mitotic spindle. Interestingly, after initial formation, the asters collapse and are either small or unrecognizable during metaphase. This collapse is transient, as the asters reappear in anaphase. Why asters collapse during metaphase is unknown and needs further investigation.

It is commonly thought that human sperm centrioles are essential for pronuclear migration, based on studies on abnormal sperm asters in the zygote. Immunofluorescence analysis of fertilized zygotes with arrested development has shown disorganized and diminished sperm aster microtubule arrays, along with the lack of pronuclear formation and/or migration (Asch et al., 1995; Van Blerkom, 1996). These concurrent findings suggest that the sperm aster may be responsible for normal pronuclear development. These studies are limited by the fact that microtubules are also nucleated by non-centriolar microtubule-organizing centers, and that, in many of these studies, a defect in the centriole was not found or studied, making the specific role of the centriole and sperm aster in the zygote unclear.

After entering the egg, the PC is thought to be released from the sperm neck structures before recruiting PCM and forming astral microtubules, a process proposed to be mediated by proteasomes (Wojcik et al., 2000; Rawe et al., 2008; Sutovsky, 2018), but it is unknown if the DC is detached from the neck structures. Spermatozoan proteasomes have been localized to the neck region/midpiece in close association with the centrioles; however, relatively little is known about their function. Spermatozoa from humans and bovine, preloaded with function-blocking anti-proteasome antibody, resulted in disrupted sperm aster formation and pronuclear development/apposition of human oocytes, despite the lack of observable centriole structural deficits (Rawe et al., 2008). This suggests that spermatozoan proteasomes may play an important role in centriole contribution to zygote development. More pharmacological and genetic studies should be done to investigate the mechanism and the precise role of the proteasome in sperm and zygote centrioles.

EPIDEMIOLOGICAL EVIDENCE FOR CENTRIOLE CONTRIBUTION TO HUMAN FERTILITY

Sperm with impaired centrioles were long thought to result in embryos with abnormal cleavage and infertility (Sathananthan, 1994; Schatten, 1994). This idea is now widely accepted and is supported by some epidemiological studies using artificial insemination to overcome barriers to fertilization in defective sperm samples. However, this idea is based on few studies, which analyzed 1–10 patients and few fertile donors as a control (**Table 1**). The phenotypes observed in these studies are diverse, providing opportunity for many inferences but making direct correlation with centriole phenotype difficult. Also, many studies are complicated by the presence of other defects in the sperm (in addition to the centriole), which may have a significant impact on the embryo phenotype. In particular, one can expect that some forms of centriolar defect may originate early in germline development and will result in abnormal DNA content due to abnormities in mitosis or meiosis in addition to the centriole defect, as was found for the mutation in the centriolar protein Centrobin (Liška et al., 2009). Unfortunately, these drawbacks negatively impact the confidence that we have in inferring the role of the sperm centriole in embryo development. However, the totality of these studies suggests that sperm centrioles are likely essential for normal embryo development.

Intracytoplasmic sperm injection is a useful treatment for male infertility due to interference with sperm translocation to the egg and fusion with it, but not for infertility due to dysfunction of sperm components that are needed after fusion (Palermo et al., 1992). Indeed, ICSI allows successful fertilization for many couples, but this may require multiple attempts, and, in many other couples, this fails [reviewed in Neri et al. (2014)].

TABLE 1 | Parameters of various studies of direct sperm phenotype dysfunctions.

Study	Male patient (n)	Female partner	Control men (n)	Sperm morphology and method	Total sperm count (million)	Sperm volume (mL)	Sperm concentration (million/mL)	Sperm motility (%)	Progressive motility (%)	Sperm viability (%)
Normal sperm reference values World Health Organization [WHO], 2010				>4	>39	>1.5	>15	>40	>32	>58
Nakamura et al., 2002	1 man 38-year-old		2	90% **Globozoospermic:** IF		2.5	12	41.7		
Chemes et al., 1999	10 sterile men			**Head-neck defect**: TEM; nine patients had 75–100% spermatozoa with minute cephalic ends and 0–25% abnormal head-middle piece attachments.			Oligozoospermia	Ranged from normal to severe asthenozoospermia (3–60% total motility		
Rawe et al., 2002	1 man 36-year-old	31-year-old, normal ovarian function	1	**Head-neck defect**: TEM				Total asthenozoospermia		
Porcu et al., 2003	2 brothers #1: 25 and #2: 36-year-old	#1: 24-year-old, irregular menses, normal hysterosalpingography and hormonal assessment #2: 31-year-old, regular menses, normal hysterosalpingography and hormonal assessment	2	#1: 100% **teratozoospermia**; 71% tail-less heads #2: 98–100% **teratozoospermia:** TEM + IF; 45–83% of isolated heads; 6–29% with head-tail misalignment;	#1:		#1: 1–1.7 normal sperm + 7.9–16.8 acephalic sperm #2: 4.5 normal sperm); + 0.5 tail-less heads) + 4.5–34 isolated motile tails	#1: 15–30 #2: 10–20	#1: no progressive motility #2: no progressive motility	
Emery et al., 2004	1 man 50-year-old	45-year-old, possible decreased ovarian reserve	1	**Easily decapitated sperm:** TEM; 23% normal head forms and 2% normal tail forms		2.5	33		13	
Sha et al., 2017	1 man 30-year-old		few	**MMAF:** Teratozoospermia		2.9	20	1.8 Asthenozoospermia		
Fonttis et al., 2002	1 man 39-year-old	31-year-old, healthy with no prior pregnancy	0	13% normal; 93% axonemal alterations (TEM); 90% abnormal mitochondrial sheaths (IF)		3	64^{6}	15 **Asthenozoospermia;**	5	
Terada et al., 2009	1 man 35-year-old	31-year-old, normal fertility	3	normal	12	2	6	27 **Oligoasthenozoospermia**		

(Continued)

TABLE 1 | Continued

Study	Male patient (n)	Female partner	Control men (n)	Sperm morphology and method	Total sperm count (million)	Sperm volume (mL)	Sperm concentration (million/mL)	Sperm motility (%)	Progressive motility (%)	Sperm viability (%)
Moretti et al., 2019	1 man-year-old		2	**Globozoospermia**						
Garanina et al., 2019	2 men #1 41-year-old #2 34-year-old	Normal	5	**Unexplained**; normal	Normal	Normal	Normal	Normal	Normal	Normal
Moretti et al., 2017	1 man 37-year-old	35-year-old Normal	1	55% **head-tail defect**: TEM + IF; 26% completely detached heads; 19% isolated tails		2.5–3.5	12–16	0		

IF, immunofluorescence; TEM, transmission electron microscopy.

This suggests that in these failed cases, infertility may be caused by processes downstream of gamete fusion that depend on the male contribution. However, the multifactorial nature of reduced semen quality has prevented many of the underlying contributory molecular mechanisms from being fully elucidated.

The only routine clinical assay to assess sperm phenotype is semen analysis, and this assay by itself cannot implicate the sperm centriole in infertility. Semen analysis compares the quality of the patient's semen and sperm against several standardized parameters and helps identify specific defects in the male which are seen in up to one-third of infertile couples (Isidori et al., 2006) (**Table 1**). One group of sperm defects with several phenotypes that could originate from centriolar defect is idiopathic male factors (male infertility due to a sperm defect that has no explanation, i.e., when the male is infertile despite having normal semen analysis, history, and physical examination, and when female factor infertility has been ruled out) (Chemes and Rawe, 2010). For example, it was suggested that abnormal centrioles will form an abnormal sperm tail (which is one phenotype of teratozoospermia, defined as presence of sperm with abnormal morphology), a defective sperm axoneme resulting in poor motility (asthenozoospermia), or a combination of the two (asthenoteratozoospermia). Some of these cases of male factor infertility may be due to a subtle sperm centriolar defect–a hypothesis that will be examined in the following sections.

Asthenoteratozoospermia

Extremely abnormal sperm morphology can inhibit spermatozoan movement through the female reproductive tract and prevent fusion with the oocyte. These morphological abnormalities have many causes and take many forms, and their definition is controversial, but they can be present in ~10% of infertile men (Khan et al., 2011). As described below, some of these cases are suggested to be caused by or accompanied by a centriolar defect, but these defects have not been fully elucidated.

Head-Neck Defect

Head-neck defects characterized by separated heads and tails provide the strongest evidence that human centrioles are essential for fertility; however, this evidence does have some limitations. In mice, injection of the sperm nucleus without the sperm tail results in a fertilized egg that produces offspring, suggesting that mouse sperm centrioles are dispensable (Kuretake et al., 1996). In contrast, in humans, injection of the sperm nucleus without the sperm tail is insufficient to produce offspring (Palermo et al., 1997; Emery et al., 2004). This may suggest that centriolar absence is the reason for infertility, but this interpretation is limited by the fact that other components in the tail may be essential for embryo development in humans. For example, it was recently shown that MicroRNA-34c localizes to the sperm neck and is required for the first cleavage division (Liu W.-M. et al., 2012; Fereshteh et al., 2018). Therefore, it is not possible in these types of experiments to disentangle the phenotypical consequences of not providing paternal centrioles from that of not delivering other factors essential in the zygote.

The centriole-containing sperm neck is the mechanically weakest part of the sperm. Externally applied pressure may cause the sperm neck to break, forming two fragments: a head fragment and a neck-tail fragment (Firat-Karalar et al., 2014). Indeed, decapitated sperm often breaks between the head and tail and only more rarely at the midpiece (Baccetti et al., 1989; Rawe et al., 2002; Porcu et al., 2003; Gambera et al., 2010). Another rare form of break is caused by disassociation between the PC and DC (Holstein et al., 1986). A variety of structural abnormalities have been observed in sperm with head-neck defect, but their causes are still not well understood. Easily decapitated sperm syndrome is one of the mildest subtypes of head-neck defect teratozoospermia, as some heads and tails in the ejaculate remain connected (Perotti et al., 1981; Toyama et al., 2000). Electron microscopy of decapitated sperm often reveals an absent basal plate and/or implantation fossa with observable breaks between the head and tail (Baccetti et al., 1989) (**Figure 2**). Injection of individual or separated sperm parts allows oocyte activation and pronucleus formation but does not facilitate pronuclear migration and fusion, leading to abnormal embryos (Colombero et al., 1996). Embryos injected with dissected isolated sperm tails or separated heads and tails show chromosome mosaicism, suggesting centrosome and centriole dysfunction (Palermo et al., 1997). However, overall, ICSI has mixed outcomes with easily decapitated sperm, sometimes overcoming infertility but many other times failing despite good embryo morphology (Kamal et al., 1999; Saias-Magnan et al., 1999).

Chemes et al. (1999; **Table 1**) used electron microscopy of testicular biopsies from patients with this defect to show that the forming sperm tail developed uncharacteristically independent of the nucleus, a phenomenon which can be caused by a centriolar defect. Rawe et al. (2002; **Table 1**) used immunofluorescence of human spermatozoa with this defect injected into bovine oocytes to show scarce centrosome-associated microtubules and arrested sperm asters, as compared to fertile donor controls that formed sperm asters in a majority of samples. Ejaculated spermatozoa from patients were also injected into human metaphase II oocytes and analyzed by immunofluorescence. No pronuclei fusion or zygote cleavage occurred with the first attempt. The following three attempts selectively injected sperm with near-normal head-neck alignment; they resulted in fusion and cleavage, but the embryos failed to develop into pregnancy. Emery et al. (2004; **Table 1**) performed ICSI with easily decapitated sperm and reported a successful birth when the separated tails were placed immediately next to the sperm head within the oocyte. The authors surmised that careful integration of all parts of the sperm (head and tail) during ICSI ensured that centrioles, which are likely lost in other less delicate techniques, are included and ultimately allow normal development of the oocyte. Indeed (**Table 1**), successful pregnancies can be achieved by ICSI using intact sperm from men with abnormal head-tail junction (Porcu et al., 2003; Gambera et al., 2010).

ICSI With Sperm Tail Abnormality (MMAF)

Multiple morphological abnormalities of the flagella (MMAF) is a rare form of asthenoteratozoospermia known to cause male infertility (Wang et al., 2019). MMAF is caused by mutations in proteins of the axoneme or transport the mechanism that forms it [e.g., inner-arm heavy chain DNAH1 (Ben Khelifa et al., 2014), or the intraflagellar transport (IFT)-associated protein TTC21A (Liu et al., 2019)] an estimated 50% or more of the molecular mechanisms behind MMAF are yet to be identified. Recently, a sporadic defect in the centriolar protein CEP135 was found to contribute to MMAF (**Table 1**). Sha et al. (2017) identified an inherited missense homozygous mutation in CEP135 in an infertile male with MMAF. Immunofluorescence analysis showed that CEP135 localized to the PC in normal spermatozoa, while the patient's mutated proteins localized elsewhere in the sperm, forming ectopic aggregates in the sperm neck and flagella (**Figure 2**). Following ICSI, embryos demonstrated pronucleus formation and cleavage, but ultimately the mother failed to become pregnant. This suggests that a centriole abnormality can produce a phenotype that is exhibited later in embryogenesis.

Dysplasia of the Fibrous Sheath

The fibrous sheath is a structure surrounding the axoneme in the flagellar principle piece (**Figure 2**). Dysplasia of the fibrous sheath is a rare condition of immotile sperm, which have morphological deformities in the neck, midpiece, and tail and exhibit centriolar dysfunction. Microscopy of dysplastic sperm reveals an increased and disorganized fibrous sheath with disruption of the underlying axoneme (Chemes et al., 1987a). Immunofluorescence with the centriolar protein Centrin-1 shows frequent abnormal positioning of the centrioles, sometimes with duplication, resulting in two nucleus-implantation sites (Moretti et al., 2017). Initial attempts at ICSI with dysplastic sperm were unsuccessful at achieving pregnancy, due to failure of either fertilization or embryo development (Chemes and Rawe, 2003). Nakamura et al. (2005) used bovine oocytes for heterologous ICSI and found that the vast majority of injected oocytes showed no immunocytochemical evidence of sperm aster formation or cytoplasmic microtubule organization. This is consistent with the observation that only 2% of the dysplastic sperm expressed the centriolar protein centrin at the midpiece. Failure to form sperm asters in the setting of severely diminished centrin expression strongly suggests that the sperm centrioles are either abnormal or missing. Therefore, it seems likely that centriole abnormality is contributing to infertility in some of these patients.

Globozoospermia

Globozoospermia is a rare condition describing spermatozoa with a round head and disorganized mid-piece that lack both a functional acrosome and acrosomal enzymes (Singh, 1992). An absent acrosome prevents penetration of the oocyte zona pellucida, and was originally believed to be the sole cause of infertility in affected spermatozoa (Rybouchkin et al., 1996). The rate of successful fertilization with ICSI for men with globozoospermia is lower than the general ICSI success rate [reviewed in Dam et al. (2007)], suggesting that there may be additional problems with reproductive machinery that are not overcome by ICSI. Centriole dysfunction may help explain this discrepancy. Indeed, globozoospermic sperm appear to have centriole dysfunction, based on heterologous

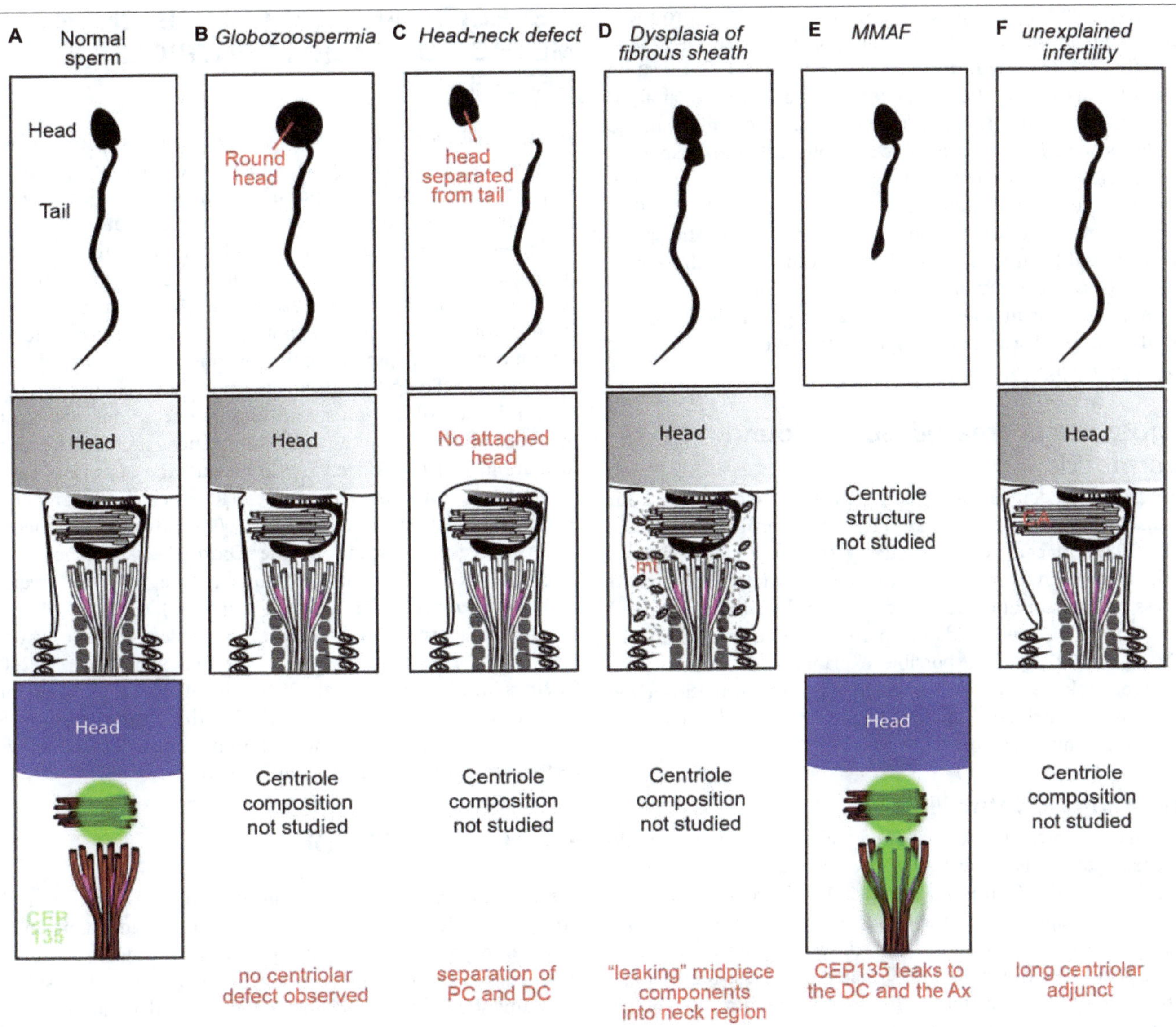

FIGURE 2 | Examples of spermatozoan morphology, structure, and protein distributions in a fertile donor **(A)**, oligospermia **(B)**, head-neck defect **(C)**, DFS **(D)**, MMAF **(E)**, and unexplained infertility **(F)**.

ICSI with bovine oocytes [reviewed in Dam et al. (2007)] (**Table 1**) as well as bio-fluorescent staining of Centrin-1 (Moretti et al., 2019). For example, Nakamura et al. (2002) found that globozoospermic sperm demonstrated a significantly lower rate of sperm aster formation compared to control fertile donor sperm, suggesting a centrosome dysfunction. However, these also showed a significantly lower rate of male pronucleus formation and a significantly higher rate of prematurely condensed chromosomes, suggesting a more pleiotropic mechanism. Many papers show that globozoospermic sperm centrioles have normal ultrastructure, but the composition has yet to be fully investigated. However, due to the heterologous nature of globozoospermia, the discovery of the atypical DC, and the functional data showing poor aster formation in globozoospermia embryos, we propose that more work is necessary to test whether or not malformed centrioles may be implicated in this disease.

Asthenozoospermia

Poor sperm motility seen in asthenozoospermia impedes proper transport of spermatozoa to the oocyte for penetration and membrane fusion. Theoretically, this infertility should be completely resolved by ICSI since the spermatozoa are artificially transported to within the oocyte. However, the low rate of successful pregnancies with ICSI in the setting of complete asthenozoospermia suggests the presence of additional factors (Nagy et al., 1995; Casper et al., 1996; Kahraman et al., 1996; Nijs et al., 1996; Cayan et al., 2001; Fonttis et al., 2002; Chatzimeletiou et al., 2007; Terada et al., 2009). Immunocytochemical analysis of oocytes which had failed fertilization by an asthenozoospermic donor showed several phenotypes, including two pronuclei without the presence of recognizable sperm aster formation, suggesting centrosomal dysfunction had caused fertilization arrest (Terada et al., 2009). Western blot and ELISA analysis found that the centriolar protein centrin and the centriolar and flagellar protein Tektin 2 are reduced in oligoasthenozoospermic men, suggesting that their lower levels can result in lower pregnancy percentage after ICSI (Hinduja et al., 2008, 2010; Bhilawadikar et al., 2013). Also, recently, the base of the sperm tail was found to function as an atypical centriole in the zygote (Avidor-Reiss and Fishman, 2018). Thus, centriolar dysfunction may not only impair sperm motility as originally believed but may also cause a disruption of zygotic intracellular processes that ICSI cannot remedy.

Azoospermia Treated Using Round Spermatids

Azoospermia is defined as the complete absence of sperm from the ejaculate and is present in ~15% of infertile men (Jarow et al., 1989). It can be treated using spermatids or testicular spermatozoa. However, the use of round spermatids has limited success, and fertilization rates were lower than those obtained using elongating spermatids or spermatozoa [discussed in Liu X.-Y. et al. (2012)]. One possible explanation is that the two sperm centrioles are not yet remodeled in round spermatids. How the status of centriolar remodeling affects embryo development needs further investigation.

Unexplained Infertility

Unexplained infertility, the absence of any observable male or female factor, is known to cause infertility in 10–30% of cases (Hart, 2003; Gunn and Bates, 2016). Recently, Garanina et al. (2019) suggested that a longer sperm centriolar adjunct is associated with unexplained infertility. They found through transmission electron microscopy that the average total length of the PC and its centriolar adjunct was significantly longer in the spermatozoa of two unexplained infertility patients than in the spermatozoa of five healthy donors. The two affected patients displayed repeated zygotic arrest after *in vitro* fertilization. One patient had a centriolar adjunct nearly double the length seen in healthy donors and failed all fertility treatments. The second patient with intermediate findings (~1.5 longer) finally conceived a healthy baby that was delivered at 40 weeks of gestation. Ultimately, the function of the centriolar adjunct is still unknown. In all mammals except for human, the centriolar adjunct is a transient structure present during spermiogenesis but absent in the mature spermatozoon (**Figure 2**). In human spermatozoa, the centriolar adjunct is present and was postulated to be characteristic of relative immaturity of the human sperm (Zamboni and Stefanini, 1971). Therefore, it is unclear if centriolar adjuncts are essential only in humans, if a long centriolar adjunct causes a problem, or if the long adjunct is a marker for other defects in the centrioles. Further study of the association between centriolar adjuncts and fertility outcome is needed.

A SPECIFIC AND RAPID ASSESSMENT METHOD OF SPERM CENTRIOLES IS NEEDED

Several assays for studying typical sperm centrioles are available. However, the technology is either insufficiently specific or inappropriately laborious. Sperm cell centrioles has been assessed by electron microscopy, a laborious technique that is inadequate for large-scale studies and is inaccessible in most clinical settings (Chemes et al., 1987b; Moretti et al., 2016). Sperm centriolar protein content has been assessed by Western blot, which studied total protein and is not specific to the centriole and cannot conclusively implicate the centriole in infertility (Hinduja et al., 2010). Sperm centriole function has been assessed by microinjection of human sperm into bovine, rabbit, or hamster oocytes followed by immunofluorescence staining for aster formation, which has been useful in studying abnormal sperm centrioles in some infertility cases (Rawe et al., 2002; Terada et al., 2004; Yoshimoto-Kakoi et al., 2008). However, this method is now illegal according to the Dickey-Wicker amendment (the U.S. federal bill that prohibits funding for the creation of human embryos for research purposes). Because of these limitations, sperm centriole defect in infertile men has only been demonstrated in small case studies (Nanassy and Carrell, 2008; Chemes, 2012; Moretti et al., 2016; Sha et al., 2017). Therefore, there is a need for a specific and high-throughput method for assessing sperm centrioles and determining their association with certain embryonic phenotypes and outcomes.

FUTURE DIRECTIONS

Previous animal and epidemiological studies of sperm centrioles provide a basis for a correlation between centriole abnormality and embryo development pathology; however, further investigation is needed for conclusiveness on this subject. This investigation should include new model mammals and more conclusive clinical research.

Since mice do not have detectable centrioles in the sperm and early embryo, other mammalian models with these centrioles should be developed. For instance, centriole inheritance in rabbits resembles that of humans, and they are suitable models because they are the smallest non-murine mammal with established genetic engineering (Liu et al., 2004; Terada, 2007). The generation of a model rabbit for studying centriole-based infertility would be very useful; however, to do so, the tools necessary for specifically interfering with the sperm centriole must first be identified. Characterizing the mechanisms of sperm centriole formation and function as well as their unique properties will provide the insights necessary to develop these tools. CRISPR/Cas9 editing can be used to alter sperm-specific sequences, which will enable the development of a specific model animal.

Despite the correlation between centriole dysfunction and infertility that has been proposed in the epidemiological literature, the extent and significance of this relationship is still not known. The main reason is that most human studies to date have not demonstrated a clear case of specific centriole dysfunction. Therefore, a diagnostic test should be developed to better identify sperm with specific centriolar defect. Also, because such defect is likely to affect only a small fraction of all infertility cases, the diagnostic test needs to be easy and rapid. One additional approach for improving epidemiological studies is to include advanced semen analysis that examines DNA and egg activation factors, followed by testing sperm that have only centriolar defect. Ultimately, these efforts should lead to more conclusive clinical research, such as large prospective cohort studies and randomized controlled trials.

Sperm centriole defect may be mediated by genetic, environmental, or infectious factors; however, no directed effort has been made to identify these factors. Therefore, there is a need to identify sperm centriole defect in human, to find their cause, and to characterize its impact on male infertility.

AUTHOR CONTRIBUTIONS

TA-R conceived, supervised, and wrote the manuscript. MM wrote the manuscript and searched the literature. EF prepared the figures. PS performed the clinical perspective.

FUNDING

This work was supported by grants R03 HD087429 and R21 HD092700 from the Eunice Kennedy Shriver National Institute of Child Health and Human Development (NICHD).

ACKNOWLEDGMENTS

We would like to thank Nahshon Puente and Katerina Turner for assistance in preparing the manuscript.

REFERENCES

Asch, R., Simerly, C., Ord, T., Ord, V. A., and Schatten, G. (1995). The stages at which human fertilization arrests: microtubule and chromosome configurations in inseminated oocytes which failed to complete fertilization and development in humans. *Hum. Reprod.* 10, 1897–1906. doi: 10.1093/oxfordjournals.humrep.a136204

Avidor-Reiss, T., and Fishman, E. L. (2018). It takes two (centrioles) to tango. *Reproduction* doi: 10.1530/REP-18-0350 [Epub ahead of print].

Avidor-Reiss, T., and Gopalakrishnan, J. (2013). Building a centriole. *Curr. Opin. Cell Biol.* 25, 72–77. doi: 10.1016/j.ceb.2012.10.016

Avidor-Reiss, T., and Leroux, M. R. (2015). Shared and distinct mechanisms of compartmentalized and cytosolic ciliogenesis. *Curr. Biol.* 25, R1143–R1150. doi: 10.1016/j.cub.2015.11.001

Baccetti, B., Burrini, A. G., Collodel, G., Magnano, A. R., Piomboni, P., Renieri, T., et al. (1989). Morphogenesis of the decapitated and decaudated sperm defect in two brothers. *Gamete Res.* 23, 181–188. doi: 10.1002/mrd.1120230205

Bangs, F. K., Schrode, N., Hadjantonakis, A.-K., and Anderson, K. V. (2015). Lineage specificity of primary cilia in the mouse embryo. *Nat. Cell Biol.* 17, 113–122. doi: 10.1038/ncb3091

Basiri, M. L., Ha, A., Chadha, A., Clark, N. M., Polyanovsky, A., Cook, B., et al. (2014). A migrating ciliary gate compartmentalizes the site of axoneme assembly in *Drosophila* spermatids. *Curr. Biol.* 24, 2622–2631. doi: 10.1016/j.cub.2014.09.047

Ben Khelifa, M., Coutton, C., Zouari, R., Karaouzene, T., Rendu, J., Bidart, M., et al. (2014). Mutations in DNAH1, which encodes an inner arm heavy chain dynein, lead to male infertility from multiple morphological abnormalities of the sperm flagella. *Am. J. Hum. Genet.* 94, 95–104. doi: 10.1016/j.ajhg.2013.11.017

Bettencourt-Dias, M., Hildebrandt, F., Pellman, D., Woods, G., and Godinho, S. A. (2011). Centrosomes and cilia in human disease. *Trends Genet.* 27, 307–315. doi: 10.1016/j.tig.2011.05.004

Bhak, J.-S., Lee, S.-L., Ock, S.-A., Choe, S.-Y., and Rho, G.-J. (2006). Developmental rate and ploidy of embryos produced by nuclear transfer with different activation treatments in cattle. *Animal Reprod. Sci.* 92, 37–49. doi: 10.1016/j.anireprosci.2005.04.016

Bhilawadikar, R., Zaveri, K., Mukadam, L., Naik, S., Kamble, K., Modi, D., et al. (2013). Levels of Tektin 2 and CatSper 2 in normozoospermic and oligoasthenozoospermic men and its association with motility, fertilization rate, embryo quality and pregnancy rate. *J. Assist. Reprod. Genet.* 30, 513–523. doi: 10.1007/s10815-013-9972-6

Blachon, S., Khire, A., and Avidor-Reiss, T. (2014). The origin of the second centriole in the zygote of *Drosophila melanogaster*. *Genetics* 197, 199–205. doi: 10.1534/genetics.113.160523

Bobinnec, Y., Khodjakov, A., Mir, L. M., Rieder, C. L., Edde, B., and Bornens, M. (1998). Centriole disassembly in vivo and its effect on centrosome structure and function in vertebrate cells. *J. Cell Biol.* 143, 1575–1589. doi: 10.1083/jcb.143.6.1575

Breed, W. G., Leigh, C. M., Aplin, K. P., Shahin, A. A., and Avenant, N. L. (2014). Morphological diversity and evolution of the spermatozoon in the mouse-related clade of rodents. *J. Morphol.* 275, 540–547. doi: 10.1002/jmor.20236

Brevini, T., Pennarossa, G., Vanelli, A., Maffei, S., and Gandolfi, F. (2012). Parthenogenesis in non-rodent species: developmental competence and differentiation plasticity. *Theriogenology* 77, 766–772. doi: 10.1016/j.theriogenology.2011.11.010

Calarco, P. G., Donahue, R. P., and Szollosi, D. (1972). Germinal vesicle breakdown in the mouse oocyte. *J. Cell Sci.* 10, 369–385.

Carvalho-Santos, Z., Azimzadeh, J., Pereira-Leal, J. B., and Bettencourt-Dias, M. (2011). Evolution: tracing the origins of centrioles, cilia, and flagella. *J. Cell Biol.* 194, 165–175. doi: 10.1083/jcb.201011152

Casper, R. F., Meriano, J. S., Jarvi, K. A., Cowan, L., and Lucato, M. L. (1996). The hypo-osmotic swelling test for selection of viable sperm for intracytoplasmic sperm injection in men with complete asthenozoospermia. *Fertil. Steril.* 65, 972–976. doi: 10.1016/s0015-0282(16)58271-5

Cayan, S., Conaghan, J., Schriock, E. D., Ryan, I. P., Black, L. D., and Turek, P. J. (2001). Birth after intracytoplasmic sperm injection with use of testicular sperm from men with Kartagener/immotile cilia syndrome. *Fertil. Steril.* 76, 612–614. doi: 10.1016/s0015-0282(01)01974-4

Chatzimeletiou, K., Rutherford, A., Griffin, D. K., and Handyside, A. H. (2007). Is the sperm centrosome to blame for the complex polyploid chromosome patterns observed in cleavage stage embryos from an OAT patient? *Zygote* 15,81–90.

Chemes, E. H., and Rawe, Y. V. (2003). Sperm pathology: a step beyond descriptive morphology. Origin, characterization and fertility potential of abnormal sperm phenotypes in infertile men. *Hum. Reprod. Update* 9, 405–428. doi: 10.1093/humupd/dmg034

Chemes, H. E. (2012). "Sperm centrioles and their dual role in flagellogenesis and cell cycle of the Zygote," in *The Centrosome: Cell and Molecular Mechanisms of Functions and Dysfunctions in Disease*, ed. H. Schatten, (Totowa, NJ: Humana Press), 33–48. doi: 10.1007/978-1-62703-035-9_2

Chemes, H. E., Brugo, S., Zanchetti, F., Carrere, C., and Lavieri, J. C. (1987a). Dysplasia of the fibrous sheath: an ultrastructural defect of human spermatozoa associated with sperm immotility and primary sterility. *Fertil. Steril.* 48, 664–669. doi: 10.1016/s0015-0282(16)59482-5

Chemes, H. E., Carizza, C., Scarinci, F., Brugo, S., Neuspiller, N., and Schwarsztein, L. (1987b). Lack of a head in human spermatozoa from sterile patients: a syndrome associated with impaired fertilization. *Fertil. Steril.* 47, 310–316. doi: 10.1016/s0015-0282(16)50011-9

Chemes, H. E., Puigdomenech, E. T., Carizza, C., Olmedo, S. B., Zanchetti, F., and Hermes, R. (1999). Acephalic spermatozoa and abnormal development of the head-neck attachment: a human syndrome of genetic origin. *Hum. Reprod.* 14, 1811–1818. doi: 10.1093/humrep/14.7.1811

Chemes, H. E., and Rawe, V. Y. (2010). The making of abnormal spermatozoa: cellular and molecular mechanisms underlying pathological spermiogenesis. *Cell Tissue Res.* 341, 349–357. doi: 10.1007/s00441-010-1007-3

Colombero, L., Moomjy, M., Rosenwaks, Z., and Palermo, G. (1996). Indirect evidence of centrosome and spindle development in embryos generated by sperm segments. *Hum. Reprod.* 11, 21–22.

Comizzoli, P., Wildt, D. E., and Pukazhenthi, B. S. (2006). Poor centrosomal function of cat testicular spermatozoa impairs embryo development in vitro after intracytoplasmic sperm injection. *Biol. Reprod.* 75, 252–260. doi: 10.1095/biolreprod.106.051342

Connolly, J. A., Kiosses, B. W., and Kalnins, V. I. (1986). Centrioles are lost as embryonic myoblasts fuse into myotubes in vitro. *Eur. J. Cell Biol.* 39, 341–345.

Cox, L. J., Larman, M. G., Saunders, C. M., Hashimoto, K., Swann, K., and Lai, F. A. (2002). Sperm phospholipase Czeta from humans and cynomolgus monkeys triggers Ca2+ oscillations, activation and development of mouse oocytes. *Reproduction* 124, 611–623. doi: 10.1530/reprod/124.5.611

Crozet, N. (1990). Behavior of the sperm centriole during sheep oocyte fertilization. *Eur. J. Cell Biol.* 53, 326–332.

Crozet, N., Dahirel, M., and Chesne, P. (2000). Centrosome inheritance in sheep zygotes: centrioles are contributed by the sperm. *Microsc. Res. Tech.* 49, 445–450. doi: 10.1002/(SICI)1097-0029(20000601)49:5<445::AID-JEMT6>3.0.CO;2-B

Cummins, J., and Woodall, P. (1985). On mammalian sperm dimensions. *Reproduction* 75, 153–175. doi: 10.1530/jrf.0.0750153

Dallai, R., Mercati, D., Lino-Neto, J., Dias, G., and Lupetti, P. (2017). Evidence of a procentriole during spermiogenesis in the coccinellid insect *Adalia decempunctata* (L): an ultrastructural study. *Arthropod. Struct. Dev.* 46, 815–823. doi: 10.1016/j.asd.2017.10.004

Dam, A. H., Feenstra, I., Westphal, J. R., Ramos, L., van Golde, R. J., Kremer, J. A. (2007). Globozoospermia revisited. *Hum. Reprod. Update* 13, 63–75. doi: 10.1093/humupd/dml047

Emery, B. R., Thorp, C., Malo, J. W., and Carrell, D. T. (2004). Pregnancy from intracytoplasmic sperm injection of a sperm head and detached tail. *Fertil. Steril.* 81, 686–688. doi: 10.1016/j.fertnstert.2003.07.025

Fawcett, D. W. (1975). The mammalian spermatozoon. *Dev. Biol.* 44, 394–436. doi: 10.1016/0012-1606(75)90411-x

Fawcett, D. W., and Phillips, D. M. (1969). The fine structure and development of the neck region of the mammalian spermatozoon. *Anat. Rec.* 165, 153–164. doi: 10.1002/ar.1091650204

Fereshteh, Z., Schmidt, S. A., Al-Dossary, A. A., Accerbi, M., Arighi, C., Cowart, J., et al. (2018). Murine Oviductosomes (OVS) microRNA profiling during the estrous cycle: Delivery of OVS-borne microRNAs to sperm where miR-34c-5p localizes at the centrosome. *Sci. Rep.* 8:16094. doi: 10.1038/s41598-018-34409-4

Firat-Karalar, E. N., Sante, J., Elliott, S., and Stearns, T. (2014). Proteomic analysis of mammalian sperm cells identifies new components of the centrosome. *J. Cell Sci.* 127, 4128–4133. doi: 10.1242/jcs.157008

Fishman, E., Jo, K., Ha, A., Royfman, R., Zinn, A., Krishnamurthy, M., et al. (2017). Atypical centrioles are present in *Tribolium* sperm. *Open. Biol.* 7:160334. doi: 10.1098/rsob.160334

Fishman, E. L., Jo, K., Nguyen, Q. P., Kong, D., Royfman, R., Cekic, A. R., et al. (2018). A novel atypical sperm centriole is functional during human fertilization. *Nat. Commun.* 9:2210. doi: 10.1038/s41467-018-04678-8

Fonttis, A. A., Napolitano, R., and Tomas, M. (2002). Successful ICSI in a case of severe asthenozoospermia due to 93% non-specific axonemal alterations and 90% abnormal or absent mitochondrial sheaths. *Reprod. Biomed. Online* 5, 270–272. doi: 10.1016/s1472-6483(10)61831-7

Fukasawa, K. (2007). Oncogenes and tumour suppressors take on centrosomes. *Nat. Rev. Cancer* 7, 911–924. doi: 10.1038/nrc2249

Gambera, L., Falcone, P., Mencaglia, L., Collodel, G., Serafini, F., De Leo, V., et al. (2010). Intracytoplasmic sperm injection and pregnancy with decapitated sperm. *Fertil. Steril.* 93, 1347.e7–1347.e12. doi: 10.1016/j.fertnstert.2008.12.087

Garanina, A. S., Alieva, I. B., Bragina, E. E., Blanchard, E., Arbeille, B., Guerif, F., et al. (2019). The centriolar adjunct–appearance and disassembly in spermiogenesis and the potential impact on fertility. *Cells* 8:180. doi: 10.3390/cells8020180

Godinho, S., and Pellman, D. (2014). Causes and consequences of centrosome abnormalities in cancer. *Philos. Trans. R. Soc. B Biol. Sci.* 369:20130467. doi: 10.1098/rstb.2013.0467

Gomendio, M., and Roldan, E. R. (2008). Implications of diversity in sperm size and function for sperm competition and fertility. *Int. J. Dev. Biol.* 52, 439–447. doi: 10.1387/ijdb.082595mg

Gottardo, M., Callaini, G., and Riparbelli, M. G. (2015). Structural characterization of procentrioles in *Drosophila* spermatids. *Cytoskeleton* 72, 576–584. doi: 10.1002/cm.21260

Gueth-Hallonet, C., Antony, C., Aghion, J., Santa-Maria, A., Lajoie-Mazenc, I., Wright, M., et al. (1993). gamma-Tubulin is present in acentriolar MTOCs during early mouse development. *J. Cell Sci.* 105 (Pt 1), 157–166.

Gunn, D. D., and Bates, G. W. (2016). Evidence-based approach to unexplained infertility: a systematic review. *Fertil. Steril.* 105, 1566e1–1174e1. doi: 10.1016/j.fertnstert.2016.02.001

Hart, R. (2003). Unexplained infertility, endometriosis, and fibroids. *BMJ* 327, 721–724. doi: 10.1136/bmj.327.7417.721

Hertig, A. T., and Adams, E. C. (1967). Studies on the human oocyte and its follicle. I. Ultrastructural and histochemical observations on the primordial follicle stage. *J. Cell Biol.* 34, 647–675. doi: 10.1083/jcb.34.2.647

Hewitson, L., Haavisto, A., Simerly, C., Jones, J., and Schatten, G. (1997). Microtubule organization and chromatin configurations in hamster oocytes during fertilization and parthenogenetic activation, and after insemination with human sperm. *Biol. Reprod.* 57, 967–975. doi: 10.1095/biolreprod57.5.967

Hinchcliffe, E. H. (2011). The centrosome and bipolar spindle assembly: does one have anything to do with the other? *Cell Cycle* 10, 3841–3848. doi: 10.4161/cc.10.22.18293

Hinduja, I., Baliga, N. B., and Zaveri, K. (2010). Correlation of human sperm centrosomal proteins with fertility. *J. Hum. Reprod. Sci.* 3, 95–101. doi: 10.4103/0974-1208.69344

Hinduja, I., Zaveri, K., and Baliga, N. (2008). Human sperm centrin levels & outcome of intracytoplasmic sperm injection (ICSI)–A pilot study. *Indian J. Med. Res.* 128, 606–610.

Holstein, A., Schill, W., and Breucker, H. (1986). Dissociated centriole development as a cause of spermatid malformation in man. *Reproduction* 78, 719–725. doi: 10.1530/jrf.0.0780719

Isidori, A. M., Pozza, C., Gianfrilli, D., and Isidori, A. (2006). Medical treatment to improve sperm quality. *Reprod. Biomed. Online* 12, 704–714. doi: 10.1016/s1472-6483(10)61082-6

Jarow, J. P., Espeland, M. A., and Lipshultz, L. I. (1989). Evaluation of the azoospermic patient. *J. Urol.* 142, 62–65. doi: 10.1016/s0022-5347(17)38662-7

Joshi, H. C., and Palevitz, B. A. (1996). gamma-Tubulin and microtubule organization in plants. *Trends Cell Biol.* 6, 41–44. doi: 10.1016/0962-8924(96)81008-7

Kahraman, S., Tasdemir, M., Tasdemir, I., Vicdan, K., Ozgur, S., Polat, G., et al. (1996). Pregnancies achieved with testicular and ejaculated spermatozoa in combination with intracytoplasmic sperm injection in men with totally or initially immotile spermatozoa in the ejaculate. *Hum. Reprod.* 11, 1343–1346. doi: 10.1093/oxfordjournals.humrep.a019384

Kai, Y., Iwata, K., Iba, Y., and Mio, Y. (2015). Diagnosis of abnormal human fertilization status based on pronuclear origin and/or centrosome number. *J. Assist. Reprod. Genet.* 32, 1589–1595. doi: 10.1007/s10815-015-0568-1

Kamal, A., Mansour, R., Fahmy, I., Serour, G., Rhodes, C., and Aboulghar, M. (1999). Easily decapitated spermatozoa defect: a possible cause of unexplained infertility. *Hum. Reprod.* 14, 2791–2795. doi: 10.1093/humrep/14.11.2791

Khan, M. S., Deepa, F., Ahmed, Z., Tahir, F., and Khan, M. A. (2011). Assessment of male reproductive health by conventional method of semen analysis. *J. Ayub Med. Coll. Abbottabad* 23, 84–88.

Khire, A., Jo, K. H., Kong, D., Akhshi, T., Blachon, S., Cekic, A. R., et al. (2016). Centriole remodeling during spermiogenesis in *Drosophila*. *Curr. Biol.* 26, 3183–3189. doi: 10.1016/j.cub.2016.07.006

Kim, N. H., Simerly, C., Funahashi, H., Schatten, G., and Day, B. N. (1996). Microtubule organization in porcine oocytes during fertilization and parthenogenesis. *Biol. Reprod.* 54, 1397–1404. doi: 10.1095/biolreprod54.6.1397

Kono, T. (2006). Genomic imprinting is a barrier to parthenogenesis in mammals. *Cytogenet. Genome Res.* 113, 31–35. doi: 10.1159/000090812

Kovacic, B., and Vlaisavljevic, V. (2000). Configuration of maternal and paternal chromatin and pertaining microtubules in human oocytes failing to fertilize after intracytoplasmic sperm injection. *Mol. Reprod. Dev.* 55, 197–204. doi: 10.1002/(SICI)1098-2795(200002)55:2<197::AID-MRD9<3.0.CO;2-Q

Kuretake, S., Kimura, Y., Hoshi, K., and Yanagimachi, R. (1996). Fertilization and development of mouse oocytes injected with isolated sperm heads. *Biol. Reprod.* 55, 789–795. doi: 10.1095/biolreprod55.4.789

Lange, B. M., and Gull, K. (1996). Structure and function of the centriole in animal cells: progress and questions. *Trends Cell Biol.* 6, 348–352. doi: 10.1016/0962-8924(96)10033-7

Le Guen, P., and Crozet, N. (1989). Microtubule and centrosome distribution during sheep fertilization. *Eur. J. Cell Biol.* 48, 239–249.

Lehti, M. S., and Sironen, A. (2016). Formation and function of the manchette and flagellum during spermatogenesis. *Reproduction* 151, R43–R54. doi: 10.1530/REP-15-0310

Leidel, S., and Gonczy, P. (2005). Centrosome duplication and nematodes: recent insights from an old relationship. *Dev. Cell* 9, 317–325. doi: 10.1016/j.devcel.2005.08.004

Liška, F., Gosele, C., Rivkin, E., Tres, L., Cardoso, M. C., Domaing, P., et al. (2009). Rat hd mutation reveals an essential role of centrobin in spermatid head shaping and assembly of the head-tail coupling apparatus. *Biol. Reprod.* 81, 1196–1205. doi: 10.1095/biolreprod.109.078980

Liu, J.-L., Kusakabe, H., Chang, C.-C., Suzuki, H., Schmidt, D. W., Julian, M., et al. (2004). Freeze-dried sperm fertilization leads to full-term development in rabbits. *Biol. Reprod.* 70, 1776–1781. doi: 10.1095/biolreprod.103.025957

Liu, W., He, X., Yang, S., Zouari, R., Wang, J., Wu, H., et al. (2019). Bi-allelic mutations in TTC21A induce Asthenoteratospermia in humans and mice. *Am. J. Hum. Genet.* 104, 738–748. doi: 10.1016/j.ajhg.2019.02.020

Liu, W.-M., Pang, R. T., Chiu, P. C., Wong, B. P., Lao, K., Lee, K.-F., et al. (2012). Sperm-borne microRNA-34c is required for the first cleavage division in mouse. *Proc. Natl. Acad. Sci.* 109, 490–494. doi: 10.1073/pnas.1110368109

Liu, X.-Y., Miao, Y.-L., Zhang, J., Qiu, J.-H., Cui, X.-Z., Gao, W.-Q., et al. (2012). Effects of activation on functional aster formation, microtubule assembly, and blastocyst development of goat oocytes injected with round spermatids. *Cell. Reprogram.* 14, 436–447. doi: 10.1089/cell.2012.0029

Loncarek, J., and Bettencourt-Dias, M. (2018). Building the right centriole for each cell type. *J. Cell Biol.* 217, 823–835. doi: 10.1083/jcb.201704093

Loncarek, J., and Khodjakov, A. (2009). Ab ovo or de novo? Mechanisms of centriole duplication. *Mol. Cells* 27, 135–142. doi: 10.1007/s10059-009-0017-z

Long, C. R., Pinto-Correia, C., Duby, R. T., Ponce de Leon, F. A., Boland, M. P., Roche, J. F., et al. (1993). Chromatin and microtubule morphology during the first cell cycle in bovine zygotes. *Mol. Reprod. Dev.* 36, 23–32. doi: 10.1002/mrd.1080360105

Longo, F. J. (1976). Sperm aster in rabbit zygotes: its structure and function. *J. Cell Biol.* 69, 539–547. doi: 10.1083/jcb.69.3.539

Manandhar, G., Schatten, H., and Sutovsky, P. (2005). Centrosome reduction during gametogenesis and its significance. *Biol. Reprod.* 72, 2–13. doi: 10.1095/biolreprod.104.031245

Manandhar, G., Sutovsky, P., Joshi, H. C., Stearns, T., and Schatten, G. (1998). Centrosome reduction during mouse spermiogenesis. *Dev. Biol.* 203, 424–434. doi: 10.1006/dbio.1998.8947

Mennella, V., Keszthelyi, B., McDonald, K. L., Chhun, B., Kan, F., Rogers, G. C., et al. (2012). Subdiffraction-resolution fluorescence microscopy reveals a domain of the centrosome critical for pericentriolar material organization. *Nat. Cell Biol.* 14, 1159–1168. doi: 10.1038/ncb2597

Miller, K. L., Rico, S. C., Muletz-Wolz, C. R., Campana, M. G., McInerney, N., Augustine, L., et al. (2019). Parthenogenesis in a captive Asian water dragon (*Physignathus cocincinus*) identified with novel microsatellites. *PLoS One* 14:e0217489. doi: 10.1371/journal.pone.0217489

Moretti, E., Collodel, G., Salvatici, M. C., Belmonte, G., and Signorini, C. (2019). New insights into sperm with total globozoospermia: increased fatty acid oxidation and centrin1 alteration. *Syst. Biol. Reprod. Med.* doi: 10.1080/19396368.2019.1626934 [Epub ahead of print].

Moretti, E., Pascarelli, N. A., Belmonte, G., Renieri, T., and Collodel, G. (2016). Sperm with fibrous sheath dysplasia and anomalies in head-neck junction: focus on centriole and centrin 1. *Andrologia* 49:e12701. doi: 10.1111/and.12701

Moretti, E., Pascarelli, N. A., Belmonte, G., Renieri, T., and Collodel, G. (2017). Sperm with fibrous sheath dysplasia and anomalies in head-neck junction: focus on centriole and centrin 1. *Andrologia* 49:e12701. doi: 10.1111/and.12701

Nagy, Z. P., Liu, J., Joris, H., Verheyen, G., Tournaye, H., Camus, M., et al. (1995). The result of intracytoplasmic sperm injection is not related to any of the three basic sperm parameters. *Hum. Reprod.* 10, 1123–1129. doi: 10.1093/oxfordjournals.humrep.a136104

Nakamura, S., Terada, Y., Horiuchi, T., Emuta, C., Murakami, T., Yaegashi, N., et al. (2002). Analysis of the human sperm centrosomal function and the oocyte activation ability in a case of globozoospermia, by ICSI into bovine oocytes. *Hum. Reprod.* 17, 2930–2934. doi: 10.1093/humrep/17.11.2930

Nakamura, S., Terada, Y., Rawe, V. Y., Uehara, S., Morito, Y., Yoshimoto, T., et al. (2005). A trial to restore defective human sperm centrosomal function. *Hum. Reprod.* 20, 1933–1937. doi: 10.1093/humrep/deh899

Nanassy, L., and Carrell, D. T. (2008). Paternal effects on early embryogenesis. *J. Exp. Clin. Assist. Reprod.* 5:2. doi: 10.1186/1743-1050-5-2

Navara, C. S., First, N. L., and Schatten, G. (1994). Microtubule organization in the cow during fertilization, polyspermy, parthenogenesis, and nuclear transfer: the role of the sperm aster. *Dev. Biol.* 162, 29–40. doi: 10.1006/dbio.1994.1064

Neri, Q. V., Lee, B., Rosenwaks, Z., Machaca, K., and Palermo, G. D. (2014). Understanding fertilization through intracytoplasmic sperm injection (ICSI). *Cell Calcium* 55, 24–37. doi: 10.1016/j.ceca.2013.10.006

Nigg, E. A., and Holland, A. J. (2018). Once and only once: mechanisms of centriole duplication and their deregulation in disease. *Nat. Rev. Mol. Cell Biol.* 19, 297–312. doi: 10.1038/nrm.2017.127

Nigg, E. A., and Raff, J. W. (2009). Centrioles, centrosomes, and cilia in health and disease. *Cell* 139, 663–678. doi: 10.1016/j.cell.2009.10.036

Nijs, M., Vanderzwalmen, P., Vandamme, B., Segal-Bertin, G., Lejeune, B., Segal, L., et al. (1996). Fertilizing ability of immotile spermatozoa after intracytoplasmic sperm injection. *Hum. Reprod.* 11, 2180–2185. doi: 10.1093/oxfordjournals.humrep.a019073

Ounjai, P., Kim, K. D., Lishko, P. V., and Downing, K. H. (2012). Three-dimensional structure of the bovine sperm connecting piece revealed by electron cryotomography. *Biol. Reprod.* 87:73. doi: 10.1016/0014-5793(85)80430-0

Palermo, G., Joris, H., Devroey, P., and Van Steirteghem, A. C. (1992). Pregnancies after intracytoplasmic injection of single spermatozoon into an oocyte. *Lancet* 340, 17–18. doi: 10.1016/0140-6736(92)92425-f

Palermo, G. D., Colombero, L. T., and Rosenwaks, Z. (1997). The human sperm centrosome is responsible for normal syngamy and early embryonic development. *Rev. Reprod.* 2, 19–27. doi: 10.1530/revreprod/2.1.19

Perotti, M. E., Giarola, A., and Gioria, M. (1981). Ultrastructural study of the decapitated sperm defect in an infertile man. *J. Reprod. Fertil.* 63, 543–549. doi: 10.1530/jrf.0.0630543

Phillips, K. A., Bales, K. L., Capitanio, J. P., Conley, A., Czoty, P. W., t Hart, B. A., et al. (2014). Why primate models matter. *Am. J. Primatol.* 76, 801–827. doi: 10.1002/ajp.22281

Pickering, S. J., Johnson, M. H., Braude, P. R., and Houliston, E. (1988). Cytoskeletal organization in fresh, aged and spontaneously activated human oocytes. *Hum. Reprod.* 3, 978–989. doi: 10.1093/oxfordjournals.humrep.a136828

Pimenta-Marques, A., Bento, I., Lopes, C. A., Duarte, P., Jana, S. C., and Bettencourt-Dias, M. (2016). A mechanism for the elimination of the female gamete centrosome in *Drosophila melanogaster*. *Science* 353:aaf4866. doi: 10.1126/science.aaf4866

Pinto-Correia, C., Poccia, D. L., Chang, T., and Robl, J. M. (1994). Dephosphorylation of sperm midpiece antigens initiates aster formation in rabbit oocytes. *Proc. Natl. Acad. Sci. U.S.A.* 91, 7894–7898. doi: 10.1073/pnas.91.17.7894

Porcu, G., Mercier, G., Boyer, P., Achard, V., Banet, J., Vasserot, M., et al. (2003). Pregnancies after ICSI using sperm with abnormal head-tail junction from two brothers: case report. *Hum. Reprod.* 18, 562–567. doi: 10.1093/humrep/deg121

Preble, A. M., Giddings, T. M., Jr., and Dutcher, S. K. (2000). Basal bodies and centrioles: their function and structure. *Curr. Top. Dev. Biol.* 49, 207–233. doi: 10.1016/s0070-2153(99)49010-6

Rawe, V. Y., Diaz, E. S., Abdelmassih, R., Wojcik, C., Morales, P., Sutovsky, P., et al. (2008). The role of sperm proteasomes during sperm aster formation and early zygote development: implications for fertilization failure in humans. *Hum. Reprod.* 23, 573–580. doi: 10.1093/humrep/dem385

Rawe, V. Y., Terada, Y., Nakamura, S., Chillik, C. F., Olmedo, S. B., and Chemes, H. E. (2002). A pathology of the sperm centriole responsible for defective sperm aster formation, syngamy and cleavage. *Hum. Reprod.* 17, 2344–2349. doi: 10.1093/humrep/17.9.2344

Riparbelli, M. G., and Callaini, G. (2011). Male gametogenesis without centrioles. *Dev. Biol.* 349, 427–439. doi: 10.1016/j.ydbio.2010.10.021

Rybouchkin, A., Dozortsev, D., Pelinck, M. J., De Sutter, P., and Dhont, M. (1996). Analysis of the oocyte activating capacity and chromosomal complement of round-headed human spermatozoa by their injection into mouse oocytes. *Hum. Reprod.* 11, 2170–2175. doi: 10.1093/oxfordjournals.humrep.a019071

Saias-Magnan, J., Metzler-Guillemain, C., Mercier, G., Carles-Marcorelles, F., Grillo, J. M., and Guichaoua, M. R. (1999). Failure of pregnancy after intracytoplasmic sperm injection with decapitated spermatozoa: case report. *Hum. Reprod.* 14, 1989–1992. doi: 10.1093/humrep/14.8.1989

Sathananthan, A. H. (1994). Functional competence of abnormal spermatozoa. *Baillieres Clin. Obstet. Gynaecol.* 8, 141–156. doi: 10.1016/s0950-3552(05)80029-x

Sathananthan, A. H., Kola, I., Osborne, J., Trounson, A., Ng, S. C., Bongso, A., et al. (1991). Centrioles in the beginning of human development. *Proc. Natl. Acad. Sci. U.S.A.* 88, 4806–4810. doi: 10.1073/pnas.88.11.4806

Sathananthan, A. H., Ng, S. C., Chia, C. M., Law, H. Y., Edirisinghe, W. R., and Ratnam, S. S. (1985). The origin and distribution of cortical granules in human oocytes with reference to Golgi, nucleolar, and microfilament activity. *Ann. N. Y. Acad. Sci.* 442, 251–264. doi: 10.1111/j.1749-6632.1985.tb37526.x

Sathananthan, A. H., Ratnam, S. S., Ng, S. C., Tarin, J. J., Gianaroli, L., and Trounson, A. (1996). The sperm centriole: its inheritance, replication and perpetuation in early human embryos. *Hum. Reprod.* 11, 345–356. doi: 10.1093/humrep/11.2.345

Sathananthan, A. H., Selvaraj, K., Girijashankar, M. L., Ganesh, V., Selvaraj, P., and Trounson, A. O. (2006). From oogonia to mature oocytes: inactivation of the maternal centrosome in humans. *Microsc. Res. Tech.* 69, 396–407. doi: 10.1002/jemt.20299

Schatten, G. (1994). The centrosome and its mode of inheritance: the reduction of the centrosome during gametogenesis and its restoration during fertilization. *Dev. Biol.* 165, 299–335. doi: 10.1006/dbio.1994.1256

Schatten, G., Simerly, C., and Schatten, H. (1985). Microtubule configurations during fertilization, mitosis, and early development in the mouse and the requirement for egg microtubule-mediated motility during mammalian fertilization. *Proc. Natl. Acad. Sci. U.S.A.* 82, 4152–4156. doi: 10.1073/pnas.82.12.4152

Schatten, G., Simerly, C., and Schatten, H. (1991). Maternal inheritance of centrosomes in mammals? Studies on parthenogenesis and polyspermy in mice. *Proc. Natl. Acad. Sci. U.S.A.* 88, 6785–6789. doi: 10.1073/pnas.88.15.6785

Schatten, H., Schatten, G., Mazia, D., Balczon, R., and Simerly, C. (1986). Behavior of centrosomes during fertilization and cell division in mouse oocytes and in sea urchin eggs. *Proc. Natl. Acad. Sci. U.S.A.* 83, 105–109. doi: 10.1073/pnas.83.1.105

Schatten, H., and Sun, Q. Y. (2010). The role of centrosomes in fertilization, cell division and establishment of asymmetry during embryo development. *Semin. Cell Dev. Biol.* 21, 174–184. doi: 10.1016/j.semcdb.2010.01.012

Severson, A. F., von Dassow, G., and Bowerman, B. (2016). Oocyte meiotic spindle assembly and function. *Curr. Top. Dev. Biol.* 116, 65–98. doi: 10.1016/bs.ctdb.2015.11.031

Sha, Y. W., Xu, X., Mei, L. B., Li, P., Su, Z. Y., He, X. Q., et al. (2017). A homozygous CEP135 mutation is associated with multiple morphological abnormalities of the sperm flagella (MMAF). *Gene* 633, 48–53. doi: 10.1016/j.gene.2017.08.033

Shahid, U., and Singh, P. (2018). Emerging Picture of deuterosome-dependent centriole amplification in MCCs. *Cells* 7:152. doi: 10.3390/cells7100152

Simerly, C., Wu, G. J., Zoran, S., Ord, T., Rawlins, R., Jones, J., et al. (1995). The paternal inheritance of the centrosome, the cell's microtubule-organizing center, in humans, and the implications for infertility. *Nat. Med.* 1, 47–52. doi: 10.1038/nm0195-47

Simerly, C., Zoran, S. S., Payne, C., Dominko, T., Sutovsky, P., Navara, C. S., et al. (1999). Biparental inheritance of gamma-tubulin during human fertilization: molecular reconstitution of functional zygotic centrosomes in inseminated human oocytes and in cell-free extracts nucleated by human sperm. *Mol. Biol. Cell* 10, 2955–2969. doi: 10.1091/mbc.10.9.2955

Singh, G. (1992). Ultrastructural features of round-headed human spermatozoa. *Int. J. Fertil.* 37, 99–102.

Sir, J.-H., Pütz, M., Daly, O., Morrison, C. G., Dunning, M., Kilmartin, J. V., et al. (2013). Loss of centrioles causes chromosomal instability in vertebrate somatic cells. *J. Cell Biol.* 203, 747–756. doi: 10.1083/jcb.201309038

Sutovsky, P. (2018). Sperm–oocyte interactions and their implications for bull fertility, with emphasis on the ubiquitin–proteasome system. *Animal* 12, s121–s132. doi: 10.1017/s1751731118000253

Sutovsky, P., Navara, C. S., and Schatten, G. (1996). Fate of the sperm mitochondria, and the incorporation, conversion, and disassembly of the sperm tail structures during bovine fertilization. *Biol. Reprod.* 55, 1195–1205. doi: 10.1095/biolreprod55.6.1195

Sutovsky, P., and Schatten, G. (1997). Depletion of glutathione during bovine oocyte maturation reversibly blocks the decondensation of the male pronucleus and pronuclear apposition during fertilization. *Biol. Reprod.* 56, 1503–1512. doi: 10.1095/biolreprod56.6.1503

Szollosi, D., and Ozil, J. P. (1991). De novo formation of centrioles in parthenogenetically activated, diploidized rabbit embryos. *Biol. Cell* 72, 61–66. doi: 10.1016/0248-4900(91)90079-3

Terada, Y. (2007). Functional analyses of the sperm centrosome in human reproduction: implications for assisted reproductive technique. *Soc. Reprod. Fertil. Suppl.* 63, 507–513.

Terada, Y., Hasegawa, H., Takahashi, A., Ugajin, T., Yaegashi, N., and Okamura, K. (2009). Successful pregnancy after oocyte activation by a calcium ionophore for a patient with recurrent intracytoplasmic sperm injection failure, with an assessment of oocyte activation and sperm centrosomal function using bovine eggs. *Fertil. Steril.* 91, 935.e11–935.e14. doi: 10.1016/j.fertnstert.2008.09.043

Terada, Y., Nakamura, S., Morita, J., Tachibana, M., Morito, Y., Ito, K., et al. (2004). Use of Mammalian eggs for assessment of human sperm function: molecular and cellular analyses of fertilization by intracytoplasmic sperm injection. *Am. J. Reprod. Immunol.* 51, 290–293. doi: 10.1111/j.1600-0897.2004.00158.x

Terada, Y., Simerly, C. R., Hewitson, L., and Schatten, G. (2000). Sperm aster formation and pronuclear decondensation during rabbit fertilization and development of a functional assay for human sperm. *Biol. Reprod.* 62, 557–563. doi: 10.1095/biolreprod62.3.557

Toyama, Y., Iwamoto, T., Yajima, M., Baba, K., and Yuasa, S. (2000). Decapitated and decaudated spermatozoa in man, and pathogenesis based on the ultrastructure. *Int. J. Androl.* 23, 109–115. doi: 10.1046/j.1365-2605.2000.t01-1-00217.x

Van Blerkom, J. (1996). Sperm centrosome dysfunction: a possible new class of male factor infertility in the human. *Mol. Hum. Reprod.* 2, 349–354. doi: 10.1093/molehr/2.5.349

Vorobjev, I. A., and Chentsov Yu, S. (1982). Centrioles in the cell cycle. I. Epithelial cells. *J. Cell Biol.* 93, 938–949. doi: 10.1083/jcb.93.3.938

Wang, W.-L., Tu, C.-F., and Tan, Y.-Q. (2019). Insight on multiple morphological abnormalities of sperm flagella in male infertility: what is new? *Asian J. Androl.* doi: 10.4103/aja.aja_53_19 [Epub ahead of print].

World Health Organization [WHO] (2010). *WHO Laboratory Manual for the Examination and Processing of Human Semen*, 5th Edn. (Geneva: World Health Organization), 7–113.

Winey, M., and O'Toole, E. (2014). Centriole structure. *Philos. Trans. R. Soc. Lond. B Biol. Sci.* 369:20130457. doi: 10.1098/rstb.2013.0457

Wininger, J. D. (2004). "Parthenogenetic stem cells," in *Handbook of Stem Cells*, ed. R. P. Lanza, (Amsterdam: Elsevier). 635–637. doi: 10.1016/b978-012436643-5/50072-9

Wojcik, C., Benchaib, M., Lornage, J., Czyba, J. C., and Guerin, J. F. (2000). Proteasomes in human spermatozoa. *Int. J. Androl.* 23, 169–177. doi: 10.1046/j.1365-2605.2000.00223.x

Wu, G. J., Simerly, C., Zoran, S. S., Funte, L. R., and Schatten, G. (1996). Microtubule and chromatin dynamics during fertilization and early development in rhesus monkeys, and regulation by intracellular calcium ions. *Biol. Reprod.* 55, 260–270. doi: 10.1095/biolreprod55.2.260

Yabe, T., Ge, X., and Pelegri, F. (2007). The zebrafish maternal-effect gene cellular atoll encodes the centriolar component sas-6 and defects in its paternal function promote whole genome duplication. *Dev. Biol.* 312, 44–60. doi: 10.1016/j.ydbio.2007.08.054

Yan, W., Morozumi, K., Zhang, J., Ro, S., Park, C., and Yanagimachi, R. (2008). Birth of mice after intracytoplasmic injection of single purified sperm nuclei and detection of messenger RNAs and MicroRNAs in the sperm nuclei. *Biol. Reprod.* 78, 896–902. doi: 10.1095/biolreprod.107.067033

Yllera-Fernandez, M. M., Crozet, N., and Ahmed-Ali, M. (1992). Microtubule distribution during fertilization in the rabbit. *Mol. Reprod. Dev.* 32, 271–276. doi: 10.1002/mrd.1080320313

Yoon, S. Y., Jellerette, T., Salicioni, A. M., Lee, H. C., Yoo, M. S., Coward, K., et al. (2008). Human sperm devoid of PLC, zeta 1 fail to induce Ca(2+) release and are unable to initiate the first step of embryo development. *J. Clin. Invest.* 118, 3671–3681. doi: 10.1172/JCI36942

Yoshimoto-Kakoi, T., Terada, Y., Tachibana, M., Murakami, T., Yaegashi, N., and Okamura, K. (2008). Assessing centrosomal function of infertile males using heterologous ICSI. *Syst. Biol. Reprod. Med.* 54, 135–142. doi: 10.1080/19396360802043091

Zamboni, L., and Stefanini, M. (1971). The fine structure of the neck of mammalian spermatozoa. *Anatomical. Record.* 169, 155–172. doi: 10.1002/ar.1091690203

8

Toward Development of the Male Pill: A Decade of Potential Non-hormonal Contraceptive Targets

Katarzyna Kent[1,2,3], Madelaine Johnston[1,3], Natasha Strump[1,3] and Thomas X. Garcia[1,2,3]*

[1] Department of Pathology & Immunology, Baylor College of Medicine, Houston, TX, United States, [2] Department of Biology and Biotechnology, University of Houston–Clear Lake, Houston, TX, United States, [3] Center for Drug Discovery, Baylor College of Medicine, Houston, TX, United States

***Correspondence:**
Thomas X. Garcia
thomas.garcia@bcm.edu

With the continued steep rise of the global human population, and the paucity of safe and practical contraceptive options available to men, the need for development of effective and reversible non-hormonal methods of male fertility control is widely recognized. Currently there are several contraceptive options available to men, however, none of the non-hormonal alternatives have been clinically approved. To advance progress in the development of a safe and reversible contraceptive for men, further identification of novel reproductive tract-specific druggable protein targets is required. Here we provide an overview of genes/proteins identified in the last decade as specific or highly expressed in the male reproductive tract, with deletion phenotypes leading to complete male infertility in mice. These phenotypes include arrest of spermatogenesis and/or spermiogenesis, abnormal spermiation, abnormal spermatid morphology, abnormal sperm motility, azoospermia, globozoospermia, asthenozoospermia, and/or teratozoospermia, which are all desirable outcomes for a novel male contraceptive. We also consider other associated deletion phenotypes that could impact the desirability of a potential contraceptive. We further discuss novel contraceptive targets underscoring promising leads with the objective of presenting data for potential druggability and whether collateral effects may exist from paralogs with close sequence similarity.

Keywords: contraception, drug target, knockout mouse, spermatozoa, druggability

INTRODUCTION

Currently, fertility control approaches for men fall into one of two categories: hormonal and non-hormonal. Several approaches have been investigated involving injectable or transdermal regimes using testosterone alone or combined with other molecules (Bagatell et al., 1993; Ilani et al., 2012). Although claims of total reversibility and full recovery to fertility have been made with hormonal contraception in males (Pasztor et al., 2017), prolonged use of exogenous hormones is associated with off-target effects, such as decreased high density lipoprotein cholesterol levels and potential cardiovascular risk in otherwise healthy men (Meriggiola et al., 1995). Therefore, there has been considerable interest in alternative methods for safe and reversible fertility control. Several non-hormonal methods are currently under development including gel-based obstruction of vas deferens, contraceptive vaccines, sperm-specific calcium ion channel blockers, and anti-spermatogenic indenopyridines with varied effectiveness and risks involved (Aitken, 2002; Hild et al., 2007; Morakinyo et al., 2009; Baggelaar et al., 2019).

THE 'POPULAR' PROTEINS: WHAT HAS BEEN TARGETED SO FAR?

Past efforts on the development of a safe non-hormonal contraceptive for men has resided on a diverse array of targets identified through both forward and reverse approaches. Forward approaches include identification of a target protein prior to drug development, while reverse approaches identify a drug with contraceptive effect prior to identification of the target protein. Often reverse approaches fail to identify specific drug targets with minimal side effects as discussed below.

Targets Involved in Sertoli-Germ Cell Interactions

Adjudin, a derivative of 1H-indazole-3-carboxylic acid, was shown to have potent anti-spermatogenic activity in rats, rabbits, and dogs prior to identification of its targets (Mok et al., 2011). Through further studies, it was later found to disrupt the Sertoli-germ cell junction proteins ACTB, ITGA6, ITGB1, MYH11, and OCLN (Mok et al., 2011, 2012; Mruk and Cheng, 2011). Unsurprisingly, administration of this drug resulted in significant toxicity, including effects on liver and skeletal muscle (Mruk et al., 2006) necessitating efforts to lower systemic toxicity by developing a conjugate capable of delivering Adjudin directly to the testis (Mruk et al., 2006), and by utilizing different formulations of the drug for its oral use to reduce the effective dose (Chen et al., 2016a). However, the efficacy of these approaches has yet to be determined.

H2-Gamendazole, an additional indazole carboxylic acid analog, blocks spermatogenesis by inhibiting production of inhibin B by primary Sertoli cells (Tash et al., 2008a), inhibiting HSP90AB1 and EEF1A1, and increasing Interleukin 1 Alpha expression in Sertoli cells (Tash et al., 2008b), which is a known disruptor of Sertoli cell-spermatid junction integrity (Nilsson et al., 1998). Although Gamendazole was shown to induce significant loss of spermatids (Tash et al., 2008b) and cause complete infertility after just a single dose, the damages to the seminiferous epithelium were not fully reversible (Tash et al., 2008a). The failure of some animals to regain fertility may have resulted from the combined effects of this drug on EEF1A1 and HSP90 in less differentiated spermatogenic cells. Therefore, further progress on this drug has been halted until these issues can be addressed. Generation of potentially safer analogs of gamendazole are currently under development (Kanishchev and Dolbier, 2018).

Targets That Reside on the Testis Side of the Blood–Testis Barrier

One major obstacle in the development of a safe, reversible, and non-hormonal male contraceptive is identifying small molecule inhibitors that can penetrate the highly selective blood–testis barrier (BTB), or Sertoli cell barrier (SCB). Established through a strong network of tight junction proteins between adjacent Sertoli cells, the BTB/SCB partitions the seminiferous epithelium into two compartments: basal and adluminal (lumen-facing) (Franca et al., 2016). The basal compartment contains the undifferentiated spermatogonia, differentiating spermatogonia, and early differentiating spermatocytes. Meanwhile, the lumen-facing compartment contains differentiated spermatocytes, and round and elongated spermatids that—due to homologous recombination during meiosis—are no longer recognized by the immune system and thus require an immune privileged location. Many molecules have been shown to not cross the BTB/SCB and are thus used as molecular tools for measuring an intact BTB/SCB in manipulated animal models (Chen et al., 2018).

To the best of our knowledge, the small-molecule inhibitor JQ1, which inhibits the bromodomain-containing, testis-specific protein, BRDT, is currently the only molecule that has been shown to be present beyond the BTB/SCB (Matzuk et al., 2012). By binding to the BRDT acetyl-lysine binding pocket, JQ1 disrupts spermatogenesis at the spermatocyte and round spermatid stages, producing a reversible contraceptive effect in mice (Matzuk et al., 2012) that phenocopies the male infertility phenotype of BRDT knockout mice (Shang et al., 2007). Development of JQ1 was done in a target-based drug discovery approach focused on finding inhibitors of BRD4, a close paralog of BRDT. JQ1 blocks the production of sperm in the testes by inhibiting BRDT, however, it also acts on other bromodomains (BRD) of the bromo-and-extra-terminal (BET) proteins known to regulate transcription and DNA repair, which include important BRDT paralogs with oncogenic effects (French et al., 2008). BRD4, has become known as an important therapeutic target in several types of cancers, including breast and prostate cancers, as well as glioblastoma multiforme (GMB) (Shi et al., 2014; Zhou et al., 2016; Wen et al., 2019). JQ1 possesses anti-tumor effects (Shao et al., 2014; Das et al., 2015) and has been identified as a promising inhibitor for treating GBM (Wen et al., 2019). Along with other related pan-BET BRD compounds JQ1 was also associated with improvement of associated memory and enhancement of special memory precision in mice, showing potential for treatment of dementia (Benito et al., 2017). Given the therapeutic potential of JQ1 significant efforts have been made to understand the mechanisms of its action on the BET BRD family, giving insight into the intricate protein–protein interactions (PPI) with transcriptional complexes, and most importantly, providing means for enhancing inhibition specificity for a single BET (Lambert et al., 2019).

Sperm Maturation in the Epididymis

The epididymis is a prime target for the development of a male contraceptive. This is because sperm leaving the testis are neither motile nor able to recognize or fertilize an egg; they must transit through the epididymis to acquire these abilities (Sullivan and Mieusset, 2016). Knockout mice of several epididymis-specific proteins have confirmed that the epididymis is essential for sperm maturation in the mouse (Davies et al., 2004; Roberts et al., 2006; Sipila et al., 2009). To the best of our knowledge, inhibitors that target an epididymis-specific protein do not yet exist. However, one of the most promising reversible, non-hormonal male contraceptives developed thus far has been against EPPIN (epididymal protease inhibitor; SPINLW1), which was developed through a reverse approach. EPPIN is a protein secreted by Sertoli cells and epithelial cells of the epididymis that gets deposited on the surface of maturing spermatozoa (Silva et al., 2012). The small molecule inhibitor EP055, which targets EPPIN, causes reversible infertility in primates (Silva et al., 2012) most likely by targeting the testes and epididymis where the drug can be found (O'Rand et al., 2018). In fact, deposition of EPPIN on the sperm surface appears to be greatest in the epididymis, indicating that the drug primarily acts in the epididymis (O'Rand et al., 2018). Current efforts are focused on increasing the half-life of the drug molecule (O'Rand et al., 2018).

Additionally, the inhibitors cyclosporine A and FK506, which are used as immunosuppressant drugs, target the sperm calcineurin subunits PPP3CC and PPP3R2 in the epididymis causing reversible effects on sperm morphology and motility (Miyata et al., 2015). Treatment of mice with cyclosporine A or FK506 creates phenocopies of the sperm motility and morphological defects apparent in knockout mice, which appear within 4 to 5 days of treatment and are reversed a week after discontinuation (Miyata et al., 2015). Unfortunately, cyclosporine A and FK506 are undesirable candidates due to their immunosuppressive effect (Stucker and Ackermann, 2011).

FACTORS THAT MAKE A PROMISING CANDIDATE TARGET

When evaluating potential druggability in a target-based drug discovery process, one must consider the protein properties that are required for safe and effective inhibition. Among the most significant is tissue expression specificity to minimize potential adverse effects; protein function and whether protein activity or interaction with other proteins is potentially druggable; sequence similarity to closely related paralogs that may be ubiquitously expressed; whether genetically manipulated animal models demonstrate a functional requirement for the target of interest; and other considerations as discussed below.

Male Reproductive Tract Specificity

By ensuring in the first steps of development that candidate drug targets are near exclusively expressed in the male reproductive tract, the potential for off-target effects in humans is minimized. Gamendazole, for example, targets HSP90AB1 and EEF1A1, which are highly expressed in non-reproductive tissues (Djureinovic et al., 2014; Uhlen et al., 2015). Therefore, significant toxicity as evidenced through previous studies (Tash et al., 2008a,b) could have been predicted based on target gene expression analysis. Likewise, the toxicity of Adjudin has resulted in attempts to target the drug specifically to the testes through conjugation with FSH (Chen et al., 2016a), a complicated approach which may minimize, but not completely remove, off-target effects. Since the identified molecular targets of Adjudin are ACTB, ITGA6, ITGB1, MYH11, and OCLN (Mruk and Cheng, 2011; Mok et al., 2012), which are all widely expressed in non-reproductive organs (Djureinovic et al., 2014; Uhlen et al., 2015), likewise, the toxicity of Adjudin could have been predicted and avoided had the drug's development began with a target-based discovery approach.

Protein Druggability

Protein druggability is often based on the protein family for which other members are known drug targets (Hopkins and Groom, 2002). For instance, an enzyme with a known binding site might be an easier target when compared to a novel protein that has not already been categorized. The development of an inhibiting drug for an uncategorized protein might seem challenging, however, disrupting PPI has recently been gaining attention as one of the possible methods. Generally, PPI are considered to be more challenging than traditional drug targets due to the smaller protein interfaces and difficulty with finding a sufficiently binding ligand capable of interrupting the interaction site at a suitable concentration (Whitty and Kumaravel, 2006). However, PPI targets are not deemed undruggable, based on the discovery of small molecules capable of deeper and higher affinity binding within the contact surfaces of the target protein (Wells and McClendon, 2007). Therefore, although not initially compelling, uncategorized genes have the likelihood of becoming potential drug targets by using druglike compounds that can modulate the PPI at multiple interface sites—increasing the ligand binding affinity—and consequently lowering the necessary drug dose administered (Fuller et al., 2009). **Table 1** presents the list of male reproductive tract-specific genes expressed at various stages of spermatogenesis with assigned categories of protein families. Besides a handful of enzymes (HFM1, MOV10L1, PGK2, PRSS37, and LRGUK), two transcription factors (SOX30 and TERB1), a few epigenetically active proteins (SCML2 and TDRD5) and a sperm specific ion channel KCNU1, most of the proteins discussed in this review belong to an unknown category. However, the contraceptive potential of these genes should not be overseen, but rather investigated for the identification of a high-affinity small molecule that can either (1) interfere with PPI, or (2) target the protein specifically for degradation as discussed below.

Many of the potential drug targets, such as non-enzymatic proteins, are uncategorized and identified as "undruggable" due to various challenges with existing targeting approaches. However, an emerging targeted protein degradation method called Proteolysis Targeting Chimeras (PROTACs) is a promising technique that can address these issues. The traditional approach to most enzymatic proteins serves to interfere with the functional aspect of the protein target, whereas PROTACs eliminate the protein through utilization of the ubiquitin-proteasome system to promote selective degradation (Bondeson et al., 2015; Lu et al., 2015; Olson et al., 2018). Thus, PROTACs do not require that an identified small molecule both bind with high affinity and reduce activity of the target protein (through interference of the binding pocket, etc.). PROTACs only requires that the identified small molecule bind with high affinity to the protein target. Additional design and chemistry are conducted to conjugate the small molecule to a high affinity E3 ubiquitin ligase ligand that results in target protein ubiquitination. There are currently various combinations of PROTACs developed to overcome the limitations of cell permeability, stability, solubility, selectivity, and tissue distribution (Brooks et al., 2005;

TABLE 1 | Recently identified reproductive tract-specific genes with male infertility phenotypes in mice: potential non-hormonal male contraceptive drug targets.

Gene Symbol (Mouse/Human)	Drug Target Type	Spermatogenic Site of Expression	MW (kDa) Mouse	MW (kDa) Human	# TM	Secreted	Conditions underlying male infertility in mouse	Reduced testis size in mouse	References
Asz1/ASZ1	Unknown	Spermatogonia	53	53.5	0	No	increased hypomethylation of retrotransposons, germ cell loss due to apoptosis, Sertoli cell only phenotype	Yes	Ma et al., 2009
Mov10l1/MOV10L1	Enzyme	Spermatogonia	132.8	135.3	0	No	Abnormal spermatocyte morphology, arrest of male meiosis	Yes	Frost et al., 2010
Scml2/SCML2	Epigenetic	Spermatogonia	80.1	77.3	0	No	Abnormal spermiogenesis	Yes	Hasegawa et al., 2015
Tex101/TEX101	Unknown	Spermatogonia	21.1	26.7	0	No	Abnormal sperm physiology	No	Li et al., 2013
4930447C04Rik/ C14orf39	Unknown	Spermatocytes	66.9	68.2	0	No	Azoospermia	Yes	Gomez et al., 2016
Boll/BOLL	Unknown	Spermatocytes	30.9	31.3	0	No	Azoospermia, abnormal male germ cell apoptosis, abnormal spermatogenesis	Yes	VanGompel and Xu, 2010
Btbd18/BTBD18	Unknown	Spermatocytes	79.5	77.9	0	No	Abnormal spermatid morphology, arrest of spermiogenesis	Yes	Zhou et al., 2017
Ccdc155/CCDC155	Unknown	Spermatocytes	72.4	62.8	0	No	Abnormal chromosomal synapsis, abnormal double-strand DNA break repair, abnormal meiotic attachment of telomere to nuclear envelope	Yes	Horn et al., 2013
Ccdc63/CCDC63	Unknown	Spermatocytes	65.2	66.3	0	No	Shortened sperm flagella	No	Young et al., 2015
Cnbd2/CNBD2	Unknown	Spermatocytes	77.9	67.5	0	No	Abnormal sperm midpiece morphology, abnormal sperm motility	Yes	Krahling et al., 2013
Fbxo43/FBXO43	Unknown	Spermatocytes	71.2	78.4	0	No	Arrest of male meiosis	Yes	Gopinathan et al., 2017
Hfm1/HFM1	Enzyme	Spermatocytes	161.4	162.6	0	No	Abnormal chiasmata formation, abnormal chromosomal synapsis, arrest of male meiosis	Yes	Guiraldelli et al., 2013
Hormad2/HORMAD2	Unknown	Spermatocytes	34.8	35.3	0	No	Abnormal chiasmata formation, arrest of spermatogenesis	Yes	Kogo et al., 2012a
Insl6/INSL6	Unknown	Spermatocytes	22.2	22.5	0	Yes	Azoospermia, abnormal male germ cell morphology	Yes	Burnicka-Turek et al., 2009
Ly6k/LY6K	Unknown	Spermatocytes	11.7	14.2	0	Yes	Abnormal sperm physiology	No	Fujihara et al., 2014
Mcmdc2/MCMDC2	Unknown	Spermatocytes	76	76.2	0	No	Abnormal double-strand DNA break repair, abnormal synaptonemal complex	Yes	Finsterbusch et al., 2016
Meiob/MEIOB	Unknown	Spermatocytes	53	49.3	0	No	Abnormal double-strand DNA break repair, abnormal meiosis, arrest of spermatogenesis	Yes	Luo et al., 2013; Souquet et al., 2013
Meioc/MEIOC	Unknown	Spermatocytes	108.9	107.6	0	No	Abnormal double-strand DNA break repair, abnormal synaptonemal complex	Yes	Abby et al., 2016
Nup210l/NUP210L	Unknown	Spermatocytes	205.1	206.6	1	Yes	Abnormal acrosome morphology, abnormal sperm midpiece morphology	Unknown	Walters et al., 2009
Pgk2/PGK2	Kinase	Spermatocytes	44.9	44.7	0	No	Asthenozoospermia	No	Danshina et al., 2010
Pih1h3b/PIH1D3	Unknown	Spermatocytes	24.5	24.1	0	No	Abnormal sperm axoneme morphology, abnormal sperm flagellum morphology	Yes	Dong et al., 2014
Rad21l/RAD21L1	Unknown	Spermatocytes	62.7	63.3	0	No	Azzospermia, abnormal male meiosis	Yes	Herran et al., 2011
Sox30/SOX30	TF	Spermatocytes	83.9	82.9	0	No	Abnormal spermatid morphology, arrest of spermiogenesis	Yes	Feng et al., 2017
Spata22/SPATA22	Unknown	Spermatocytes	40.2	41.3	0	No	Abnormal chromosomal synapsis, abnormal double-strand DNA break repair, abnormal synaptonemal complex	Yes	La Salle et al., 2012
Spdya/SPDYA	Unknown	Spermatocytes	36.1	36.5	0	No	Abnormal chiasmata formation, abnormal chromosomal synapsis, abnormal synaptonemal complex	Yes	Tu et al., 2017
Syce3/SYCE3	Unknown	Spermatocytes	10.5	10.6	0	No	Abnormal chromosomal synapsis, abnormal synaptonemal complex	Yes	Schramm et al., 2011
Tdrd5/TDRD5	Epigenetic	Spermatocytes	116	109.7	0	No	Globozoospermia, abnormal acrosome morphology, abnormal spermatocyte morphology, arrest of male meiosis	Yes	Yabuta et al., 2011

(Continued)

TABLE 1 | Continued

Gene Symbol (Mouse/Human)	Drug Target Type	Spermatogenic Site of Expression	MW (kDa)		# TM	Secreted	Conditions underlying male infertility in mouse	Reduced testis size in mouse	References
			Mouse	Human					
Terb1/TERB1	TF	Spermatocytes	86.8	83.1	0	No	Abnormal X-Y chromosome synapsis during male meiosis	Yes	Shibuya et al., 2014
Topaz1/TOPAZ1	Unknown	Spermatocytes	185.5	191	0	No	Abnormal male germ cell morphology, arrest of male meiosis	Yes	Luangpraseuth-Prosper et al., 2015
Calr3/CALR3	Unknown	Spermatids	42.2	42.9	0	Yes	Abnormal sperm physiology	No	Ikawa et al., 2011
Ccdc42/CCDC42	Unknown	Spermatids	38	38	0	No	Abnormal sperm axoneme morphology, abnormal sperm head morphology, absent sperm flagellum, detached acrosome	No	Pasek et al., 2016
Ccdc62/CCDC62	Unknown	Spermatids	79.3	77.7	0	No	Abnormal sperm head morphology, abnormal sperm midpiece morphology, abnormal sperm motility, absent acrosome	No	Li et al., 2017
Lrguk/LRGUK	Enzyme	Spermatids	93.2	124.9	1	No	Oligoasthenoteratospermia, manchette dysfunction, abnormal sperm head shaping	Yes	Liu et al., 2015
Prss37/PRSS37	Enzyme	Spermatids	24.7	24.3	0	Yes	Abnormal sperm physiology, abnormal spermiogenesis, impaired fertilization	Yes	Shen et al., 2013
Rimbp3/RIMBP3B	Unknown	Spermatids	177.3	181	0	No	Detached acrosome, detached sperm flagellum, ectopic manchette	No	Zhou et al., 2009
Spaca1/SPACA1	Unknown	Spermatids	30.6	29.3	1	Yes	Abnormal acrosome morphology, abnormal sperm head morphology, coiled sperm flagellum	No	Fujihara et al., 2012
Tcte1/TCTE1	Unknown	Spermatids	55.5	55.6	1	No	Axoneme dysfunction, abnormal sperm motility	No	Castaneda et al., 2017
Tdrd12/TDRD12	Epigenetic	Spermatids	137.6	132.6	0	No	Abnormal spermatid morphology, arrest of male meiosis	Yes	Asano et al., 2009; Pandey et al., 2013
Atp1a4/ATP1A4	Transporter	Spermatozoa	114.9	114.2	10	No	Impaired sperm capacitation, kinked sperm flagellum	No	Jimenez et al., 2011
Catsperd/CATSPERD	Unknown	Spermatozoa	89.5	90.4	1	Yes	Abnormal germ cell morphology, reduced hyperactivated sperm motility	No	Chung et al., 2011
Cfap54/CFAP54	Unknown	Spermatozoa	353.8	352	0	No	Abnormal sperm axoneme morphology, absent sperm flagellum, short sperm flagellum	No	McKenzie et al., 2015
Kcnu1/KCNU1	IC	Spermatozoa	126.9	129.5	7	No	Impaired acrosome reaction, impaired fertilization, impaired sperm capacitation	No	Santi et al., 2010; Zeng et al., 2011
Pmis2/PMIS2	Unknown	Spermatozoa	11	15.8	2	No	Abnormal sperm physiology	Unknown	Yamaguchi et al., 2012
Rsph6a/RSPH6A	Unknown	Spermatozoa	80.2	80.9	0	No	Abnormal manchette morphology, abnormal sperm axoneme morphology, abnormal sperm fibrous sheath morphology	No	Abbasi et al., 2018
Sun5/SUN5	Unknown	Spermatozoa	42.7	43.1	2	No	Globozoospermia, sperm head detachment	No	Shang et al., 2017

TM, transmembrane.

Bechara and Sagan, 2013; Ottis et al., 2017; Bondeson et al., 2018). Therefore, PROTACs technology provides the potential to greatly promote the development of contraceptive drugs against the "undruggable" non-enzymatic protein targets.

Sequence Similarity to Known Paralogs

The probability of two or more paralogs sharing a specific function increases with the percentage of sequence similarity (Zallot et al., 2016). If a reproductive tract-specific target is found to have high sequence similarity to a ubiquitously expressed protein or paralog, especially in the potentially druggable domain, this would make the target a poor choice for contraceptive development due to potential off-target effects. However, if a reproductive tract-specific protein has one or more ubiquitously expressed paralogs with low sequence similarity, this indicates that the function of the expressed proteins in the reproductive tract could be disrupted without significant off-target risks. Considerably high contraceptive potential resides in genes without a confirmed paralog; however, one must remain cautious in assuming a complete lack of paralogs as the druggable domain may be present in completely unrelated proteins, and further investigation should be conducted before proceeding to contraceptive drug development.

Validation Through Ablation – Creating Functional Knockouts to Verify Contraceptive Potential

Mice serve as one of the most efficient and effective models to understanding human physiology for a variety of reasons. The mouse genome is very well-characterized with almost all genes sharing similar functions to human orthologs (Cheng et al., 2014; Lin et al., 2014). Mice are biologically very similar, yet because they are small and have very short lifespans compared to humans, developmental processes can be studied economically and at an accelerated rate. Genetically manipulated knockout mouse models have significantly advanced our understanding of male gamete differentiation and the molecular mechanisms underlying male fertility. Nevertheless, there is still much to be learned about these intricate processes considering only approximately half of the protein coding genes have been individually ablated in mice (Dickinson et al., 2016; Smith et al., 2018). By ensuring that a knockout animal model of an individual protein target of interest leads to a complete male infertility phenotype, not subfertility, confidence in potential drug efficacy is established.

The current popularity of CRISPR-generated knockout mouse models as a method to study the function of a gene *in vivo* has dominated over other approaches. While knockout methods lead to a complete depletion of gene expression, or complete elimination of gene function, methods involving gene knockdowns lead to reduction in protein expression, the results of which may yield valuable information. RNA interference (RNAi) was found to be useful for silencing gene expression in mammals and employed to study the functional relevance of genes in a relatively fast and easy way. Past reproductive studies have utilized short interfering RNA (siRNA) to determine functional significance of genes in male mouse fertility and has, in some cases, resulted in impaired or complete infertility phenotype in viable mice (Nagai et al., 2011; Welborn et al., 2015). Several interesting experiments that compared the phenotypes resulting from knocking-out and knocking-down mouse genes have revealed that the two methods are complimentary in conducting gene functional studies (De Souza et al., 2006). The focus of this review, however, lies in male reproductive genes whose functional relevance was determined through knockout mouse models, since incisive genetic approaches provide a more definitive foundation for establishing the contraceptive potential of a novel reproductive tract-specific gene. A variable and indeterminate level of off-target effects introduced from transfection or lentivirus-mediated infection cannot be excluded as confounding variables in knockdown experiments.

Many reproductive tract-specific genes have been identified as dispensable for male fertility when individually ablated in mice (Miyata et al., 2016; Holcomb et al., 2020; Lu et al., 2019). Functional compensation through upregulation of other functionally similar genes or molecular pathways may explain the lack of phenotype (Marschang et al., 2004; Hanada et al., 2009; Kashiwabara et al., 2016). Therefore, identifying a small molecule inhibitor against an individually dispensable target would yield no contraceptive effect.

As previously discussed, BRDT is a testis-specific gene that when individually ablated in mice results in arrest of male meiosis, azoospermia, and complete male infertility (Barda et al., 2016). Since BRDT has enough sequence dissimilarity—$>55\%$ sequence dissimilarity with its closest paralogs that are ubiquitously expressed, BRD4 and BRD2, development of BRDT inhibitors with enhanced specificity and drug selectivity is feasible and currently underway (Matzuk et al., 2012; Miller et al., 2016). On the other end of the spectrum, GJA1 is an example of a gene that when conditionally ablated in the Sertoli cells of male mice leads to male infertility (Brehm et al., 2007). However, because the gene is not exclusively expressed in the reproductive tract and (Djureinovic et al., 2014; Uhlen et al., 2015) other knockout animal models of this gene display a variety of non-reproductive phenotypes including severe heart abnormalities (Gutstein et al., 2001; Liao et al., 2001), thus demonstrating that this target is not suitable for the development of a safe male contraceptive.

Human Mutations Implicated in Male Infertility

Mutations causing male infertility in humans might also be informative in the context of contraception and should be taken into consideration in the search for a potential non-hormonal target. There are 1,517 human genes associated with male infertility and/or either azoospermia, globozospermia, or oligospermia as reported by GeneCards and MalaCards (Stelzer et al., 2016; Rappaport et al., 2017). Of these 1,517 genes, 202 genes are reproductive tract-specific in humans as reported through the CITDBase Contraceptive Target Database (GTEx Consortium, 2013; Djureinovic et al., 2014; Uhlen et al., 2015; Schmidt et al., 2017; Lee, 2019; Samaras et al., 2019) and/or Djureinovic et al. (2014) and Uhlen et al. (2015) (**Figure 1**). Of these 202 genes, 21 genes do not have a corresponding mouse ortholog and 3 of these genes (*KLK2*, *CDY2A*, and *RHOXF2*) may be of potential interest for further study as they encode an enzyme, an epigenetic protein, and a transcription factor, respectively; all proteins with potential druggable activity (**Supplementary Table S1**). The remaining 18 genes without a corresponding mouse ortholog encode proteins of unknown drug target type (**Supplementary Table S1**). Of the 202 reproductive tract-specific human genes associated with human infertility, 78 genes have a corresponding mouse ortholog displaying male infertility in the mouse (**Figure 1** and **Supplementary Table S1**). The remaining 124 genes either (1) have a single mouse ortholog each and none have been knocked-out in the mouse, (2) have two or more mouse ortholog genes, whereby none or an incomplete number of orthologs have been knocked-out, and of those that have been knocked-out, none display a male infertility phenotype, (3) have a single mouse ortholog or multiple mouse orthologs that when individually ablated all lack a male infertility phenotype, or (4) have multiple mouse orthologs that have all been knocked out and that individually do not display a male infertility phenotype (**Figure 1** and **Supplementary Table S1**). While the first two categories (categories 1 and 2) require further study for functional validation of the contraceptive potential of these genes, the latter categories (categories 3 and 4) do not require any further study. Genes listed in the first two categories (47 genes total) encode 2 enzymes (*KLK3* and *SPAM1*), 1 kinase (*TSSK2*), 3 transcription factors (*HSFY1*, *TGIF2LX*, and *TGIF2LY*), and 41 proteins of unknown drug target type (**Supplementary Table S1**). Of the 202 reproductive tract-specific human genes associated with human infertility, 32 genes are mentioned in **Figure 2**, and four genes (*BOLL*, *KCNU*, *SPATA22*, and *TEX101*) are discussed in further detail within this review.

Site of Target Expression

Potential contraceptives could hit targets expressed along various stages of sperm development in the testis and epididymis, including targets active during the maintenance of the progenitor spermatogonia pool, entry into and passage through the various stages of meiosis, spermatid development and release, and sperm maturation through the epididymis. The contraceptive potential at these various stages varies in advantages and disadvantages. Targeting genes involved in early sperm development, for instance, could potentially be more effective, as suggested by several previous reviews identifying groups of male reproductive tract-expressed genes as promising drug targets (Schultz et al., 2003; Archambeault and Matzuk, 2014; Payne and Goldberg, 2014; O'Rand et al., 2016). However, disrupting the early stages of spermatogenesis poses the risk of testicular atrophy, longer recovery, and an increased

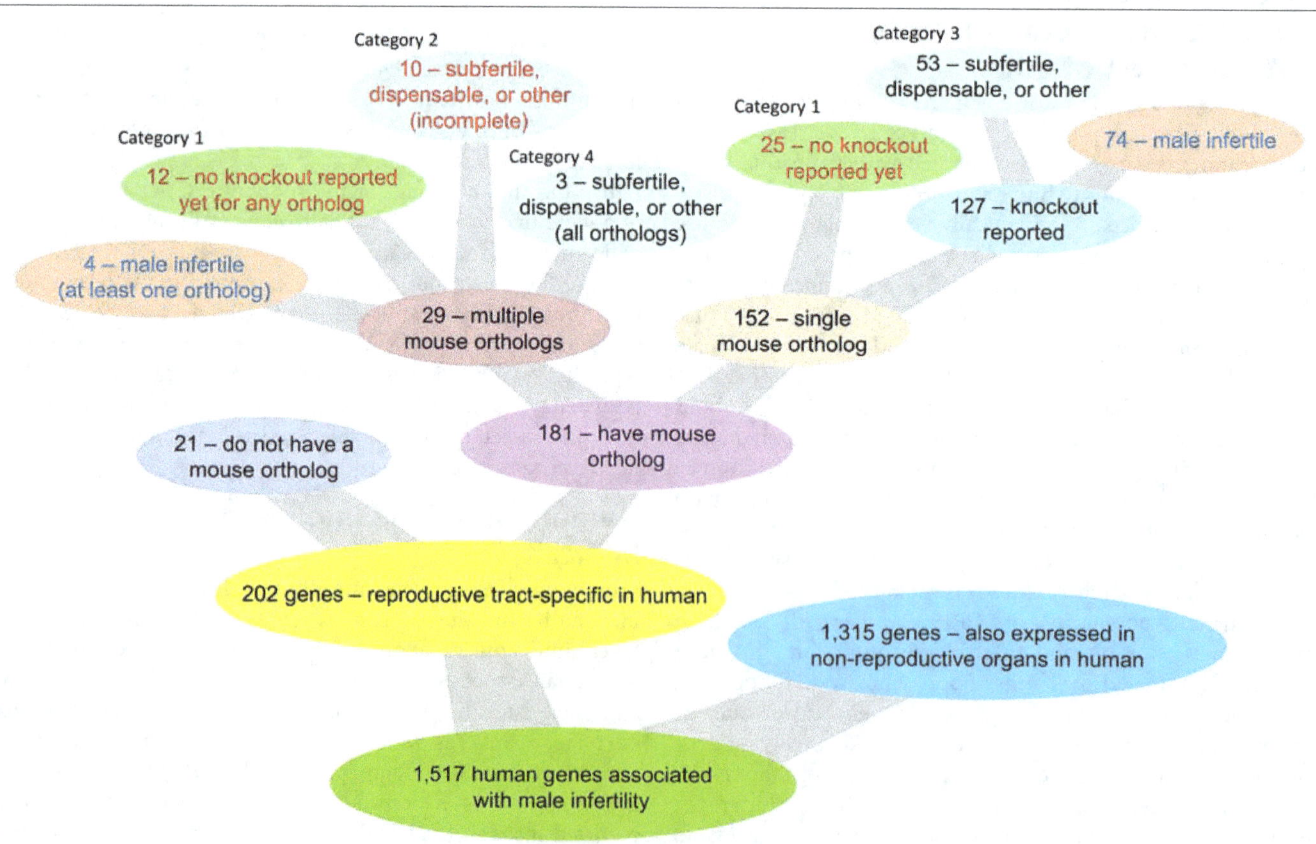

FIGURE 1 | Knockout mouse model availability and phenotype outcome of single and multiple mouse ortholog genes corresponding to 202 reproductive tract-specific human genes associated with male infertility and/or either azoospermia, globozospermia, or oligospermia as reported by GeneCards and MalaCards (Stelzer et al., 2016; Rappaport et al., 2017).

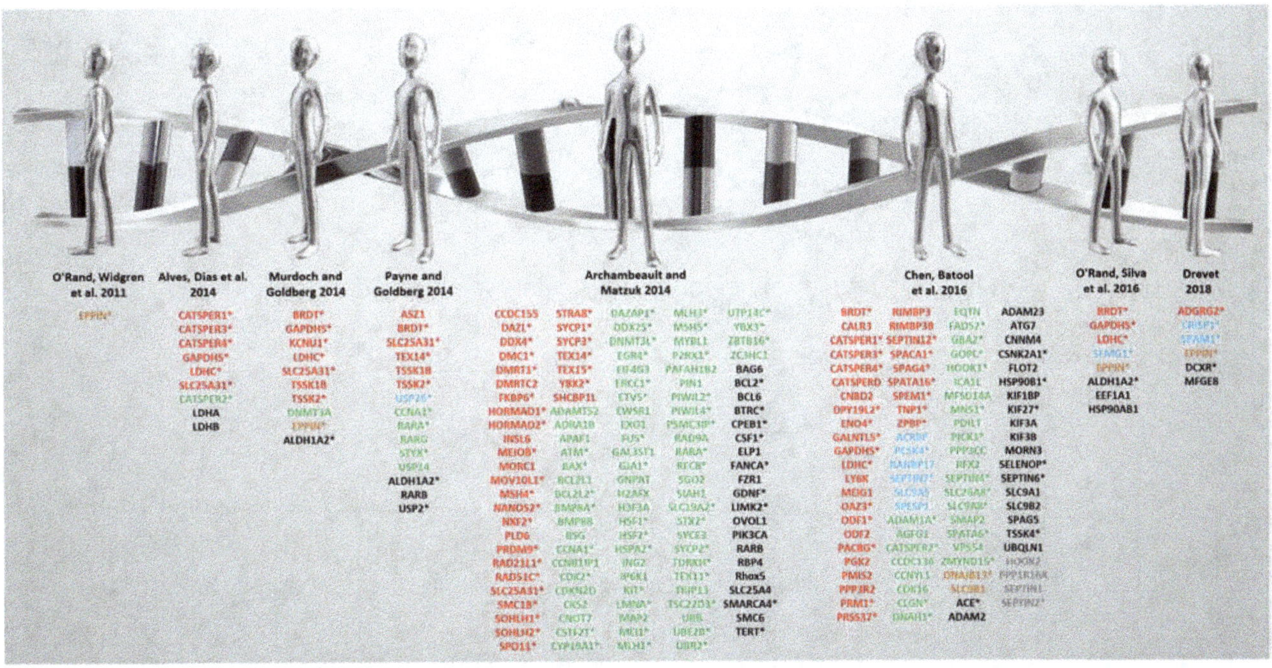

FIGURE 2 | A review of reviews from the past decade. Targets identified by the listed reviews are color-coded based on reproductive tract-specificity and fertility phenotype as follows: **red** = reproductive tract-specific displaying male infertility phenotype; **green** = non-reproductive tract-expressed and male infertility phenotype; **blue** = reproductive tract-specific displaying fertile or subfertile phenotype; **orange** = reproductive tract-specific with unknown fertility phenotype; **black** = non-reproductive tract-expressed displaying fertile or subfertile phenotype; **gray** = non-reproductive tract-expressed with unknown fertility phenotype. Expression and phenotype data obtained from Contraceptive Infertility Target DataBase (CITDBase), Human Protein Atlas (HPA), Ensembl Biomart, Mouse Genome Informatics (MGI), and the International Mouse Phenotyping Consortium (IMPC). *denotes genes implicated in human male infertility according to GeneCards and MalaCards.

possibility of irreversibility. Genes involved in later phases of spermatogenesis, namely spermiogenesis, acrosome and flagella formation, spermiation, and sperm maturation, would be more desirable contraceptive targets because testicular size would most likely remain unaffected, with a quicker, more reliable return to full fertility. Functional analysis of the expression patterns and specificity of male reproductive tract genes is imperative as it often provides additional insight into the molecular mechanisms of various stages of spermatogenesis, understanding of which is necessary in the process of developing a safe and effective non-hormonal male contraceptive.

Other Considerations

Identification of a drug-like small molecule that can effectively modulate the activity of a given target should also be assessed based on protein properties such as structure, size, and complexity (Kozakov et al., 2015). Targets that contain transmembrane helices could increase the difficulty of obtaining a properly folded and soluble protein for drug selection purposes. Likewise, due to glycosylation and processing through the secretory pathway, secreted proteins require protein production in eukaryotic expression systems, which could increase the difficulty of obtaining suitable quantities of purified protein. Therefore, whether drug development is feasible resides on careful consideration of the biophysical properties of the protein.

TARGET GENES

Previously Reviewed 'Novel' Target Genes

Several notable reviews published in the last decade have mentioned promising, non-hormonal, contraceptive leads that include both meiotically and post-meiotically expressed genes that are testis-specific or epididymis-specific genes required for sperm maturation (O'Rand et al., 2011; Alves et al., 2014; Archambeault and Matzuk, 2014; Murdoch and Goldberg, 2014; Payne and Goldberg, 2014; Chen et al., 2016b; O'Rand et al., 2016; Drevet, 2018) (**Figure 2**). Some are, in fact, not reproductive tract-specific, but are still required for fertility, while others that are indeed reproductive tract-specific, lead to subfertility, not infertility, which is an ineffective and highly undesirable outcome for a contraceptive. Thus, the genes in **Figure 2** are color-coded according to reproductive tract-specificity and infertility phenotype in the mouse. It is worth noting that while the reviews were restricted to the past decade, the reproductive tract-specific genes mentioned in these reviews were first identified beyond the past decade including some that were reported in 2006 and earlier, such as TNP1 (Yu et al., 2000), CATSPER1 (Ren et al., 2001), and TEX14 (Greenbaum et al., 2006).

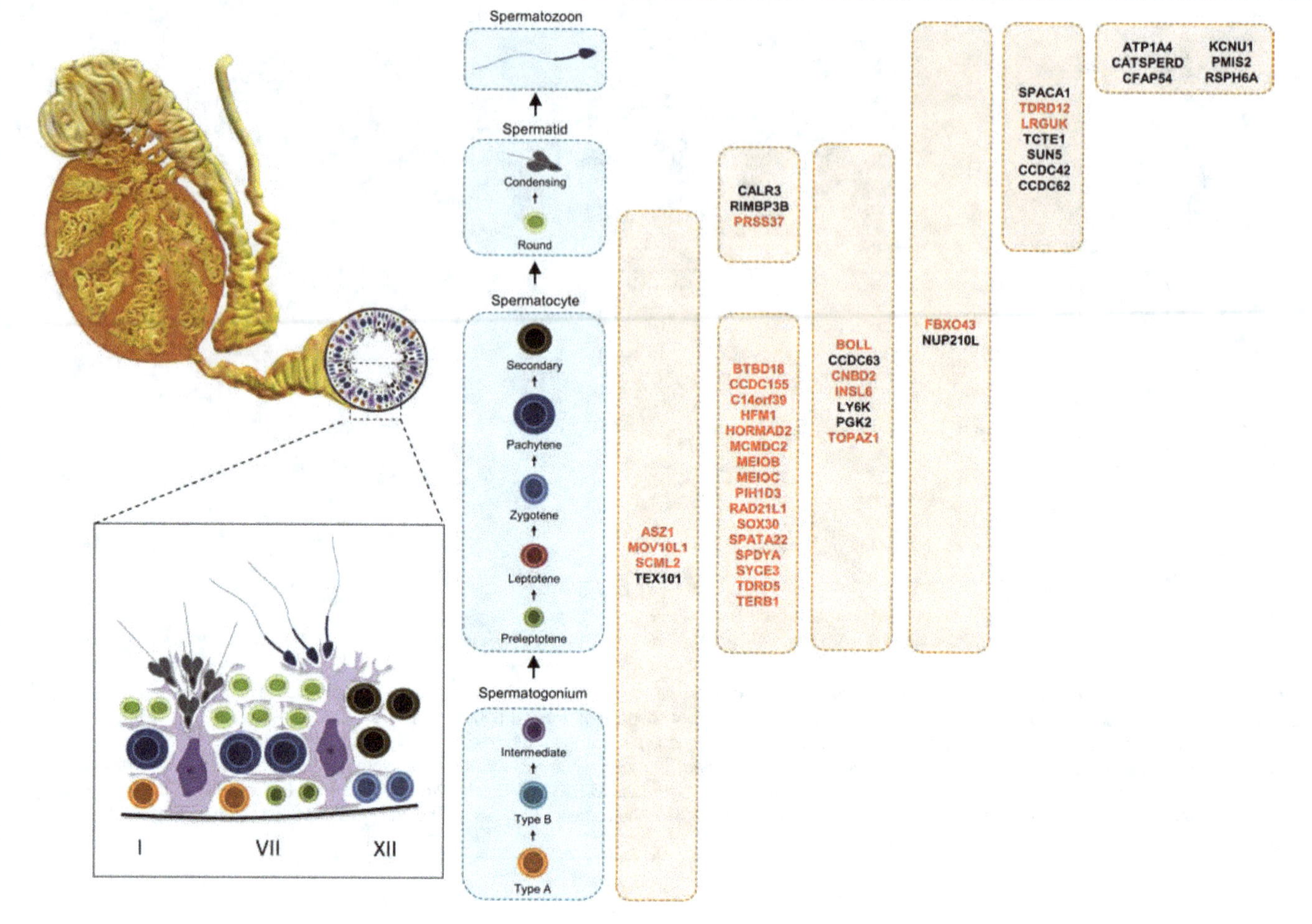

FIGURE 3 | Diagrammatic representation of germ cells along the spermatogenic pathway showing the cell types displaying expression of the potential targets. Targets in red display decreased testes size in mice.

In This Review

In this review, 45 genes are discussed in further detail as they were identified in the last decade as required for male fertility through knockout mouse studies, whereby many of these genes were not discussed or discussed minimally in any previous male contraceptive drug target review. Henceforth, these 45 genes will be listed according to their published expression patterns (**Figure 3**), which is an important criterium that should be considered in the selection of a safe and/or desirable contraceptive target. It is worth noting that nearly all of the genes mentioned below are male reproductive tract-specific or highly enriched as reported in the literature and with additional confirmation through the published expression data from CITDBase (GTEx Consortium, 2013; Uhlen et al., 2015; Schmidt et al., 2017; Lee, 2019; Samaras et al., 2019) and/or the Human Protein Atlas (Djureinovic et al., 2014; Uhlen et al., 2015). A graphical summary of the RNAseq-based expression data for these 45 genes is depicted in **Figure 4**. Those that are not reproductive tract-specific are identified as such through the level of non-reproductive tissue expression. The following discussion provides detailed information about individual genes with focus on determining the contraceptive potential of each. Additional relevant information for these genes is listed in **Table 1**.

Spermatogonia

In the last decade, only four reproductive tract-specific genes with infertile mouse models have been identified that fit the criteria of being expressed as early as the spermatogonia stage: *ASZ1* (Ma et al., 2009), *MOV10L1* (Frost et al., 2010; Zheng et al., 2010), *SCML2* (Hasegawa et al., 2015), and *TEX101* (Fujihara et al., 2013; Li et al., 2013) (**Table 1**). With expression as early as the spermatogonia stage (Teng et al., 2006; Ma et al., 2009; Frost et al., 2010; Maezawa et al., 2018), a deficiency of these genes' functions will likely require at least 2 months prior to a contraceptive effect, at least 2 months for recovery, and in some cases, depending on the gene, the potential for irreversibility of the contraceptive effect. Nevertheless, since this form of contraceptive may be considered desirable due to the permanence of the effect, and the need for a compound that can traverse the BTB is not required, these genes are worthy of consideration. Since the conserved domains of human ASZ1, MOV10L1, and TEX101 show sequence similarity below 40%

	Max Repro	Max Normal	Fold
PGK2	346.1	0	TS
PPP3R2	137.1	0	TS
ACTL7B	58.9	0	TS
SPACA1	51.2	0	TS
SUN5	41.0	0	TS
ASZ1	18.7	0	TS
TCTE3	17.2	0	TS
ODF4	17.1	0	TS
CATSPERD	16.0	0	TS
FBXO47	7.2	0	TS
TOPAZ1	6.5	0	TS
SPATA16	105.7	0.1	1057.0
RAD21L1	21.7	0.1	217.0
ODF1	418.3	0.2	2091.5
CALR3	98.8	0.2	494.0
NXF2	23.3	0.2	116.5
NUTM1	22.5	0.2	112.5
INSL6	21.6	0.2	108.0
FAM170A	21.0	0.2	105.0
CCDC42	128.6	0.3	428.7
SMC1B	57.3	0.3	191.0
PRSS37	55.3	0.3	184.3
C11orf94	20.7	0.3	69.0
C3orf20	10.4	0.3	34.7
CCDC155	56.9	0.4	142.3
NUP210L	47.8	0.4	119.5
RIMBP3C	15.7	0.4	39.3
KCNU1	13.5	0.4	33.8
RIMBP3B	12.1	0.4	30.3
DNAH17	10.3	0.4	25.8
FBXO43	9.8	0.5	19.6
BTBD18	4.0	0.5	8.0
LRGUK	8.4	0.6	14.0
SOX30	144.4	0.7	206.3
CCDC62	116.0	0.7	165.7
ADAD2	32.3	0.7	46.1
MEIKIN	13.4	0.7	19.1
MEIG1	13.0	0.8	16.3
PNLDC1	12.2	0.9	13.6
CCDC63	29.6	1.0	29.6
MEIOB	71.4	1.1	64.9
TDRD5	42.6	1.1	38.7
TERB1	25.0	1.1	22.7
RIMBP3	45.4	1.2	37.8
BOLL	87.9	1.3	67.6
ADGB	58.5	1.4	41.8
SPATA22	415.6	1.5	277.1
HORMAD2	35.2	1.5	23.5
TEX101	173.9	1.6	108.7
MEIOC	86.2	1.6	53.9
SPDYA	58.6	1.9	30.8
PIH1D3	13.8	1.9	7.3
TEX38	260.8	2.0	130.4
TDRD12	33.5	2.0	16.8
ARRDC5	18.2	2.3	7.9
MOV10L1	39.9	2.4	16.6
C14orf39	19.7	2.4	8.2
HFM1	25.0	2.7	9.3
CFAP54	11.0	2.9	3.8
SYCE3	116.7	3.0	38.9
MCMDC2	21.6	3.2	6.8
C16orf92	22.9	3.4	6.7
ENO4	6.8	3.4	2.0
M1AP	14.8	3.5	4.2
RSPH6A	30.4	4.5	6.8
PHF7	2183.4	5.0	436.7
SCML2	19.2	5.0	3.8
LY6K	29.0	5.9	4.9
CNBD2	38.0	6.5	5.8
SPINK2	6416.1	8.1	792.1
ATP1A4	18.2	8.6	2.1
HORMAD1	224.9	8.8	25.6
GAPDH	942.3	9889.6	0.1

FIGURE 4 | Digital PCR (heatmap) depicting the average transcripts per million (TPM) value per tissue per gene from human RNAseq data published by the Human Protein Atlas (Djureinovic et al., 2014; Uhlen et al., 2015). White = 0 TPM, Black ≥ 30 TPM. The genes are ordered from most reproductive tract-specific to least based on the level of non-reproductive tissue expression. "Fold" = testis/max normal. The data was obtained from a tab-separated file including Ensembl gene identifier, analyzed sample, and TPM value per gene that was downloaded from the Human Protein Atlas website. The expression profile of the housekeeping genes, *GAPDH,* is included.

to their respective, non-reproductive tract expressed paralogs, ANKRD34C, CT55, and CD177, then these protein targets have a reasonable potential for drug specificity with a low risk of collateral effects. However, as it has been previously reported that human SCML2 is expressed ubiquitously at low levels (Bonasio et al., 2014) (**Figure 4**), low but potentially physiologically relevant expression of *SCML2* across many non-reproductive tissues may therefore be of concern in the process of drug development. Additionally, the closest paralog to SCML2, SCMH1, is ubiquitously expressed and shows 60% sequence similarity in its conserved domain. Based on this information, human SCML2 may not be an ideal contraceptive target.

Spermatocytes

The genes discussed here are expressed in spermatocytes during preleptotene, leptotene, zygotene, pachytene, and/or diplotene stages and typically serve an essential role in meiosis I or meiosis II. A deficiency of these early stage genes results in male infertility typically due to meiotic arrest, which indicates a strong contraceptive potential. Important to note: although these genes may not directly impact spermatogonial stem cell self-renewal, and a healthy pool of spermatogonial stem cells may still remain for the regeneration of spermatogenesis, recovery time following cessation of targeting these genes may still take considerably longer than drugs targeting later stages of spermatogenesis or sperm. Consistently, the onset of a reliable contraceptive effect could take weeks, which may be an undesirable timeframe for drug action.

In the last decade, at least twenty-five reproductive tract-specific genes with infertile mouse models have been identified that fit the criteria of being expressed in spermatocytes (**Table 1**). Of these, seven genes—*MEIOB*, *MEIOC*, *PIH1D3*, *SPATA22*, *SYCE3*, *TERB1*, and *TOPAZ1*—encode the most promising target candidates as they do not have an associated paralog, or conserved domain with sequence similarity to any known protein, and thus these proteins bear the lowest risks of generating off-target effects from inhibiting compounds. Additionally, HORMAD2 is also an attractive target considering it only has one paralog, HORMAD1, which is also highly enriched in the male reproductive tract and leads to male infertility phenotype when ablated in mice (Shin et al., 2010; Daniel et al., 2011; Kogo et al., 2012b). Although *HORMAD1* shows low, but appreciable gene expression in two non-reproductive tissues (**Figure 4**) this fact may be offset by the sequence dissimilarity between HORMAD1 and HORMAD2 (50% whole protein and 40% conserved domain) which can aid in the identification of a selective inhibitor with careful drug selection and design. C14orf39 and CNBD2 would both be attractive candidates because they also lack paralogs, however both have tissue specificity issues of concern (**Figure 4**), and *Cnbd2* null mice display incomplete penetrance (Krahling et al., 2013), which may translate to potential ineffectiveness in humans. Therefore, while MEIOB, MEIOC, PIH1D3, SPATA22, SYCE3, TERB1, and TOPAZ1 are ideal candidates, C14orf39 and CNBD2 are not.

The next most promising candidates (another six genes)—*BTBD18*, *CCDC63*, *CCDC155*, *HFM1*, *MCMDC2*, and *TDRD5*—encode proteins that show sequence similarity below 40% to their respective, non-reproductive tract expressed paralogs, and within the conserved domains of their paralogs, KLHL26, SSH2, CCDC114, SNRNP200, MCM3, and TDRD1; thus, these potential targets have a reasonable potential for drug specificity with a low risk of collateral effects. However, the following six candidates—BOLL, FBXO43, INSL6, NUP210L, SOX30, and SPDYA—may require careful drug selection and design since the conserved domains of these proteins are 48–60% similar to the conserved domains of their respective, non-reproductive tract expressed paralogs, DAZ4, FBXO5, RLN1, NUP210, SOX7, and SPDYC. With respect to NUP210L, spermatid-Sertoli cell interaction was severely impaired in the knockout mouse model, resulting in Sertoli cell degeneration (Walters et al., 2009). Since this may cause irreversible disruption of spermatogenesis, this candidate may pose potential irreversibility issues. LY6K would be an attractive candidate because its closest ubiquitously expressed paralog, GML, has only 28% sequence similarity to LY6K; however, low, but appreciable expression of *LY6K* in non-reproductive tissues is of concern (**Figure 4**).

The most difficult spermatocyte-expressed candidates to target specifically are RAD21L1 and PGK2, which have ubiquitously expressed paralogs, RAD21 and PGK1, that have 83 and 87% similarity in their respective conserved domains. Since human mutations in RAD21 and PGK1 are characterized by significant disorders affecting numerous organ systems—Cornelia de Lange syndrome 4 (Deardorff et al., 2012), Mungan syndrome (Bonora et al., 2015), and phosphoglycerate kinase 1 deficiency (Fermo et al., 2012)—extraordinary effort would need to be made to generate specific drug molecules against RAD21L1 and PGK2.

Round and Elongated Spermatids

The proteins discussed here are expressed during the later stages of spermatogenesis and sperm maturation (**Table 1**). These proteins are found in round or elongating spermatids, either in the acrosome, acroplaxome, basal body, manchette, or flagellum during spermiogenesis, and these proteins function in either proper sperm head formation and attachment, midpiece formation, acrosome formation and attachment, generating sperm with normal motility, or generating sperm capable of normal sperm-zona binding. Targeting genes at these post-meiotic stages is more likely to act within a faster timeframe and lead to better and potentially faster recovery of fertility upon cessation of drug.

In the last decade, at least nine reproductive tract-specific genes with infertile mouse models have been identified that fit the criteria of being expressed in spermatids (**Table 1**). Again, the most attractive candidates are those that show excellent reproductive tract-specificity and that do not have any ubiquitously expressed paralogs, or that have ubiquitously expressed paralogs with low sequence similarity. CCDC62, SPACA1, and TCTE1 do not have any paralogs and TDRD12, CCDC42, PRSS37, and LRGUK have ubiquitously expressed paralogs, TDRD15, CFAP73, KLK15, and PPP1R42, that share less than 40% sequence similarity at the whole protein and conserved domain level. CALR3 has a ubiquitously expressed paralog, CALR, that shows 51% and 55% sequence similarity at the whole protein and conserved domain level, respectively, which may necessitate careful drug selection and design to ensure off-target effects are minimized. RIMBP3, RIMBP3B, and RIMBP3C in humans are all testis-specific and RIMBP3B and RIMBP3C share conserved domains with identical protein sequences, indicating a strong evolutionary requirement for the function of these proteins and high likelihood of targeting more than one isoform with one small molecule inhibitor. However, the closest ubiquitously expressed paralog to these proteins is RIMBP2, which shares 76% sequence similarity in its conserved domain, which may be of concern in finding a specific drug molecule that targets this region.

Spermatozoa

Genes in this group are highly expressed in spermatozoa and disrupting their function would most likely affect spermatozoa maturation as they pass through the epididymis, while still maintaining the pool of testicular spermatogonia and spermatocytes, or inhibit proper spermatozoa function after sperm maturation. These targets are typically localized to the neck, principal piece, flagellum, or the central microtubule apparatus of mature spermatozoa. Since these targets act late, it is important to note that some—depending on the binding kinetics of the drugs and if the drugs are reversible or irreversible inhibitors—may only provide a momentary decrease in sperm function while in the male reproductive tract, and shortly thereafter, but not indefinitely in the female reproductive tract after ejaculation as the drug concentration invariably decreases over time. Thus, although this category of drug may be the most desirable due to having fastest onset of drug action, fastest recovery after cessation of drug, and no effect on testicular size, there may be additional challenges to address during drug development to ensure contraceptive efficacy.

In the last decade, at least seven reproductive tract-specific genes with infertile mouse models have been identified that fit the criteria of being present in mature sperm (**Table 1**). CATSPERD, KCNU1, PMIS2, and SUN5 show the lowest potentials for off-target effects as their closest ubiquitously expressed paralogs, CASC4, KCNMA1, SYNDIG1L, and SUN1, have less than 50% similarity at the whole protein and conserved domain level. After that, RSPH6A, has 52% (whole) and 63% (CD) similarity to its closest ubiquitously expressed paralog, RSPH4A, which may make it a promising lead with additional attention during drug selection and design to minimize off-target effects. Although, CFAP54 would be an excellent candidate with less than 22% similarity (whole and CD) to its closest ubiquitously expressed paralog, NPBWR2, expression in cilia of the respiratory epithelium (Djureinovic et al., 2014; Uhlen et al., 2015) and additional low but potentially physiologically relevant expression across many non-reproductive tissues (**Figure 4**) indicate targeting this candidate may yield side effects. Likewise, ATP1A4 is not an ideal candidate due to having high sequence similarity—81% similarity (whole and CD)—to its closest ubiquitously expressed paralog, ATP1A2, and also having low but potentially physiologically relevant expression levels across many non-reproductive tissues (**Figure 4**).

Additional Potential Targets

Not discussed in terms of potential drug target specificity, however of additional potential interest are the following genes that are also reproductive tract-specific in humans according to CITDBase (GTEx Consortium, 2013; Uhlen et al., 2015; Schmidt et al., 2017; Lee, 2019; Samaras et al., 2019) with mouse models displaying male infertility phenotype published in peer-reviewed journals in the last 10 years: 3 genes encoding enzymes [*ENO4* (Nakamura et al., 2013), *PNLDC1* (Nishimura et al., 2018), and *SPINK2* (Lee et al., 2011)] and 8 genes encoding proteins of unknown drug target type [*M1AP* (Arango et al., 2013), *MEIG1* (Zhang et al., 2009), *MEIKIN* (Kim et al., 2015), *NXF2* (Pan et al., 2009), *ODF1* (Yang et al., 2012), *PPP3R2* (Miyata et al., 2015), *SMC1B* (Revenkova et al., 2010), and *SPATA16* (Fujihara et al., 2017)]. Furthermore, the following genes are reproductive tract-specific in humans according to CITDBase (GTEx Consortium, 2013; Uhlen et al., 2015; Schmidt et al., 2017; Lee, 2019; Samaras et al., 2019) with mouse models displaying male infertility phenotypes as reported by the International Mouse Phenotyping Consortium (IMPC) (Munoz-Fuentes et al., 2018): 1 gene encoding an enzyme (*ADAD2*); 1 gene encoding an epigenetic-related protein (*PHF7*); and 11 genes encoding proteins of unknown drug target type (*ACTL7B, ADGB, ARRDC5, C11orf94, C16orf92, C3orf20, DNAH17, FBXO47, NUTM1, ODF4, TEX38*). The expression pattern of these additional individually published and IMPC-reported genes are listed in **Figure 4**.

CONCLUSION

Global demand for the development of a "male pill" is at an all-time high with the exponential growth of the human population. Efforts to reduce unplanned pregnancies are recognized as the search for a safe and effective method of male contraception has been a decades-long quest (Prasad and Rajalakshmi, 1976; Frick and Aulitzky, 1988; Herndon, 1992; Waites, 1993; Gottwald et al., 2006; Mruk, 2008). Identification of reproductive tract-specific targets through transcriptomic and proteomic approaches followed by validation of their functional requirement using knockout mice models has helped advance this quest. In this review, we discuss novel reproductive tract-specific protein targets that have been identified in the past 10 years, their potential druggability, the factors that contribute to their druggability and why they should be taken into consideration when selecting male contraceptive targets. We direct the reader to consider that optimal gene targets are those that contribute to the later phases of spermatogenesis as disrupting genes in the earlier phases could potentially lead to permanent infertility. Additionally, the reader is directed to consider the potential adverse effects that may exist when targets whose protein sequences bear high sequence similarity to other ubiquitously expressed proteins. This information can be valuable in future studies since off-target effects can considerably hamper development of a safe, non-hormonal male contraceptive. Continued persistence in the search for an optimal protein target should lead to a clinically approved, affordable product.

AUTHOR CONTRIBUTIONS

KK and TG designed the research and wrote the manuscript. KK, MJ, NS, and TG performed the research and analyzed the data.

FUNDING

This research was supported by the Eunice Kennedy Shriver National Institute of Child Health and Human Development (R01HD095341 to TG).

SUPPLEMENTARY MATERIAL

TABLE S1 | Orthologous mouse genes and mouse model information of 202 reproductive tract-specific human genes associated with male infertility in humans. Mouse ortholog gene symbols and phenotype information collected from Ensembl BioMart and MGI. For publication references refer to MGI. "Incomplete mouse data available" means not all orthologs have been knocked-out. ‡Genes that have been knocked-out are indicated in bold. *In instances where more than one mouse ortholog exists, the male infertile mouse ortholog is indicated in bold.

REFERENCES

Abbasi, F., Miyata, H., Shimada, K., Morohoshi, A., Nozawa, K., Matsumura, T., et al. (2018). RSPH6A is required for sperm flagellum formation and male fertility in mice. *J. Cell Sci.* 131:jcs221648. doi: 10.1242/jcs.221648

Abby, E., Tourpin, S., Ribeiro, J., Daniel, K., Messiaen, S., Moison, D., et al. (2016). Implementation of meiosis prophase I programme requires a conserved retinoid-independent stabilizer of meiotic transcripts. *Nat. Commun.* 7:10324. doi: 10.1038/ncomms10324

Aitken, R. J. (2002). Immunocontraceptive vaccines for human use. *J. Reprod. Immunol.* 57, 273–287. doi: 10.1016/s0165-0378(02)00010-4

Alves, M. G., Dias, T. R., Silva, B. M., and Oliveira, P. F. (2014). Metabolic cooperation in testis as a pharmacological target: from disease to contraception. *Curr. Mol. Pharmacol.* 7, 83–95. doi: 10.2174/1874467208666150126153830

Arango, N. A., Li, L., Dabir, D., Nicolau, F., Pieretti-Vanmarcke, R., Koehler, C., et al. (2013). Meiosis I arrest abnormalities lead to severe oligozoospermia in meiosis 1 arresting protein (M1ap)-deficient mice. *Biol. Reprod.* 88:76. doi: 10.1095/biolreprod.111.098673

Archambeault, D. R., and Matzuk, M. M. (2014). Disrupting the male germ line to find infertility and contraception targets. *Ann. Endocrinol.* 75, 101–108. doi: 10.1016/j.ando.2014.04.006

Asano, Y., Akiyama, K., Tsuji, T., Takahashi, S., Noguchi, J., and Kunieda, T. (2009). Characterization and linkage mapping of an ENU-induced mutant mouse with defective spermatogenesis. *Exp. Anim.* 58, 525–532. doi: 10.1538/expanim.58.525

Bagatell, C. J., Matsumoto, A. M., Christensen, R. B., Rivier, J. E., and Bremner, W. J. (1993). Comparison of a gonadotropin releasing-hormone antagonist plus testosterone (T) versus T alone as potential male contraceptive regimens. *J. Clin. Endocrinol. Metab.* 77, 427–432. doi: 10.1210/jcem.77.2.8345047

Baggelaar, M. P., den Dulk, H., Florea, B. I., Fazio, D., Bernabo, N., Raspa, M., et al. (2019). ABHD2 inhibitor identified by activity-based protein profiling reduces acrosome reaction. *ACS Chem. Biol.* 14, 2295–2304. doi: 10.1021/acschembio.9b00640

Barda, S., Yogev, L., Paz, G., Yavetz, H., Hauser, R., Breitbart, H., et al. (2016). New insights into the role of the Brdt protein in the regulation of development and spermatogenesis in the mouse. *Gene Expr. Patterns* 20, 130–137. doi: 10.1016/j.gep.2016.03.003

Bechara, C., and Sagan, S. (2013). Cell-penetrating peptides: 20 years later, where do we stand? *FEBS Lett.* 587, 1693–1702. doi: 10.1016/j.febslet.2013.04.031

Benito, E., Ramachandran, B., Schroeder, H., Schmidt, G., Urbanke, H., Burkhardt, S., et al. (2017). The BET/BRD inhibitor JQ1 improves brain plasticity in WT and APP mice. *Transl. Psychiatry* 7:e1239. doi: 10.1038/tp.2017.202

Bonasio, R., Lecona, E., Narendra, V., Voigt, P., Parisi, F., Kluger, Y., et al. (2014). Interactions with RNA direct the Polycomb group protein SCML2 to chromatin where it represses target genes. *eLife* 3:e02637. doi: 10.7554/eLife.02637

Bondeson, D. P., Mares, A., Smith, I. E., Ko, E., Campos, S., Miah, A. H., et al. (2015). Catalytic in vivo protein knockdown by small-molecule PROTACs. *Nat. Chem. Biol.* 11, 611–617. doi: 10.1038/nchembio.1858

Bondeson, D. P., Smith, B. E., Burslem, G. M., Buhimschi, A. D., Hines, J., Jaime-Figueroa, S., et al. (2018). Lessons in PROTAC design from selective degradation with a promiscuous warhead. *Cell Chem. Biol.* 25, 78.e5–87.e5. doi: 10.1016/j.chembiol.2017.09.010

Bonora, E., Bianco, F., Cordeddu, L., Bamshad, M., Francescatto, L., Dowless, D., et al. (2015). Mutations in RAD21 disrupt regulation of APOB in patients with chronic intestinal pseudo-obstruction. *Gastroenterology* 148, 771.e11–782.e11. doi: 10.1053/j.gastro.2014.12.034

Brehm, R., Zeiler, M., Ruttinger, C., Herde, K., Kibschull, M., Winterhager, E., et al. (2007). A sertoli cell-specific knockout of connexin43 prevents initiation of spermatogenesis. *Am. J. Pathol.* 171, 19–31. doi: 10.2353/ajpath.2007.061171

Brooks, H., Lebleu, B., and Vives, E. (2005). Tat peptide-mediated cellular delivery: back to basics. *Adv. Drug Deliv. Rev.* 57, 559–577. doi: 10.1016/j.addr.2004.12.001

Burnicka-Turek, O., Shirneshan, K., Paprotta, I., Grzmil, P., Meinhardt, A., Engel, W., et al. (2009). Inactivation of insulin-like factor 6 disrupts the progression of spermatogenesis at late meiotic prophase. *Endocrinology* 150, 4348–4357. doi: 10.1210/en.2009-0201

Castaneda, J. M., Hua, R., Miyata, H., Oji, A., Guo, Y., Cheng, Y., et al. (2017). TCTE1 is a conserved component of the dynein regulatory complex and is required for motility and metabolism in mouse spermatozoa. *Proc. Natl. Acad. Sci. U.S.A.* 114, E5370–E5378. doi: 10.1073/pnas.1621279114

Chen, H., Lui, W. Y., Mruk, D. D., Xiao, X., Ge, R., Lian, Q., et al. (2018). Monitoring the integrity of the blood-testis barrier (BTB): an *in vivo* assay. *Methods Mol. Biol.* 1748, 245–252. doi: 10.1007/978-1-4939-7698-0_17

Chen, H., Mruk, D. D., Xia, W., Bonanomi, M., Silvestrini, B., and Cheng, C. Y. (2016a). Effective delivery of male contraceptives behind the blood-testis barrier (BTB) - lesson from adjudin. *Curr. Med. Chem.* 23, 701–713. doi: 10.2174/0929867323666160112122724

Chen, S. R., Batool, A., Wang, Y. Q., Hao, X. X., Chang, C. S., Cheng, C. Y., et al. (2016b). The control of male fertility by spermatid-specific factors: searching for contraceptive targets from spermatozoon's head to tail. *Cell Death Dis.* 7:e2472. doi: 10.1038/cddis.2016.344

Cheng, Y., Ma, Z., Kim, B. H., Wu, W., Cayting, P., Boyle, A. P., et al. (2014). Principles of regulatory information conservation between mouse and human. *Nature* 515, 371–375. doi: 10.1038/nature13985

Chung, J. J., Navarro, B., Krapivinsky, G., Krapivinsky, L., and Clapham, D. E. (2011). A novel gene required for male fertility and functional CATSPER channel formation in spermatozoa. *Nat. Commun.* 2:153. doi: 10.1038/ncomms1153

Daniel, K., Lange, J., Hached, K., Fu, J., Anastassiadis, K., Roig, I., et al. (2011). Meiotic homologue alignment and its quality surveillance are controlled by mouse HORMAD1. *Nat. Cell Biol.* 13, 599–610. doi: 10.1038/ncb2213

Danshina, P. V., Geyer, C. B., Dai, Q., Goulding, E. H., Willis, W. D., Kitto, G. B., et al. (2010). Phosphoglycerate kinase 2 (PGK2) is essential for sperm function and male fertility in mice. *Biol. Reprod.* 82, 136–145. doi: 10.1095/biolreprod.109.079699

Das, A., Chai, J. C., Yang, C. S., Lee, Y. S., Das, N. D., Jung, K. H., et al. (2015). Dual transcriptome sequencing reveals resistance of TLR4 ligand-activated bone marrow-derived macrophages to inflammation mediated by the BET inhibitor JQ1. *Sci. Rep.* 5:16932. doi: 10.1038/srep16932

Davies, B., Baumann, C., Kirchhoff, C., Ivell, R., Nubbemeyer, R., Habenicht, U. F., et al. (2004). Targeted deletion of the epididymal receptor HE6 results in fluid dysregulation and male infertility. *Mol. Cell Biol.* 24, 8642–8648. doi: 10.1128/MCB.24.19.8642-8648.2004

De Souza, A. T., Dai, X., Spencer, A. G., Reppen, T., Menzie, A., Roesch, P. L., et al. (2006). Transcriptional and phenotypic comparisons of Ppara knockout and siRNA knockdown mice. *Nucleic Acids Res.* 34, 4486–4494. doi: 10.1093/nar/gkl609

Deardorff, M. A., Wilde, J. J., Albrecht, M., Dickinson, E., Tennstedt, S., Braunholz, D., et al. (2012). RAD21 mutations cause a human cohesinopathy. *Am. J. Hum. Genet.* 90, 1014–1027. doi: 10.1016/j.ajhg.2012.04.019

Dickinson, M. E., Flenniken, A. M., Ji, X., Teboul, L., Wong, M. D., White, J. K., et al. (2016). High-throughput discovery of novel developmental phenotypes. *Nature* 537, 508–514. doi: 10.1038/nature19356

Djureinovic, D., Fagerberg, L., Hallstrom, B., Danielsson, A., Lindskog, C., Uhlen, M., et al. (2014). The human testis-specific proteome defined by transcriptomics and antibody-based profiling. *Mol. Hum. Reprod.* 20, 476–488. doi: 10.1093/molehr/gau018

Dong, F., Shinohara, K., Botilde, Y., Nabeshima, R., Asai, Y., Fukumoto, A., et al. (2014). Pih1d3 is required for cytoplasmic preassembly of axonemal dynein in mouse sperm. *J. Cell Biol.* 204, 203–213. doi: 10.1083/jcb.201304076

Drevet, J. R. (2018). Epididymal approaches to male contraception. *Basic Clin. Androl.* 28:12. doi: 10.1186/s12610-018-0078-y

Feng, C. A., Spiller, C., Merriner, D. J., O'Bryan, M. K., Bowles, J., and Koopman, P. (2017). SOX30 is required for male fertility in mice. *Sci. Rep.* 7:17619. doi: 10.1038/s41598-017-17854-5

Fermo, E., Bianchi, P., Chiarelli, L. R., Maggi, M., Mandara, G. M., Vercellati, C., et al. (2012). A new variant of phosphoglycerate kinase deficiency (p.*I371K*) with multiple tissue involvement: molecular and functional characterization. *Mol. Genet. Metab.* 106, 455–461. doi: 10.1016/j.ymgme.2012.05.015

Finsterbusch, F., Ravindranathan, R., Dereli, I., Stanzione, M., Trankner, D., and Toth, A. (2016). Alignment of homologous chromosomes and effective repair of programmed DNA double-strand breaks during mouse meiosis require the minichromosome maintenance domain containing 2 (MCMDC2) protein. *PLoS Genet.* 12:e1006393. doi: 10.1371/journal.pgen.1006393

Franca, L. R., Hess, R. A., Dufour, J. M., Hofmann, M. C., and Griswold, M. D. (2016). The Sertoli cell: one hundred fifty years of beauty and plasticity. *Andrology* 4, 189–212. doi: 10.1111/andr.12165

French, C. A., Ramirez, C. L., Kolmakova, J., Hickman, T. T., Cameron, M. J., Thyne, M. E., et al. (2008). BRD-NUT oncoproteins: a family of closely related nuclear proteins that block epithelial differentiation and maintain the growth of carcinoma cells. *Oncogene* 27, 2237–2242. doi: 10.1038/sj.onc.1210852

Frick, J., and Aulitzky, W. (1988). Male contraception. *Hum. Reprod.* 3, 147–151. doi: 10.1093/oxfordjournals.humrep.a136664

Frost, R. J., Hamra, F. K., Richardson, J. A., Qi, X., Bassel-Duby, R., and Olson, E. N. (2010). MOV10L1 is necessary for protection of spermatocytes against retrotransposons by Piwi-interacting RNAs. *Proc. Natl. Acad. Sci. U.S.A.* 107, 11847–11852. doi: 10.1073/pnas.1007158107

Fujihara, Y., Oji, A., Larasati, T., Kojima-Kita, K., and Ikawa, M. (2017). Human globozoospermia-related gene Spata16 is required for sperm formation revealed by CRISPR/Cas9-mediated mouse models. *Int. J. Mol. Sci.* 18:2208. doi: 10.3390/ijms18102208

Fujihara, Y., Okabe, M., and Ikawa, M. (2014). GPI-anchored protein complex, LY6K/TEX101, is required for sperm migration into the oviduct and male fertility in mice. *Biol. Reprod.* 90:60. doi: 10.1095/biolreprod.113.112888

Fujihara, Y., Satouh, Y., Inoue, N., Isotani, A., Ikawa, M., and Okabe, M. (2012). SPACA1-deficient male mice are infertile with abnormally shaped sperm heads reminiscent of globozoospermia. *Development* 139, 3583–3589. doi: 10.1242/dev.081778

Fujihara, Y., Tokuhiro, K., Muro, Y., Kondoh, G., Araki, Y., Ikawa, M., et al. (2013). Expression of TEX101, regulated by ACE, is essential for the production of fertile mouse spermatozoa. *Proc. Natl. Acad. Sci. U.S.A.* 110, 8111–8116. doi: 10.1073/pnas.1222166110

Fuller, J. C., Burgoyne, N. J., and Jackson, R. M. (2009). Predicting druggable binding sites at the protein-protein interface. *Drug Discov. Today* 14, 155–161. doi: 10.1016/j.drudis.2008.10.009

Gomez, H. L., Felipe-Medina, N., Sanchez-Martin, M., Davies, O. R., Ramos, I., Garcia-Tunon, I., et al. (2016). C14ORF39/SIX6OS1 is a constituent of the synaptonemal complex and is essential for mouse fertility. *Nat. Commun.* 7:13298. doi: 10.1038/ncomms13298

Gopinathan, L., Szmyd, R., Low, D., Diril, M. K., Chang, H. Y., Coppola, V., et al. (2017). Emi2 is essential for mouse spermatogenesis. *Cell Rep.* 20, 697–708. doi: 10.1016/j.celrep.2017.06.033

Gottwald, U., Davies, B., Fritsch, M., and Habenicht, U. F. (2006). New approaches for male fertility control: HE6 as an example of a putative target. *Mol. Cell. Endocrinol.* 250, 49–57. doi: 10.1016/j.mce.2005.12.024

Greenbaum, M. P., Yan, W., Wu, M. H., Lin, Y. N., Agno, J. E., Sharma, M., et al. (2006). TEX14 is essential for intercellular bridges and fertility in male mice. *Proc. Natl. Acad. Sci. U.S.A.* 103, 4982–4987. doi: 10.1073/pnas.0505123103

GTEx Consortium (2013). The genotype-tissue expression (GTEx) project. *Nat. Genet.* 45, 580–585. doi: 10.1038/ng.2653

Guiraldelli, M. F., Eyster, C., Wilkerson, J. L., Dresser, M. E., and Pezza, R. J. (2013). Mouse HFM1/Mer3 is required for crossover formation and complete synapsis of homologous chromosomes during meiosis. *PLoS Genet.* 9:e1003383. doi: 10.1371/journal.pgen.1003383

Gutstein, D. E., Morley, G. E., Tamaddon, H., Vaidya, D., Schneider, M. D., Chen, J., et al. (2001). Conduction slowing and sudden arrhythmic death in mice with cardiac-restricted inactivation of connexin43. *Circ. Res.* 88, 333–339. doi: 10.1161/01.res.88.3.333

Hanada, K., Kuromori, T., Myouga, F., Toyoda, T., Li, W. H., and Shinozaki, K. (2009). Evolutionary persistence of functional compensation by duplicate genes in *Arabidopsis*. *Genome Biol. Evol.* 1, 409–414. doi: 10.1093/gbe/evp043

Hasegawa, K., Sin, H. S., Maezawa, S., Broering, T. J., Kartashov, A. V., Alavattam, K. G., et al. (2015). SCML2 establishes the male germline epigenome through regulation of histone H2A ubiquitination. *Dev. Cell* 32, 574–588. doi: 10.1016/j.devcel.2015.01.014

Herndon, N. (1992). Looking for the "male pill". *Netw. Res. Triangle Park N. C.* 13, 20–23.

Herran, Y., Gutierrez-Caballero, C., Sanchez-Martin, M., Hernandez, T., Viera, A., Barbero, J. L., et al. (2011). The cohesin subunit RAD21L functions in meiotic synapsis and exhibits sexual dimorphism in fertility. *EMBO J.* 30, 3091–3105. doi: 10.1038/emboj.2011.222

Hild, S. A., Reel, J. R., Dykstra, M. J., Mann, P. C., and Marshall, G. R. (2007). Acute adverse effects of the indenopyridine CDB-4022 on the ultrastructure of sertoli cells, spermatocytes, and spermatids in rat testes: comparison to the known sertoli cell toxicant Di-n-pentylphthalate (DPP). *J. Androl.* 28, 621–629. doi: 10.2164/jandrol.106.002295

Holcomb, R. J., Oura, S., Nozawa, K., Kent, K., Yu, Z., Robertson, M. J., et al. (2020). The testis-specific serine proteases Prss44, Prss46, and Prss54 are dispensable for male mouse fertility†. *Biol. Reprod.* 102, 84–91. doi: 10.1093/biolre/ioz158

Hopkins, A. L., and Groom, C. R. (2002). The druggable genome. *Nat. Rev. Drug Discov.* 1, 727–730. doi: 10.1038/nrd892

Horn, H. F., Kim, D. I., Wright, G. D., Wong, E. S., Stewart, C. L., Burke, B., et al. (2013). A mammalian KASH domain protein coupling meiotic chromosomes to the cytoskeleton. *J. Cell Biol.* 202, 1023–1039. doi: 10.1083/jcb.201304004

Ikawa, M., Tokuhiro, K., Yamaguchi, R., Benham, A. M., Tamura, T., Wada, I., et al. (2011). Calsperin is a testis-specific chaperone required for sperm fertility. *J. Biol. Chem.* 286, 5639–5646. doi: 10.1074/jbc.M110.140152

Ilani, N., Roth, M. Y., Amory, J. K., Swerdloff, R. S., Dart, C., Page, S. T., et al. (2012). A new combination of testosterone and nestorone transdermal gels for male hormonal contraception. *J. Clin. Endocrinol. Metab.* 97, 3476–3486. doi: 10.1210/jc.2012-1384

Jimenez, T., McDermott, J. P., Sanchez, G., and Blanco, G. (2011). Na,K-ATPase alpha4 isoform is essential for sperm fertility. *Proc. Natl. Acad. Sci. U.S.A.* 108, 644–649. doi: 10.1073/pnas.1016902108

Kanishchev, O. S., and Dolbier, W. R. (2018). Synthesis of 6-SF5-indazoles and an SF5-analog of gamendazole. *Org. Biomol. Chem.* 16, 5793–5799. doi: 10.1039/c8ob01460d

Kashiwabara, S., Tsuruta, S., Okada, K., Saegusa, A., Miyagaki, Y., and Baba, T. (2016). Functional compensation for the loss of testis-specific poly(A)-binding protein, PABPC2, during mouse spermatogenesis. *J. Reprod. Dev.* 62, 305–310. doi: 10.1262/jrd.2016-023

Kim, J., Ishiguro, K., Nambu, A., Akiyoshi, B., Yokobayashi, S., Kagami, A., et al. (2015). Meikin is a conserved regulator of meiosis-I-specific kinetochore function. *Nature* 517, 466–471. doi: 10.1038/nature14097

Kogo, H., Tsutsumi, M., Inagaki, H., Ohye, T., Kiyonari, H., and Kurahashi, H. (2012a). HORMAD2 is essential for synapsis surveillance during meiotic prophase via the recruitment of ATR activity. *Genes Cells* 17, 897–912. doi: 10.1111/gtc.12005

Kogo, H., Tsutsumi, M., Ohye, T., Inagaki, H., Abe, T., and Kurahashi, H. (2012b). HORMAD1-dependent checkpoint/surveillance mechanism eliminates asynaptic oocytes. *Genes Cells* 17, 439–454. doi: 10.1111/j.1365-2443.2012.01600.x

Kozakov, D., Hall, D. R., Napoleon, R. L., Yueh, C., Whitty, A., and Vajda, S. (2015). New frontiers in druggability. *J. Med. Chem.* 58, 9063–9088. doi: 10.1021/acs.jmedchem.5b00586

Krahling, A. M., Alvarez, L., Debowski, K., Van, Q., Gunkel, M., Irsen, S., et al. (2013). CRIS-a novel cAMP-binding protein controlling spermiogenesis and the development of flagellar bending. *PLoS Genet.* 9:e1003960. doi: 10.1371/journal.pgen.1003960

La Salle, S., Palmer, K., O'Brien, M., Schimenti, J. C., Eppig, J., and Handel, M. A. (2012). Spata22, a novel vertebrate-specific gene, is required for meiotic progress in mouse germ cells. *Biol. Reprod.* 86:45. doi: 10.1095/biolreprod.111.095752

Lambert, J. P., Picaud, S., Fujisawa, T., Hou, H., Savitsky, P., Uuskula-Reimand, L., et al. (2019). Interactome rewiring following pharmacological targeting of BET bromodomains. *Mol. Cell* 73, 621.e17–638.e17. doi: 10.1016/j.molcel.2018.11.006

Lee, B., Park, I., Jin, S., Choi, H., Kwon, J. T., Kim, J., et al. (2011). Impaired spermatogenesis and fertility in mice carrying a mutation in the Spink2 gene expressed predominantly in testes. *J. Biol. Chem.* 286, 29108–29117. doi: 10.1074/jbc.M111.244905

Lee, M. S. (2019). *CITDBase: Contraceptive Infertility Target DataBase*. Available: https://www.citdbase.org/ (accessed October, 2019).

Li, W., Guo, X. J., Teng, F., Hou, X. J., Lv, Z., Zhou, S. Y., et al. (2013). Tex101 is essential for male fertility by affecting sperm migration into the oviduct in mice. *J. Mol. Cell Biol.* 5, 345–347. doi: 10.1093/jmcb/mjt031

Li, Y., Li, C., Lin, S., Yang, B., Huang, W., Wu, H., et al. (2017). A nonsense mutation in Ccdc62 gene is responsible for spermiogenesis defects and male infertility in repro29/repro29 mice. *Biol. Reprod.* 96, 587–597. doi: 10.1095/biolreprod.116.141408

Liao, Y., Day, K. H., Damon, D. N., and Duling, B. R. (2001). Endothelial cell-specific knockout of connexin 43 causes hypotension and bradycardia in mice. *Proc. Natl. Acad. Sci. U.S.A.* 98, 9989–9994. doi: 10.1073/pnas.171305298

Lin, S., Lin, Y., Nery, J. R., Urich, M. A., Breschi, A., Davis, C. A., et al. (2014). Comparison of the transcriptional landscapes between human and mouse tissues. *Proc. Natl. Acad. Sci. U.S.A.* 111, 17224–17229. doi: 10.1073/pnas.1413624111

Liu, Y., DeBoer, K., de Kretser, D. M., O'Donnell, L., O'Connor, A. E., Merriner, D. J., et al. (2015). LRGUK-1 is required for basal body and manchette function during spermatogenesis and male fertility. *PLoS Genet.* 11:e1005090. doi: 10.1371/journal.pgen.1005090

Lu, J., Qian, Y., Altieri, M., Dong, H., Wang, J., Raina, K., et al. (2015). Hijacking the E3 ubiquitin ligase cereblon to efficiently target BRD4. *Chem. Biol.* 22, 755–763. doi: 10.1016/j.chembiol.2015.05.009

Lu, Y., Oura, S., Matsumura, T., Oji, A., Sakurai, N., Fujihara, Y., et al. (2019). CRISPR/Cas9-mediated genome editing reveals 30 testis-enriched genes dispensable for male fertility in mice. *Biol. Reprod.* 101, 501–511. doi: 10.1093/biolre/ioz103

Luangpraseuth-Prosper, A., Lesueur, E., Jouneau, L., Pailhoux, E., Cotinot, C., and Mandon-Pepin, B. (2015). TOPAZ1, a germ cell specific factor, is essential for male meiotic progression. *Dev. Biol.* 406, 158–171. doi: 10.1016/j.ydbio.2015.09.002

Luo, M., Yang, F., Leu, N. A., Landaiche, J., Handel, M. A., Benavente, R., et al. (2013). MEIOB exhibits single-stranded DNA-binding and exonuclease activities and is essential for meiotic recombination. *Nat. Commun.* 4:2788. doi: 10.1038/ncomms3788

Ma, L., Buchold, G. M., Greenbaum, M. P., Roy, A., Burns, K. H., Zhu, H., et al. (2009). GASZ is essential for male meiosis and suppression of retrotransposon expression in the male germline. *PLoS Genet.* 5:e1000635. doi: 10.1371/journal.pgen.1000635

Maezawa, S., Hasegawa, K., Yukawa, M., Kubo, N., Sakashita, A., Alavattam, K. G., et al. (2018). Polycomb protein SCML2 facilitates H3K27me3 to establish bivalent domains in the male germline. *Proc. Natl. Acad. Sci. U.S.A.* 115, 4957–4962. doi: 10.1073/pnas.1804512115

Marschang, P., Brich, J., Weeber, E. J., Sweatt, J. D., Shelton, J. M., Richardson, J. A., et al. (2004). Normal development and fertility of knockout mice lacking the tumor suppressor gene LRP1b suggest functional compensation by LRP1. *Mol. Cell Biol.* 24, 3782–3793. doi: 10.1128/mcb.24.9.3782-3793.2004

Matzuk, M. M., McKeown, M. R., Filippakopoulos, P., Li, Q., Ma, L., Agno, J. E., et al. (2012). Small-molecule inhibition of BRDT for male contraception. *Cell* 150, 673–684. doi: 10.1016/j.cell.2012.06.045

McKenzie, C. W., Craige, B., Kroeger, T. V., Finn, R., Wyatt, T. A., Sisson, J. H., et al. (2015). CFAP54 is required for proper ciliary motility and assembly of the central pair apparatus in mice. *Mol. Biol. Cell* 26, 3140–3149. doi: 10.1091/mbc.E15-02-0121

Meriggiola, M. C., Marcovina, S., Paulsen, C. A., and Bremner, W. J. (1995). Testosterone enanthate at a dose of 200 mg/week decreases HDL-cholesterol levels in healthy men. *Int. J. Androl.* 18, 237–242. doi: 10.1111/ijan.1995.18.5.237

Miller, T. C., Simon, B., Rybin, V., Grotsch, H., Curtet, S., Khochbin, S., et al. (2016). A bromodomain-DNA interaction facilitates acetylation-dependent bivalent nucleosome recognition by the BET protein BRDT. *Nat. Commun.* 7:13855. doi: 10.1038/ncomms13855

Miyata, H., Castaneda, J. M., Fujihara, Y., Yu, Z., Archambeault, D. R., Isotani, A., et al. (2016). Genome engineering uncovers 54 evolutionarily conserved and testis-enriched genes that are not required for male fertility in mice. *Proc. Natl. Acad. Sci. U.S.A.* 113, 7704–7710. doi: 10.1073/pnas.1608458113

Miyata, H., Satouh, Y., Mashiko, D., Muto, M., Nozawa, K., Shiba, K., et al. (2015). Sperm calcineurin inhibition prevents mouse fertility with implications for male contraceptive. *Science* 350, 442–445. doi: 10.1126/science.aad0836

Mok, K. W., Lie, P. P. Y., Mruk, D. D., Mannu, J., Mathur, P. P., Silvestrini, B., et al. (2012). The apical ectoplasmic specialization-blood-testis barrier functional axis is a novel target for male contraception. *Adv. Exp. Med. Biol.* 763, 334–355. doi: 10.1007/978-1-4614-4711-5_17

Mok, K. W., Mruk, D. D., Lie, P. P., Lui, W. Y., and Cheng, C. Y. (2011). Adjudin, a potential male contraceptive, exerts its effects locally in the seminiferous epithelium of mammalian testes. *Reproduction* 141, 571–580. doi: 10.1530/REP-10-0464

Morakinyo, A. O., Iranloye, B. O., and Adegoke, O. A. (2009). Antireproductive effect of calcium channel blockers on male rats. *Reprod. Med. Biol.* 8, 97–102. doi: 10.1007/s12522-009-0018-9

Mruk, D. D. (2008). New perspectives in non-hormonal male contraception. *Trends Endocrinol. Metab.* 19, 57–64. doi: 10.1016/j.tem.2007.11.002

Mruk, D. D., and Cheng, C. Y. (2011). Testin and actin are key molecular targets of adjudin, an anti-spermatogenic agent, in the testis. *Spermatogenesis* 1, 137–146. doi: 10.4161/spmg.1.2.16449

Mruk, D. D., Wong, C. H., Silvestrini, B., and Cheng, C. Y. (2006). A male contraceptive targeting germ cell adhesion. *Nat. Med.* 12, 1323–1328. doi: 10.1038/nm1420

Munoz-Fuentes, V., Cacheiro, P., Meehan, T. F., Aguilar-Pimentel, J. A., Brown, S. D. M., Flenniken, A. M., et al. (2018). The international mouse phenotyping consortium (IMPC): a functional catalogue of the mammalian genome that informs conservation. *Conserv. Genet.* 19, 995–1005. doi: 10.1007/s10592-018-1072-9

Murdoch, F. E., and Goldberg, E. (2014). Male contraception: another Holy Grail. *Bioorg. Med. Chem. Lett.* 24, 419–424. doi: 10.1016/j.bmcl.2013.12.004

Nagai, M., Moriyama, T., Mehmood, R., Tokuhiro, K., Ikawa, M., Okabe, M., et al. (2011). Mice lacking Ran binding protein 1 are viable and show male infertility. *FEBS Lett.* 585, 791–796. doi: 10.1016/j.febslet.2011.02.002

Nakamura, N., Dai, Q., Williams, J., Goulding, E. H., Willis, W. D., Brown, P. R., et al. (2013). Disruption of a spermatogenic cell-specific mouse enolase 4 (eno4) gene causes sperm structural defects and male infertility. *Biol. Reprod.* 88:90. doi: 10.1095/biolreprod.112.107128

Nilsson, M., Husmark, J., Bjorkman, U., and Ericson, L. E. (1998). Cytokines and thyroid epithelial integrity: interleukin-1alpha induces dissociation of the junctional complex and paracellular leakage in filter-cultured human thyrocytes. *J. Clin. Endocrinol. Metab.* 83, 945–952. doi: 10.1210/jcem.83.3.4626

Nishimura, T., Nagamori, I., Nakatani, T., Izumi, N., Tomari, Y., Kuramochi-Miyagawa, S., et al. (2018). PNLDC1, mouse pre-piRNA Trimmer, is required for meiotic and post-meiotic male germ cell development. *EMBO Rep.* 19:e44957. doi: 10.15252/embr.201744957

Olson, C. M., Jiang, B., Erb, M. A., Liang, Y., Doctor, Z. M., Zhang, Z., et al. (2018). Pharmacological perturbation of CDK9 using selective CDK9 inhibition or degradation. *Nat. Chem. Biol.* 14, 163–170. doi: 10.1038/nchembio.2538

O'Rand, M. G., Hamil, K. G., Adevai, T., and Zelinski, M. (2018). Inhibition of sperm motility in male macaques with EP055, a potential non-hormonal male contraceptive. *PLoS One* 13:e0195953. doi: 10.1371/journal.pone.0195953

O'Rand, M. G., Silva, E. J., and Hamil, K. G. (2016). Non-hormonal male contraception: a review and development of an Eppin based contraceptive. *Pharmacol. Ther.* 157, 105–111. doi: 10.1016/j.pharmthera.2015.11.004

O'Rand, M. G., Widgren, E. E., Hamil, K. G., Silva, E. J., and Richardson, R. T. (2011). Epididymal protein targets: a brief history of the development of epididymal protease inhibitor as a contraceptive. *J. Androl.* 32, 698–704. doi: 10.2164/jandrol.110.012781

Ottis, P., Toure, M., Cromm, P. M., Ko, E., Gustafson, J. L., and Crews, C. M. (2017). Assessing different E3 ligases for small molecule induced protein ubiquitination and degradation. *ACS Chem. Biol.* 12, 2570–2578. doi: 10.1021/acschembio.7b00485

Pan, J., Eckardt, S., Leu, N. A., Buffone, M. G., Zhou, J., Gerton, G. L., et al. (2009). Inactivation of Nxf2 causes defects in male meiosis and age-dependent depletion of spermatogonia. *Dev. Biol.* 330, 167–174. doi: 10.1016/j.ydbio.2009.03.022

Pandey, R. R., Tokuzawa, Y., Yang, Z., Hayashi, E., Ichisaka, T., Kajita, S., et al. (2013). Tudor domain containing 12 (TDRD12) is essential for secondary PIWI interacting RNA biogenesis in mice. *Proc. Natl. Acad. Sci. U.S.A.* 110, 16492–16497. doi: 10.1073/pnas.1316316110

Pasek, R. C., Malarkey, E., Berbari, N. F., Sharma, N., Kesterson, R. A., Tres, L. L., et al. (2016). Coiled-coil domain containing 42 (Ccdc42) is necessary for proper sperm development and male fertility in the mouse. *Dev. Biol.* 412, 208–218. doi: 10.1016/j.ydbio.2016.01.042

Pasztor, N., Hegyi, B. E., Bado, A., and Nemeth, G. (2017). [Male hormonal contraception: past, present, future]. *Orv. Hetil.* 158, 1819–1830. doi: 10.1556/650.2017.30876

Payne, C., and Goldberg, E. (2014). Male contraception: past, present and future. *Curr. Mol. Pharmacol.* 7, 175–181.

Prasad, M. R., and Rajalakshmi, M. (1976). Target sites for suppressing fertility in the male. *Adv. Sex. Horm. Res.* 2, 263–287.

Rappaport, N., Twik, M., Plaschkes, I., Nudel, R., Iny Stein, T., Levitt, J., et al. (2017). MalaCards: an amalgamated human disease compendium with diverse clinical and genetic annotation and structured search. *Nucleic Acids Res.* 45, D877–D887. doi: 10.1093/nar/gkw1012

Ren, D., Navarro, B., Perez, G., Jackson, A. C., Hsu, S., Shi, Q., et al. (2001). A sperm ion channel required for sperm motility and male fertility. *Nature* 413, 603–609. doi: 10.1038/35098027

Revenkova, E., Herrmann, K., Adelfalk, C., and Jessberger, R. (2010). Oocyte cohesin expression restricted to predictyate stages provides full fertility and prevents aneuploidy. *Curr. Biol.* 20, 1529–1533. doi: 10.1016/j.cub.2010.08.024

Roberts, K. P., Ensrud, K. M., Wooters, J. L., Nolan, M. A., Johnston, D. S., and Hamilton, D. W. (2006). Epididymal secreted protein Crisp-1 and sperm function. *Mol. Cell. Endocrinol.* 250, 122–127. doi: 10.1016/j.mce.2005.12.034

Samaras, P., Schmidt, T., Frejno, M., Gessulat, S., Reinecke, M., Jarzab, A., et al. (2019). ProteomicsDB: a multi-omics and multi-organism resource for life science research. *Nucleic Acids Res.* 48, D1153–D1163. doi: 10.1093/nar/gkz974

Santi, C. M., Martinez-Lopez, P., de la Vega-Beltran, J. L., Butler, A., Alisio, A., and Darszon, A. (2010). The SLO3 sperm-specific potassium channel plays a vital role in male fertility. *FEBS Lett.* 584, 1041–1046. doi: 10.1016/j.febslet.2010.02.005

Schmidt, T., Samaras, P., Frejno, M., Gessulat, S., Barnert, M., Kienegger, H., et al. (2017). ProteomicsDB. *Nucleic Acids Res.* 46, D1271–D1281. doi: 10.1093/nar/gkx1029

Schramm, S., Fraune, J., Naumann, R., Hernandez-Hernandez, A., Hoog, C., Cooke, H. J., et al. (2011). A novel mouse synaptonemal complex protein is essential for loading of central element proteins, recombination, and fertility. *PLoS Genet.* 7:e1002088. doi: 10.1371/journal.pgen.1002088

Schultz, N., Hamra, F. K., and Garbers, D. L. (2003). A multitude of genes expressed solely in meiotic or postmeiotic spermatogenic cells offers a myriad of contraceptive targets. *Proc. Natl. Acad. Sci. U.S.A.* 100, 12201–12206. doi: 10.1073/pnas.1635054100

Shang, E., Nickerson, H. D., Wen, D., Wang, X., and Wolgemuth, D. J. (2007). The first bromodomain of Brdt, a testis-specific member of the BET sub-family of double-bromodomain-containing proteins, is essential for male germ cell differentiation. *Development* 134, 3507–3515. doi: 10.1242/dev.004481

Shang, Y., Zhu, F., Wang, L., Ouyang, Y. C., Dong, M. Z., Liu, C., et al. (2017). Essential role for SUN5 in anchoring sperm head to the tail. *eLife* 6:e28199. doi: 10.7554/eLife.28199

Shao, Q., Kannan, A., Lin, Z., Stack, B. C. Jr., Suen, J. Y., and Gao, L. (2014). BET protein inhibitor JQ1 attenuates Myc-amplified MCC tumor growth in vivo. *Cancer Res.* 74, 7090–7102. doi: 10.1158/0008-5472.CAN-14-0305

Shen, C., Kuang, Y., Liu, J., Feng, J., Chen, X., Wu, W., et al. (2013). Prss37 is required for male fertility in the mouse. *Biol. Reprod.* 88:123. doi: 10.1095/biolreprod.112.107086

Shi, J., Wang, Y., Zeng, L., Wu, Y., Deng, J., Zhang, Q., et al. (2014). Disrupting the interaction of BRD4 with diacetylated Twist suppresses tumorigenesis in basal-like breast cancer. *Cancer Cell* 25, 210–225. doi: 10.1016/j.ccr.2014.01.028

Shibuya, H., Ishiguro, K., and Watanabe, Y. (2014). The TRF1-binding protein TERB1 promotes chromosome movement and telomere rigidity in meiosis. *Nat. Cell Biol.* 16, 145–156. doi: 10.1038/ncb2896

Shin, Y. H., Choi, Y., Erdin, S. U., Yatsenko, S. A., Kloc, M., Yang, F., et al. (2010). Hormad1 mutation disrupts synaptonemal complex formation, recombination, and chromosome segregation in mammalian meiosis. *PLoS Genet.* 6:e1001190. doi: 10.1371/journal.pgen.1001190

Silva, E. J., Patrao, M. T., Tsuruta, J. K., O'Rand, M. G., and Avellar, M. C. (2012). Epididymal protease inhibitor (EPPIN) is differentially expressed in the male rat reproductive tract and immunolocalized in maturing spermatozoa. *Mol. Reprod. Dev.* 79, 832–842. doi: 10.1002/mrd.22119

Sipila, P., Jalkanen, J., Huhtaniemi, I. T., and Poutanen, M. (2009). Novel epididymal proteins as targets for the development of post-testicular male contraception. *Reproduction* 137, 379–389. doi: 10.1530/REP-08-0132

Smith, C. L., Blake, J. A., Kadin, J. A., Richardson, J. E., Bult, C. J., and Mouse Genome Database Group, (2018). Mouse genome database (MGD)-2018: knowledgebase for the laboratory mouse. *Nucleic Acids Res.* 46, D836–D842. doi: 10.1093/nar/gkx1006

Souquet, B., Abby, E., Herve, R., Finsterbusch, F., Tourpin, S., Le Bouffant, R., et al. (2013). MEIOB targets single-strand DNA and is necessary for meiotic recombination. *PLoS Genet.* 9:e1003784. doi: 10.1371/journal.pgen.1003784

Stelzer, G., Rosen, N., Plaschkes, I., Zimmerman, S., Twik, M., Fishilevich, S., et al. (2016). The GeneCards suite: from gene data mining to disease genome sequence analyses. *Curr. Protoc. Bioinform.* 54, 1.30.1–1.30.33. doi: 10.1002/cpbi.5

Stucker, F., and Ackermann, D. (2011). [Immunosuppressive drugs - how they work, their side effects and interactions]. *Ther. Umsch.* 68, 679–686. doi: 10.1024/0040-5930/a000230

Sullivan, R., and Mieusset, R. (2016). The human epididymis: its function in sperm maturation. *Hum. Reprod. Update* 22, 574–587. doi: 10.1093/humupd/dmw015

Tash, J. S., Attardi, B., Hild, S. A., Chakrasali, R., Jakkaraj, S. R., and Georg, G. I. (2008a). A novel potent indazole carboxylic acid derivative blocks spermatogenesis and is contraceptive in rats after a single oral dose. *Biol. Reprod.* 78, 1127–1138. doi: 10.1095/biolreprod.106.057810

Tash, J. S., Chakrasali, R., Jakkaraj, S. R., Hughes, J., Smith, S. K., Hornbaker, K., et al. (2008b). Gamendazole, an orally active indazole carboxylic acid male contraceptive agent, targets HSP90AB1 (HSP90BETA) and EEF1A1 (eEF1A), and stimulates Il1a transcription in rat Sertoli cells. *Biol. Reprod.* 78, 1139–1152. doi: 10.1095/biolreprod.107.062679

Teng, X., Yang, J., Xie, Y., Ni, Z., Hu, R., Shi, L., et al. (2006). A novel spermatogenesis-specific uPAR gene expressed in human and mouse testis. *Biochem. Biophys. Res. Commun.* 342, 1223–1227. doi: 10.1016/j.bbrc.2006.01.175

Tu, Z., Bayazit, M. B., Liu, H., Zhang, J., Busayavalasa, K., Risal, S., et al. (2017). Speedy A-Cdk2 binding mediates initial telomere-nuclear envelope attachment during meiotic prophase I independent of Cdk2 activation. *Proc. Natl. Acad. Sci. U.S.A.* 114, 592–597. doi: 10.1073/pnas.1618465114

Uhlen, M., Fagerberg, L., Hallstrom, B. M., Lindskog, C., Oksvold, P., Mardinoglu, A., et al. (2015). Tissue-based map of the human proteome. *Science* 347:1260419. doi: 10.1126/science.1260419

VanGompel, M. J., and Xu, E. Y. (2010). A novel requirement in mammalian spermatid differentiation for the DAZ-family protein Boule. *Hum. Mol. Genet.* 19, 2360–2369. doi: 10.1093/hmg/ddq109

Waites, G. M. (1993). Male fertility regulation: the challenges for the year 2000. *Br. Med. Bull.* 49, 210–221. doi: 10.1093/oxfordjournals.bmb.a072599

Walters, E. M., Bauer, B. A., Franklin, C. L., Evans, T. J., Bryda, E. C., Riley, L. K., et al. (2009). Mutational insertion of a ROSA26-EGFP transgene leads to defects in spermiogenesis and male infertility in mice. *Comp. Med.* 59, 545–552.

Welborn, J. P., Davis, M. G., Ebers, S. D., Stodden, G. R., Hayashi, K., Cheatwood, J. L., et al. (2015). Rhox8 ablation in the sertoli cells using a tissue-specific RNAi approach results in impaired male fertility in mice. *Biol. Reprod.* 93:8. doi: 10.1095/biolreprod.114.124834

Wells, J. A., and McClendon, C. L. (2007). Reaching for high-hanging fruit in drug discovery at protein-protein interfaces. *Nature* 450, 1001–1009. doi: 10.1038/nature06526

Wen, N., Guo, B., Zheng, H., Xu, L., Liang, H., Wang, Q., et al. (2019). Bromodomain inhibitor jq1 induces cell cycle arrest and apoptosis of glioma stem cells through the VEGF/PI3K/AKT signaling pathway. *Int. J. Oncol.* 55, 879–895. doi: 10.3892/ijo.2019.4863

Whitty, A., and Kumaravel, G. (2006). Between a rock and a hard place? *Nat. Chem. Biol.* 2, 112–118. doi: 10.1038/nchembio0306-112

Yabuta, Y., Ohta, H., Abe, T., Kurimoto, K., Chuma, S., and Saitou, M. (2011). TDRD5 is required for retrotransposon silencing, chromatoid body assembly, and spermiogenesis in mice. *J. Cell Biol.* 192, 781–795. doi: 10.1083/jcb.201009043

Yamaguchi, R., Fujihara, Y., Ikawa, M., and Okabe, M. (2012). Mice expressing aberrant sperm-specific protein PMIS2 produce normal-looking but fertilization-incompetent spermatozoa. *Mol. Biol. Cell* 23, 2671–2679. doi: 10.1091/mbc.E11-12-1025

Yang, K., Meinhardt, A., Zhang, B., Grzmil, P., Adham, I. M., and Hoyer-Fender, S. (2012). The small heat shock protein ODF1/HSPB10 is essential for tight linkage of sperm head to tail and male fertility in mice. *Mol. Cell Biol.* 32, 216–225. doi: 10.1128/MCB.06158-11

Young, S. A., Miyata, H., Satouh, Y., Kato, H., Nozawa, K., Isotani, A., et al. (2015). CRISPR/Cas9-mediated rapid generation of multiple mouse lines identified Ccdc63 as essential for spermiogenesis. *Int. J. Mol. Sci.* 16, 24732–24750. doi: 10.3390/ijms161024732

Yu, Y. E., Zhang, Y., Unni, E., Shirley, C. R., Deng, J. M., Russell, L. D., et al. (2000). Abnormal spermatogenesis and reduced fertility in transition nuclear protein 1-deficient mice. *Proc. Natl. Acad. Sci. U.S.A.* 97, 4683–4688. doi: 10.1073/pnas.97.9.4683

Zallot, R., Harrison, K. J., Kolaczkowski, B., and de Crecy-Lagard, V. (2016). Functional annotations of paralogs: a blessing and a curse. *Life* 6:39. doi: 10.3390/life6030039

Zeng, X. H., Yang, C., Kim, S. T., Lingle, C. J., and Xia, X. M. (2011). Deletion of the Slo3 gene abolishes alkalization-activated K+ current in mouse spermatozoa. *Proc. Natl. Acad. Sci. U.S.A.* 108, 5879–5884. doi: 10.1073/pnas.1100240108

Zhang, Z., Shen, X., Gude, D. R., Wilkinson, B. M., Justice, M. J., Flickinger, C. J., et al. (2009). MEIG1 is essential for spermiogenesis in mice. *Proc. Natl. Acad. Sci. U.S.A.* 106, 17055–17060. doi: 10.1073/pnas.0906414106

Zheng, K., Xiol, J., Reuter, M., Eckardt, S., Leu, N. A., McLaughlin, K. J., et al. (2010). Mouse MOV10L1 associates with Piwi proteins and is an essential component of the Piwi-interacting RNA (piRNA) pathway. *Proc. Natl. Acad. Sci. U.S.A.* 107, 11841–11846. doi: 10.1073/pnas.1003953107

Zhou, J., Du, Y. R., Qin, W. H., Hu, Y. G., Huang, Y. N., Bao, L., et al. (2009). RIM-BP3 is a manchette-associated protein essential for spermiogenesis. *Development* 136, 373–382. doi: 10.1242/dev.030858

Zhou, J., Li, W., Guo, J., Li, G., Chen, F., and Zhou, J. (2016). Downregulation of miR-329 promotes cell invasion by regulating BRD4 and predicts poor prognosis in hepatocellular carcinoma. *Tumour Biol.* 37, 3561–3569. doi: 10.1007/s13277-015-4109-4

Zhou, L., Canagarajah, B., Zhao, Y., Baibakov, B., Tokuhiro, K., Maric, D., et al. (2017). BTBD18 regulates a subset of piRNA-generating loci through transcription elongation in mice. *Dev. Cell* 40, 453.e5–466.e5. doi: 10.1016/j.devcel.2017.02.007

9

Membrane Potential Assessment by Fluorimetry as a Predictor Tool of Human Sperm Fertilizing Capacity

Carolina Baro Graf[1,2†]*, Carla Ritagliati*[1†]*, Valentina Torres-Monserrat*[3]*, Cintia Stival*[1]*, Carlos Carizza*[3]*, Mariano G. Buffone*[4*] *and Dario Krapf*[1,2*]

[1] Laboratory of Cell Signal Transduction Networks, Instituto de Biología Molecular y Celular de Rosario (IBR), CONICET-UNR, Rosario, Argentina, [2] Laboratorio de Medicina Reproductiva, Facultad de Ciencias Bioquímicas y Farmacéuticas, Universidad Nacional de Rosario, Rosario, Argentina, [3] Fertya, Medicina Reproductiva, Rosario, Argentina, [4] Instituto de Biología y Medicina Experimental (IBYME), CONICET, Buenos Aires, Argentina

***Correspondence:**
Mariano G. Buffone
mgbuffone@ibyme.conicet.gov.ar
Dario Krapf
krapf@ibr-conicet.gov.ar

† These authors share first authorship

Mammalian sperm acquire the ability to fertilize eggs by undergoing a process known as capacitation. Capacitation is triggered as the sperm travels through the female reproductive tract. This process involves specific physiological changes such as rearrangement of the cell plasma membrane, post-translational modifications of certain proteins, and changes in the cellular permeability to ions – with the subsequent impact on the plasma membrane potential (*Em*). Capacitation-associated *Em* hyperpolarization has been well studied in mouse sperm, and shown to be both necessary and sufficient to promote the acrosome reaction (AR) and fertilize the egg. However, the relevance of the sperm *Em* upon capacitation on human fertility has not been thoroughly characterized. Here, we performed an extensive study of the *Em* change during capacitation in human sperm samples using a potentiometric dye in a fluorimetric assay. Normospermic donors showed significant *Em* hyperpolarization after capacitation. *Em* values from capacitated samples correlated significantly with the sperm ability to undergo induced AR, highlighting the role of hyperpolarization in acrosomal responsiveness, and with successful *in vitro* fertilization (IVF) rates. These results show that *Em* hyperpolarization could be an indicator of human sperm fertilizing capacity, setting the basis for the use of *Em* values as a robust predictor of the success rate of IVF.

Keywords: membrane potential, sperm capacitation, *in vitro* fertilization, acrosome reaction, human infertility

INTRODUCTION

Infertility is a worldwide public health problem affecting ~1 in 7, or ~80 million couples worldwide (Slama et al., 2012; Datta et al., 2016). Although the causes of infertility are heterogeneous, the male factor is now conceived as important as the female etiology, accounting for at least 50% of cases (HFEA, 2014). Infertile couples rely on assisted reproductive technology (ART) to conceive, which include: IUI (intra-uterine insemination), *in vitro* fertilization (IVF), and ICSI (intra-cytoplasmic sperm injection). These treatments are expensive, invasive and risky. Excluding the female contribution, the decision on which treatment to choose often relies on general parameters of sperm in their basal state (i.e., non-capacitated sperm). However, these parameters are not true indicators of treatment success. Thus, a detailed understanding of how both normal and dysfunctional spermatozoa behave is necessary to develop a platform for new diagnostic tools and to infer best treatment options (Barratt et al., 2017, 2018).

Immediately after ejaculation the mammalian sperm is unable to fertilize the egg until it goes through a maturation process known as capacitation. Two capacitation events are essential for successful sperm penetration into oocytes: a vigorous motility called hyperactivation (HA) and the ability to undergo the acrosome reaction (AR) in response to a physiological agonist (Yanagimachi, 1994a,b). In addition, a series of sequential and concomitant biochemical processes must occur during capacitation, including the hyperpolarization of the plasma membrane (Zeng et al., 1995; Arnoult et al., 1999; Muñoz-Garay et al., 2001; Demarco et al., 2003; Ritagliati et al., 2018). In sperm, as in most cells, the internal ion concentrations are markedly different from those in the extracellular medium. At rest, the balance of ion fluxes, gradients, and permeabilities results in an electric potential, known as the resting *Em* (Visconti et al., 2011; Stival et al., 2016). Mammalian sperm encounter environments with very different ionic composition on their journey to meet the egg. Sperm must regulate their *Em* and adapt to the changes of external ion concentration. In turn, *Em* modulates membrane ion channels and transporters, including the sperm-specific Ca^{2+} channel CatSper and voltage-gated proton channel Hv1 (Darszon et al., 2011; Lishko et al., 2012). Ion channels and ionic gradients play key roles in orchestrating intracellular signaling pathways.

Hyperpolarization of the plasma membrane during capacitation has been thoroughly studied in mouse sperm. Initially, mouse sperm are relatively depolarized (*Em* between −35 and −45 mV) and become hyperpolarized (*Em* around −70 mV) upon capacitation (Zeng et al., 1995; Arnoult et al., 1999; Stival et al., 2015; Ritagliati et al., 2018). This hyperpolarization has been shown to be both necessary and sufficient for sperm to undergo $[Ca^{2+}]_i$ increases and the AR in response to an agonist (De La Vega-Beltran et al., 2012). Despite the different roles that membrane hyperpolarization might play during capacitation, *Em* changes have not been extensively studied in human sperm. Linares-Hernández et al. (1998) reported that the *Em* of non-capacitated sperm is around −40 mV, whereas Patrat et al. (2005) reported that capacitated sperm exhibit an *Em* of about −58 mV. On the other hand, López-González et al. (2014) used a potentiometric dye in a flow cytometry assay to show that a subpopulation of human sperm undergoes *Em* hyperpolarization upon capacitation, which correlated with an increase in intracellular pH and Ca^{2+} concentration. However, they determined relative membrane potentials through the median fluorescence observed in each condition and not absolute values. Furthermore, the physiological relevance of *Em* hyperpolarization has not been elucidated yet.

Mouse sperm lacking either the K^+ channel Slo3 or its auxiliary subunit Lrrc52 have markedly reduced fertility (Santi et al., 2010; Zeng et al., 2011, 2015). Thus, it could be hypothesized that malfunction of K^+ channels in human sperm might also contribute to the occurrence of subfertility in men. Brown et al. (2016) used whole-cell patch-clamp electrophysiology to assess the biophysical characteristics of sperm from men undergoing fertility treatments and compared to those from fertile, healthy donors. In approximately 10% of the samples from infertile patients there was either a negligible outward conductance or an enhanced inward current, both of which caused *Em* depolarization. Analysis of clinical data from IVF patients showed a significant association of depolarized *Em* assessed by patch-clamp with low fertilization rate (Brown et al., 2016). These results point toward the correlation of the *Em* value of a sperm sample with its fertilizing capacity. However, patch-clamp is a complex, laborious and time-consuming technique, not compatible with prediction tools needed for the clinic. In addition, in view of the heterogeneity of sperm populations, it is highly possible that values acquired by patch-clamp techniques from a few cells would not be representative of those undergoing capacitation, which could lead to incorrect conclusions.

We aimed to analyze in depth human sperm *Em* during capacitation, its role in the acquisition of HA and AR, and its association with fertilization competence. Therefore, we characterized the *Em* upon capacitation in 60 human sperm samples using a potentiometric dye in a fluorimetric assay (Baro Graf et al., 2019). Sperm from normospermic donors showed a significant *Em* hyperpolarization during capacitation. In addition, *Em* values from capacitated sperm correlated significantly with the sperm capacity to undergo induced AR, underlying the essential role of hyperpolarization in acrosomal responsiveness. More importantly, this study shows that *Em* hyperpolarization is associated with successful IVF rates. Our results pave the way for the application of *Em* measurement as a useful tool to predict the success rate of IVF procedures.

MATERIALS AND METHODS

Ethical Approval

Volunteer donors and patients were provided with written information about the study prior to giving informed consent. The study protocol was approved by the Bioethics Committee of the *Facultad de Ciencias Bioquímicas y Farmacéuticas, Universidad Nacional de Rosario*, protocol #564/2018. The studies are in compliance with the Declaration of Helsinki principles.

Human Sperm Preparation

Semen samples were obtained by masturbation from healthy donors after 2–5 days of abstinence and analyzed following WHO recommendations (World Health Organization, 2010). Samples that fulfilled semen parameters (total fluid volume, sperm concentration, motility, viability and morphology) according to WHO normality criteria, were considered as normospermic and those that did not fulfilled any of them as non-normospermic. Samples were allowed to liquefy for 1 h at room temperature, then, sperm ejaculates were allowed to swim-up in non-capacitating media at 37°C for 1 h. The non-capacitating medium used was HEPES-buffered human tubal fluid (HTF) containing 90.7 mM NaCl, 4.7 mM KCl, 0.3 mM KH_2PO_4, 1.2 mM $MgSO_4$, 2.8 mM glucose, 3.4 mM sodium pyruvate, 1.6 mM $CaCl_2$, 60 mM sodium lactate and 23.8 mM HEPES (pH 7.4), which was supplemented with 20 mM bicarbonate and 5 mg/ml BSA to obtain the capacitating medium. Cells were left to capacitate at 37°C as detailed for each experiment, in the same procedure as that used to prepare spermatozoa for IVF.

In Fertya (Assisted Reproduction Medical Clinic), commercially available HTF media was used for sperm preparation. The spermatozoa were separated from semen by two-layer density gradient centrifugation (Irvine Scientific Isolate) and then washed and concentrated with Quinn's Advantage Medium with HEPES (Sage) which was supplemented with 10% Serum Protein Substitute (Sage). Washed spermatozoa were incubated to capacitate at 37°C pH 7.4 for 3–4 h prior to performing the IVF.

Membrane Potential Assay in Cell Populations

Cells were loaded with 1 μM of the membrane-potential-sensitive dye $DISC_3(5)$ (Molecular Probes) for at least 5 min. No mitochondrial un-couplers were used because their contribution to the resting potential has been determined to be insignificant (Guzmán-Grenfell et al., 2000). Sperm were then transferred to a gently stirred cuvette at 37°C, and the fluorescence was monitored with a Varian Cary Eclipse fluorescence spectrophotometer at 620/670 nm excitation/emission wavelengths. Recordings were initiated when steady-state fluorescence was reached and calibration was performed at the end of each measure by adding 1 μM valinomycin and sequential additions of KCl for internal calibration curves, as previously described (Ritagliati et al., 2018; Baro Graf et al., 2019). Sperm *Em* was obtained from the initial fluorescence (measured as Arbitrary Fluorescence Units) by linearly interpolating it in the theoretical *Em* values from the calibration curve against arbitrary fluorescence units of each trace. This internal calibration for each determination compensates for variables that influence the absolute fluorescence values.

Acrosome Status Assay

After incubation in the respective conditions, progesterone (21 μM) was added and incubated for another 30 min. Alternatively, in the NC_0 condition, 1 μM valinomycin was added 5 min before the progesterone. Cells were seeded on eight-well glass slides. After air-drying, sperm were fixed with 3.7% formaldehyde in PBS for 15 min at room temperature, permeabilized with 0.5% Triton X-100 for 5 min, washed with PBS and incubated with PBS containing 1% BSA and FITC-conjugated pisum sativum lectin (1/200) for 1 h at room temperature. Before mounting, samples were washed with PBS (four times for 5 min each time). Epifluorescence microscopy was used to assess acrosome status. At least 200 sperm were analyzed in each condition.

Sperm Motility Analysis

Sperm suspensions were loaded on a 30-μm deep slide and placed on a microscope stage at 37°C. Sperm movements were examined using computer-assisted semen analysis (CASA) system (IVOS Sperm Analyzer, Hamilton Thorn). Thirty frames were acquired at a rate of 60 Hz. At least 200 sperm were analyzed in each condition. The following parameters were measured: mean path velocity (VAP, μm/sec), curvilinear velocity (VCL, μm/sec), straight-line velocity (VSL, μm/sec), linearity (LIN, %), amplitude of lateral head displacement (ALH, μm), and straightness (STR, %). Sperm were considered hyperactivated when presenting VCL $\geq$ 150 μm/sec, LIN $<$ 50%, and ALH $\geq$ 5 μm. At the time of the analysis, 0.5 mg/ml BSA was added to non-capacitated conditions to avoid sperm adherence to the slide.

Fertilization Rate at IVF

In vitro fertilization was performed 3–4 h post sperm preparation in 4-well dishes (Oosafe) with 0.5 ml of Quinn's Advantage Fertilization medium supplemented with 10% Serum Protein Substitute (Sage) and covered with 0.5 ml of tissue culture oil (Sage). In order to assure good oocyte quality, this study only involved female patients with no detected female factors. All patients were below 38 years old. One thousand sperm were incubated per cumulus-oocyte complex. A maximum of five cumulus-oocyte complex were incubated per well in K-System G185 incubator (37°C, 6.2% CO_2, 5% O_2) during 4 h. After this period, oocytes were denudated and incubated in individual drops in QA Protein plus Cleavage medium (SAGE®) covered with 0.5 ml of tissue culture oil (Sage) in the same conditions as described above. At 18 h post insemination, fertilization was analyzed with an inverted microscope. Successful fertilization was considered when two pronuclei (2PN) and two distinct or fragmented polar bodies were observed. When at least 60% of eggs were fertilized, the IVF procedure was classified as successful, according to local regulations.

Statistical Analyses

Data are expressed as mean ± standard deviation (SD) or standard error of the mean (SEM), as indicated in each figure, of at least six independent experiments for all determinations. Statistical analyses were performed using the GraphPad Prism 6 software (La Jolla, CA, United States). Student's *t* test was used to compare mean values between control and tested groups, while the difference between mean values of multiple groups was analyzed by one-way analysis of variance (ANOVA) with multiple comparison tests. A probability (p) value $p < 0.05$ was considered statistically significant.

RESULTS

Human Sperm Hyperpolarize During Capacitation

In this work, we performed a fluorimetric population assay to determine the absolute *Em* values of non-capacitated and capacitated sperm. When constant concentrations of sperm and probe are used, this method provides a highly reproducible value of plasma membrane potential after calibration using valinomycin (a K^+ ionophore) and sequential additions of KCl (Baro Graf et al., 2019) (**Figure 1A**). A total of 60 sperm samples were analyzed, among which 49 corresponded to normospermic and 11 to non-normospermic donors, as categorized on the basis of total sperm number, ejaculate volume and motility

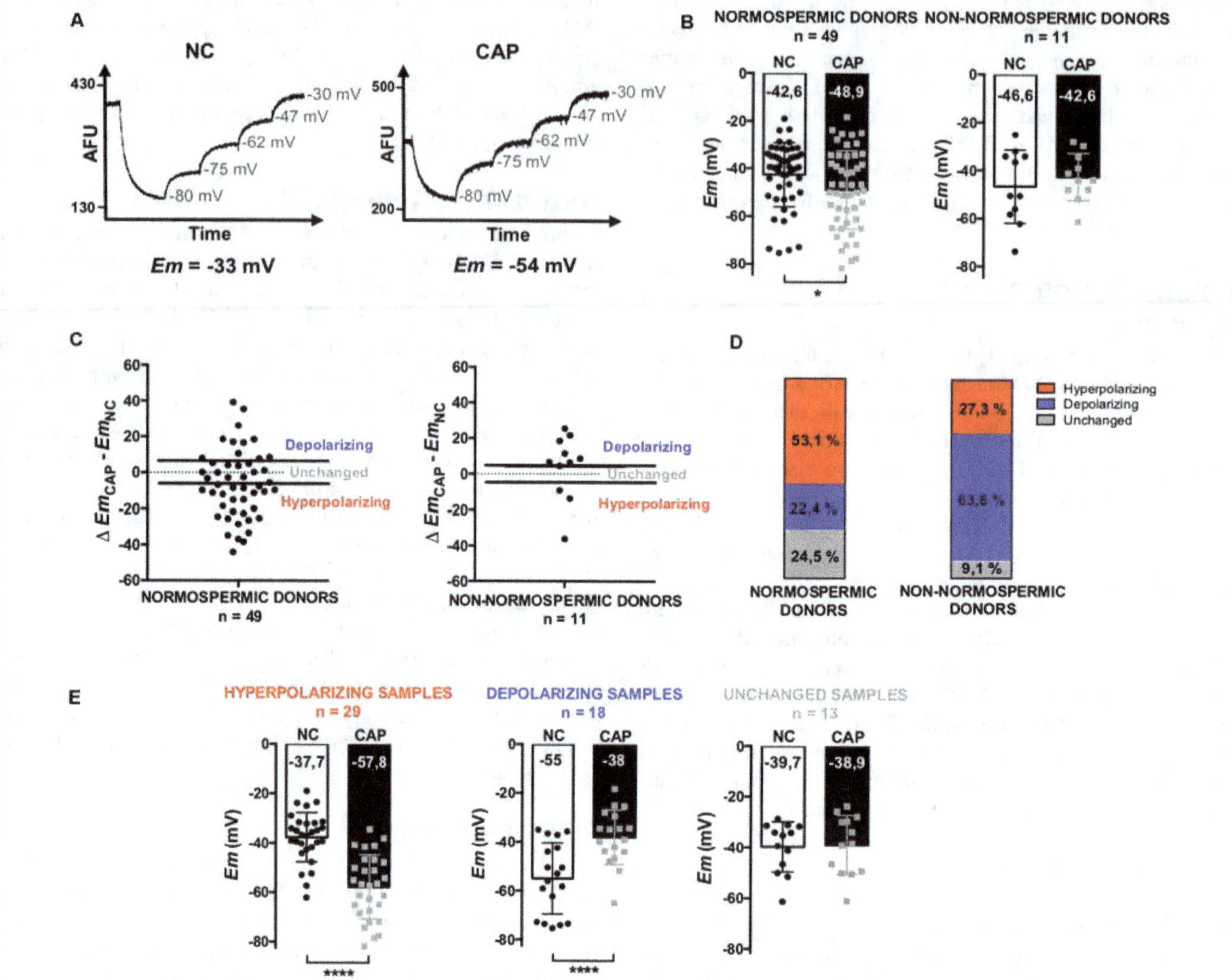

FIGURE 1 | Determination of the *Em* of sperm samples by a fluorimetric assay. Non-capacitated (NC) and capacitated (CAP) human sperm from normospermic (n = 49) and non-normospermic (n = 11) donors. **(A)** Representative fluorescence traces showing *Em* values. **(B)** Distribution and mean *Em* values obtained in each condition. **(C)** Plots of the change on *Em* obtained upon capacitation ($\Delta\ Em_{CAP} - Em_{NC}$). The samples with a positive difference were classified as depolarizing, the ones with a negative difference as hyperpolarizing and those which did not change or with a difference under 5 mV where classified as unchanged. **(D)** Representation of the three types of behaviors among normospermic and non-normospermic donors. **(E)** Pooled *Em* values from hyperpolarizing (n = 29), depolarizing (n = 18) and unchanged (n = 13) samples. Data represent mean ± SD. Paired Student's t test was performed between NC and CAP: $^{*}p < 0.05$, $^{****}p < 0.0001$.

according to WHO guidelines (see section "Materials and Methods" for details). Consistent with previous observations using flow cytometry (López-González et al., 2014), we found a large heterogeneity among *Em* values of samples from different individuals. However, normal sperm samples exhibited a significant hyperpolarization after capacitation, while sub-normal samples did not (**Figure 1B**). The *Em* changes ($Em_{CAP} - Em_{NC}$) were also very variable between individuals. Both in normospermic and non-normospermic donors we could identify samples with depolarizing, hyperpolarizing or unchanged behaviors (**Figure 1C**). However, while in normospermic donors the majority of the samples (53.6%) hyperpolarized, among donors with sub-normal parameters, only 27.3% hyperpolarized and 63.6% depolarized (**Figure 1D**). When samples with different behaviors were pooled and further analyzed, *Em* changes became more evident. These results demonstrate that in most normospermic individuals there is a capacitation-induced hyperpolarization, with an initial non-capacitated *Em* value of −37.7 ± 9.9 mV, that shifts to -57.8 ± 12.9 mV upon capacitation (**Figure 1E**).

Hyperpolarization Correlates With Acrosomal Responsiveness

The AR is a key step in fertilization. In mammalian sperm, the AR is mediated by intracellular calcium fluxes. Since Ca^{2+} channels in sperm cells are voltage-dependent, it has been hypothesized that gating might be controlled by *Em*.

We evaluated the role of the *Em* in the acquisition of acrosomal responsiveness to progesterone (Pg) in samples from normospermic donors. Both *Em* and AR were evaluated immediately after swim-up (NC_0), as well as after 5 h in either non-capacitating (NC_5) or capacitating (CAP) media. For AR analysis, cells were further incubated for 30 min in the absence or presence of Pg. Non-capacitated sperm obtained after swim-up (NC_0) did not increase the percentage of acrosome reacted sperm in the presence of Pg. However, they acquired acrosomal responsiveness after pharmacological hyperpolarization with valinomycin (1 μM for 5 min) (**Figures 2B,C**). These results point toward the pharmacological hyperpolarization sufficiency for acrosomal responsiveness, in agreement to previous results in mouse sperm (De La Vega-Beltran et al., 2012). On the other hand, capacitated human sperm hyperpolarized (**Figure 2A**) and showed significantly increased induced AR (**Figures 2B,C**). Furthermore, a correlation analysis between *Em* change upon capacitation ($Em_{CAP} - Em_{NC0}$) and the induced AR (induced – spontaneous), although not statistically significant ($p = 0.06$), showed a clear negative correlation ($r = -0.6337$) (**Figure 2D**). Interestingly, as observed in the correlation analysis between absolute *Em* values and induced AR for each condition (**Figures 2E,F**), there is a strong negative correlation for sperm incubated in capacitating ($r = -0.8234$) media, but not in NC_0 ($r = 0.0025$).

Role of *Em* in Hyperactivated Motility

Hyperactivation is essential for mammalian sperm to fertilize the oocyte (White and Aitken, 1989; Suarez et al., 1993); we therefore aimed to determine if hyperpolarization of human sperm would affect their motility. Hyperactivated motility is defined by an increase in the VCL and the ALH and a decreased LIN: VCL $\geq$ 150 μm/s, LIN $\leq$ 50% and ALH $\geq$ 5 μm/s, being VCL the most characteristic parameter. **Figure 3** shows *Em* values (**Figure 3A**), percentage of hyperactivated sperm (**Figure 3B**) and VCL (**Figure 3C**) of sperm incubated in either non-capacitated or capacitated conditions at different time points. As can be observed, sperm progressively hyperpolarized in time with a maximum at 5 h (which was the longest time assayed), while the maximum HA rate and VCL were at 3 h (**Figures 3A–C**). In order to assess the role of hyperpolarization in sperm motility, we performed a correlation analysis of *Em* values with HA and

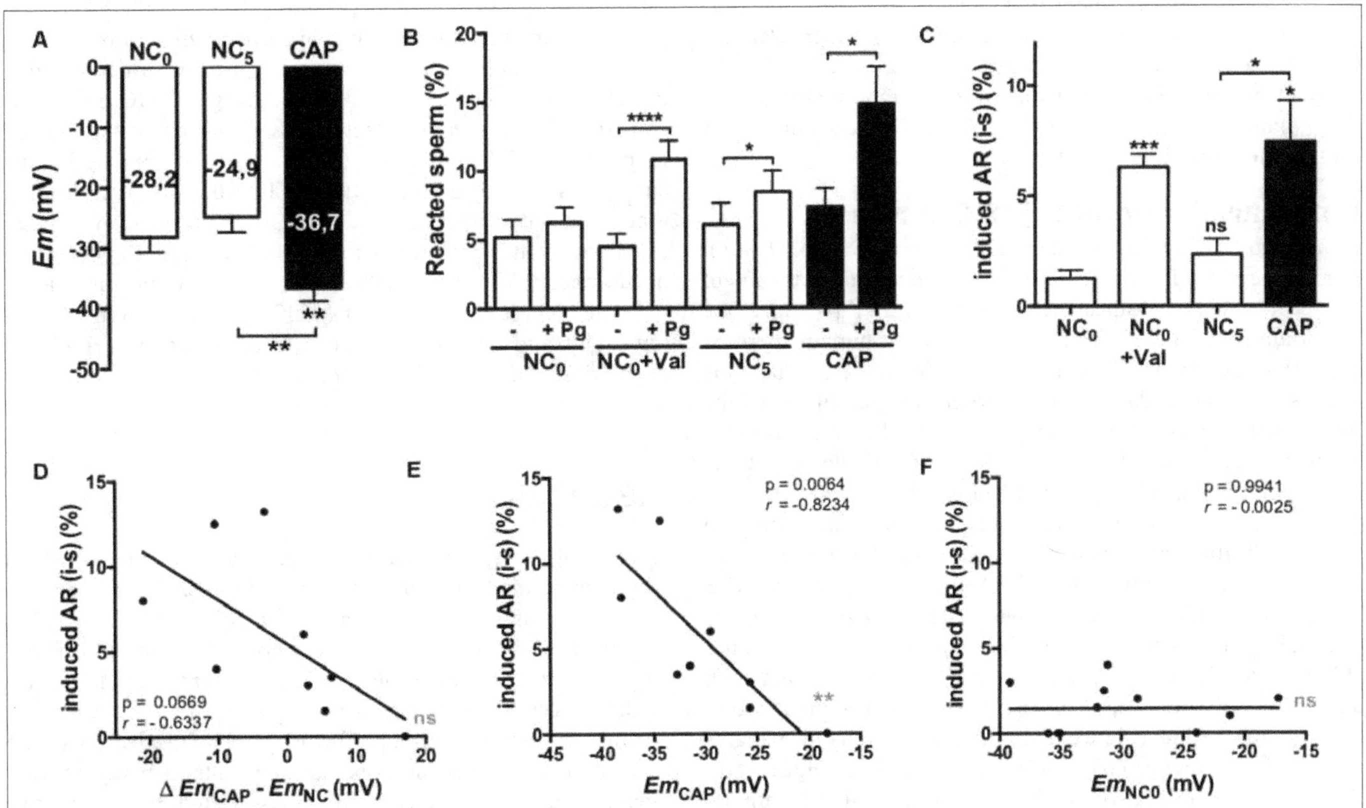

FIGURE 2 | Hyperpolarized membrane potentials correlate with acrosomal responsiveness. Sperm samples from normospermic donors obtained after swim-up (NC_0) and upon 5 h incubation in non-capacitating (NC_5) and capacitating (CAP) media were analyzed. **(A)** *Em* measurements. **(B,C)** Cells were further incubated for 30 min in the absence (-) or presence (+) of 21 μM progesterone (Pg). The percentage of acrosome reacted sperm was assessed by FITC-PSA staining as described in section "Materials and Methods." Data represent mean ± SEM from at least six independent experiments. Paired Student's *t* test was performed. Statistically significant differences between the indicated conditions or with the control NC_0 (asterisks on each column bar) are as follows: *$p < 0.05$, **$p < 0.01$, ***$p < 0.005$, ****$p < 0.0001$. **(D–F)** Correlation analysis between the change on *Em* (**D**, $\Delta\ Em_{CAP} - Em_{NC0}$) or the *Em* values in CAP **(E)** and NC_0 **(F)** and the induced AR. The correlation coefficients (*r*) and *p* values are indicated.

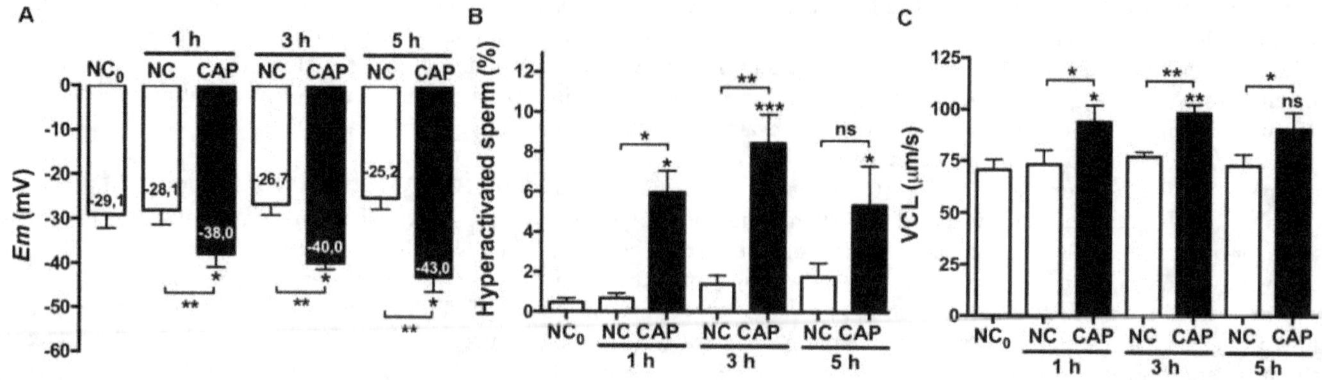

FIGURE 3 | Hyperpolarization and HA. Sperm samples from normospermic donors obtained after swim-up (NC_0) and upon incubation in non-capacitating (NC) and capacitating (CAP) media for 1, 3, and 5 h were analyzed. **(A)** *Em* measurements. **(B,C)** The percentage of hyperactivated sperm **(B)** and VCL **(C)** were obtained using CASA software. Data represent mean ± SEM from at least six independent experiments. Paired Student's *t* test was performed. Statistically significant differences between the indicated conditions or with the control NC_0 (asterisks on each column bar) are as follows: $^*p < 0.05$, $^{**}p < 0.01$, $^{***}p < 0.005$.

VCL after 3 and 5 h of capacitation (**Supplementary Figure S1**). Though not significant, there is a tendency in the correlation between *Em* at 3 h of capacitation and VCL (**Supplementary Figure S1A**). On the other hand, the correlation was weaker at 5 h of capacitation (**Supplementary Figure S1B**), which can be explained by the fact that at 5 h sperm further hyperpolarized, while HA did not continue increasing (**Figure 3**). Finally, the analysis between *Em* change upon capacitation (Em_{CAP3} – Em_{NC0}) and the VCL or HA values, showed a weak correlation (**Supplementary Figure S1C**).

Em Analysis Predicts IVF Outcome

Aiming to further investigate the biological role of *Em* on human sperm fertilization competence, we determined the *Em* of non-capacitated and capacitated sperm from IVF patients. One important drawback in correlation analyses of human sperm is the biological variation between samples obtained from the same donors on different days. Thus, in order to avoid this issue, the fluorimetric *Em* measurements were performed on aliquots of the ejaculate used on the day of the IVF treatment, allowing direct comparison of *Em* values with fertilization success.

In vitro fertilization patients were classified according to their fertilization rate, satisfying local clinical parameters for successful (fertilization rate ≥ 60%) and unsuccessful IVF procedures (fertilization rate < 60%). These two groups showed significant differences between their mean IVF success rates (**Figure 4A**). In a retrospective analysis, sperm samples with successful IVF rates exhibited a significant *Em* hyperpolarization during capacitation (**Figure 4B**). On the other hand, patients with IVF rates under 60% did not hyperpolarize (**Figure 4B**). As can be seen in **Figure 4C**, 78.6% of successful IVF samples hyperpolarized during capacitation. However, the majority of samples from poor IVF rate patients (66.7%) showed a depolarizing behavior. These results indicate that the IVF outcome might be dependent on a capacitation-associated hyperpolarization. To test this hypothesis, we performed correlation analysis of absolute *Em* values obtained after capacitation and IVF rates (**Figure 4D**), and also of *Em* changes upon capacitation (Em_{CAP} – Em_{NC}) against IVF rates (**Figure 4E**). In agreement with our previous results (**Figure 2**) where we observed a correlation between capacitated sperm *Em* and induced AR, there was a significant correlation between capacitated sperm *Em* (Em_{CAP}) and IVF rate. Interestingly, a predictive analysis showed that hyperpolarizing samples have significantly higher IVF rates in comparison with depolarizing samples, as depicted in **Figure 4F**. Finally, a ROC curve was constructed to assess the effectiveness of capacitated sperm *Em* in predicting IVF outcomes (**Figure 5**). The area under the curve was 0.8571 ± 0.098 (95% CI = 0.6647-1), indicating that capacitated sperm *Em* (Em_{CAP}) is a good parameter to discriminate between successful IVF rate (>60%) and unsuccessful IVF rate (<60%). The cut off value for Em_{CAP} with the highest sensitivity and specificity was −48.6 mV (100% sensitivity and 71.4% specificity). Considering our results, a depolarized *Em* could be related to IVF failure in idiopathic subfertile patients.

DISCUSSION

A total of 60 sperm samples were analyzed, among which 49 corresponded to normospermic donors. These samples exhibited a significant *Em* hyperpolarization after incubation in capacitating media, while sub-normal samples did not hyperpolarize. This raises the question whether functional defects in the capacitation-associated hyperpolarization relate to sub-normal parameters. Although further work is needed regarding more non-normospermic donors, our results may suggest that normal semen parameters can be associated to the relative permeability of the plasma membrane, ion channels regulation and metabolic state of the sperm resulting in their ability to hyperpolarize in capacitating conditions.

The AR, a key step in fertilization, is strictly dependent on an increase in intracellular Ca^{2+} (Romarowski et al., 2016). In 1998, a voltage-dependent Ca^{2+} influx caused by sperm depolarization was described in human sperm, which was enhanced when

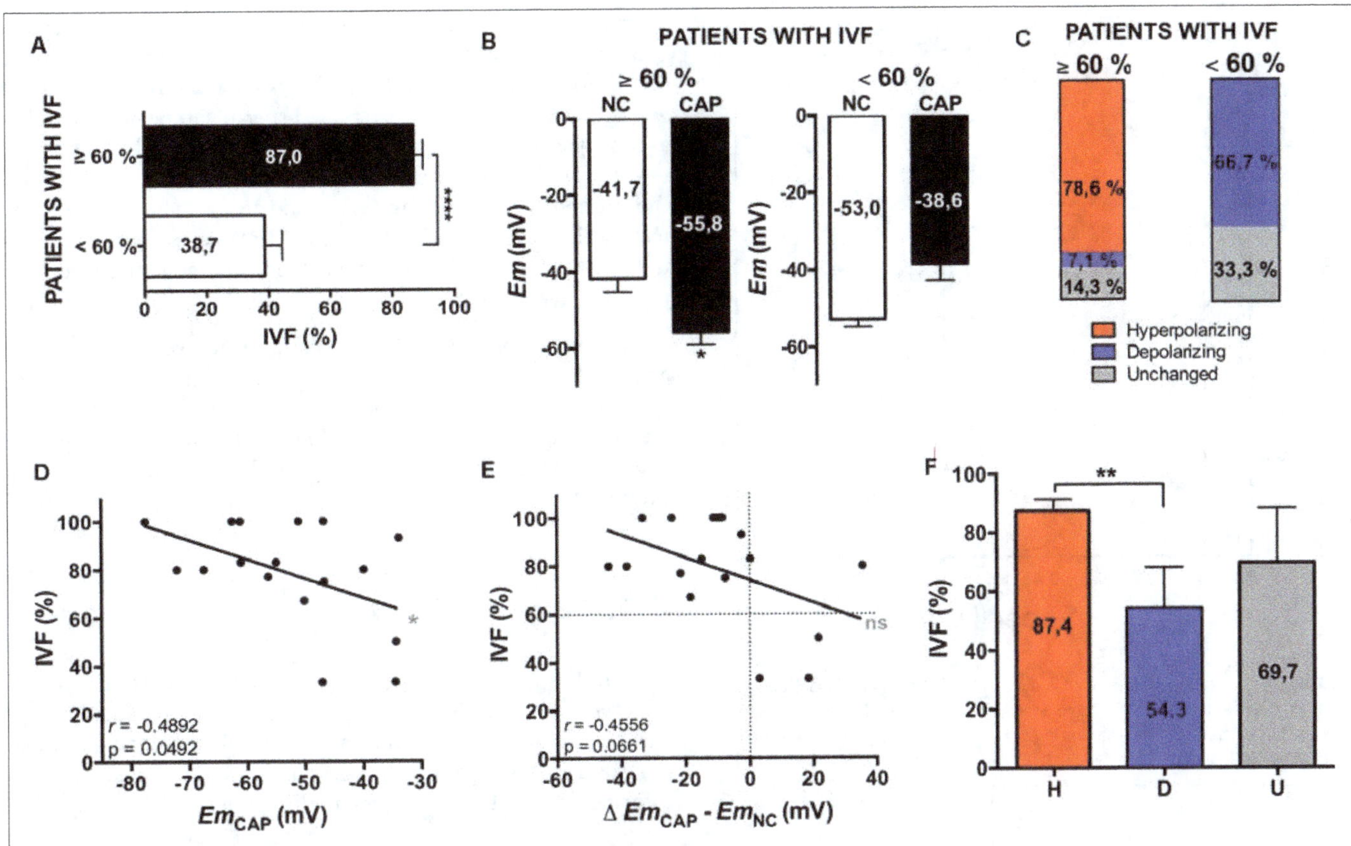

FIGURE 4 | *Em* hyperpolarization correlates with higher IVF rates. **(A)** IVF patients were classified according to their fertilization rate: ≥60% and <60% of fertilized oocytes. Data represent mean ± SEM, an unpaired Student's *t* test was performed: $^{****}p < 0.0001$. **(B)** *Em* measurements from patients' samples. Data represent mean ± SEM, a paired Student's *t* test was performed: $^{*}p < 0.05$. **(C)** Representation of the percentages of each type of behavior: hyperpolarizing (red), depolarizing (blue) and unchanged (gray). **(D,E)** Correlation analysis between the percentage of IVF and the *Em* in CAP **(D)** and the change on *Em* ($\Delta\ Em_{CAP} - Em_{NCO}$) **(E)**. The correlation coefficients (*r*) and *p* values are indicated. **(F)** Mean IVF rates of hyperpolarizing (H, red), depolarizing (D, blue), and unchanged (U, gray) samples. Data represent mean ± SEM, an unpaired Student's *t* test was performed: $^{**}p < 0.01$.

depolarization was preceded by hyperpolarization (Linares-Hernández et al., 1998). This was consistent with a hypothesis stating that capacitation-associated hyperpolarization is required to remove voltage Ca^{2+} channels inactivation. Furthermore, the steroid hormone progesterone, which is the only well-characterized biological agonist of the AR in human sperm, activates CatSper, induces Ca^{2+} influx, membrane depolarization and AR (Aitken, 1997; Kirkman-Brown et al., 2000; Patrat et al., 2005; Lishko et al., 2011). In mouse sperm it has been shown that *Em* hyperpolarization is necessary and sufficient for cells to acquire acrosomal responsiveness (De La Vega-Beltran et al., 2012). However, in human sperm, the correlation between *Em* and acrosomal responsiveness had not been thoroughly demonstrated yet. The results presented herein indicate that *Em* hyperpolarization plays an important role in human sperm AR. We have shown that: (1) capacitated sperm exhibit significant *Em* hyperpolarization and induced AR; (2) non-capacitated depolarized sperm only gain acrosomal responsiveness after pharmacological hyperpolarization; and (3) there is a strong and significant negative correlation between *Em* and induced AR in capacitated sperm. Altogether, these data support an important role of *Em* hyperpolarization for the acquisition of acrosomal responsiveness.

It is generally accepted that good sperm motility is a central component of male fertility. Individuals with poorly motile or immotile sperm are considered infertile or subfertile, and in need of ART procedures. In fact, asthenozoospermia is the commonest problem underlying male subfertility (Van Der Steeg et al., 2011) and because the root cause of this condition is usually not known, treatments for this problem are non-specific. In this context, we aimed to understand whether human sperm *Em* hyperpolarization and HA were linked. A correlation tendency was observed at 3 h between both parameters. It is well established that intracellular calcium plays a pivotal role in sperm motility regulation. Alasmari et al. (2013) showed that defects in Ca^{2+} signaling lead to poor HA and that the ability to undergo Ca^{2+} -induced HA affects sperm fertilizing capacity. This is in agreement with our results and with the hypothesis that the *Em* might play a role in regulating Ca^{2+} channels and, consequently, in intracellular calcium and indirectly in sperm motility (reviewed in Ritagliati et al., 2018).

Regardless the amount of work invested toward understanding the molecular basis of sperm capacitation,

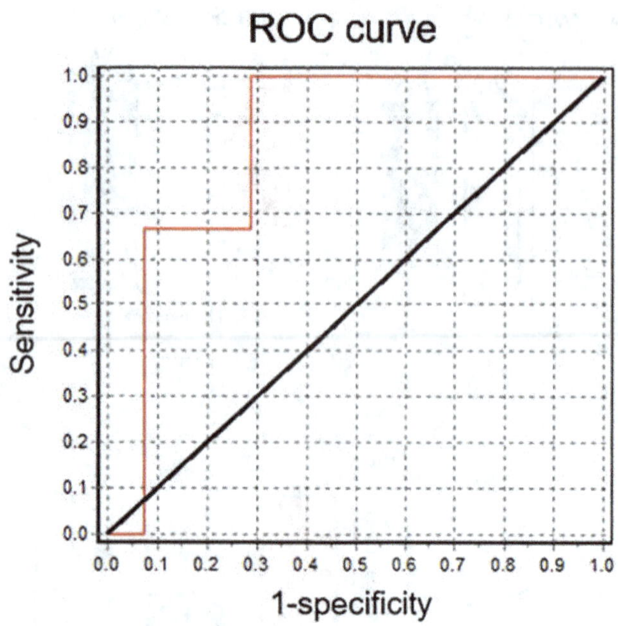

FIGURE 5 | Capacitated sperm *Em* is a good predictor for IVF. Receiver operating characteristic (ROC) curve analysis for capacitated sperm *Em* values. The reference line is marked in black. The area under the curve is 0.8571 ± 0.098 (95% CI = 0.6647; 1).

studies of male factor issues attending reproductive clinics seem to be completely dissociated from basic science knowledge. Regretfully, semen diagnostic analysis hardly involves sperm function evaluation, i.e., capacitation parameters required for fertilization. With this in mind, we aimed to analyze whether *Em* hyperpolarization relates to human sperm fertilizing capacity. It has been recently proposed that a certain degree of *Em* shift is associated with normal sperm function, as assessed by electrophysiology and IVF outcome (Brown et al., 2016). However, this study involved laborious techniques that hampered the analysis of many cells per patient. Thus, we pursued the study of sperm *Em* from patients attending a fertility clinic using a robust and relatively simple technique. In the fluorimetric population assay, the sample's behavior is followed throughout the experiment and is performed in the physiological working conditions allowing more accurate correlations (Baro Graf et al., 2019). *Em* measurements were performed on aliquots of the same samples used in IVF procedures. Our data show that almost 80% of successful IVF samples hyperpolarized. On the other hand, there was no hyperpolarization in samples with unsuccessful IVF rates. In fact, the majority of these samples (66.7%) depolarized during incubation in capacitating conditions. Accordingly, there is a significant strong correlation between capacitated sperm *Em* and IVF rate. These data strongly suggest that human sperm *Em* changes have an implication in sperm fertilizing capacity. Interestingly, in a predictive study, samples that depolarized upon capacitation exhibited lower fertilization rates. After a ROC analysis we determined that the *Em* absolute value from capacitated sperm can be considered as a good parameter to predict IVF rates, with a cut-off value of −48.6 mV. Although further work is needed in order to increase the number of patients analyzed, and to evaluate whether this technical approach could also predict IUI success, this study has the potential to add diagnostic tools to help predict the success of reproductive techniques.

During preparation of this manuscript, we contacted the group of Dr. Celia Santi at Washington University School of Medicine in Saint Louis, who independently achieved the same results using a different methodology. Both this manuscript and Santi's work are intended to be published concurrently (Puga Molina et al., 2020).

ETHICS STATEMENT

The studies involving human participants were reviewed and approved by the Bioethics Committee of the Facultad de Ciencias Bioquímicas y Farmacéuticas, Universidad Nacional de Rosario. The patients/participants provided their written informed consent to participate in this study.

AUTHOR CONTRIBUTIONS

CB, CR, and CS conducted the experiments. VT-M and CC designed and conducted the IVF procedures. CB, CR, MB, and DK conceived the study. CB, CR, and DK wrote the manuscript. All authors analyzed the data and revised the final version of the manuscript.

FUNDING

This work was supported by grants from the Agencia Nacional de Promoción Científica y Tecnológica de Argentina PICT 2015-3164 and PICT 2017-3217 (awarded to DK). CB, CR, and CS are recipients of a fellowship from CONICET, Argentina.

ACKNOWLEDGMENTS

We thank the Male Contraceptive Initiative for support granted to CB and the Statistics and Data Processing Department from Facultad de Ciencias Bioquímicas y Farmacéuticas, Universidad Nacional de Rosario, Argentina.

REFERENCES

Aitken, R. (1997). Molecular mechanisms regulating human sperm function. *Mol. Hum. Reprod.* 3, 169–173. doi: 10.1093/molehr/3.3.169

Alasmari, W., Barratt, C. L. R., Publicover, S. J., Whalley, K. M., Foster, E., Kay, V., et al. (2013). The clinical significance of calcium-signalling pathways mediating human sperm hyperactivation. *Hum. Reprod.* 28, 866–876. doi: 10.1093/humrep/des467

Arnoult, C., Kazam, I. G., Visconti, P. E., Kopf, G. S., Villaz, M., and Florman, H. M. (1999). Control of the low voltage-activated calcium channel of mouse sperm by egg ZP3 and by membrane hyperpolarization during capacitation. *Proc. Natl. Acad. Sci. U.S.A.* 96, 6757–6762. doi: 10.1073/pnas.96.12.6757

Baro Graf, C., Ritagliati, C., Stival, C., Balestrini, P. A., Buffone, M. G., and Krapf, D. (2019). Determination of a robust assay for human sperm membrane potential analysis. *Front. Cell Dev. Biol.* 7:101. doi: 10.3389/fcell.2019.00101

Barratt, C. L. R., Björndahl, L., De Jonge, C. J., Lamb, D. J., Martini, F. O., McLachlan, R., et al. (2017). The diagnosis of male infertility: an analysis of the evidence to support the development of global WHO guidance-challenges and future research opportunities. *Hum. Reprod. Update* 23, 660–680. doi: 10.1093/humupd/dmx021

Barratt, C. L. R., De Jonge, C. J., and Sharpe, R. M. (2018). "Man Up": the importance and strategy for placing male reproductive health centre stage in the political and research agenda. *Hum. Reprod.* 33, 541–545. doi: 10.1093/humrep/dey020

Brown, S. G., Publicover, S. J., Mansell, S. A., Lishko, P. V., Williams, H. L., Ramalingam, M., et al. (2016). Depolarization of sperm membrane potential is a common feature of men with subfertility and is associated with low fertilization rate at IVF. *Hum. Reprod.* 31, 1147–1157. doi: 10.1093/humrep/dew056

Darszon, A., Nishigaki, T., Beltran, C., and Treviño, C. L. (2011). Calcium channels in the development, maturation, and function of spermatozoa. *Physiol. Rev.* 91, 1305–1355. doi: 10.1152/physrev.00028.2010

Datta, J., Palmer, M. J., Tanton, C., Gibson, L. J., Jones, K. G., Macdowall, W., et al. (2016). Prevalence of infertilityand help seeking among 15 000 women and men. *Hum. Reprod.* 31, 2108–2118. doi: 10.1093/humrep/dew123

De La Vega-Beltran, J. L., Sánchez-Cárdenas, C., Krapf, D., Hernandez-González, E. O., Wertheimer, E., Treviño, C. L., et al. (2012). Mouse sperm membrane potential hyperpolarization is necessary and sufficient to prepare sperm for the acrosome reaction. *J. Biol. Chem.* 287, 44384–44393. doi: 10.1074/jbc.M112.393488

Demarco, I. A., Espinosa, F., Edwards, J., Sosnik, J., De la Vega-Beltrán, J. L., Hockensmith, J. W., et al. (2003). Involvement of a Na+/HCO3- cotransporter in mouse sperm capacitation. *J. Biol. Chem.* 278, 7001–7009. doi: 10.1074/jbc.M206284200

Guzmán-Grenfell, A. M., Bonilla-Hernández, M. A., and González-Martínez, M. T. (2000). Glucose induces a Na+,K+-ATPase-dependent transient hyperpolarization in human sperm. I. Induction of changes in plasma membrane potential by the proton ionophore CCCP. *Biochim. Biophys. Acta Biomembr.* 1464, 188–198. doi: 10.1016/S0005-2736(99)00247-3

HFEA (2014). *Fertility Treatment in 2013: Trends and Figures*. London: HFEA.

Kirkman-Brown, J. C., Bray, C., Stewart, P. M., Barratt, C. L. R., and Publicover, S. J. (2000). Biphasic elevation of [Ca 2+](i) in individual human spermatozoa exposed to progesterone. *Dev. Biol.* 222, 326–335. doi: 10.1006/dbio.2000.9729

Linares-Hernández, L., Guzmán-Grenfell, A. M., Hicks-Gomez, J. J., and González-Martínez, M. T. (1998). Voltage-dependent calcium influx in human sperm assessed by simultaneous optical detection of intracellular calcium and membrane potential. *Biochim. Biophys. Acta Biomembr.* 1372, 1–12. doi: 10.1016/S0005-2736(98)00035-2

Lishko, P. V., Botchkina, I. L., and Kirichok, Y. (2011). Progesterone activates the principal Ca2+ channel of human sperm. *Nature* 471, 387–392. doi: 10.1038/nature09767

Lishko, P. V., Kirichok, Y., Ren, D., Navarro, B., Chung, J.-J., and Clapham, D. E. (2012). The control of male fertility by spermatozoan ion channels. *Annu. Rev. Physiol.* 74, 453–475. doi: 10.1146/annurev-physiol-020911-153258

López-González, I., Torres-Rodríguez, P., Sánchez-Carranza, O., Solís-López, A., Santi, C. M., Darszon, A., et al. (2014). Membrane hyperpolarization during human sperm capacitation. *Mol. Hum. Reprod.* 20, 619–629. doi: 10.1093/molehr/gau029

Muñoz-Garay, C., De la Vega-Beltrán, J. L., Delgado, R., Labarca, P., Felix, R., and Darszon, A. (2001). Inwardly rectifying K(+) channels in spermatogenic cells: functional expression and implication in sperm capacitation. *Dev. Biol.* 234, 261–274. doi: 10.1006/dbio.2001.0196

Patrat, C., Serres, C., and Jouannet, P. (2005). Progesterone induces hyperpolarization after a transient depolarization phase in human spermatozoa1. *Biol. Reprod.* 66, 1775–1780. doi: 10.1095/biolreprod66.6.1775

Puga Molina, L. C., Gunderson, S., Riley, J., Lybaert, P., Borrego-Alvarez, A., Jungheim, E. S., et al. (2020). Membrane potential determined by flow cytometry predicts fertilizing ability of human sperm. *Front. Cell Dev. Biol.* 7:387. doi: 10.3389/fcell.2019.00387

Ritagliati, C., Baro Graf, C., Stival, C., and Krapf, D. (2018). Regulation mechanisms and implications of sperm membrane hyperpolarization. *Mech. Dev.* 154, 33–43. doi: 10.1016/j.mod.2018.04.004

Romarowski, A., Sánchez-Cárdenas, C., Ramírez-Gómez, H. V., Puga Molina, L., del, C., Treviño, C. L., et al. (2016). A specific transitory increase in intracellular calcium induced by progesterone promotes acrosomal exocytosis in mouse sperm1. *Biol. Reprod.* 94:63. doi: 10.1095/biolreprod.115.136085

Santi, C. M., Martínez-López, P., de la Vega-Beltrán, J. L., Butler, A., Alisio, A., Darszon, A., et al. (2010). The SLO3 sperm-specific potassium channel plays a vital role in male fertility. *FEBS Lett.* 584, 1041–1046. doi: 10.1016/j.febslet.2010.02.005

Slama, R., Hansen, O. K. H., Ducot, B., Bohet, A., Sorensen, D., Giorgis Allemand, L., et al. (2012). Estimation of the frequency of involuntary infertility on a nation-wide basis. *Hum. Reprod.* 27, 1489–1498. doi: 10.1093/humrep/des070

Stival, C., La Spina, F. A., Graf, C. B., Arcelay, E., Arranz, S. E., Ferreira, J. J., et al. (2015). Src kinase is the connecting player between Protein Kinase A (PKA) activation and hyperpolarization through SLO3 potassium channel regulation in mouse sperm. *J. Biol. Chem.* 290, 18855–18864. doi: 10.1074/jbc.M115.640326

Stival, C., Puga Molina, L. D. C., Paudel, B., Buffone, M. G., Visconti, P. E., and Krapf, D. (2016). Sperm capacitation and acrosome reaction in mammalian sperm. *Adv. Anat. Embryol. Cell Biol.* 220, 93–106. doi: 10.1007/978-3-319-30567-7_5

Suarez, S. S., Varosi, S. M., and Dai, X. (1993). Intracellular calcium increases with hyperactivation in intact, moving hamster sperm and oscillates with the flagellar beat cycle. *Cell Biol.* 90, 4660–4664. doi: 10.1073/pnas.90.10.4660

Van Der Steeg, J. W., Steures, P., Eijkemans, M. J. C., Habbema, J. D. F., Hompes, P. G. A., Kremer, J. A. M., et al. (2011). Role of semen analysis in subfertile couples. *Fertil. Steril.* 95, 1013–1019. doi: 10.1016/j.fertnstert.2010.02.024

Visconti, P. E., Krapf, D., de la Vega-Beltrán, J. L., Acevedo, J. J., and Darszon, A. (2011). Ion channels, phosphorylation and mammalian sperm capacitation. *Asian J. Androl.* 13, 395–405. doi: 10.1038/aja.2010.69

White, D. R., and Aitken, R. J. (1989). Relationship between calcium, cyclic AMP, ATP, and intracellular pH and the capacity of hamster spermatozoa to express hyperactivated motility. *Gamete Res.* 22, 163–177. doi: 10.1002/mrd.1120220205

World Health Organization (2010). *WHO Laboratory Manual for the Examination and Processing of Human Semen*. Geneva: World Health Organisation.

Yanagimachi, R. (1994a). Fertility of mammalian spermatozoa: its development and relativity. *Zygote* 2, 371–372. doi: 10.1017/s0967199400002240

Yanagimachi, R. (1994b). "Mammalian fertilization", in *The Physiology of Reproduction*, eds E. Knobil, and J. D. Neill, (New York, NY: Raven Press), 189–317.

Zeng, X.-H., Yang, C., Kim, S. T., Lingle, C. J., and Xia, X.-M. (2011). Deletion of the Slo3 gene abolishes alkalization-activated K+ current in mouse spermatozoa. *Proc. Natl. Acad. Sci. U.S.A.* 108, 5879–5884. doi: 10.1073/pnas.1100240108

Zeng, X.-H., Yang, C., Xia, X.-M., Liu, M., and Lingle, C. J. (2015). SLO3 auxiliary subunit LRRC52 controls gating of sperm KSPER currents and is critical for normal fertility. *Proc. Natl. Acad. Sci. U.S.A.* 112, 2599–2604. doi: 10.1073/pnas.1423869112

Zeng, Y., Clark, E., and Hm, F. (1995). Sperm membrane potential: hyperpolarization during capacitation regulates zona pellucida-dependent acrosomal secretion. *Dev. Biol.* 171, 554–563. doi: 10.1006/dbio.1995.1304

10

Novel Techniques of Sperm Selection for Improving IVF and ICSI Outcomes

Iván Oseguera-López[1†], Sara Ruiz-Díaz[2,3†], Priscila Ramos-Ibeas[3] and Serafín Pérez-Cerezales[3]*

[1] *Unidad Iztapalapa, Universidad Autónoma Metropolitana, Mexico City, Mexico,* [2] *Mistral Fertility Clinics S.L., Clínica Tambre, Madrid, Spain,* [3] *Department of Animal Reproduction, Instituto Nacional de Investigación y Tecnología Agraria y Alimentaria, Madrid, Spain*

Correspondence:
Serafín Pérez-Cerezales
perez.serafin@inia.es;
s.perez.cerezales@gmail.com

† These authors have contributed equally to this work

Almost 50% of the infertility cases are due to male factors. Assisted reproductive technologies (ARTs) allow to overcome the incapacity of these patients' spermatozoa to fertilize the oocyte and produce a viable and healthy offspring, but the efficiency of the different techniques has still the potential to improve. According to the latest reports of the European Society of Human Reproduction and Embryology (ESHRE) and the Centers for Disease Control and Prevention of the United States (CDC), the percentages of deliveries per ART cycle in 2014 and 2016 were 21 and 22%, respectively. Among the reasons for this relatively low efficiency, the quality of the spermatozoa has been pointed out as critical, and the presence of high percentages of DNA-damaged spermatozoa in patients' ejaculates is possibly one of the main factors reducing the ARTs outcomes. Thus, one of the main challenges in reproductive medicine is to ensure the highest quality of the spermatozoa used in ARTs, and specifically, in terms of genetic integrity. The latest techniques for the preparation and selection of human spermatozoa are herein discussed focusing on those proven to improve one or several of the following parameters: sperm genetic integrity, fertilization capacity, embryo production, and *in vitro* survival, as well as pregnancy and delivery rates following *in vitro* fertilization (IVF) and intracytoplasmic sperm injection (ICSI). In addition, we discuss the potential of techniques developed in non-human mammals that could be further transferred to the clinic.

Keywords: sperm selection, ICSI, IVF, ARTs, sperm quality

INTRODUCTION

Current Efficiency of ARTs

According to the World Health Organization, infertility is defined as "a disease characterized by the failure to establish a clinical pregnancy after 12 months of regular, unprotected sexual intercourse or due to an impairment of a person's capacity to reproduce either as an individual or with his/her partner" (Zegers-Hochschild et al., 2017). Around 15–20% of couples within the reproductive age are infertile and in ~50% of the cases, the male factor is present. Furthermore, in 30–40% of cases, the male infertility is idiopathic (Katz et al., 2017). In order to overcome infertility, a number of clinical treatments have been successfully developed and are englobed in what is known as assisted reproductive technologies (ARTs). These involve *in vitro* handling of oocytes, sperm, and embryos for their use in reproduction and comprise *in vitro* fertilization (IVF), embryo transfer, intracytoplasmic sperm injection (ICSI), embryo biopsy, preimplantation genetic testing, and gamete and embryo cryopreservation. The use of ARTs has been steadily rising in the developed countries in last decades (Ferraretti et al., 2017) and from 1997 to 2014, at least 1.5 million babies have been conceived by these techniques in Europe (De Geyter et al., 2018). ARTs are also used in the veterinarian clinical practice and livestock production. However, assisted insemination (AI) is still the preferential reproductive procedure in breeding programs because of its simplicity and effectiveness (Hansen, 2014; Knox, 2016). In cattle embryo production, because of its high efficiency, IVF is intensively used in routine breeding management and millions of calves have been born by this technique (Sirard, 2018). In contrast, ARTs are not applied in sheep and goat farming although the technology has already been developed (Paramio and Izquierdo, 2014). In porcine, the main disadvantage when producing embryos by IVF is the high level of polyspermy (Nagai et al., 2006). This problem can be bypassed by ICSI since normal blastocysts can be produced by this technique with the same efficiency than IVF (Wu et al., 2001). In livestock species, ICSI is not used to overcome male infertility unless the male has a high value, as for endangered species or stallion (Galli et al., 2014; Herrick, 2019), because of the low efficiencies of embryo production achieved in farm animals with this technique (Salamone et al., 2017). In stallion, only two foals have been reported to born following IVF using *in vivo* matured oocytes. As a result in this species, ICSI is the only alternative and has allowed the production of foals from *in vitro* matured oocytes mainly in the clinical management of infertile individuals (Galli et al., 2014).

Despite the wide use of ARTs in the last decades, their efficiency still has the potential to improve. Using both techniques (ICSI or IVF), the latest efficiencies reported by the American and European societies of reproduction and fertility are around 37% of pregnancies and 25% of deliveries per embryo transfer (CDC, 2018; De Geyter et al., 2018). These percentages were higher when fresh oocytes from donors were used, reporting 54 and 38% of pregnancies and deliveries per embryo transfer, respectively. In livestock species, ARTs and specially ICSI are also inefficient (García-Roselló et al., 2009; Salamone et al., 2017) or have not been successfully developed, as in the case of IVF in horse (Leemans et al., 2016) and ICSI in cattle (Li et al., 2004). These low efficiencies can be due to multiple factors such as suboptimal *in vitro* conditions, injuries associated to gametes and embryo manipulation, subjacent male and female factors, etc. We overview herein the different methods recently developed in order to improve ARTs, focusing on the strategy of spermatozoa selection.

Why It Is Important to Select the Spermatozoa? Semen Quality and ARTs Outcome

After the copula, from the millions of spermatozoa ejaculated, only a small number of about few hundreds make it to the region of the oviduct (ampulla), where they encounter the egg and fertilization occurs (Williams et al., 1993; Hino et al., 2016). Presumably, this subpopulation has been selected through the oviduct in a way that only those with the highest fertilization capability and the best features for supporting embryo development get the opportunity to fertilize the egg (Sakkas et al., 2015; Pérez-Cerezales et al., 2017). Thus, it has been proposed that one of the reasons for the relatively low efficiency of ARTs is that we currently lack an effective methodology to separate this specific sperm subpopulation for its use in ARTs (Sakkas et al., 2015; Pérez-Cerezales et al., 2017). This is especially relevant if we consider that both IVF and ICSI bypass the sperm selection operating *in vivo*, increasing the risk of fertilizing the oocyte with defective spermatozoa that could lead to developmental failure and even affect the offspring in the long run (Fernandez-Gonzalez et al., 2008). This risk could be higher in the clinical practice since the incidence of sperm abnormalities, including DNA fragmentation, is higher in infertile men (Saleh et al., 2003; Ozmen et al., 2007; Schulte et al., 2010).

The extent to which the initial quality of the sperm sample affects ARTs success is not clear. It has been generally accepted that depending on the nature of the male factor, IVF or ICSI should be followed as a preferable treatment. In contrast to IVF, ICSI bypasses the last barriers that the spermatozoa have to overcome during fertilization, increasing the risk of fertilizing the oocyte with defective spermatozoa. Therefore, the recommendation is to use always IVF as first choice and ICSI only in the following cases: testicular and epididymal spermatozoa, immotile but viable spermatozoa, asthenozoospermia, globozoospermia, teratozoospermia, and with frozen spermatozoa (Tournaye, 2012). However, because ICSI has been proven to report the same efficiencies as IVF (Schwarze et al., 2017), nowadays this is the most used technique in fertility treatments in developed countries, replacing IVF as the first choice (71.3 and 72% of total cycles were performed by ICSI in Europe in 2014 and in United States in 2016, respectively) (CDC, 2018; De Geyter et al., 2018). This goes against the effectiveness of the last spermatozoa selection barriers imposed by the oocyte during IVF. In a former study, Jones et al. (1998) reported a negative correlation between the presence of male infertility factor and the IVF outcome in terms of blastocyst production. However, in this study and another one conducted by Boulet et al. (2015), no differences were found in final ratios of live births among patients with or without male factor using IVF or ICSI (Jones et al., 1998; Boulet et al., 2015). Recently, Chapuis et al. (2017) reported that using ICSI, patients showing severe oligospermia showed reduced blastulation rate, whereas a reduced progressive motility affected the fertilization and cleavage rates when IVF was performed. Pregnancy rates also decreased in both IVF and ICSI when the father was older than 51, although female age could also have conditioned these results.

Chromatin integrity is the most studied parameter out of the classical and routinely evaluated features of spermatozoa. However, its power to predict ARTs outcome is also under discussion and there are a number of publications showing opposite results as reviewed by Schulte et al. (2010). Latter reviews including a meta-analysis from existing literature corroborate that abnormal chromatin is associated to male infertility and suggest a negative correlation with the probability of ARTs to succeed (Simon et al., 2017b,c). Recent works proved that sperm DNA fragmentation delays embryo cleavage when donated oocytes are used for ICSI but does not affect the final quality of the embryo (Esbert et al., 2018; Casanovas et al., 2019). Also recently, Jerre et al. (2019) retrospectively analyzed the use of semen with different degrees of chromatin packaging for IVF and ICSI in 1602 pregnancies and found that, above certain threshold, spermatozoa porting immature chromatin slightly increased the risk of early miscarriage. The contradictory results reported in the literature could be related to the different methods used for evaluating genetic integrity, all susceptible of variability between different labs. For further insight into the principles of the methods employed for the determination of chromatin integrity, their advantages and disadvantages, and their correlation with male infertility, we address the reader to specific reviews available in the literature (Raheem and Walsh, 2016; Majzoub et al., 2019).

The difficulties to establish a clear correlation among the presence of male factor, sperm chromatin status, and ARTs success could be due to the multifactorial nature of fertility, where the oocyte, spermatozoid, endometrial environment, etc., are individually determinant on pregnancy failure. An under-evaluation of the sperm quality could also be withholding this correlation, since different features are currently not taken into consideration in andrology laboratories as a routine, due to the complexity of the required analysis and to the lack of basic research on molecular markers of sperm quality. Recent studies have also revealed the complex composition of the ejaculate at different levels including epigenetics, indicating that a number of sperm subpopulations with a wide diversity of features coexist (see the next section). Thus, further research should be done to identify additional markers in the spermatozoa related to ARTs success that could serve to isolate the sperm subpopulation whose features support a better embryo development and pregnancy to term.

Sperm Heterogeneity

Any given sperm sample shows a complex heterogeneity revealed at different levels. The most obvious intra-sample diversity can be directly seen under the bright field microscope as different motions are shown by each spermatozoon. A closest examination also reveals a mosaic of subpopulations regarding various morphological features. This heterogeneity of the sperm motility and morphology is objectively confirmed by automatized techniques of sperm tracking and analysis (i.e., CASA and CAMA) that classify the spermatozoa into different subpopulations according to specific kinetical parameters (Martínez-Pastor et al., 2011) and morphologies (Yániz et al., 2015; Soler et al., 2016). Moreover, the composition of sperm subpopulations regarding motility is dynamic throughout time. For instance, *in vitro* conditions for capacitation cause time-dependent changes in the spermatozoa at the cellular level that can be recorded as changes in motility, such as the acquisition of the hyperactive motility. This motility type involves vigorous movements under low-viscous conditions produced by asymmetrical and high-amplitude waves in the flagella and resulting in erratic swimming trajectories (Suarez, 2008). However, not all the spermatozoa acquire the hyperactive motility under capacitation conditions, reaching a maximum of around 20% in humans (Burkman, 1984). Furthermore, human spermatozoa also show a heterogeneous response to chemical inductors of hyperactivation. Ooi et al. (2014), following a single cell analysis by high-speed video recording of adhered human spermatozoa, showed that in response to the potent hyperactivation inducer 4-aminopyridine (4AP), multiple patterns of flagellar beating are produced in each spermatozoa, configuring complex and heterogeneous responses to this type of stimulus. Moreover, using the chemoattractant progesterone, another inductor of hyperactivation, Armon and Eisenbach (2011) showed a variety of responses of individual spermatozoa within few seconds immediately after the sperm–progesterone interaction. These observations suggest the existence of different sperm subpopulations, each with a specific sensitivity to respond by chemotaxis, a mechanism leading the spermatozoa to orient their swimming within a chemical gradient (Eisenbach, 1999). In accordance, only 2–12% of the human spermatozoa are able to align the direction of their swimming toward follicular fluid in a chemotactical response (Cohen-Dayag et al., 1994) and only ~5% of human spermatozoa migrate toward the warmer temperature in response to thermotaxis (Bahat et al., 2012), a mechanism leading the spermatozoa to orient their swimming within a temperature gradient (Bahat et al., 2003).

Sperm heterogeneity has been reported at every level and it can be noticed almost in any study and analysis. Accordingly, a number of research studies hypothesize that only a small subpopulation of spermatozoa within the ejaculate retain the ability to achieve fertilization (Holt and Fazeli, 2015; Sakkas et al., 2015; Pérez-Cerezales et al., 2017). This determines that a high number of spermatozoa are needed to be placed directly onto the oocyte for achieving fertilization *in vitro*. The standard ratio for IVF in humans is 50,000 or more motile sperm per oocyte (Stephens et al., 2013); however, the lower limits of this ratio for achieving fertilization depend on the sperm quality. For example, in a study with subfertile male patients showing diverse sperm qualities, the use of 5000 sperm/oocyte resulted in 37% of zygotes from total oocytes, a percentage that was significantly increased to 60% when using 20,000 sperm/oocyte (Tournaye et al., 2002). The meta-analysis conducted on available publications reporting randomized controlled trials for the treatment of male subfertility evidences a large variability of fertilization ratios, ranging from 50,000 to 10×10^6 sperm/oocyte for IVF (Tournaye et al., 2002). In mice, this limit was reduced to 5 motile sperm/oocyte achieving 60% of fertilization by prolonging the capacitated status of the spermatozoa via creatine supplementation of the medium (Umehara et al., 2018). Therefore, these results also indicate a transient availability of capacitated and "fertile spermatozoa" within the semen. Overall, these data indicate that from the whole spermatozoa population, only a small fraction is susceptible of acquiring the capacity to achieve fertilization at a given time point under *in vitro* conditions.

This observable intra-sample heterogeneity is surely determined by underlying differences among spermatozoa at the cellular and molecular levels. Using discontinuous Percoll gradient, Buffone et al. (2004) found at the different fractions (45, 65, and 90% of Percoll) that human spermatozoa possessed different characteristics regarding quality (motility and morphology) and capacity to show hyperactive motility and protein tyrosine phosphorylation in response to incubation under capacitating conditions. A recent study on bull sperm reported that within two different sperm populations separated by density gradient centrifugation (DGC), there were 31 proteins more abundant in low motile spermatozoa, while 80 proteins were more abundant in the high motile population (D'Amours et al., 2018). Following discontinuous gradient centrifugation of spermatozoa from normozoospermic men, Jenkins et al. (2014) proved the existence of differentially methylated regions in the DNA between high-quality and low-quality fractions. Immunocytological studies on the location of opsins in human and mouse spermatozoa revealed heterogeneous staining patterns for each of the studied proteins involved in the thermotaxis response (Pérez-Cerezales et al., 2015) and reported that a specific subpopulation (~15% of the ejaculate) showing rhodopsin at a specific cellular location is the one with the capability of migrating toward the higher temperature within a gradient (Pérez-Cerezales et al., 2018).

The heterogeneity of the spermatozoa is also reflected at the genetic and epigenetic levels. Thus, single cell analysis of DNA fragmentation by the Comet assay reveals high intra-sample heterogeneity in human spermatozoa, as described by Simon et al. (2017a). We have observed as well that the level of DNA fragmentation of individual spermatozoa ranged from 0 to 70% in normozoospermic men and from 0 to 65% in epididymal mouse spermatozoa (Pérez-Cerezales et al., 2018). The sperm sample also shows various subpopulations at the chromatin packaging level, as evaluated by the sperm chromatin structure assay (SCSA). This assay discriminates subpopulations with high and low chromatin compaction, with different degrees among individual spermatozoids (Evenson, 2016). Moreover, about 9% of the human spermatozoa port some chromosomic alteration (Martin, 2008) and a high percentage of them carries punctual mutations (Wang et al., 2012). In addition, single cell analysis of the telomere length of human spermatozoa also revealed intra-sample heterogeneity with no differences between normal or abnormal spermatozoa (Antunes et al., 2015). These new findings included in the -omics fields reveal the high level of complexity of the ejaculate and the intimate association between these features and male infertility (for a comprehensive review on sperm -omics, we direct the reader to Sinha et al., 2017). The deep study of the genome, epigenome, transcriptome, proteome, and metabolome at the single cell level or in specific sperm subpopulations is expected to reveal higher levels of complexity than the currently known. This type of analyses could help to identify and correlate the presence/absence of specific sperm subpopulations with fertility, and these subpopulations could also be selected for improving ARTs outcome.

In conclusion, it is widely accepted that not all the spermatozoa from an ejaculate are equally good for achieving fertilization *in vivo* or *in vitro* (Holt and Fazeli, 2015). Due to the heterogeneity of the ejaculate, sperm selection prior to ARTs has been considered an important step for ensuring a successful outcome and a strategy to improve ARTs efficiency.

ROUTINE PREPARATION OF SEMEN FOR ARTs

Sperm selection/preparation techniques should be operatively simple and economic in order to fit in the routines of the human and veterinary clinics. Also, they always must ensure the enrichment of the sample in high-quality spermatozoa in the shortest time possible. Besides removing low quality spermatozoa, including those immotile, sperm preparation techniques should allow to eliminate other cells such as leukocytes and bacteria, as well as toxic or bioactive substances like reactive oxygen species (ROS) (Henkel and Schill, 2003).

Because they satisfy all these requirements, swim-up (SU) and DGC (**Figure 1**) are the most extended techniques for the preparation of spermatozoa (Henkel and Schill, 2003). SU was first described by Mahadevan and Baker (1984) and the general principle is the recovery of motile spermatozoa that migrate toward a cells-free medium usually placed above the sperm sample. Different variants of SU are available involving centrifugation (Mahadevan and Baker, 1984), straight migration from unprocessed semen (Aitken and Clarkson, 1988), recovery of spermatozoa from non-resuspended pellet (Carreras et al., 1990), or spermatozoa sedimentation by gravity prior to SU [migration sedimentation (MS) method] (Kiratli et al., 2018). On the other hand, DGC is based on the capacity of motile spermatozoa to progress through a gradient of density constituted by colloidal particles during centrifugation (Henkel and Schill, 2003). Variants of the method consist in different types of gradient: continuous or discontinuous (Henkel and Schill, 2003) and substances used to generate the gradient of density: ficoll (Harrison, 1976), PVP-coated silica particles or Percoll, or the current commercial variants such as IxaPrep® (MediCult, Copenhagen, Denmark), SilSelect® (FertiPro N.V., Beernem, Belgium), PureSperm® (NidaCon Laboratories AB, Gothenburg, Sweden), or ISolate® (Irvine Scientific, Santa Ana, CA, United States) (Henkel and Schill, 2003) used in human clinics to substitute Percoll due to its toxicity (Mousset-Siméon et al., 2004) and side effects on the sperm function (Strehler et al., 1998). In all the SU and DGC variants, it has been shown that the recovered sample is enriched in motile spermatozoa showing normal morphology. It has even been observed that both techniques select those spermatozoa with the longest telomeres (Zhao et al., 2016), this being an indicator of correct spermatogenesis (Rocca et al., 2016).

A number of studies have tried to clarify which of these two methods is more efficient; however, the results available in the literature are multiple and contradictory. In a first study approaching sperm selection for ICSI in patients with cryptozoospermia or severe oligoasthenoteratozoospermia (OAT), Sanchez et al. (1996) showed that the MS method (a type of SU) yielded a sperm fraction with better motility, vitality,

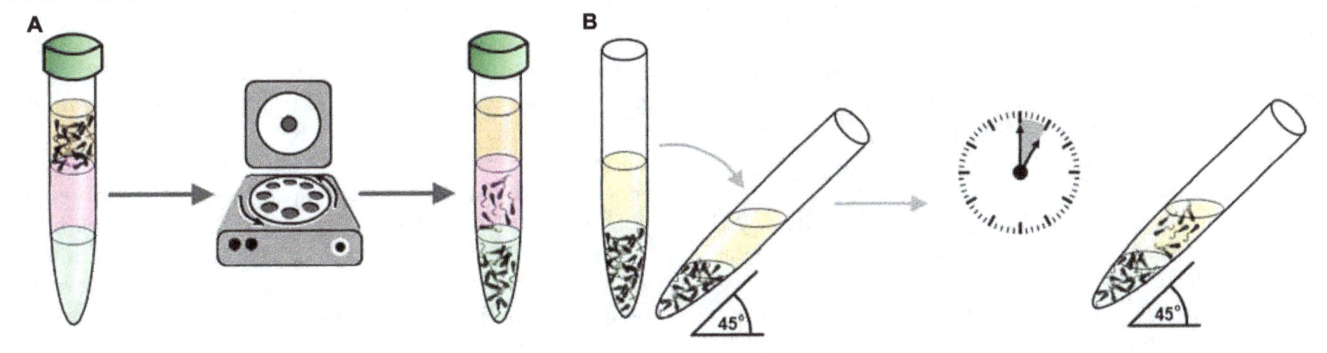

FIGURE 1 | Methods for routine sperm preparation for ARTs. **(A)** Example of sperm selection by density gradient centrifugation (DGC): Semen is placed on top a gradient of colloid (e.g., silica particles coated with silane) prepared in a centrifuge tube and then subject to centrifugation. Subsequently, motile spermatozoa are recovered from the tube bottom containing the fraction with higher density of colloid. **(B)** Example of sperm selection by swim-up (SU): In a centrifuge tube, a medium free of cells (yellow in the figure) is placed on top of the seminal sample (green in the figure). The tube is then inclined 45° and incubated for about 1 h allowing motile spermatozoa to swim-up towards the medium free of cells where they are collected for downstream applications.

morphology, and chromatin condensation than when using minipercoll (a type of DGC), achieving 39.7% of pregnancies (n = 159 cycles). Also, Zini et al. (2000) showed that DGC is less efficient than SU for the separation out of spermatozoa with less DNA integrity. These results were contradictory to those reported by Sakkas et al. (2000) indicating the opposite. Amiri et al. (2012) reported that spermatozoa from normozoospermic donors selected by DGC showed less DNA fragmentation, higher normal morphology, and higher motility than when selected by SU (24 vs 32%, 28 vs 14%, and 76 vs 52%, respectively). Supporting these results, Wang et al. (2014) proved that DGC reduces DNA fragmentation in patients with oligozoospermia and astenozoospermia. Karamahmutoglu et al. (2014) reported that the use of spermatozoa of subfertile patients selected by DCG for intrauterine insemination significantly improved the pregnancy rate compared to the use of SU (18 vs 7%). In contrast, Oguz et al. (2018) reported that SU enriched the sample in spermatozoa with less DNA fragmentation in patients with mild or idiopathic male factor, while DGC did not allow such enrichment in those same patients. A variant of SU, the direct micro-SU, has shown comparable fertilization percentages by ICSI to those of DCG but higher blastocyst development *in vitro* and pregnancy rates (42 vs 26%, respectively), also reducing the abortion rate (13 vs 29%, respectively) (Palini et al., 2017).

In livestock species, SU and DGC are also the most used techniques for sperm selection (Arias et al., 2017) and although Percoll is currently avoided in human ART because of safety issues, as above indicated, it is still a method of choice for animal ART (Cesari et al., 2006). In rams, it has been reported that SU gives better results in terms of reducing the presence of apoptotic spermatozoa vs DGC with Percoll (67 vs 72%, respectively). However, DGC with Percoll delivered a higher percentage of capacitated spermatozoa than the SU method (Martí et al., 2006). In bovine, when comparing DGC (BoviPure^{TM}) (Nidacon, Sweden) vs SU for selecting frozen-thawed spermatozoa, BoviPure^{TM} resulted in spermatozoa showing a greater progressive motility and viability, as well as a higher blastocyst yield (31.79 vs 21.91%, respectively) (Samardzija et al., 2006). Arias et al. (2017) reported that Percoll gradient recovered more spermatozoa with intact plasma and acrosomal membranes (89.8 and 87.5%) than BoviPure gradient (83.3 and 80.4%), but ROS levels were higher with Percoll separation. In addition, Percoll gradient resulted in lower blastocyst yield in comparison to BoviPure^{TM} (~20 vs 30%, respectively) using frozen-thawed semen (Lee et al., 2009). Thus, BoviPure^{TM} should be considered the best frozen-thawed sperm selection technique for *in vitro* production of bovine embryos.

Both SU and DGC are regularly used in laboratories around the world prior to IVF and ICSI but, as discussed in the section "Introduction," the success rates of both techniques should be improved in both human and veterinary practices. Both methodologies for sperm selection are exclusively based on the motile capacity of sperm, which does not mean that all motile sperm are of the highest quality. For instance, it has been pointed that both SU and DGC are not efficient methods to select spermatozoa in terms of apoptosis, DNA integrity, membrane maturation, and sperm ultrastructure (Said and Land, 2011). Furthermore, centrifugation steps inherent to both techniques generate ROS, which have a detrimental effect on sperm quality (Aitken and Clarkson, 1988; Henkel and Schill, 2003). Therefore, new sperm selection methods should be based on sperm characteristics that are better connected to fertilization ability and quality of the spermatozoa, as well as on their contribution to support embryo development to term.

DIRECT SELECTION OF IMMOTILE SPERM

It is important to note that samples in which spermatozoa are immotile, or where the percentage of motile spermatozoa is low, are not suitable for SU and DGC methodologies. This is the case of sperm samples obtained by testicular sperm extraction (TESE) in azoospermic (AO) patients. Nowadays, in the routine practice of fertility clinics, only vague and subjective morphological criteria are followed to select the immotile spermatozoa prior to ICSI, like the identification of spermatozoa with normal head and tail. However, in the last decades, a number of efforts have been made in order to find a selection method for this type of sample, aiming to discriminate viable spermatozoa directly under the micromanipulator irrespectively of their motility.

Marques de Oliveira et al. (2004) proposed the mechanical touch technique (MTT). According to these authors, MTT allows to identify immotile but viable spermatozoa because their tail is flexible when applying a lateral force to the flagella with the ICSI micropipette. In contrast, flagella of non-viable spermatozoa remain rigid to the same force. These authors conducted the only published clinical trial of MTT and found no differences in the ICSI outcome, including deliveries, between motile spermatozoa, and those immotile selected by MTT, in both fresh or frozen samples (Marques de Oliveira et al., 2004). Unfortunately, this study was never corroborated and completed by others. It would be desirable to report as well the comparison between the use of viable vs non-viable spermatozoa selected by MTT for ICSI. Without this information, it is difficult to envisage the actual utility of this technique.

Another sperm selection method that has been investigated is the hipo-osmotic swelling (HOS) test. This technique is based on the fundament that the tails of viable spermatozoa swell or curl under hypo-osmotic conditions due to normal membrane function, thus allowing their identification and recovery under the microscope, potentially for their use for ICSI (Verheyen et al., 1997). Sallam et al. (2005) conducted a randomized study with 79 couples following TESE-ICSI. In this study, where both frozen and fresh samples with total absence of sperm motility were used, pregnancy rates were 20.5% for the 44 couples following HOS and 2.9% for the 35 couples following morphological evaluation (normal head and tail) prior to ICSI. Fertilization and grade I and II embryos rates were also significantly higher in the HOS group. However, when data were analyzed separately, considering the type of sperm sample (fresh or frozen), pregnancy results were not significantly different.

Under polarized light microscopy, the head of viable spermatozoa is birefringent. On this basis, Baccetti (2004) proposed to use this property as a parameter for sperm selection. Indeed, the selection of immotile spermatozoa with birefringent head for ICSI has shown to increase clinical pregnancy and implantation rates compared to control immotile spermatozoa (58 vs 9% and 42 vs 12%, respectively) (Gianaroli et al., 2008) and to increase clinical pregnancy when compared to those selected by HOS (45 vs 11%, respectively) (Ghosh et al., 2012).

The use of chemical inducers of sperm motility has also been investigated. Thus, phosphodiesterase inhibitors of the xanthine family, such as pentoxifylline (PTF), demethylxanthine theophylline (TPF), and papverine have shown to activate the motility in a fraction of immotile testicular sperm (Taşdemir et al., 1998; Ebner et al., 2011; Terriou et al., 2015). The use of this motile fraction, whether using PTF, TPF, or papverine, has allowed to achieve normal fertilization, pregnancy, and birth after ICSI (Terriou et al., 2000; Kovačič et al., 2006; Amer et al., 2013; Sandi-Monroy et al., 2019). Furthermore, Mangoli et al. (2011) showed that the use of PTF compared with HOS selected spermatozoa, yielded higher fertilization rate, and doubled clinical pregnancies (32 and 16%, respectively, $n = 25$). Interestingly, the successful treatment of male infertility associated to the Kartagener's syndrome has been reported with both PTF and HOS, achieving the delivery of healthy babies in ICSI cycles (Hattori et al., 2011; Montjean et al., 2015). These findings show the therapeutic potential of both methodologies that could be useful for the treatment of other male infertility cases.

Motility of immotile but vital spermatozoa can also be induced with a single laser shot to the tip of the flagellum (Aktan et al., 2004). Thus, the laser-assisted immotile sperm selection (LAISS) has been proposed as an alternative to the use of chemicals like xanthines, avoiding in this way their potential toxic effects. This method has shown to significantly increase cleavage and birth rates after ICSI using both testicular and ejaculated sperm when compared to control groups (Aktan et al., 2004; Nordhoff et al., 2013). Moreover, LAISS has shown its utility to restore fertility following ICSI in specific cases of male patients showing primary cilia dyskinesia (Gerber et al., 2008) and the Kartagener's syndrome (Ozkavukcu et al., 2018). Despite the potential of this technique, its complexity and cost have possibly prevented its use in clinical routines and explain the scarce number of published studies.

In addition to these specific procedures, the methodologies described in the following sections, that do not require sperm motility, in principle are also suitable for sperm selection in immotile samples, although their efficiency for this type of samples should be further explored.

SPERM SELECTION BASED ON MEMBRANE CHARACTERISTICS

The outer membrane of the spermatozoa is crucial for their functionality as it takes part in a number of basic processes such as cell metabolism, capacitation, ova binding, acrosome reaction, etc. Its accessibility and relation with sperm vitality and quality make this organelle, its integrity, and variable characteristics, a logic target for the development of selection methods of high-quality spermatozoa for their use in ARTs.

Annexin V Magnetic Activated Cell Sorting (AV-MACS)

Magnetic activated cell sorting (MACS) is a method that allows the separation of cell populations based on their surface antigens (Plouffe et al., 2015). Coating magnetic nanoparticles with a molecule with affinity for these antigens allows the trapping of the desired cell subpopulation and its separation within a column subject to a strong magnetic field. Thus, cells expressing the antigen stay in the column while other cells flow through for downstream applications. The loss of membrane integrity is an early event of the apoptotic response

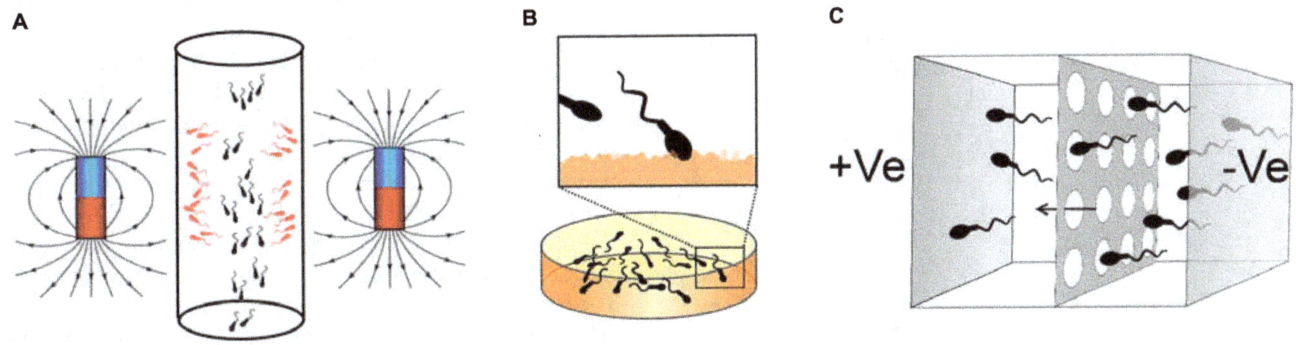

FIGURE 2 | Methods for sperm selection based on membrane characteristics. **(A)** Example of Annexin V magnetic activated cell sorting (AV-MACS): Apoptotic spermatozoa (red in the figure) are bound to magnetic nanoparticles coated with Annexin V and affinity to the externalized phosphatidylserine in this sperm population. Semen is then passed through a column with magnetos on the side, thus apoptotic spermatozoa are retained and non-apoptotic are washed out for downstream applications. **(B)** Example of method for sperm selection based on hyaluronic acid-binding. Spermatozoa are placed on a dish coated with hyaluronic acid (HA, orange in the figure). Matured spermatozoa bind to the surface due to their interaction with the HA. These spermatozoa can be then recovered for ICSI using a micromanipulation system. **(C)** Example of sperm selection by the Z-method developed by Ainsworth et al. (2005): Spermatozoa are placed in a well isolated from another adjacent well by a porous membrane and filled with a medium free of cells. An electric field is then applied with the anode in the well free of cells and the cathode in the well containing the sperm suspension. Due to the negative charge of the sperm membrane, spermatozoa migrate towards the compartment free of cells passing through the porous membrane. Spermatozoa can be then collected for downstream applications.

and leads to the externalization of phosphatidylserine (Elmore, 2007). On this basis, magnetic nanoparticles coated with Annexin V, a molecule showing high affinity for phosphatidylserine (Vermes et al., 1995), bind to apoptotic spermatozoa that are retained in the MACS column, allowing the recovery of non-apoptotic spermatozoa for their use in ARTs (Gil et al., 2013) (**Figure 2A**).

The use of Annexin V MACS (AV-MACS) for sperm selection in the human clinical practice was first reported by Grunewald et al. (2001), demonstrating the utility of this technique for the enrichment of the sample with non-apoptotic spermatozoa retaining membrane integrity. Since then, a number of studies have shown the enrichment of high-quality spermatozoa with reduced levels of DNA fragmentation using AV-MACS (**Table 1**). Said et al. (2006) employed AV-MACS for the selection of semen from 35 healthy donors, reporting an enrichment of spermatozoa with lower DNA fragmentation and higher oocyte penetration capacity. Using this method, Zahedi et al. (2013) also reported an enrichment of spermatozoa with lower DNA fragmentation in both fertile and infertile (terato- and asthenozoospermic) patients. Additionally, Lee et al. (2010) and Degheidy et al. (2015) proved that spermatozoa selected by AV-MACS from idiopathic infertile patients and patients diagnosed with varicocele showed lower DNA fragmentation than the original sample and kept intact sperm motility. However, a number of studies comparing AV-MACS with SU and DGC question the actual utility of this technique for the enrichment in spermatozoa with higher quality. Therefore, Tavalaee et al. (2012) found that combined AV-MACS followed by DGC on semen from infertile patients with different etiologies was more efficient at enriching the sample in spermatozoa with lower DNA fragmentation than both procedures autonomously or DGC followed by AV-MACS. Nadalini et al. (2014) obtained better results with DGC followed by SU than with DGC followed by AV-MACS in terms of sperm quality as determined by motility, morphology, and DNA fragmentation. Cakar et al. (2016) did not find significant differences in any of the analysis of sperm quality, including DNA fragmentation, by using AV-MACS, SU, DG, SU/AV-MACS, and DG/AV-MACS, perhaps due to the low sample size of the study. In contrast, Berteli et al. (2017) found a better quality in terms of motility and DNA fragmentation in spermatozoa selected by AV-MACS followed by DCG than with the other combinations tested: DCG and AV-MACS alone or DCG followed by AV-MACS. Similar to these results, Zhang et al. (2018) reported that the combination of DCG followed by AV-MACS in immotile sperm samples resulted in the recovery of a sperm population with lower DNA fragmentation compared to DGC alone. In agreement, Esbert et al. (2017) reported that DGC followed by AV-MACS reduced the number of spermatozoa porting chromosomal abnormalities.

Regarding the use of the spermatozoa selected by AV-MACS for ARTs, reported results are scarce and unclear (**Table 2**). An early study employing 196 oligoasthenozoospermic patients reported an increase of cleavage and pregnancy rates when AV-MACS was applied prior to ICSI in comparison to DGC (Dirican et al., 2008). However, another study registering 237 infertile couples following ICSI with donated oocytes did not find significant differences in terms of embryo quality and in the ratios of fertilization, implantation, pregnancy, and live birth when the semen was cryopreserved and then selected by SU or SU followed by AV-MACS (Romany et al., 2014). García-Ferreyra et al. (2014) reported higher, but not statically significant pregnancy and implantation rates when semen showing basal high DNA fragmentation was selected by AV-MACS followed by DGC, compared to DGC alone in ICSI treatments. These results are supported by those reported by Stimpfel et al. (2018) in couples of teratozoospermic patients and women over 30 years old undergoing ICSI, showing higher quality blastocysts when

TABLE 1 | DNA fragmentation of spermatozoa selected by AV-MACS.

Groups compared	DNA fragmentation (%)	Type of male donors/patients (*n*)	References
Unsorted	14.4 ± 13.2^a	Donors (35)	Said et al., 2006
Annexin positive	21 ± 13.6^b		
Annexin negative	9.7 ± 10.6^c		
DGC	13.5 ± 5.6	Normozoospermic (60)	Lee et al., 2010
DGC/AV-MACS	$9.9 \pm 3.6^{***}$		
Unsorted	$29,72 \pm 3.41^a$	Infertile, various etiologies (15)	Tavalaee et al., 2012
DGC	$21,27 \pm 3.47^b$		
AV-MACS	$21,72 \pm 3.41^b$		
DGC/AV-MACS	$17,63 \pm 3.72^c$		
AV-MACS/DGC	$15,27 \pm 3.49^c$		
Unsorted	17.7 ± 1.6	Fertile (10), infertile (26): terato- and asthenozoospermia	Zahedi et al., 2013
MACS	$12.1 \pm 1.7^*$		
Unsorted	3.48 ± 4.54^a	Infertile, various etiologies (25)	Nadalini et al., 2014
DGC/AV-MACS	2.41 ± 2.72^b		
DGC/SU	2.1 ± 2.75^c		
Unsorted	12.43 ± 6.29	Infertile, vaticocele (36)	Degheidy et al., 2015
AV-MACS	$9.61 \pm 5.62^*$		
SU	21.4 ± 16.6	Normozoospermic (10)	Cakar et al., 2016
SU/AV-MACS	15 ± 4.9		
DGC	18.6 ± 5.8		
DGC/AV-MACS	21 ± 6.4		
SU	12 ± 16.6	Oligozoospermic (10)	
SU/AV-MACS	9.4 ± 9.9		
DGC	10.6 ± 8.4		
DGC/AV-MACS	8.4 ± 6.3		
Unsorted	24 (9–26)	Normozoospermic (15)	Berteli et al., 2017
DGC	10 (5–16)		
DGC/AV-MACS	6 (3–11)		
AV-MACS/DGC	4 (2–7)		
AV-MACS	8 (6–16)		
Unsorted	9.56 ± 3.39^a	Asthenozoospermic (16)	Zhang et al., 2018
DGC	5.25 ± 1.61^b		
DGC/AV-MACS	2.75 ± 1.2^c		

*DNA fragmentation was analyzed in all cases by TUNEL. Values of % DNA fragmentation are expressed as % ± SEM, SD or (interquartile range). *$P < 0.05$, ***$P < 0.001$ and different letters indicate differences between groups ($P < 0.05$).*

spermatozoa were selected by DGC/SU followed by AV-MACS, compared to DGC/SU. Recently, Ziarati et al. (2019) reported a significant increase in the percentage of high-quality embryos and clinical pregnancies employing DGC followed by MACS in 80 infertile couples showing male factor and undergoing ICSI when compared to DGC itself.

Studies conducted in livestock species using MACS are missing. In rabbits, AV-MACS did not show a clear enrichment in non-apoptotic spermatozoa and did not affect the reproductive outcome when the selected semen was used for AI (Vasicek et al., 2014).

These studies collectively show that the combination of DGC and MACS might provide slight benefits in patients with male factor undergoing ICSI in terms of clinical pregnancy. However, it is not clear to which extent live birth rate is actually improved. Thus, the type of donor or patient and the combination of AV-MACS with other sperm preparation methods could be determinant for improving ARTs. More experiments, registering larger number of patients, and exploring the different variables involved, are needed in order to certificate the utility of AV-MACS for the human clinical practice.

Hyaluronic Acid (HA) Binding

The hyaluronic acid (HA) is one of the main components of the extracellular matrix surrounding the cumulus-oocyte complex (COC) (Dandekar et al., 1992), and those spermatozoa that follow an adequate spermatogenesis and maturation exhibit binding sites to it (Cayli et al., 2003; Huszar et al., 2006). Therefore, two methodologies of sperm selection have been developed based on the spermatozoa-HA interaction: (i) recovering those spermatozoa trapped on the surface of HA coated dishes (Huszar et al., 2006) (**Figure 2B**) and (ii) picking up those spermatozoa moving slow when swimming in a medium containing HA in solution (Barak et al., 2001).

According to published data, both methods have shown their capacity to select spermatozoa with lower DNA fragmentation (**Table 3**). In an early work, Nasr-Esfahani et al. (2008), employing HA-coated dishes, reported a significant inverse correlation among the percentage of HA-bounded spermatozoa and protamine deficiency, DNA fragmentation, and abnormal sperm morphology in the original sample. While Razavi et al. (2010) reported that spermatozoa recovered from HA-coated dishes show the same level of DNA fragmentation than the unselected ones, other laboratories reported higher DNA integrity in spermatozoa selected by HA-binding methods (Parmegiani et al., 2010a; Yagci et al., 2010; Mongkolchaipak and Vutyavanich, 2013) Furthermore, Parmegiani et al. (2010a) and Huang et al. (2015) showed lower DNA fragmentation in spermatozoa selected in HA solution compared to SU, and by HA coated dishes compared to DGC, respectively. However, both studies reported similar levels of DNA fragmentation when compared to spermatozoa selected under the microscope regarding motility and morphological features. Similarly, Mongkolchaipak and Vutyavanich (2013) did not find any difference between DGC/HA coated dishes and DGC/intracytoplasmic morphologically selected sperm injection

TABLE 2 | Reproductive outcomes of ARTs employing spermatozoa selected by AV-MACS.

Sperm origin	Oocyte origin	Sperm groups	Fertilization rate (%)	Cleavage (%)	Blastocyst (%)	Embryos transferred (*n*)	Clinical pregnancy (%)	Live birth rate/ET (%)	References
Fresh. oligoastheno-zoospermic	ND	DGC	69.9	88.2	85	ND	36.49	ND	Dirican et al., 2008
		AV-MACS	69.52	97.2*	84.9		48.36*		
Cryopreserved	Donors	SU/AV-MACS	75.3 (71.6–78.9)	ND	ND	123	64.2 (55.4–72.1)	48.4 (39.6–57.1)	Romany et al., 2014
		SU	72.1 (68.6–75.7)			114	71.1 (62.1–78.6)	56.4 (47.3–65.5)	
Fresh. high DNA fragmentation	Donors	DGC	76.5	89.1	41.1	146	45.5	ND	García-Ferreyra et al., 2014
		DGC/AV-MACS	74.5	98.3	50.8	107	63.2		
Fresh. infertile, at least two abnormal parameters	Donors	DGC	74.78 + 3.41	ND	ND	33	24.24	ND	Ziarati et al., 2019
		MACS + DGC	76.13 + 4.38			22	54.54**		
Fresh. teratozoospermic	Patients. women aged ≤ 30 years	DGC/SU	70.6	100	56.5	4	50	50	Stimpfel et al., 2018
		DGC/SU/AV-MACS	65.6	95.2	41.2	4	75	50	
	Patients. women aged ≥ 31 years	DGC/SU	79.8	97.5	41.1	5	20	20	Stimpfel et al., 2018
		DGC/SU/AV-MACS	69.5	97	41.4	12	16.7	16.7	

*All the reported cases followed ICSI. Values are expressed as % ± w/o, SEM, SD, or (interquartile range). *P < 0.05, **P < 0.01.*

(IMSI) respect to sperm DNA fragmentation. These results question the utility of sperm selection based on HA-binding.

Although the use of HA was first conceived for substituting the routinely used PVP as an agent to decrease sperm motion prior ICSI (Sbracia et al., 1997; Barak et al., 2001), the potential as a selective agent was soon explored (Cayli et al., 2003). Thus, Park et al. (2005) used HA solution to select boar spermatozoa and found a significant increase of embryos with normal chromosomal counts and less chromosome abnormalities when compared to conventional ICSI. Few months later, similar results were reported in humans showing that sperm selection by HA led to a reduction of chromosomal disomy frequencies, diploidy, and sex chromosome disomy; all abnormalities associated to embryos produced by ICSI (Jakab et al., 2005). All these publications did not report clear effects on ICSI outcomes; however, this was possibly not carefully studied until 2008. Since then, a number of publications have specifically checked the capability of sperm selection by HA-binding for improving ICSI outcome (**Table 4**). In a first attempt, Nasr-Esfahani et al. (2008) found an increase of the fertilization rate using HA-coated dishes but there was no detectable effect on pregnancy or implantation rates. Parmegiani et al. (2010b) studied the reproductive outcome in 331 patients undergoing ICSI using HA solution (293 patients) or conventional ICSI (86), finding no differences in clinical pregnancies or live birth ratios but an improvement in embryo quality and implantation rate. In another study, the same authors reported comparable results employing 206 oligozoospermic patients (Parmegiani et al., 2010a). Similar results were reported in subsequent studies using either HA-coated dishes or HA solution (Choe et al., 2012; Parmegiani et al., 2012; Majumdar and Majumdar, 2013; Mokánszki et al., 2014). In contrast, Worrilow et al. (2013) reported that the use of HA-coated dishes significantly increased pregnancy (Worrilow et al., 2013; Mokánszki et al., 2014) and live birth rate (Mokánszki et al., 2014) for those patients undergoing ICSI which semen showed a HA-binding capacity $\leq$ 65%, as measured by the Hyaluronan binding assay. This effect proves that the method could be useful only in specific cases and indicates the need of a preliminary semen analysis for determining the suitability of the technique. Therefore, Erberelli et al. (2017) reported a significant improvement of ICSI using HA-coated dishes in patients with various categories of male factor. Their results also suggested that the benefit of this method could be higher for teratozoospermic patients. In a randomized study employing a large number of patients (2772 couples), Miller et al. (2019) did not find any significant benefit of HA-coated dishes compared to conventional ICSI and either detected an association between results of Hyaluronan binding assay and ICSI outcomes, contradicting previous works above described. These results collectively show a poor capacity of HA binding methods for improving ICSI; however, more studies are needed to identify the types of patients that could benefit from this procedure.

Zeta Method

Sperm membrane is negatively charged (Engelmann et al., 1988). On this basis, methods for separating X- and Y-bearing

TABLE 3 | DNA fragmentation of spermatozoa selected by hyaluronic acid.

Groups compared	DNA fragmentation (%)	Type of male donors/patients (*n*)	DNA fragmentation technique	References
Unsorted	32.87 ± 8.65	Patients (77): Severe (13%), moderate (61%), and normospermic (26%)	SCD	Razavi et al., 2010
PICSI	30.94 ± 8.7			
Unsorted	16.5[a]	Patients (20): Normozoospermic (12) and oligozoospermic (8)	SCD	Parmegiani et al., 2010a,b
SU	11[b]			
Microscopically selected	11[c]			
Sperm slow	5.3[d]			
Unsorted	45 ± 1.9	Patients (50)	AOF	Yagci et al., 2010
PICSI	0.9 ± 1.9**			
DGC	26,8	Donors (50)	TUNEL	Mongkolchaipak and Vutyavanich, 2013
DGC/PICSI	2.6			
DGC/IMSI	1.7			
DGC	33.2[a]	Patients (46)	AOF	Huang et al., 2015
Microscopically selected	17.9[b]			
PICSI	16.1[b]			

*Analysis of DNA fragmentation was conducted by Sperm Chromatin Dispersion (SCD) test, Acridin Orange fluorescence (AOF), or TUNEL. Values of % of DNA fragmentation are expressed as % ± SEM. **$P < 0.01$ and different letters indicate differences between groups ($P < 0.05$).*

TABLE 4 | Reproductive outcomes of ARTs spermatozoa selected by hyaluronic acid.

Sperm origin	Oocyte origin	Number of couples	Sperm groups	Fertilization rate (%)	Cleavage (%)	Blastocyst (%)	Embryos transferred (n)	Clinical pregnancy (%)	Live birth rate/ET (%)	References
Patients: wide range of sperm quality	Patients. different conditions	50	HA coated dishes	79.4 ± 26	ND	ND	ND	40	ND	Nasr-Esfahani et al., 2008
			PVP	67.7 ± 23.5				55		
Patients: oligozoospermic	Patients: average age of 37–38 years	112	HA solution	91.6	ND	ND	125	24.8	23.2	Parmegiani et al., 2010a
		94	PVP	85.8			105	20.9	18	
Patients	Patients: age ≤ 39 years	293	HA coated dishes	93.4	ND	ND	326	32.8	16.3	Parmegiani et al., 2010b
		86	PVP	87.1			96	21.6	18.8	
Patients: normozoospermic	Patients: ages ranged from 30 to 42 years	18	HA solution	75.7	72.9	22.9	ND	ND	ND	Choe et al., 2012
			PVP	83	83	24				
Patients: motility ≥ 5%, total sperm number ≥ 1 × 10^6	Patients: age ≤ 40 years	50	HA coated dishes	82	ND	ND	49	42.9	18	Parmegiani et al., 2012
		50	HA solution	82			50	40	15	
Patients	Patients: age < 38 and other selection criteria	71	HA coated dishes	64.7	ND	ND	177	35.2	12.4	Majumdar and Majumdar, 2013
		80	PVP	65.7			192	35	10.9	
Patients	Patients: (age < 40 years)	63	HA coated dishes	ND	ND	ND	ND	50.8*	ND	Worrilow et al., 2013
		58	PVP					37.9		
Patients	Patients (age < 40 years)	102	HA coated dishes	55.7	ND	ND	ND	39.3**	0.49***	Mokánszki et al., 2014
		42	PVP	52.8				26.6	0.27	
Patients: various male factors included	ND	19	HA coated dishes	71.93	95.12	ND	19	42.1***	ND	Erberelli et al., 2017
		37	PVP	64.14	95.27		37	16.21		
Patients: able to produce freshly ejaculate (ages 18–55 years)	Patients: age (18–43)	1387	HA coated dishes	66	ND	ND	1381	35.2	27.4	Miller et al., 2019
		1385	PVP	69			1371	35.7	25.2	

All the reported cases followed ICSI. Values are expressed as % ± w/o, SEM, SD, or (interquartile range). $^{*}P < 0.05$, $^{**}P < 0.01$, $^{***}P < 0.001$.

spermatozoa (Engelmann et al., 1988) and for the separation of pure sperm heads from disintegrated mammalian spermatozoa (Chaudhuri and Datta, 1994) were developed decades ago. Later, the methods developed by Chan et al. (2006) and Ainsworth et al. (2005) (**Figure 2C**) allowed to collect the charged spermatozoa adhered to the wall of a centrifuge tube or migrating within an electric field, respectively. With both methodologies, downstream analysis of the selected spermatozoa revealed an increased percentage of spermatozoa with higher quality and porting high-integrity DNA (Kheirollahi-Kouhestani et al., 2009; Razavi et al., 2010; Zarei-Kheirabadi et al., 2012; Zahedi et al., 2013) (**Table 5**). This procedure, known as Zeta method, has allowed the selection of spermatozoa with lower DNA fragmentation compared to the HA-coated dish selection (Razavi et al., 2010). Also, sperm DNA fragmentation has been proven to be lower using DGC-Zeta than DGC by itself (Zarei-Kheirabadi et al., 2012) or MACS-DGZ (Zahedi et al., 2013). However, despite these promising results, only one randomized study has been published using spermatozoa selected by Zeta method in patients undergoing ICSI (Esfahani et al., 2016). In this research, significant increases in top quality embryos [45.83 ± 3.11% vs 35.38 ± 4.64% (P = 0.04)] and pregnancy rates [39.2 vs 21.8% (P = 0.009)] were obtained with DGC/Zeta compared to DGC, respectively. However, further analysis is needed to know the potential of Zeta method for improving ARTs.

Future of Sperm Selection Based on Membrane Characteristics

As exposed above, sperm selection by AV-MACS and HA does not seem to contribute in general terms to a significant improvement of ARTs outcome, and Zeta method needs to proof its efficiency in larger studies. However, the use of the properties of the plasma membrane for sperm selection could really improve ARTs if markers with higher potential for discriminating high-quality spermatozoa are discovered. Thus, new antigens could be used as targets for selection by MACS, by coated plates or even by fluorescence-activated cell sorting (Funaro et al., 2013). However, this research direction is currently poorly explored, possibly because of the lack of basic knowledge about markers discriminating the various sperm populations contained in the ejaculate. Heidari et al. (2018) explored three surface proteins, HSPA2, Dj-1, and serum amyloid P, as biomarkers of sperm DNA integrity and found that the abundance of these three

TABLE 5 | DNA fragmentation of spermatozoa selected by Zeta method.

Groups compared	DNA fragmentation (%)	Type of male donors/patients (n)	Fragmentation technique	References
Unsorted	19 ± 0.1	Patients (8)	AOF	Chan et al., 2006
Zeta	11 ± 0.1*			
Unsorted	8 ± 2*	Donors (6)	TUNEL	Ainsworth et al., 2005
Zeta	3 ± 2			
Unsorted	49.65 ± 15.1[a]	Patients (60)	AOF	Kheirollahi-Kouhestani et al., 2009
DGC	32.65 ± 14.38[b]			
Zeta	28.85 ± 15.83[c]			
Unsorted	15.83 ± 8.14[a]	Patients (55)	TUNEL	
DGC	8.17 ± 4.23[b]			
Zeta	5.89 ± 3.92[c]			
Unsorted	50.43 ± 15.58[a]	Patients (51)	SCD	
DGC	33.58 ± 16.24[b]			
Zeta	29.21 ± 14.95[c]			
Unsorted	32.87 ± 8.65[a]	Patients (77), 13, 61, and 26% (severe, moderate, and normospermic respectively)	SCD	Razavi et al., 2010
HA coated dish	30.94 ± 8.7[ab]			
Zeta	18.19 ± 8.64[b]			
Unsorted	21.97 ± 3.84[a]	Patients (30)	TUNEL	Zarei-Kheirabadi et al., 2012
DGC	17.47 ± 3.52[b]			
DGC-Zeta	6.98 ± 1.45[c]			
Unsorted	17.7 ± 1.6[a]	Fertile (10), infertile (26): terato- and asthenozoospermia	TUNEL	Zahedi et al., 2013
MACS-DGC	12.1 ± 1.7[b]			
DGC-Zeta	9.8 ± 1.2[b]			

*Analysis of DNA fragmentation was conducted by Sperm Chromatin Dispersion (SCD) test, Acridin Orange fluorescence (AOF), or TUNEL. Values of % of DNA fragmentation are expressed as % ± SEM or SD. *P < 0.05 and different letters indicate differences between groups (P < 0.05).*

proteins in the semen was directly correlated to sperm quality, DNA integrity, and embryo quality. Mostek et al. (2018) found that high-quality bull ejaculates showed higher abundance of extracellular sperm surface proteins and that sperm proteins in low-quality ejaculates are characterized by high carbonylation levels. All these membrane features and new ones yet to be discovered could be used with the aim of improving ARTs through sperm selection.

SPERM SELECTION BASED ON SPERM MORPHOLOGY – INTRACYTOPLASMIC MORPHOLOGICALLY SELECTED SPERM INJECTION (IMSI)

The morphometric evaluation of spermatozoa is widely applied to analyze sperm quality due to its correlation to fertility (Yániz et al., 2015; Soler et al., 2016). Furthermore, the introduction of computer-enhanced digital microscopy has enabled the analysis and quantification of detailed features of the cell that applied to motile spermatozoa configure the "Motile Sperm Organelle Morphology Examination" (MSOME) (Bartoov et al., 2002). The use of MSOME for selecting spermatozoa for ICSI is known as IMSI. This technique consists in the selection and direct capture of those spermatozoa with a low number of vacuoles and a nucleus of normal morphology under a microscope equipped with a micromanipulation system and a magnification system of 6300x (Bartoov et al., 2002) (**Figure 3**). The power of selecting spermatozoa with higher DNA integrity has been proved by different authors, although contradictory results are also present in the literature (**Table 6**). Using this methodology, Franco et al. (2008) revealed that the presence of large vacuoles in the sperm nucleus is associated with a higher DNA fragmentation compared to those spermatozoa with normal nucleus. The correlation between the presence of vacuoles, as detected by MSOME, and DNA fragmentation was later confirmed by Wilding et al. (2011). However, Leandri et al. (2013) did not find significant differences in this respect between the spermatozoa selected by IMSI and those selected as conventionally done during regular ICSI. Other authors have suggested that IMSI could be useful only in specific cases of male infertility. Accordingly, when spermatozoa from infertile donors showing more than 13% of DNA fragmentation were selected by IMSI, those showing normal morphology under high magnification delivered less DNA fragmentation than those classified as motile and normal using conventional magnification of 200x (Hammoud et al., 2013). Moreover, the authors reported in the same work that those selected under lower magnification showed the same DNA fragmentation than the unsorted spermatozoa. Results reported by Lavolpe et al. (2015) suggest that in patients whose semen scored $\leq$ 4% according to the strict morphology index, the presence of vacuoles in the nucleus of the spermatozoa was less related to DNA fragmentation and chromatin compaction than in those patients with strict morphology index $\geq$ 14%.

Recently, in the largest study reported to date where 873 sperm samples were analyzed by MSOSE, the presence of head vacuoles was not associated to sperm DNA fragmentation and live birth rate (Fortunato et al., 2016). Authors claim that vacuoles are physiological features that do not alter sperm functionality. The controversy about the convenience of IMSI for improving ARTs exists from the first moment the method was described. We address here the reader to an excellent systematic review on the literature published between 2001 and 2013, where the authors conclude that IMSI was only proven to improve reproductive outcome in cases of recurrent implantation failure following ICSI (Boitrelle et al., 2014). The same year, other authors published a meta-analysis on 13 publications confronting IMSI vs conventional ICSI in cases with previous ICSI failures and when the male factor was the cause of infertility, and concluded that in both cases, IMSI improved the reproductive outcome (Setti et al., 2014). However, authors pointed to the lack of randomized studies to corroborate their conclusions. Since then, together with the study of Fortunato et al. (2016), others have shown the failure of IMSI for improving ARTs (**Table 7**). Thus, Leandri et al. (2013), having examined 458 couples, did not find significant differences between IMSI or ICSI in the reproductive outcome, regardless of the initial characteristics of semen regarding DNA fragmentation, chromatin compaction, morphology, or motility. Setti et al. (2015) showed no benefits of IMSI for couples with poor ovarian response. In contrast, Shalom-Paz et al. (2015) reported that IMSI significantly increased implantation and clinical pregnancy rates in patients with repeated IVF-ICSI failure. However, Gatimel et al. (2016) failed in confirming these results. Kim et al. (2014) and Goswami et al. (2018) showed that IMSI applied to OAT patients of various severities resulted in significantly higher implantation, pregnancy rates, and live birth rates when compared to a previous ICSI cycle performed to the same patients, suggesting an actual utility of IMSI for these specific cases. Also, in another study on 170 patients,

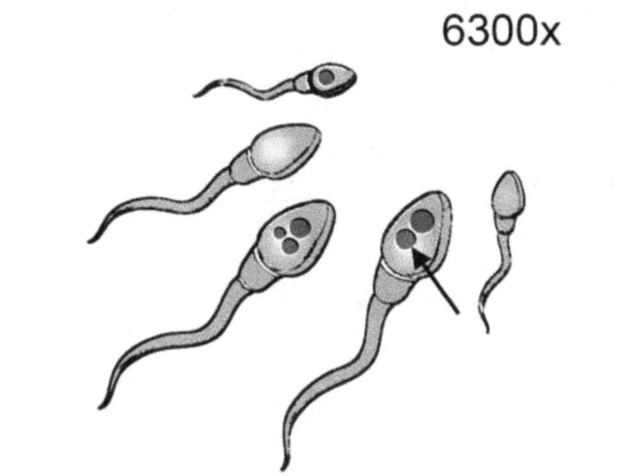

FIGURE 3 | Intracytoplasmic morphologically selected sperm injection (IMSI). Spermatozoa are examined under a magnification system of 6300x in order to discriminate those spermatozoa lacking vacuoles (arrow) and showing normal morphology. These spermatozoa are collected with the micromanipulation system for their use in ICSI.

TABLE 6 | DNA fragmentation of spermatozoa selected by IMSI.

Groups compared	DNA fragmentation (%)	Type of male donors/patients (*n*)	Fragmentation technique	References
Normal nucleus	15.9//33.1	Patients (30)	TUNEL//AOF	Franco et al., 2008
Large vacuoles	29.1***//67.9***			
ICSI	16.2 ± 8.8	Patients: ICSI (139), IMSI (116)	TUNEL	Leandri et al., 2013
IMSI	16.4 ± 9.5			
Unsorted	26.1 ± 1.5[a]	Infertile donors (8) (more than 13% of fragmented DNA spermatozoa)	TUNEL	Hammoud et al., 2013
Motile 200x	20.8 ± 2.7[ab]			
Motile and normal Spermatozoa 200x	18.7 ± 2.7[ab]			
Motile and normal spermatozoa 6300x	4.1 ± 1.1[c]			
Morphometrically normal with anterior/posterior vacuoles 6300x	15.9 ± 2.9[b]/ 22.5 ± 3.6[ab]			
IMSI no vacuoles	20.1//17.8	Strict morphology index ≤ 4% (26)	AOF//TUNEL	Lavolpe et al., 2015
IMSI vacuoles	22.6–35.2*//18.2–25.4			
IMSI No vacuoles	6.1//3.6	Strict morphology index ≥ 14% (20)	AOF//TUNEL	
IMSI Vacuoles	4.9–36.2*//5.2–16.2*			

*Analyses of DNA fragmentation were conducted by, Acridin Orange fluorescence (AOF) or TUNEL. Values of % of DNA fragmentation are expressed as % ± SEM or SD. Values separated by double slash indicate correspondence to the employed method of DNA fragmentation in that column. In Lavolpe et al. (2015) % of DNA fragmentation are intervals according to different patterns of vacuole number, morphology, and distribution. *$P < 0.05$, ***$P < 0.001$ and different letters indicate differences between groups ($P < 0.05$).*

the results suggest that IMSI can improve pregnancy rates in patients with severe sperm pathologies affecting various sperm parameters (Schachter- Safrai et al., 2019). Overall, although the literature dissuades the routine use of IMSI, it seems that it could be highly indicated for the treatment of severe cases of male factor. Larger head-to-head randomized studies discriminating seminal parameters in infertile pathologies are still needed in order to elucidate under which circumstances IMSI could benefit reproductive outcome in the human clinical practice.

SPERM SELECTION BASED ON GUIDANCE MECHANISMS

As we discussed in the section "Introduction," guidance within the female genital tract has been suggested as a physiological mechanism for the selection of those spermatozoa able to fertilize the egg and ensuring the ulterior embryo development to term (Pérez-Cerezales et al., 2017). Hence, a strategy to develop new sperm selection methodologies is to employ *in vitro* the same principles that govern the sperm selection operating within the female genital tract. Consequently, there are three known mechanisms that have been proposed to guide the spermatozoa within the oviduct and they have been tested accordingly for their capacity to select spermatozoa with the aim of improving ARTs.

Rheotaxis

Miki and Clapham (2013) proved for the first time that both human and mice spermatozoa orientate their swimming against a fluid flow, process known as rheotaxis. Latter, El-Sherry et al. (2014) and Romero-Aguirregomezcorta et al. (2018) confirmed the occurrence of this phenomenon also in bovine, stallion, and ram spermatozoa, suggesting rheotaxis as a conserved feature of mammalian spermatozoa. Furthermore, the existence in mice of oviductal flow toward the uterus intensified after copula supports rheotaxis as a long-distance guidance mechanism within the oviduct (Miki and Clapham, 2013).

De Martin et al. (2017) conducted a first study employing rheotaxis to select spermatozoa from normozoospermic donors and reported an enrichment in spermatozoa with higher chromatin compaction (99%) compared to the sample before selection (71%) and to spermatozoa selected by DCG (83%). Zaferani et al. (2018) reported the design of a microfluidic device for selecting motile spermatozoa on the basis of rheotaxis; however, these authors did not

TABLE 7 | Reproductive outcomes of ARTs spermatozoa selected by IMSI.

Sperm origin	Oocyte origin	Couples (*n*)	Sperm groups	Fertilization rate (%)	Cleavage%	Blastocyst (%)	Embryos transferred (*n*)	Clinical pregnancy (%)	Live birth rate/ET (%)	References
≥3 millions of spermatozoa in the ejaculate, ≤1 million of motile after DGC, whatever sperm morphology	Younger than 39 years and FSH under of 9 UI/L	458	IMSI	56	ND	ND	ND	31	27	Leandri et al., 2013
			ICSI	63				33	30	
Oligo-astheno-teratozoospermia	Patients	66	ICSI	65 ± 21.1	ND	ND	64	6.3	ND	Kim et al., 2014
			IMSI	67.7 ± 19.9			66	27.3		
At least one sperm pathology	Infertile Women	42	IMSI	51.4	95.3	ND	ND	41.3*	34.7**	Shalom-Paz et al., 2015
			ICSI	53.2	92			10.5	0	
Patients	Normo response (> 4 oocytes retrieved)	324	ICSI	75.9 ± 18.9	ND	30.9 ± 28.1	ND	39,4	ND	Setti et al., 2015
			IMSI	72.3 ± 21.2		29.3 ± 25.7		34,1		
	Poor response (< four oocytes retrieved)	90	ICSI	79.8 ± 29.3	ND	9.8 ± 21.1	ND	11.8	ND	
			IMSI	53.9 ± 36.7		13.9 ± 33		22.2		
Couples with two previous ICSI failures		216	IMSI	54	ND	ND	119	27	20	Gatimel et al., 2016
			ICSI	61			86	28	19	
OAT/severe OAT (SOAT) or teratozoospermia	Patients	57	IMSI	52**	ND	ND	ND	68.5***	62.4***	Goswami et al., 2018
			ICSI	30				30.2	0	
Mild to severe oligo, astheno, and/or teratozoospermia	Donors	848	IMSI	82	70	42	511		63,79	Gaspard et al., 2018
			ICSI	72	69	40	923		69,33	

*Values are expressed as % ± w/o, SEM, or SD. *$P < 0.05$, **$P < 0.01$, ***$P < 0.001$.*

analyze the quality of the selected spermatozoa. Nagata et al. (2018) used another microfluidic device to select frozen bull spermatozoa by rheotaxis (**Figure 4A**). These authors reported a reduction of the level of DNA fragmentation (0.37%) in the spermatozoa selected by rheotaxis when compared to unselected semen (7%). The use of these selected bull spermatozoa for artificial insemination delivered pregnancy results similar to semen without selection, but using a 20 times lower dose (1 million sperm/insemination against 20 million sperm/insemination, respectively).

Thus, the results reported to date are promising, but the passive nature of rheotaxis, which is based on the hydrodynamics of the motile spermatozoa (Zhang et al., 2016), indicates that this mechanism has poor selective potential beyond the separation of those spermatozoa with a correct swimming behavior. As a matter of fact, half of the spermatozoa orient their swimming by rheotaxis, independently of being or not capacitated when directly observed under the microscope (Miki and Clapham, 2013). Although this is the *in vitro* situation, the *in vivo* picture could be drastically different. Moreover, it has been proposed that the planar move of non-capacitated spermatozoa would make them easier to stick to the epithelium preventing their migration by rheotaxis (Miki and Clapham, 2013) under the physiological conditions of viscosity. In contrast, the rotation along their longitudinal axis that determines the swimming of capacitated spermatozoa under a viscous medium could allow their detachment from this epithelium, allowing their free swimming against the fluid current (Miki and Clapham, 2013). In this way, rheotaxis would be part of a selection system of capacitated spermatozoa allowing only this subpopulation to migrate toward the *in vivo* fertilization site. *In vitro* developed procedures could test this hypothesis for sperm selection by rheotaxis considering these physiological conditions and then configure an effective way of selecting capacitated spermatozoa for improving ARTs.

Chemotaxis

Chemotaxis is the mechanism of navigation that the spermatozoa use in the proximity of the oocyte to orient their swimming in a gradient of chemical substances released by the COC where progesterone (P4) seems to be the main chemoattractant (Oren-Benaroya et al., 2008). It should be noted that only capacitated spermatozoa respond by chemotaxis, so this property could allow the selection of this specific subpopulation (Oren-Benaroya et al., 2008). Thus, Gatica et al. (2013) selected spermatozoa from both normozoospermic donors and subfertile patients by employing a simple device named "Sperm Selection Assay" (SSA) in which a P4 gradient was established (**Figure 4B**). In this work, it was found that in both cases, the selected spermatozoa were three times more capacitated, showed less DNA fragmentation and less oxidative stress than the semen before the selection. Li et al. (2018) also reported an improvement in the sperm quality from normozoospermic donors in terms of normal morphology, lower DNA fragmentation, and lower percentage of apoptotic spermatozoa when using another device composed of a system of microfluidic channels. Dominguez et al. (2018) proved that the use of the SSA device allows the selection of higher quality bull spermatozoa, improving cleavage rates using both sexed and unsexed semen for IVF. However, the effectiveness of sperm selection by chemotaxis in the improvement of ARTs in clinical practice has not been studied to date.

Thermotaxis

Sperm thermotaxis consists in the orientation of the spermatozoa movement toward the highest temperature in a gradient (Bahat et al., 2003). Evidence indicates that this mechanism allows sperm to orient itself in the fallopian tubes to ascend to the ampulla (Pérez-Cerezales et al., 2017). As in chemotaxis, only capacitated spermatozoa respond to thermotactic stimuli, so based on it, this subpopulation could be selected (Bahat et al.,

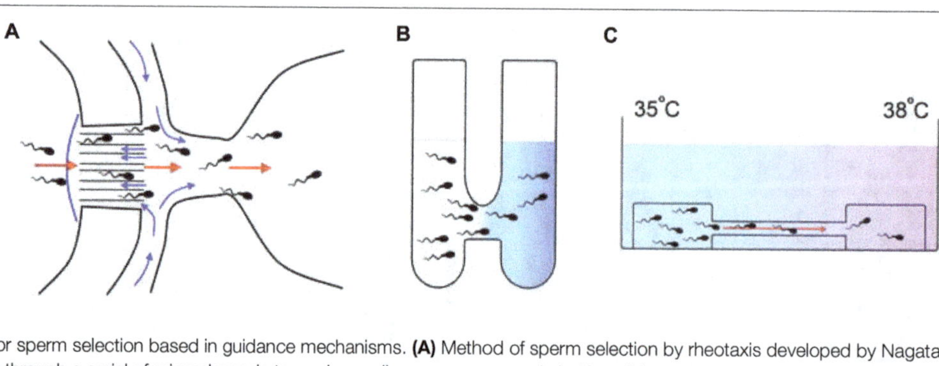

FIGURE 4 | Methods for sperm selection based in guidance mechanisms. **(A)** Method of sperm selection by rheotaxis developed by Nagata et al. (2018). A flow (blue arrows) is created through a serial of microchannels towards a well were sperm sample is placed. In response to the flow the spermatozoa swim towards it passing through the microchannels and accumulating in a receptive well where they can be collected for downstream applications (red arrows indicate migration of the sperm). **(B)** Method of sperm selection by chemotaxis developed by Gatica et al. (2013): Two wells are connected by a 2 mm length per 2.5 mm diameter tube. One of the wells is filled with a medium containing the chemoattractant molecule in solution (colored in blue) and the other well is filled with the spermatozoa suspension. The chemoattractant diffuses through the connecting tube generating a gradient and the spermatozoa respond by migrating towards the higher concentration and accumulating in the initial well free of cells where they can be collected for downstream applications. **(C)** Method of sperm selection by thermotaxis developed by Pérez-Cerezales et al. (2018). Spermatozoa are placed on a drop of a medium connected by a capillary to a second drop free of cells. A temperature gradient is generated between both drops being the highest temperature at the place of the drop free of cells. Spermatozoa respond by thermotaxis migrating towards the warmer temperature and accumulating in the second drop where they can be collected for downstream applications.

2003). In a recent publication, employing a simple method (**Figure 4C**), we showed in mice and in normozoospermic patients that spermatozoa selected by SU/thermotaxis possess higher DNA integrity compared to the seminal sample prior to selection and after selection by SU (Pérez-Cerezales et al., 2018). In addition, the use of these selected spermatozoa for ICSI in mice increased cleavage rates and blastocyst production, as well as implantation and live birth rate as opposed to the use of spermatozoa selected by SU. Although this is the only work related to the use of spermatozoa selected by thermotaxis in ARTs, a recent study carried out in bulls has shown that seminal samples delivering high pregnancy rates after artificial insemination show a greater response to thermotaxis (Mondal et al., 2016). However, as in the case of rheotaxis and chemotaxis, there are still no available publications showing the capability of sperm selection by thermotaxis to improve the ARTs efficiency in the human clinic.

SPERM SELECTION BASED ON SPERM MOTILITY (MICROFLUIDICS)

As we have seen in some of the previous methodologies, microfluidic systems are becoming transversal devices for sperm selection based on several fundaments. Therefore, microfluidic systems have been tested for sperm selection by rheotaxis (Zaferani et al., 2018), chemotaxis (Ko et al., 2018; Nagata et al., 2018), and thermotaxis (Ko et al., 2018), as well as by other physical properties that operate at small scale, allowing the selection of motile spermatozoa (**Table 8**). Nosrati et al. (2014) reported the improvement of human spermatozoa selected by a microfluidic device composed of 500 parallel microchannels in terms of reducing more than 80% DNA fragmentation. Similar results were reported by Kishi et al. (2015), showing a significant reduction of DNA fragmentation in spermatozoa selected by a commercially available device based on microfluidics and flow dynamics (Sperm Sorter Qualis®, Menicon, Kasugai, Japan) when compared to SU or unselected spermatozoa. Using the same device, Shirota et al. (2016) also reported the selection of spermatozoa with lower DNA fragmentation compared to spermatozoa selected by DGC followed by SU in healthy donors. In addition, Nagata et al. (2018) reported a robust selection of human spermatozoa porting low DNA fragmentation by utilizing a diffuser-type microfluidic sperm sorter (DMSS). Quinn et al. (2018) employed another commercially available device, a single-use chip with an inlet sample chamber connected to an outlet collection chamber by a microfluidic channel (FERTILE, Zymot, DxNow Inc., Gaithersburg, MD, United States), and showed a very effective selection of spermatozoa with low fragmented DNA compared to unselected spermatozoa or those selected by DGC-SU.

Due to the novelty of these methodologies, there is only one study that employs the selected spermatozoa in ARTs. In a recent publication in which spermatozoa were selected from 122 patients with infertility of unknown etiology using a commercial microfluidic device (61 patients) (Fertile Chip®, KOEK Biotechnology, Turkey) or by SU (61 patients), no differences were found in terms of fertilization, pregnancy, and live birth rates during ICSI between both sperm selection methods (Yetkinel et al., 2019). However, these authors observed

TABLE 8 | DNA fragmentation of spermatozoa selected by microfluidic devices.

Specie of study	Groups compared	DNA fragmentation (%)	Type of male donors/patients (*n*)	Fragmentation technique	References
Human	Control	10.9	Healthy donors (8)	SCSA	Nosrati et al., 2014
	Microfluidic radial 500 channels in parallel	4.32/3.37/2.40			
Human	Control	27.7 ± 0[a]	Donors (10) normal, oligozoospermia, and asthenozoospermia	SCD	Kishi et al., 2015
	SU	8.3 ± 0.05[b]			
	Sperm sorter qualis	5.9 ± 0.04[c]			
Human	DGC-SU	10.1 ± 8.5	Donors (37)	SCSA	Shirota et al., 2016
	Sperm sorter qualis	0.8 ± 1.9*			
Bovine	Unsorted	7.08 ± 1.06	7	TUNEL	Nagata et al., 2018
	Microfluid DMSS	0.37 ± 0.15**	12		
Human	Control	15 (11–19)***	Samples (70)	SCD	Quinn et al., 2018
	DGC-SU	6 (3–11.5)***			
	Fertile (Zymot) device	0 (0–2.4)			

*Analyses of DNA fragmentation were conducted by sperm chromatin structure assay (SCSA), sperm chromatin dispersion (SCD) test, or TUNEL. Values of % of DNA fragmentation are expressed as % ± SEM or SD. In Nosrati et al. (2014), DNA fragmentation separated by slash corresponds to the microchannel lengths 6/7.5/9 mm, respectively. Negative linear correlation between microchannel lengths was reported (R^2 = 0.99). *$P < 0.05$, **$P < 0.01$, ***$P < 0.001$. Different letters indicate differences between groups ($P < 0.005$).*

a higher quality in those embryos produced with spermatozoa selected by Fertile Chip®. Further studies are then necessary to determine under which conditions these devices are suitable for improving ARTs outcomes.

CONCLUSION

The efficiency of ARTs has a margin for improvement. Sperm selection may be an important factor for achieving higher live birth rates in ARTs, especially in infertility cases where the male factor is present. However, the methodologies developed to date have not proven to be useful for their routine application in the clinical practice and seem to be effective only in specific cases of male infertility. Some novel methods described here based on the physiological selection operating *in vivo* and on microfluidic environments have delivered promising results yet to be confirmed in large studies in the context of clinical practice. These studies should be randomized and strict in the confrontation of results with sperm samples of different qualities minimizing the female factor. It may even be necessary to combine several sperm selection methodologies to increase the efficiency of the ARTs.

AUTHOR CONTRIBUTIONS

IO-L and SR-D conducted literature review and wrote the manuscript. PR-I wrote the manuscript. SP-C defined the topic, conducted literature review, and structured and wrote the manuscript.

FUNDING

This work was supported by Grant RTI2018-096736-A-I00 from the Spanish Ministry of Science, Innovation, and Universities. IO-L and SR-D were supported by CONACYT fellowship of the Mexican Government (283833) and "doctorados industriales 2018," fellowship of Comunidad of Madrid (IND2018/BIO-9610). PR-I was supported by a Talent Attraction Fellowship from Comunidad de Madrid. SP-C was supported by a Ramón y Cajal contract from the Spanish Ministry of Science, Innovation, and Universities (RYC-2016-20147).

ACKNOWLEDGMENTS

We thank Anna Riabzev for making the drawing.

REFERENCES

Ainsworth, C., Nixon, B., and Aitken, R. J. (2005). Development of a novel electrophoretic system for the isolation of human spermatozoa. *Hum. Reprod.* 20, 2261–2270. doi: 10.1093/humrep/dei024

Aitken, R. J., and Clarkson, J. S. (1988). Significance of reactive oxygen species and antioxidants in defining the efficacy of sperm preparation techniques. *J. Androl.* 9, 367–376. doi: 10.1002/j.1939-4640.1988.tb01067.x

Aktan, T. M., Montag, M., Duman, S., Gorkemli, H., Rink, K., and Yurdakul, T. (2004). Use of a laser to detect viable but immotile spermatozoa. *Andrologia* 36, 366–369. doi: 10.1111/j.1439-0272.2004.00636.x

Amer, M., Metawae, B., Hosny, H., and Raef, A. (2013). Beneficial effect of adding pentoxifylline to processed semen samples on ICSI outcome in infertile males with mild and moderate asthenozoospermia: a randomized controlled prospective crossover study. *Int. J. Reprod. Biomed.* 11, 939–944.

Amiri, I., Ghorbani, M., and Heshmati, S. (2012). Comparison of the DNA fragmentation and the sperm parameters after processing by the density gradient and the swim up methods. *J. Clin. Diagn. Res.* 6, 1451–1453. doi: 10.7860/JCDR/2012/4198.2530

Antunes, D. M. F., Kalmbach, K. H., Wang, F., Dracxler, R. C., Seth-Smith, M. L., Kramer, Y., et al. (2015). A single-cell assay for telomere DNA content shows increasing telomere length heterogeneity, as well as increasing mean telomere length in human spermatozoa with advancing age. *J. Assist. Reprod. Genet.* 32, 1685–1690. doi: 10.1007/s10815-015-0574-3

Arias, M. E., Andara, K., Briones, E., and Felmer, R. (2017). Bovine sperm separation by Swim-up and density gradients (Percoll and BoviPure): effect on sperm quality, function and gene expression. *Reprod. Biol.* 17, 126–132. doi: 10.1016/j.repbio.2017.03.002

Armon, L., and Eisenbach, M. (2011). Behavioral mechanism during human sperm chemotaxis: involvement of hyperactivation. *PLoS One* 6:e28359. doi: 10.1371/journal.pone.0028359

Baccetti, B. (2004). Microscopical advances in assisted reproduction. *J. Submicrosc. Cytol. Pathol.* 36, 333–339.

Bahat, A., Caplan, S. R., and Eisenbach, M. (2012). Thermotaxis of human sperm cells in extraordinarily shallow temperature gradients over a wide range. *PLoS One* 7:e41915. doi: 10.1371/journal.pone.0041915

Bahat, A., Tur-Kaspa, I., Gakamsky, A., Giojalas, L. C., Breitbart, H., and Eisenbach, M. (2003). Thermotaxis of mammalian sperm cells: a potential navigation mechanism in the female genital tract. *Nat. Med.* 9, 149–150. doi: 10.1038/nm0203-149

Barak, Y., Menezo, Y., Veiga, A., and Elder, K. (2001). A physiological replacement for polyvinylpyrrolidone (PVP) in assisted reproductive technology. *Hum. Fertil.* 4, 99–103. doi: 10.1080/1464727012000199371

Bartoov, B., Berkovitz, A., Eltes, F., Kogosowski, A., Menezo, Y., and Barak, Y. (2002). Real-time fine morphology of motile human sperm cells is associated with IVF-ICSI outcome. *J. Androl.* 23, 1–8. doi: 10.1002/j.1939-4640.2002.tb02595.x

Berteli, T. S., Da Broi, M. G., Martins, W. P., Ferriani, R. A., and Navarro, P. A. (2017). Magnetic-activated cell sorting before density gradient centrifugation improves recovery of high-quality spermatozoa. *Andrology* 5, 776–782. doi: 10.1111/andr.12372

Boitrelle, F., Guthauser, B., Alter, L., Bailly, M., Bergere, M., Wainer, R., et al. (2014). High-magnification selection of spermatozoa prior to oocyte injection: confirmed and potential indications. *Reprod. Biomed. Online* 28, 6–13. doi: 10.1016/j.rbmo.2013.09.019

Boulet, S. L., Mehta, A., Kissin, D. M., Warner, L., Kawwass, J. F., and Jamieson, D. J. (2015). Trends in use of and reproductive outcomes associated with intracytoplasmic sperm injection. *JAMA* 313, 255–263. doi: 10.1001/jama.2014.17985

Buffone, M. G., Doncel, G. F., Briggiler, C. I. M., Vazquez-Levin, M. H., and Calamera, J. C. (2004). Human sperm subpopulations: relationship between functional quality and protein tyrosine phosphorylation. *Hum. Reprod.* 19, 139–146. doi: 10.1093/humrep/deh040

Burkman, L. J. (1984). Characterization of hyperactivated motility by human spermatozoa during capacitation: comparison of fertile and oligozoospermic sperm populations. *Syst. Biol. Reprod. Med.* 13, 153–165. doi: 10.3109/01485018408987514

Cakar, Z., Cetinkaya, B., Aras, D., Koca, B., Ozkavukcu, S., Kaplanoglu, İ., et al. (2016). Does combining magnetic-activated cell sorting with density gradient or swim-up improve sperm selection? *J. Assist. Reprod. Genet.* 33, 1059–1065. doi: 10.1007/s10815-016-0742-0

Carreras, A., Palma, A., and Mendoza, C. (1990). Hypoosmotic swelling test in normo-, oligo-, astheno- and oligoasthenozoospermic men before and after swim-up separation of spermatozoa. *Andrologia* 22, 313–317. doi: 10.1111/j.1439-0272.1990.tb01992.x

Casanovas, A., Ribas-Maynou, J., Lara-Cerrillo, S., Jimenez-Macedo, A. R., Hortal, O., Benet, J., et al. (2019). Double-stranded sperm DNA damage is a cause of delay in embryo development and can impair implantation rates. *Fertil. Steril.* 111, 699–707. doi: 10.1016/j.fertnstert.2018.11.035

Cayli, S., Jakab, A., Ovari, L., Delpiano, E., Celik-Ozenci, C., Sakkas, D., et al. (2003). Biochemical markers of sperm function: male fertility and sperm selection for ICSI. *Reprod. Biomed. Online* 7, 462–468. doi: 10.1016/S1472-6483(10)61891-3

CDC, (2018). *2016 - National Summary Report - Assisted Reproductive Technology.* Washington, DC: US Department of Health. Human Service.

Cesari, A., Kaiser, G. G., Mucci, N., Mutto, A., Vincenti, A., Fornés, M. W., et al. (2006). Integrated morphophysiological assessment of two methods for sperm selection in bovine embryo production in vitro. *Theriogenology* 66, 1185–1193. doi: 10.1016/j.theriogenology.2006.03.029

Chan, P. J., Jacobson, J. D., Corselli, J. U., and Patton, W. C. (2006). A simple zeta method for sperm selection based on membrane charge. *Fertil. Steril.* 85, 481–486. doi: 10.1016/j.fertnstert.2005.07.1302

Chapuis, A., Gala, A., Ferrières-Hoa, A., Mullet, T., Bringer-Deutsch, S., Vintejoux, E., et al. (2017). Sperm quality and paternal age: effect on blastocyst formation and pregnancy rates. *Basic Clin. Androl.* 27:2. doi: 10.1186/s12610-016-0045-4

Chaudhuri, A. R., and Datta, H. (1994). A novel technique for isolation of pure sperm heads from disintegrated mammalian spermatozoa. *Prep. Biochem.* 24, 185–192. doi: 10.1080/10826069408010092

Choe, S. A., Tae, J. C., Shin, M. Y., Kim, H. J., Kim, C. H., Lee, J. Y., et al. (2012). Application of sperm selection using hyaluronic acid binding in intracytoplasmic sperm injection cycles: a sibling oocyte study. *J. Korean Med. Sci.* 27, 1569–1573. doi: 10.3346/jkms.2012.27.12.1569

Cohen-Dayag, A., Ralt, D., Tur-Kaspa, I., Manor, M., Makler, A., Dor, J., et al. (1994). Sequential acquisition of chemotactic responsiveness by human spermatozoa. *Biol. Reprod.* 50, 786–790. doi: 10.1095/biolreprod50.4.786

D'Amours, O., Frenette, G., Bourassa, S., Calvo, É, Blondin, P., and Sullivan, R. (2018). Proteomic markers of functional sperm population in bovines: comparison of low- and high-density spermatozoa following cryopreservation. *J. Proteome Res.* 17, 177–188. doi: 10.1021/acs.jproteome.7b00493

Dandekar, P., Aggeler, J., and Talbot, P. (1992). Structure, distribution and composition of the extracellular matrix of human oocytes and cumulus masses. *Hum. Reprod.* 7, 391–398. doi: 10.1093/oxfordjournals.humrep.a137656

De Geyter, C., Calhaz-Jorge, C., Kupka, M. S., Wyns, C., Mocanu, E., Motrenko, T., et al. (2018). ART in Europe, 2014: results generated from European registries by ESHRE. *Hum. Reprod.* 33, 1586–1601. doi: 10.1093/humrep/dey242

De Martin, H., Cocuzza, M. S., Tiseo, B. C., Wood, G. J. A., Miranda, E. P., Monteleone, P. A. A., et al. (2017). Positive rheotaxis extended drop: a one-step procedure to select and recover sperm with mature chromatin for intracytoplasmic sperm injection. *J. Assist. Reprod. Genet.* 34, 1699–1708. doi: 10.1007/s10815-017-1024-1

Degheidy, T., Abdelfattah, H., Seif, A., Albuz, F. K., Gazi, S., and Abbas, S. (2015). Magnetic activated cell sorting: an effective method for reduction of sperm DNA fragmentation in varicocele men prior to assisted reproductive techniques. *Andrologia* 47, 892–896. doi: 10.1111/and.12343

Dirican, E. K., Özgün, O. D., Akarsu, S., Akin, K. O., Ercan, Ö, Uğurlu, M., et al. (2008). Clinical outcome of magnetic activated cell sorting of non-apoptotic spermatozoa before density gradient centrifugation for assisted reproduction. *J. Assist. Reprod. Genet.* 25, 375–381. doi: 10.1007/s10815-008-9250-1

Dominguez, E. M., Moreno-Irusta, A., Guidobaldi, H. A., Tribulo, H., and Giojalas, L. C. (2018). Improved bovine in vitro embryo production with sexed and unsexed sperm selected by chemotaxis. *Theriogenology* 122, 1–8. doi: 10.1016/j.theriogenology.2018.08.023

Ebner, T., Tews, G., Mayer, R. B., Ziehr, S., Arzt, W., Costamoling, W., et al. (2011). Pharmacological stimulation of sperm motility in frozen and thawed testicular sperm using the dimethylxanthine theophylline. *Fertil. Steril.* 96, 1331–1336. doi: 10.1016/j.fertnstert.2011.08.041

Eisenbach, M. (1999). Mammalian sperm chemotaxis and its association with capacitation. *Dev. Genet.* 25, 87–94.

Elmore, S. (2007). Apoptosis: a review of programmed cell death. *Toxicol. Pathol.* 35, 495–516. doi: 10.1080/01926230701320337

El-Sherry, T. M., Elsayed, M., Abdelhafez, H. K., and Abdelgawad, M. (2014). Characterization of rheotaxis of bull sperm using microfluidics. *Integr. Biol.* 6, 1111–1121. doi: 10.1039/c4ib00196f

Engelmann, U., Krassnigg, F., Schatz, H., and Schill, W.-B. (1988). Separation of human X and Y spermatozoa by free-flow electrophoresis. *Gamete Res.* 19, 151–160. doi: 10.1002/mrd.1120190205

Erberelli, R. F., Salgado, R. M., Pereira, D. H. M., and Wolff, P. (2017). Hyaluronan-binding system for sperm selection enhances pregnancy rates in ICSI cycles associated with male factor infertility. *J. Bras. Reprod. Assist.* 21, 2–6. doi: 10.5935/1518-0557.20170002

Esbert, M., Godo, A., Soares, S. R., Florensa, M., Amorós, D., Ballesteros, A., et al. (2017). Spermatozoa with numerical chromosomal abnormalities are more prone to be retained by Annexin V-MACS columns. *Andrology* 5, 807–813. doi: 10.1111/andr.12376

Esbert, M., Pacheco, A., Soares, S. R., Amorós, D., Florensa, M., Ballesteros, A., et al. (2018). High sperm DNA fragmentation delays human embryo kinetics when oocytes from young and healthy donors are microinjected. *Andrology* 6, 697–706. doi: 10.1111/andr.12551

Esfahani, M. H. N., Deemeh, M. R., Tavalaee, M., Sekhavati, M. H., and Gourabi, H. (2016). Zeta sperm selection improves pregnancy rate and alters sex ratio in male factor infertility patients: a double-blind, randomized clinical trial. *Int. J. Fertil. Steril.* 10, 253–260.

Evenson, D. P. (2016). The sperm chromatin structure assay (SCSA®) and other sperm DNA fragmentation tests for evaluation of sperm nuclear DNA integrity as related to fertility. *Anim. Reprod. Sci.* 169, 56–75. doi: 10.1016/j.anireprosci.2016.01.017

Fernandez-Gonzalez, R., Moreira, P. N., Pérez-Crespo, M., Sánchez-Martín, M., Ramirez, M. A., Pericuesta, E., et al. (2008). Long-term effects of mouse intracytoplasmic sperm injection with DNA-fragmented sperm on health and behavior of adult offspring. *Biol. Reprod.* 78, 761–772. doi: 10.1095/biolreprod.107.065623

Ferraretti, A. P., Nygren, K., Andersen, A. N., de Mouzon, J., Kupka, M., Calhaz-Jorge, C., et al. (2017). Trends over 15 years in ART in Europe: an analysis of 6 million cycles†. *Hum. Reprod. Open* 2017, 1–10. doi: 10.1093/hropen/hox012

Fortunato, A., Boni, R., Leo, R., Nacchia, G., Liguori, F., Casale, S., et al. (2016). Vacuoles in sperm head are not associated with head morphology, DNA damage and reproductive success. *Reprod. Biomed. Online* 32, 154–161. doi: 10.1016/j.rbmo.2015.10.009

Franco, J. G., Baruffi, R. L. R., Mauri, A. L., Petersen, C. G., Oliveira, J. B. A., and Vagnini, L. (2008). Significance of large nuclear vacuoles in human spermatozoa: implications for ICSI. *Reprod. Biomed. Online* 17, 42–45. doi: 10.1016/s1472-6483(10)60291-x

Funaro, M. G., Kim, H. H., Mazel, S., Bolyakov, A., Goldstein, M., Schlegel, P. N., et al. (2013). A novel sorting technology allows for highly efficient selection of sperm without chromatin damage. *Syst. Biol. Reprod. Med.* 59, 172–177. doi: 10.3109/19396368.2013.777135

Galli, C., Duchi, R., Colleoni, S., Lagutina, I., and Lazzari, G. (2014). Ovum pick up, intracytoplasmic sperm injection and somatic cell nuclear transfer in cattle, buffalo and horses: from the research laboratory to clinical practice. *Theriogenology* 81, 138–151. doi: 10.1016/j.theriogenology.2013.09.008

García-Ferreyra, J., Villegas, L., Romero, R., Zavala, P., Hilario, R., and Dueñas-Chacón, J. (2014). High pregnancy and implantation rates can be obtained using magnetic-activated cell sorting (MACS) to selection spermatozoa in patients with high levels of spermatic DNA fragmentation. *JFIV Reprod. Med. Genet.* 3:133. doi: 10.4172/2375-4508.1000133

García-Roselló, E., García-Mengual, E., Coy, P., Alfonso, J., and Silvestre, M. A. (2009). Intracytoplasmic sperm injection in livestock species: an update. *Reprod. Domest. Anim.* 44, 143–151. doi: 10.1111/j.1439-0531.2007.01018.x

Gaspard, O., Vanderzwalmen, P., Wirleitner, B., Ravet, S., Wenders, F., Eichel, V., et al. (2018). Impact of high magnification sperm selection on neonatal outcomes: a retrospective study. *J. Assist. Reprod. Genet.* 35, 1113–1121. doi: 10.1007/s10815-018-1167-8

Gatica, L. V., Guidobaldi, H. A., Montesinos, M. M., Teves, M. E., Moreno, A. I., Uñates, D. R., et al. (2013). Picomolar gradients of progesterone select functional human sperm even in subfertile samples. *Mol. Hum. Reprod.* 19, 559–569. doi: 10.1093/molehr/gat037

Gatimel, N., Parinaud, J., and Leandri, R. D. (2016). Intracytoplasmic morphologically selected sperm injection (IMSI) does not improve outcome in patients with two successive IVF-ICSI failures. *J. Assist. Reprod. Genet.* 33, 349–355. doi: 10.1007/s10815-015-0645-5

Gerber, P. A., Kruse, R., Hirchenhain, J., Krüssel, J. S., and Neumann, N. J. (2008). Pregnancy after laser-assisted selection of viable spermatozoa before intracytoplasmatic sperm injection in a couple with male primary cilia dyskinesia. *Fertil. Steril.* 89, 1826.e9–1826.e12. doi: 10.1016/j.fertnstert.2007.06.012

Ghosh, S., Chattopadhyay, R., Bose, G., Ganesh, A., Das, S., and Chakravarty, B. N. (2012). Selection of birefringent spermatozoa under Polscope: effect on intracytoplasmic sperm injection outcome. *Andrologia* 44, 734–738. doi: 10.1111/j.1439-0272.2011.01258.x

Gianaroli, L., Magli, M. C., Collodel, G., Moretti, E., Ferraretti, A. P., and Baccetti, B. (2008). Sperm head's birefringence: a new criterion for sperm selection. *Fertil. Steril.* 90, 104–112. doi: 10.1016/j.fertnstert.2007.05.078

Gil, M., Sar-Shalom, V., Melendez Sivira, Y., Carreras, R., and Checa, M. A. (2013). Sperm selection using magnetic activated cell sorting (MACS) in assisted reproduction: a systematic review and meta-analysis. *J. Assist. Reprod. Genet.* 30, 479–485. doi: 10.1007/s10815-013-9962-8

Goswami, G., Sharma, M., Jugga, D., and Gouri, D. (2018). Can intracytoplasmic morphologically selected spermatozoa injection be used as first choice of treatment for severe male factor infertility patients? *J. Hum. Reprod. Sci.* 11, 40–44. doi: 10.4103/jhrs.jhrs_74_17

Grunewald, S., Paasch, U., and Glander, H. J. (2001). Enrichment of non-apoptotic human spermatozoa after cryopreservation by immunomagnetic cell sorting. *Cell Tissue Bank.* 2, 127–133. doi: 10.1023/A:1020188913551

Hammoud, I., Boitrelle, F., Ferfouri, F., Vialard, F., Bergere, M., Wainer, B., et al. (2013). Selection of normal spermatozoa with a vacuole-free head (x6300) improves selection of spermatozoa with intact DNA in patients with high sperm DNA fragmentation rates. *Andrologia* 45, 163–170. doi: 10.1111/j.1439-0272.2012.01328.x

Hansen, P. J. (2014). "Current and future assisted reproductive technologies for mammalian farm animals," in *Current and Future Reproductive Technologies and World Food Production. Advances in Experimental Medicine and Biology*, eds D. Nicolas, and G. Lamb, (New York, NY: Springer).

Harrison, R. A. (1976). A highly efficient method for washing mammalian spermatozoa. *J. Reprod. Fertil.* 48, 347–353. doi: 10.1530/jrf.0.0480347

Hattori, H., Nakajo, Y., Ito, C., Toyama, Y., Toshimori, K., and Kyono, K. (2011). Birth of a healthy infant after intracytoplasmic sperm injection using pentoxifylline-activated sperm from a patient with Kartagener's syndrome. *Fertil. Steril.* 95, 2431.e9–2431.e11. doi: 10.1016/j.fertnstert.2011.03.074

Heidari, M., Darbandi, S., Darbani, M., Amirjanati, N., Bozorgmehr, M., Zeraati, H., et al. (2018). Evaluating the potential of three sperm surface antigens as egg-adhesion biomarkers for human sperm selection. *J. Reprod. Infertil.* 19, 203–210.

Henkel, R., and Schill, W.-B. (2003). Sperm preparation for ART. *Reprod. Biol. Endocrinol.* 1:108. doi: 10.1186/1477-7827-1-108

Herrick, J. R. (2019). Assisted reproductive technologies for endangered species conservation: developing sophisticated protocols with limited access to animals with unique reproductive mechanisms. *Biol. Reprod.* 100, 1158–1170. doi: 10.1093/biolre/ioz025

Hino, T., Muro, Y., Tamura-Nakano, M., Okabe, M., Tateno, H., and Yanagimachi, R. (2016). The behavior and acrosomal status of mouse spermatozoa in vitro, and within the oviduct during fertilization after natural mating. *Biol. Reprod.* 95:50. doi: 10.1095/biolreprod.116.140400

Holt, W. V., and Fazeli, A. (2015). Do sperm possess a molecular passport? Mechanistic insights into sperm selection in the female reproductive tract. *Mol. Hum. Reprod.* 21, 491–501. doi: 10.1093/molehr/gav012

Huang, M. T., Kuo-Kuang Lee, R., Lu, C. H., Chen, Y. J., Li, S. H., and Hwu, Y. M. (2015). The efficiency of conventional microscopic selection is comparable to the hyaluronic acid binding method in selecting spermatozoa for male infertility patients. *Taiwan. J. Obstet. Gynecol.* 54, 48–53. doi: 10.1016/j.tjog.2014.11.006

Huszar, G., Ozkavukcu, S., Jakab, A., Celik-Ozenci, C., Sati, G. L., and Cayli, S. (2006). Hyaluronic acid binding ability of human sperm reflects cellular maturity and fertilizing potential: selection of sperm for intracytoplasmic sperm injection. *Curr. Opin. Obstet. Gynecol.* 18, 260–267. doi: 10.1097/01.gco.0000193018.98061.2f

Jakab, A., Sakkas, D., Delpiano, E., Cayli, S., Kovanci, E., Ward, D., et al. (2005). Intracytoplasmic sperm injection: a novel selection method for sperm with normal frequency of chromosomal aneuploidies. *Fertil. Steril.* 84, 1665–1673. doi: 10.1016/j.fertnstert.2005.05.068

Jenkins, T. G., Aston, K. I., Trost, C., Farley, J., Hotaling, J. M., and Carrell, D. T. (2014). Intra-sample heterogeneity of sperm DNA methylation. *Mol. Hum. Reprod.* 21, 313–319. doi: 10.1093/molehr/gau115

Jerre, E., Bungum, M., Evenson, D., and Giwercman, A. (2019). Sperm chromatin structure assay high DNA stainability sperm as a marker of early miscarriage after intracytoplasmic sperm injection. *Fertil. Steril.* 112, 46.e2–53.e2. doi: 10.1016/j.fertnstert.2019.03.013

Jones, G. M., Trounson, A. O., Lolatgis, N., and Wood, C. (1998). Factors affecting the success of human blastocyst development and pregnancy following in vitro fertilization and embryo transfer. *Fertil. Steril.* 70, 1022–1029. doi: 10.1016/S0015-0282(98)00342-2

Karamahmutoglu, H., Erdem, A., Erdem, M., Mutlu, M. F., Bozkurt, N., Oktem, M., et al. (2014). The gradient technique improves success rates in intrauterine insemination cycles of unexplained subfertile couples when compared to swim up technique; a prospective randomized study. *J. Assist. Reprod. Genet.* 31, 1139–1145. doi: 10.1007/s10815-014-0274-4

Katz, D. J., Teloken, P., and Shoshany, O. (2017). Male infertility - the other side of the equation. *Aust. Fam. Physician.* 46, 641–646.

Kheirollahi-Kouhestani, M., Razavi, S., Tavalaee, M., Deemeh, M. R., Mardani, M., Moshtaghian, J., et al. (2009). Selection of sperm based on combined density gradient and Zeta method may improve ICSI outcome. *Hum. Reprod.* 24, 2409–2416. doi: 10.1093/humrep/dep088

Kim, H. J., Yoon, H. J., Jang, J. M., Oh, H. S., Lee, Y. J., Lee, W. D., et al. (2014). Comparison between intracytoplasmic sperm injection and intracytoplasmic morphologically selected sperm injection in oligo-astheno-teratozoospermia patients. *Clin. Exp. Reprod. Med.* 41:9. doi: 10.5653/cerm.2014.41.1.9

Kiratli, S., Yuncu, M., Kose, K., and Ozkavukcu, S. (2018). A comparative evaluation of migration sedimentation method for sperm preparation. *Syst. Biol. Reprod. Med.* 64, 122–129. doi: 10.1080/19396368.2017.1402100

Kishi, K., Ogata, H., Ogata, S., Mizusawa, Y., Okamoto, E., Matsumoto, Y., et al. (2015). Frequency of sperm DNA fragmentation according to selection method: comparison and relevance of a microfluidic device and a swim-up procedure. *J. Clin. Diagnostic Res.* 9, QC14–QC16. doi: 10.7860/JCDR/2015/10332.6811

Knox, R. V. (2016). Artificial insemination in pigs today. *Theriogenology* 85, 83–93. doi: 10.1016/j.theriogenology.2015.07.009

Ko, Y. J., Maeng, J. H., Hwang, S. Y., and Ahn, Y. (2018). Design, fabrication, and testing of a microfluidic device for thermotaxis and chemotaxis assays of sperm. *SLAS Technol.* 23, 507–515. doi: 10.1177/2472630318783948

Kovačič, B., Vlaisavljević, V., and Reljič, M. (2006). Clinical use of pentoxifylline for activation of immotile testicular sperm before ICSI in patients with azoospermia. *J. Androl.* 27, 45–52. doi: 10.2164/jandrol.05079

Lavolpe, M., Lorenzi, D., Greco, E., Nodar, F., and Alvarez Sedó, C. (2015). Relationship between sperm dna fragmentation and nuclear vacuoles. *JBRA Assist. Reprod.* 19, 70–74. doi: 10.5935/1518-0557.20150016

Leandri, R. D., Gachet, A., Pfeffer, J., Celebi, C., Rives, N., Carre-Pigeon, F., et al. (2013). Is intracytoplasmic morphologically selected sperm injection (IMSI) beneficial in the first ART cycle? A multicentric randomized controlled trial. *Andrology* 1, 692–697. doi: 10.1111/j.2047-2927.2013.00104.x

Lee, H. L., Kim, S. H., Ji, D. B., and Kim, Y. J. (2009). A comparative study of Sephadex, glass wool and Percoll separation techniques on sperm quality and IVF results for cryopreserved bovine semen. *J. Vet. Sci.* 10, 249–255. doi: 10.4142/jvs.2009.10.3.249

Lee, T. H., Liu, C. H., Shih, Y. T., Tsao, H. M., Huang, C. C., Chen, H. H., et al. (2010). Magnetic-activated cell sorting for sperm preparation reduces spermatozoa with apoptotic markers and improves the acrosome reaction in couples with unexplained infertility. *Hum. Reprod.* 25, 839–846. doi: 10.1093/humrep/deq009

Leemans, B., Gadella, B. M., Stout, T. A. E., De Schauwer, C., Nelis, H. M., Hoogewijs, M., et al. (2016). Why doesn't conventional IVF work in the horse? *Reproduction* 152, R233–R245. doi: 10.1530/REP-16-0420

Li, G.-P., Seidel, G. E., and Squires, E. L. (2004). Improved cleavage of bovine ICSI ova cultured in heparin-containing medium. *Theriogenology* 61, 1077–1084. doi: 10.1016/j.theriogenology.2003.05.005

Li, K., Li, R., Ni, Y., Sun, P., Liu, Y., Zhang, D., et al. (2018). Novel distance-progesterone-combined selection approach improves human sperm quality. *J. Transl. Med.* 16:203. doi: 10.1186/s12967-018-1575-7

Mahadevan, M., and Baker, G. (1984). "Assessment and preparation of semen for in vitro fertilization," in *Clinical In Vitro Fertilization*, eds C. Wood, and A. Trounson, (London: Springer), 83–97. doi: 10.1007/978-1-4471-3317-9_7

Majumdar, G., and Majumdar, A. (2013). A prospective randomized study to evaluate the effect of hyaluronic acid sperm selection on the intracytoplasmic sperm injection outcome of patients with unexplained infertility having normal semen parameters. *J. Assist. Reprod. Genet.* 30, 1471–1475. doi: 10.1007/s10815-013-0108-9

Majzoub, A., Agarwal, A., and Esteves, S. C. (2019). Clinical utility of sperm DNA damage in male infertility. *Panminerva Med.* 61, 118–127. doi: 10.23736/S0031-0808.18.03530-9

Mangoli, V., Mangoli, R., Dandekar, S., Suri, K., and Desai, S. (2011). Selection of viable spermatozoa from testicular biopsies: a comparative study between pentoxifylline and hypoosmotic swelling test. *Fertil. Steril.* 95, 631–634. doi: 10.1016/j.fertnstert.2010.10.007

Marques de Oliveira, N., Sánchez, R. V., Rodriguez Fiesta, S., Lopez Salgado, T., Rodríquez, R., Bethencourt, J. C. A., et al. (2004). Pregnancy with frozen-thawed and fresh testicular biopsy after motile immotile sperm microinjection, using the mechanical touch technique to assess viability. *Hum. Reprod.* 19, 262–265. doi: 10.1093/humrep/deh083

Martí, E., Pérez-Pé, R., Muiño-Blanco, T., and Cebrián-Pérez, J. A. (2006). Comparative study of four different sperm washing methods using apoptotic markers in ram spermatozoa. *J. Androl.* 27, 746–753. doi: 10.2164/jandrol.106.000109

Martin, R. H. (2008). Meiotic errors in human oogenesis and spermatogenesis. *Reprod. Biomed. Online* 16, 523–531. doi: 10.1016/S1472-6483(10)60459-2

Martínez-Pastor, F., Tizado, E. J., Garde, J. J., Anel, L., and de Paz, P. (2011). Statistical series: opportunities and challenges of sperm motility subpopulation analysis. *Theriogenology* 75, 783–795. doi: 10.1016/j.theriogenology.2010.11.034

Miki, K., and Clapham, D. E. (2013). Rheotaxis guides mammalian sperm. *Curr. Biol.* 23, 443–452. doi: 10.1016/j.cub.2013.02.007

Miller, D., Pavitt, S., Sharma, V., Forbes, G., Hooper, R., Bhattacharya, S., et al. (2019). Physiological, hyaluronan-selected intracytoplasmic sperm injection for infertility treatment (HABSelect): a parallel, two-group, randomised trial. *Lancet* 393, 416–422. doi: 10.1016/S0140-6736(18)32989-1

Mokánszki, A., Tóthné, E. V., Bodnár, B., Tándor, Z., Molnár, Z., Jakab, A., et al. (2014). Is sperm hyaluronic acid binding ability predictive for clinical success of intracytoplasmic sperm injection: PICSI vs. ICSI? *Syst. Biol. Reprod. Med.* 60, 348–354. doi: 10.3109/19396368.2014.948102

Mondal, M. A., Takagi, Y., Baba, S. A., and Hamano, K. (2016). Involvement of calcium channels and intracellular calcium in bull sperm thermotaxis. *J. Reprod. Dev.* 63, 143–148. doi: 10.1262/jrd.2016-107

Mongkolchaipak, S., and Vutyavanich, T. (2013). No difference in high-magnification morphology and hyaluronic acid binding in the selection of euploid spermatozoa with intact DNA. *Asian J. Androl.* 15, 421–424. doi: 10.1038/aja.2012.163

Montjean, D., Courageot, J., Altié, A., Amar-Hoffet, A., Rossin, B., Geoffroy-Siraudin, C., et al. (2015). Normal live birth after vitrified/warmed oocytes intracytoplasmic sperm injection with immotile spermatozoa in a patient with Kartagener's syndrome. *Andrologia* 47, 839–845. doi: 10.1111/and.12331

Mostek, A., Westfalewicz, B., Słowińska, M., Dietrich, M. A., Judycka, S., and Ciereszko, A. (2018). Differences in sperm protein abundance and carbonylation level in bull ejaculates of low and high quality. *PLoS One* 13:e0206150. doi: 10.1371/journal.pone.0206150

Mousset-Siméon, N., Rives, N., Masse, L., Chevallier, F., and Mace, B. (2004). Comparison of six density gradient media for selection of cryopreserved donor spermatozoa. *J. Androl.* 25, 881–884. doi: 10.1002/j.1939-4640.2004.tb03157.x

Nadalini, M., Tarozzi, N., Di Santo, M., and Borini, A. (2014). Annexin V magnetic-activated cell sorting versus swim-up for the selection of human sperm in ART: is the new approach better then the traditional one? *J. Assist. Reprod. Genet.* 31, 1045–1051. doi: 10.1007/s10815-014-0267-3

Nagai, T., Funahashi, H., Yoshioka, K., and Kikuchi, K. (2006). Up date of in vitro production of porcine embryo. *Front. Biosci.* 11, 2565–2573. doi: 10.2741/1991

Nagata, M. P. B., Endo, K., Ogata, K., Yamanaka, K., Egashira, J., Katafuchi, N., et al. (2018). Live births from artificial insemination of microfluidic-sorted bovine spermatozoa characterized by trajectories correlated with fertility. *Proc. Natl. Acad. Sci. U.S.A.* 115, E3087–E3096. doi: 10.1073/pnas.1717974115

Nasr-Esfahani, M. H., Razavi, S., Vahdati, A. A., Fathi, F., and Tavalaee, M. (2008). Evaluation of sperm selection procedure based on hyaluronic acid binding ability on ICSI outcome. *J. Assist. Reprod. Genet.* 25, 197–203. doi: 10.1007/s10815-008-9223-4

Nordhoff, V., Schüring, A. N., Krallmann, C., Zitzmann, M., Schlatt, S., Kiesel, L., et al. (2013). Optimizing TESE-ICSI by laser-assisted selection of immotile spermatozoa and polarization microscopy for selection of oocytes. *Andrology* 1, 67–74. doi: 10.1111/j.2047-2927.2012.00020.x

Nosrati, R., Vollmer, M., Eamer, L., San Gabriel, M. C., Zeidan, K., Zini, A., et al. (2014). Rapid selection of sperm with high DNA integrity. *Lab Chip* 14, 1142–1150. doi: 10.1039/c3lc51254a

Oguz, Y., Guler, I., Erdem, A., Mutlu, M. F., Gumuslu, S., Oktem, M., et al. (2018). The effect of swim-up and gradient sperm preparation techniques on deoxyribonucleic acid (DNA) fragmentation in subfertile patients. *J. Assist. Reprod. Genet.* 35, 1083–1089. doi: 10.1007/s10815-018-1163-z

Ooi, E. H., Smith, D. J., Gadêlha, H., Gaffney, E. A., and Kirkman-Brown, J. (2014). The mechanics of hyperactivation in adhered human sperm. *R. Soc. Open Sci.* 1:140230. doi: 10.1098/rsos.140230

Oren-Benaroya, R., Orvieto, R., Gakamsky, A., Pinchasov, M., and Eisenbach, M. (2008). The sperm chemoattractant secreted from human cumulus cells is progesterone. *Hum. Reprod.* 23, 2339–2345. doi: 10.1093/humrep/den265

Ozkavukcu, S., Celik-Ozenci, C., Konuk, E., and Atabekoglu, C. (2018). Live birth after Laser Assisted Viability Assessment (LAVA) to detect pentoxifylline resistant ejaculated immotile spermatozoa during ICSI in a couple with male Kartagener's syndrome. *Reprod. Biol. Endocrinol.* 16:10. doi: 10.1186/s12958-018-0321-6

Ozmen, B., Caglar, G. S., Koster, F., Schopper, B., Diedrich, K., and Al-Hasani, S. (2007). Relationship between sperm DNA damage, induced acrosome reaction and viability in ICSI patients. *Reprod. Biomed. Online* 15, 208–214. doi: 10.1016/s1472-6483(10)60710-9

Palini, S., De Stefani, S., Primiterra, M., Benedetti, S., Barone, S., Carli, L., et al. (2017). Comparison of in vitro fertilization outcomes in ICSI cycles after human sperm preparation by density gradient centrifugation and direct micro swim-up without centrifugation. *J. Bras. Reprod. Assist.* 21, 89–93. doi: 10.5935/1518-0557.20170022

Paramio, M. T., and Izquierdo, D. (2014). Current status of in vitro embryo production in sheep and goats. *Reprod. Domest. Anim.* 49, 37–48. doi: 10.1111/rda.12334

Park, C. Y., Uhm, S. J., Song, S. J., Kim, K. S., Hong, S. B., Chung, K. S., et al. (2005). Increase of ICSI efficiency with hyaluronic acid binding sperm for low aneuploidy frequency in pig. *Theriogenology* 64, 1158–1169. doi: 10.1016/j.theriogenology.2005.01.010

Parmegiani, L., Cognigni, G. E., Bernardi, S., Troilo, E., Ciampaglia, W., and Filicori, M. (2010a). "Physiologic ICSI": hyaluronic acid (HA) favors selection of spermatozoa without DNA fragmentation and with normal nucleus, resulting in improvement of embryo quality. *Fertil. Steril.* 93, 598–604. doi: 10.1016/j.fertnstert.2009.03.033

Parmegiani, L., Cognigni, G. E., Ciampaglia, W., Pocognoli, P., Marchi, F., and Filicori, M. (2010b). Efficiency of hyaluronic acid (HA) sperm selection. *J. Assist. Reprod. Genet.* 27, 13–16. doi: 10.1007/s10815-009-9380-0

Parmegiani, L., Cognigni, G. E., Bernardi, S., Troilo, E., Taraborrelli, S., Arnone, A., et al. (2012). Comparison of two ready-to-use systems designed for sperm-hyaluronic acid binding selection before intracytoplasmic sperm injection: PICSI vs. sperm slow: a prospective, randomized trial. *Fertil. Steril.* 98, 632–637. doi: 10.1016/j.fertnstert.2012.05.043

Pérez-Cerezales, S., Boryshpolets, S., Afanzar, O., Brandis, A., Nevo, R., Kiss, V., et al. (2015). Involvement of opsins in mammalian sperm thermotaxis. *Sci. Rep.* 5:16146. doi: 10.1038/srep16146

Pérez-Cerezales, S., Laguna-Barraza, R., De Castro, A. C. A. C., Sánchez-Calabuig, M. J. M. J., Cano-Oliva, E., De Castro-Pita, F. J. F. J., et al. (2018). Sperm selection by thermotaxis improves ICSI outcome in mice. *Sci. Rep.* 8:2902. doi: 10.1038/s41598-018-21335-8

Pérez-Cerezales, S., Ramos-Ibeas, P., Acuña, O. S., Avilés, M., Coy, P., Rizos, D., et al. (2017). The oviduct: from sperm selection to the epigenetic landscape of the embryo. *Biol. Reprod.* 98, 262–276. doi: 10.1093/biolre/iox173

Plouffe, B. D., Murthy, S. K., and Lewis, L. H. (2015). Fundamentals and application of magnetic particles in cell isolation and enrichment: a review. *Rep. Prog. Phys.* 78:016601. doi: 10.1088/0034-4885/78/1/016601

Quinn, M. M., Jalalian, L., Ribeiro, S., Ona, K., Demirci, U., Cedars, M. I., et al. (2018). Microfluidic sorting selects sperm for clinical use with reduced DNA damage compared to density gradient centrifugation with swim-up in split semen samples. *Hum. Reprod.* 33, 1388–1393. doi: 10.1093/humrep/dey239

Raheem, O. A., and Walsh, T. J. (2016). Clinical utility of sperm DNA fragmentation testing: practice recommendations based on clinical scenarios. *Transl. Androl. Urol.* 5, 935–950. doi: 10.21037/tau.2017.08.14

Razavi, S. H., Nasr-Esfahani, M. H., Deemeh, M. R., Shayesteh, M., and Tavalaee, M. (2010). Evaluation of zeta and HA-binding methods for selection of spermatozoa with normal morphology, protamine content and DNA integrity. *Andrologia* 42, 13–19. doi: 10.1111/j.1439-0272.2009.00948.x

Rocca, M. S., Speltra, E., Menegazzo, M., Garolla, A., Foresta, C., and Ferlin, A. (2016). Sperm telomere length as a parameter of sperm quality in normozoospermic men. *Hum. Reprod.* 31, 1158–1163. doi: 10.1093/humrep/dew061

Romany, L., Garrido, N., Motato, Y., Aparicio, B., Remohí, J., and Meseguer, M. (2014). Removal of annexin V-positive sperm cells for intracytoplasmic sperm injection in ovum donation cycles does not improve reproductive outcome: a controlled and randomized trial in unselected males. *Fertil. Steril.* 102, 1567–1575. doi: 10.1016/j.fertnstert.2014.09.001

Romero-Aguirregomezcorta, J., Sugrue, E., Martínez-Fresneda, L., Newport, D., and Fair, S. (2018). Hyperactivated stallion spermatozoa fail to exhibit a rheotaxis-like behaviour, unlike other species. *Sci. Rep.* 8:16897. doi: 10.1038/s41598-018-34973-9

Said, T., Agarwal, A., Grunewald, S., Rasch, M., Baumann, T., Kriegel, C., et al. (2006). Selection of nonapoptotic spermatozoa as a new tool for enhancing assisted reproduction outcomes: an in vitro model1. *Biol. Reprod.* 74, 530–537. doi: 10.1095/biolreprod.105.046607

Said, T. M., and Land, J. A. (2011). Effects of advanced selection methods on sperm quality and ART outcome: a systematic review. *Hum. Reprod. Update* 17, 719–733. doi: 10.1093/humupd/dmr032

Sakkas, D., Manicardi, G. C., Tomlinson, M., Mandrioli, M., Bizzaro, D., Bianchi, P. G., et al. (2000). The use of two density gradient centrifugation techniques and the swim-up method to separate spermatozoa with chromatin and nuclear DNA anomalies. *Hum. Reprod.* 15, 1112–1116. doi: 10.1093/humrep/15.5.1112

Sakkas, D., Ramalingam, M., Garrido, N., and Barratt, C. L. R. (2015). Sperm selection in natural conception: what can we learn from Mother Nature to improve assisted reproduction outcomes? *Hum. Reprod. Update* 21, 711–726. doi: 10.1093/humupd/dmv042

Salamone, D. F., Canel, N. G., and Rodríguez, M. B. (2017). Intracytoplasmic sperm injection in domestic and wild mammals. *Reproduction* 154, F111–F124. doi: 10.1530/REP-17-0357

Saleh, R. A., Agarwal, A., Sharma, R. K., Said, T. M., Sikka, S. C., and Thomas, A. J. (2003). Evaluation of nuclear DNA damage in spermatozoa from infertile men with varicocele. *Fertil. Steril.* 80, 1431–1436. doi: 10.1016/S0015-0282(03)02211-8

Sallam, H. N., Farrag, A., Agameya, A. F., El-Garem, Y., and Ezzeldin, F. (2005). The use of the modified hypo-osmotic swelling test for the selection of immotile testicular spermatozoa in patients treated with ICSI: a randomized controlled study. *Hum. Reprod.* 20, 3435–3440. doi: 10.1093/humrep/dei249

Samardzija, M., Karadjole, M., Getz, I., Makek, Z., Cergolj, M., and Dobranic, T. (2006). Effects of bovine spermatozoa preparation on embryonic development in vitro. *Reprod. Biol. Endocrinol.* 13:58. doi: 10.1186/1477-7827-4-58

Sanchez, R., Stalf, T., Khanaga, O., Turley, H., Gips, H., and Schill, W. B. (1996). Sperm selection methods for intracytoplasmic sperm injection (ICSI) in andrological patients. *J. Assist. Reprod. Genet.* 13, 228–233. doi: 10.1007/BF02065941

Sandi-Monroy, N. L., Musanovic, S., Zhu, D., Szabó, Z., Vogl, A., Reeka, N., et al. (2019). Use of dimethylxanthine theophylline (SpermMobil®) does not affect clinical, obstetric or perinatal outcomes. *Arch. Gynecol. Obstet.* doi: 10.1007/s00404-019-05312-8 [Epub ahead of print].

Sbracia, M., Grasso, J., Sayme, N., Stronk, J., and Huszar, G. (1997). Hyaluronic acid substantially increases the retention of motility in cryopreserved/thawed human spermatozoa. *Hum. Reprod.* 12, 1949–1954. doi: 10.1093/humrep/12.9.1949

Schachter- Safrai, N., Karavani, G., Reuveni-Salzman, A., Gil, M., and Ben-Meir, A. (2019). Which semen analysis correlates with favorable Intracytoplasmic morphologically selected sperm injection (IMSI) outcomes? *Eur. J. Obstet. Gynecol. Reprod. Biol.* 234, 85–88. doi: 10.1016/J.EJOGRB.2019.01.006

Schulte, R. T., Ohl, D. A., Sigman, M., and Smith, G. D. (2010). Sperm DNA damage in male infertility: etiologies, assays, and outcomes. *J. Assist. Reprod. Genet.* 27, 3–12. doi: 10.1007/s10815-009-9359-x

Schwarze, J.-E., Jeria, R., Crosby, J., Villa, S., Ortega, C., and Pommer, R. (2017). Is there a reason to perform ICSI in the absence of male factor? Lessons from the Latin American Registry of ART. *Hum. Reprod. Open* 2017:hox013. doi: 10.1093/hropen/hox013

Setti, A. S., Braga, D. P. A. F., Figueira, R. C. S., Iaconelli, A., and Borges, E. (2014). Intracytoplasmic morphologically selected sperm injection results in improved clinical outcomes in couples with previous ICSI failures or male factor infertility: a meta-analysis. *Eur. J. Obstet. Gynecol. Reprod. Biol.* 183, 96–103. doi: 10.1016/j.ejogrb.2014.10.008

Setti, A. S., Braga, D. P. A. F., Figueira, R. C. S., Iaconelli, A., and Borges, E. (2015). Poor-responder patients do not benefit from intracytoplasmic morphologically selected sperm injection. *J. Assist. Reprod. Genet.* 32, 445–450. doi: 10.1007/s10815-014-0422-x

Shalom-Paz, E., Anabusi, S., Michaeli, M., Karchovsky-Shoshan, E., Rothfarb, N., Shavit, T., et al. (2015). Can intra cytoplasmatic morphologically selected sperm injection (IMSI) technique improve outcome in patients with repeated IVF-ICSI failure? a comparative study. *Gynecol. Endocrinol.* 31, 247–251. doi: 10.3109/09513590.2014.982085

Shirota, K., Yotsumoto, F., Itoh, H., Obama, H., Hidaka, N., Nakajima, K., et al. (2016). Separation efficiency of a microfluidic sperm sorter to minimize sperm DNA damage. *Fertil. Steril.* 105, 315–321. doi: 10.1016/j.fertnstert.2015.10.023

Simon, L., Aston, K. I., Emery, B. R., Hotaling, J., and Carrell, D. T. (2017a). Sperm DNA damage output parameters measured by the alkaline Comet assay and their importance. *Andrologia* 49:e12608. doi: 10.1111/and.12608

Simon, L., Emery, B. R., and Carrell, D. T. (2017b). Review: diagnosis and impact of sperm DNA alterations in assisted reproduction. *Best Pract. Res. Clin. Obstet. Gynaecol.* 44, 38–56. doi: 10.1016/j.bpobgyn.2017.07.003

Simon, L., Zini, A., Dyachenko, A., Ciampi, A., and Carrell, D. (2017c). A systematic review and meta-analysis to determine the effect of sperm DNA damage on in vitro fertilization and intracytoplasmic sperm injection outcome. *Asian J. Androl.* 19, 80–90. doi: 10.4103/1008-682X.182822

Sinha, A., Singh, V., and Yadav, S. (2017). Multi-omics and male infertility: status, integration and future prospects. *Front. Biosci.* 9, 375–394. doi: 10.2741/s493

Sirard, M. A. (2018). 40 years of bovine IVF in the new genomic selection context. *Reproduction* 156, R1–R7. doi: 10.1530/REP-18-0008

Soler, C., Bono, A., Vicente-Fiel, S., Recreo, P., Santolaria, P., Carretero, T., et al. (2016). Comparison of different statistical approaches to evaluate morphometric sperm subpopulations in man. *Asian J. Androl.* 18, 819–823. doi: 10.4103/1008-682x.186872

Stephens, S. M., Arnett, D. M., and Meacham, R. B. (2013). The use of in vitro fertilization in the management of male infertility: what the urologist needs to know. *Rev Urol.* 15, 154–160. doi: 10.3909/riu0588

Stimpfel, M., Verdenik, I., Zorn, B., and Virant-Klun, I. (2018). Magnetic-activated cell sorting of non-apoptotic spermatozoa improves the quality of embryos according to female age: a prospective sibling oocyte study. *J. Assist. Reprod. Genet.* 35, 1665–1674. doi: 10.1007/s10815-018-1242-1

Strehler, E., Baccetti, B., Sterzik, K., Capitani, S., Collodel, G., De Santo, M., et al. (1998). Detrimental effects of polyvinylpyrrolidone on the ultrastructure of spermatozoa (Notulae seminologicae 13). *Hum. Reprod.* 13, 120–123. doi: 10.1093/humrep/13.1.120

Suarez, S. S. (2008). Control of hyperactivation in sperm. *Hum. Reprod. Update* 14, 647–657. doi: 10.1093/humupd/dmn029

Taşdemir, I., Taşdemir, M., and Tavukçuoğlu, Ş (1998). Effect of pentoxifylline on immotile testicular spermatozoa. *J. Assist. Reprod. Genet.* 15, 90–92. doi: 10.1007/BF02766832

Tavalaee, M., Deemeh, M. R., Arbabian, M., and Nasr-Esfahani, M. H. (2012). Density gradient centrifugation before or after magnetic-activated cell sorting: which technique is more useful for clinical sperm selection? *J. Assist. Reprod. Genet.* 29, 31–38. doi: 10.1007/s10815-011-9686-6

Terriou, P., Hans, E., Cortvrindt, R., Avon, C., Charles, O., Salzmann, J., et al. (2015). Papaverine as a replacement for pentoxifylline to select thawed testicular or epididymal spermatozoa before ICSI. *Gynécol. Obs. Fertil.* 43, 786–790. doi: 10.1016/j.gyobfe.2015.10.007

Terriou, P., Hans, E., Giorgetti, C., Spach, J. L., Salzmann, J., Urrutia, V., et al. (2000). Pentoxifylline initiates motility in spontaneously immotile epididymal and testicular spermatozoa and allows normal fertilization, pregnancy, and birth after intracytoplasmic sperm injection. *J. Assist. Reprod. Genet.* 17, 194–199. doi: 10.1023/A:1009435732258

Tournaye, H. (2012). Male factor infertility and ART. *Asian J. Androl.* 14, 103–108. doi: 10.1038/aja.2011.65

Tournaye, H., Verheyen, G., Albano, C., Camus, M., Van Landuyt, L., Devroey, P., et al. (2002). Intracytoplasmic sperm injection versus in vitro fertilization: a randomized controlled trial and a meta-analysis of the literature. *Fertil. Steril.* 78, 1030–1037. doi: 10.1016/S0015-0282(02)03377-0

Umehara, T., Kawai, T., Goto, M., Richards, J. A. S., and Shimada, M. (2018). Creatine enhances the duration of sperm capacitation: a novel factor for improving in vitro fertilization with small numbers of sperm. *Hum. Reprod.* 33, 1117–1129. doi: 10.1093/humrep/dey081

Vasicek, J., Pivko, J., and Chrenek, P. (2014). Reproductive performance of New Zealand white rabbits after depletion of apoptotic spermatozoa. *Folia Biol.* 62, 109–117. doi: 10.3409/fb62_2.109

Verheyen, G., Joris, H., Crits, K., Nagy, Z., Tournaye, H., and Van Steirteghem, A. (1997). Comparison of different hypo-osmotic swelling solutions to select viable immotile spermatozoa for potential use in intracytoplasmic sperm injection. *Hum. Reprod. Update* 3, 195–203. doi: 10.1093/humupd/3.3.195

Vermes, I., Haanen, C., Steffens-Nakken, H., and Reutellingsperger, C. (1995). A novel assay for apoptosis Flow cytometric detection of phosphatidylserine expression on early apoptotic cells using fluorescein labelled Annexin V. *J. Immunol. Methods* 184, 39–51. doi: 10.1016/0022-1759(95)00072-I

Wang, J., Fan, H. C., Behr, B., and Quake, S. R. (2012). Genome-wide single-cell analysis of recombination activity and de novo mutation rates in human sperm. *Cell* 150, 402–412. doi: 10.1016/j.cell.2012.06.030

Wang, M., Sun, J., Wang, L., Gao, X., Lu, X., Wu, Z., et al. (2014). Assessment of density gradient centrifugation (DGC) and sperm chromatin dispersion (SCD) measurements in couples with male factor infertility undergoing ICSI. *J. Assist. Reprod. Genet.* 31, 1655–1663. doi: 10.1007/s10815-014-0339-4

Wilding, M., Coppola, G., di Matteo, L., Palagiano, A., Fusco, E., and Dale, B. (2011). Intracytoplasmic injection of morphologically selected spermatozoa (IMSI) improves outcome after assisted reproduction by deselecting physiologically poor quality spermatozoa. *J. Assist. Reprod. Genet.* 28, 253–262. doi: 10.1007/s10815-010-9505-5

Williams, M., Hill, C. J., Scudamore, I., Dunphy, B., Cooke, I. D., and Barratt, C. L. (1993). Sperm numbers and distribution within the human fallopian tube around ovulation. *Hum. Reprod.* 8, 2019–2026. doi: 10.1093/oxfordjournals.humrep.a137975

Worrilow, K. C., Eid, S., Woodhouse, D., Perloe, M., Smith, S., Witmyer, J., et al. (2013). Use of hyaluronan in the selection of sperm for intracytoplasmic sperm injection (ICSI): significant improvement in clinical outcomes—multicenter, double-blinded and randomized controlled trial. *Hum. Reprod.* 28, 306–314. doi: 10.1093/humrep/des417

Wu, J., Carrell, D. T., and Wilcox, A. L. (2001). Development of in vitro-matured oocytes from porcine preantral follicles following intracytoplasmic sperm injection. *Biol. Reprod.* 66, 1579–1585. doi: 10.1095/biolreprod65.5.1579

Yagci, A., Murk, W., Stronk, J., and Huszar, G. (2010). Spermatozoa bound to solid state hyaluronic acid show chromatin structure with high DNA chain integrity: an acridine orange fluorescence study. *J. Androl.* 31, 566–572. doi: 10.2164/jandrol.109.008912

Yániz, J. L., Soler, C., and Santolaria, P. (2015). Computer assisted sperm morphometry in mammals: a review. *Anim. Reprod. Sci.* 156, 1–12. doi: 10.1016/j.anireprosci.2015.03.002

Yetkinel, S., Kilicdag, E. B., Aytac, P. C., Haydardedeoglu, B., Simsek, E., and Cok, T. (2019). Effects of the microfluidic chip technique in sperm selection for intracytoplasmic sperm injection for unexplained infertility: a prospective, randomized controlled trial. *J. Assist. Reprod. Genet.* 36, 403–409. doi: 10.1007/s10815-018-1375-2

Zaferani, M., Cheong, S. H., and Abbaspourrad, A. (2018). Rheotaxis-based separation of sperm with progressive motility using a microfluidic corral system. *Proc. Natl. Acad. Sci. U.S.A.* 115, 8272–8277. doi: 10.1073/pnas.1800819115

Zahedi, A., Tavalaee, M., Deemeh, M. R., Azadi, L., Fazilati, M., and Nasr-Esfahani, M. H. (2013). Zeta potential vs apoptotic marker: which is more suitable for ICSI sperm selection? *J. Assist. Reprod. Genet.* 30, 1181–1186. doi: 10.1007/s10815-013-0022-1

Zarei-Kheirabadi, M., Shayegan Nia, E., Tavalaee, M., Deemeh, M. R., Arabi, M., Forouzanfar, M., et al. (2012). Evaluation of ubiquitin and annexin v in sperm population selected based on density gradient centrifugation and zeta potential (DGC-Zeta). *J. Assist. Reprod. Genet.* 29, 365–371. doi: 10.1007/s10815-011-9689-3

Zegers-Hochschild, F., Adamson, G. D., Dyer, S., Racowsky, C., De Mouzon, J., Sokol, R., et al. (2017). The international glossary on infertility and fertility care, 2017. *Fertil. Steril.* 108, 393–406. doi: 10.1093/humrep/dex234

Zhang, H., Xuan, X., Yang, S., Li, X., Xu, C., and Gao, X. (2018). Selection of viable human spermatozoa with low levels of DNA fragmentation from an immotile population using density gradient centrifugation and magnetic-activated cell sorting. *Andrologia* 50:e12821. doi: 10.1111/and.12821

Zhang, Z., Liu, J., Meriano, J., Ru, C., Xie, S., Luo, J., et al. (2016). Human sperm rheotaxis: a passive physical process. *Sci. Rep.* 6:23553. doi: 10.1038/srep23553

Zhao, F., Yang, Q., Shi, S., Luo, X., and Sun, Y. (2016). Semen preparation methods and sperm telomere length: density gradient centrifugation versus the swim up procedure. *Sci. Rep.* 6:39051. doi: 10.1038/srep39051

Ziarati, N., Tavalaee, M., Bahadorani, M., and Nasr Esfahani, M. H. (2019). Clinical outcomes of magnetic activated sperm sorting in infertile men candidate for ICSI. *Hum. Fertil.* 22, 118–125. doi: 10.1080/14647273.2018.1424354

Zini, A., Finelli, A., Phang, D., and Jarvi, K. (2000). Influence of semen processing technique on human sperm DNA integrity. *Urology* 56, 1081–1084. doi: 10.1016/S0090-4295(00)00770-6

11

Membrane Potential Determined by Flow Cytometry Predicts Fertilizing Ability of Human Sperm

*Lis C. Puga Molina[1], Stephanie Gunderson[1], Joan Riley[1], Pascal Lybaert[2], Aluet Borrego-Alvarez[1], Emily S. Jungheim[1] and Celia M. Santi[1]**

[1] Department of Obstetrics & Gynecology, Washington University School of Medicine, St Louis, MO, United States, [2] Laboratory of Experimental Hormonology, School of Medicine, Université Libre de Bruxelles, Brussels, Belgium

***Correspondence:**
Celia M. Santi
santic@wustl.edu

Infertility affects 10 to 15% of couples worldwide, with a male factor contributing up to 50% of these cases. The primary tool for diagnosing male infertility is traditional semen analysis, which reveals sperm concentration, morphology, and motility. However, 25% of infertile men are diagnosed as normozoospermic, meaning that, in many cases, normal-appearing sperm fail to fertilize an egg. Thus, new information regarding the mechanisms by which sperm acquire fertilizing ability is needed to develop a clinically feasible test that can predict sperm function failure. An important feature of sperm fertilization capability in many species is plasma membrane hyperpolarization (membrane potential becoming more negative inside) in response to signals from the egg or female genital tract. In mice, this hyperpolarization is necessary for sperm to undergo the changes in motility (hyperactivation) and acrosomal exocytosis required to fertilize an egg. Human sperm also hyperpolarize during capacitation, but the physiological relevance of this event has not been determined. Here, we used flow cytometry combined with a voltage-sensitive fluorescent probe to measure absolute values of human sperm membrane potential. We found that hyperpolarization of human sperm plasma membrane correlated positively with fertilizing ability. Hyperpolarized human sperm had higher *in vitro* fertilization (IVF) ratios and higher percentages of acrosomal exocytosis and hyperactivated motility than depolarized sperm. We propose that measurements of human sperm membrane potential could be used to diagnose men with idiopathic infertility and predict IVF success in normozoospermic infertile patients. Patients with depolarized values could be guided toward intracytoplasmic sperm injection, preventing unnecessary cycles of intrauterine insemination or IVF. Conversely, patients with hyperpolarized values of sperm membrane potential could undergo only conventional IVF, avoiding the risks and costs associated with intracytoplasmic sperm injection.

Keywords: membrane potential, human, sperm, IVF, normozoospermic infertility, flow cytometry, capacitation

INTRODUCTION

Infertility, defined as the inability of a couple to achieve pregnancy after 12 months of unprotected intercourse, affects between 10 and 15% of couples around the world (Sharma et al., 2013). Many such couples turn to *in vitro* fertilization (IVF), which has been used to conceive over 6.5 million babies. Approximately 50% of infertility cases are due to a male factor (Kumar and Singh, 2015).

To diagnose these men, assisted reproduction specialists rely on semen analysis, which provides information about sperm concentration, morphology, and motility. However, this method does not reveal abnormalities in sperm from some infertile men (Bracke et al., 2018), who are then described as having normozoospermic idiopathic infertility. One possibility is that sperm from these men are unable to fertilize an egg because they are unable to capacitate, a process in which sperm become hyperactive and prepared to undergo acrosomal exocytosis. Together, hyperactivation and acrosomal exocytosis allow sperm to bind to and fuse with an oocyte (Yanagimachi, 1994). In natural pregnancies, capacitation is triggered by factors in the female reproductive tract (Austin, 1951; Chang, 1951). In IVF, sperm is capacitated by incubation in a chemically defined media containing Ca^{++}, HCO_3^-, energy sources, and a cholesterol acceptor. Given that capacitation is required for fertilization, a test that could assess the ability of sperm to undergo this process could be a valuable addition to IVF diagnostics.

In many species, sperm capacitation is accompanied by sperm plasma membrane hyperpolarization (an increase in intracellular net negative charge) (Zeng et al., 1995; Hernández-González et al., 2007; López-González et al., 2014; Escoffier et al., 2015). In mouse sperm, capacitation-associated hyperpolarization is largely driven by activation of the sperm-specific potassium (K^+) channel SLO3 (Santi et al., 2010; Chávez et al., 2013). *Slo3* knockout mice are infertile, and their sperm are unable to undergo hyperactivation or acrosomal exocytosis (Santi et al., 2010; Zeng et al., 2011). Human sperm also hyperpolarize during capacitation (López-González et al., 2014), and two studies reported that more depolarized human sperm membrane potentials values were associated with lower fertility (Calzada and Tellez, 1997; Brown et al., 2016). However, these studies did not address the effect of changes of sperm membrane potential on hyperactivation or acrosomal exocytosis. In addition, the methods used in both studies to assess membrane potential are technically difficult and not suitable to be implemented in a clinical setting. Other methods that evaluate the capacitating state of the sperm, such as the CapScore test, require staining, counting, and correctly identifying staining patterns in more than 150 individual sperm (Moody et al., 2017), which also is challenging to implement clinically.

Here, we used flow cytometry in combination with the voltage-sensitive fluorescent dye $DiSC_3(5)$ to create a calibration curve and measure absolute sperm membrane potential values. Using this method, we found that human sperm membrane hyperpolarization correlated with sperm fertility capacity in IVF patients. We propose that our method could be used clinically to diagnose male infertility and predict IVF success of normozoospermic patients.

MATERIALS AND METHODS

Reagents

All reagents to prepare non-commercial Human Tubal Fluid (HTF) and Toyoda–Yokoyama–Hosi (TYH) media, as well as valinomycin, FITC-labeled *Pisum sativum* agglutinin, Tween 20, 2′,7′-Bis-(2-Carboxyethyl)-5-(and-6)-Carboxyfluorescein, Acetoxymethyl Ester (BCECF-AM), and calcium ionophore A23187, were from Sigma (St. Louis, MO); 3, 3′-dipropyl- thiadicarbocyanine iodide [$DiSC_3(5)$] was from Invitrogen (Carlsbad, CA, United States); Hoechst 33342 was from Cayman Chemicals, (Ann Arbor, MI, United States); paraformaldehyde was from Electron Microscopy Sciences (Hatfield, PA, United States); Dulbecco's Phosphate Buffered Saline (DPBS) was from GIBCO Life Technologies (Gaithersburg, MD, United States); and Quinn's Advantage Human (HTF) fertilization media and human serum albumin were from CooperSurgical (Trumbull, CT, United States).

Mouse Samples and Ethics Statement

Washington University School of Medicine (WUSM) policy states that all research involving animals be conducted under humane conditions, with appropriate regard for animal welfare. WUSM is a registered research facility with the United States Department of Agriculture (USDA) and is committed to comply with the Guide for the Care and Use of Laboratory Animals (Department of Health and Human Services) and the provisions of the Animal Welfare Act (USDA and all applicable federal and state laws and regulations). The WUSM Animal Care and Use Committee ensures compliance with all applicable federal and state regulations for the purchase, transportation, housing, and research use of animals. WUSM has filed appropriate assurance of compliance with the Office for the Protection of Research Risks of the National Institute of Health. The WUS Animal Care and Use Committee approved the method of euthanasia for mice: CO_2 asphyxiation followed by rapid cervical dislocation. These methods are consistent with the recommendation of the panel on euthanasia of the American Veterinary Medical Association and YARC Standard Euthanasia guidelines for rodents. Caudal epididymal sperm were collected from 90-day-old *Slo3* knock-out (generated as previously described [Santi et al., 2010]) or wild-type mice.

Human Samples and Ethics Statement

This study was approved by the Washington University Institutional Review Board and was performed in collaboration with the Washington University Fertility and Reproductive Medicine Center. Semen samples were obtained via masturbation after 3–5 days of abstinence in private collection rooms at the fertility clinic. Only donors and conventional IVF patients' samples that met the World Health Organization [WHO] (2010) ($\geq$32% progressive motility; $\geq$40% total motility; $\geq 15 \times 10^6$ cells/ml). For studies involving semen donors, de-identified human sperm samples were obtained within 2 h of collection from men who were asked to have a semen analysis performed.

Couples undergoing IVF met inclusion criteria if their oocytes were subjected to conventional *in vitro* fertilization or split insemination [half intracytoplasmic sperm injection (ICSI), half conventional *in vitro* fertilization] or conventional *in vitro* fertilization, and if the female partner had a diagnosis of unexplained infertility, tubal infertility, or uterine factor infertility. Patients were excluded from this study if they had male factor infertility. Additionally, to assure good-quality oocytes for this study, patients were excluded if females had polycystic ovarian syndrome, endometriosis, anovulation, or diminished ovarian reserve. The average age of the 49 healthy men included in this study was 34.63 (range 26–48) years. On the day of oocyte retrieval, male partners gave written informed consent in accordance with the Declaration of Helsinki. At the time of consent, male partners also completed a brief health questionnaire. For IVF, around 14 × 10^6/ml sperm were incubated overnight with mature oocytes including the zona pellucida and cumulus cells. For ICSI, oocytes with zona pellucida and without cumulus cells were used. Sperm samples left over after IVF were obtained approximately 4 h after initial collection and incubated overnight at 37°C with 5% CO_2. IVF cycle data including fertilization rate were collected for analysis. The fertilization rate was calculated as the number of normally fertilized mature oocytes with two pronuclei divided by total number of inseminated mature oocytes. The Washington University Fertility and Reproductive Medicine Center defines successful IVF as a fertilization rate >70% (fertilization ratio >0.7); this cut-off is determined by calculating the mean fertilization ratio in conventional IVF cases quarterly and yearly.

For studies involving frozen human samples, five vitrified washed normozoospermic semen samples that were used to conceive a pregnancy were obtained from the Washington University Reproductive Medicine Center cryobank. The samples were produced by anonymous donors, aliquoted, frozen, and used for both intrauterine insemination and IVF. Remaining aliquots of samples that were used to conceive a pregnancy were donated for the purposes of research.

Media

Non-commercial HEPES-buffered HTF (4.67 mM KCl, 0.31 mM KH_2PO_2, 90.69 mM NaCl, 1.20 mM $MgSO_4$, 2.78 mM glucose, 1.6 mM $CaCl_2$, 0.51 mM sodium pyruvate, 60 mM sodium lactate, 23.8 mM HEPES, and 10 μg/ml Gentamicin, (pH 7.4 with NaOH) was used to measure human sperm membrane potential. Non-commercial HEPES-buffered HTF was supplemented the same day with 25 mM $NaHCO_3$ and 0.5% w/v BSA A-7906 (Sigma) for capacitating conditions, and only with 0.5% w/v BSA for non-capacitating conditions. IVF samples were processed in commercial Quinn's Advantage Human (HTF) fertilization media [CooperSurgical (Trumbull, CT, United States)] supplemented with 3 mg/ml human serum albumin (CooperSurgical) and pre-incubated overnight at 37°C with 5% CO_2 to equilibrate pH. The same media was used to capacitate IVF and donor sperm samples.

Mouse capacitating modified (TYH) medium [119.30 mM NaCl, 4.70 mM KCl, 1.71 mM $CaCl_2$, 1.20 mM KH_2PO4, 1.20 mM $MgSO_4$, 0.51 mM sodium pyruvate, 5.56 mM glucose, 20 mM HEPES, 15 mM $NaHCO_3$ and 5 mg/ml BSA A-2153 (pH 7.4 with NaOH)] was used to capacitate mouse sperm.

Human and Mouse Sperm Capacitation

Ejaculated human sperm were allowed to swim-up in commercial or non-commercial HTF capacitating medium for 1 h at 37°C with CO_2. The highly motile sperm recovered after swim up were washed, centrifuged for 5 min at 400 × *g*, and incubated overnight at 37°C with 5% CO_2. For experiments involving comparisons between non-capacitating and capacitating conditions, human sperm were allowed to swim-up in non-capacitating HTF medium at 37°C for 1 h. Then the sample was divided into two, and an equal volume of non-capacitating medium or 2-fold concentrated BSA and $NaHCO_3$ were added to prepare non-capacitating or capacitating media, respectively. Then, the samples were incubated overnight at 37°C with 5% CO_2 for capacitating conditions, or at 37°C for non-capacitating conditions.

Frozen human sperm samples were thawed for 20 min at room temperature, resuspended in 1.5 ml final volume of commercial Quinn's Advantage Human (HTF) fertilization media (CooperSurgical) medium and washed twice with centrifugation at 400 × *g* for 5 min. Sperm were allowed to swim-up in 300 μl of media with 5% CO_2 at 37°C for 1 h. Highly motile sperm were recovered from the supernatant. Half were used to determine membrane potential, and half were incubated overnight with 5% CO_2 at 37°C for to determine membrane potential after capacitation.

Mice were euthanized, and cauda epididymal sperm were placed in 1 ml of modified TYH medium. After 15 min at 37°C (swim-out), suspended sperm were collected. Sperm concentration was adjusted to a final maximum concentration of 10 × 10^6 cells/ml and incubated for 75 min at 37°C for capacitation.

Determination of Membrane Potential by Flow Cytometry

After overnight incubation, human sperm samples were centrifuged at 400 × *g* for 5 min and resuspended in non-capacitating HTF medium and 0.1 μM BCECF-AM. The samples were covered to be protected from light, incubated at 37°C for 10 min, washed again to eliminate non-incorporated dye, and resuspended in non-capacitating HTF media with 25 mM $NaHCO_3$. Before recording, 5 nM $DiSC_3(5)$ was added, and data were recorded as individual cellular events on a FACSCanto II TM cytometer (Becton Dickinson). Forward scatter area (FSC-A) and side-scatter area (SSC-A) data were collected from 20,000 events per recording. Threshold levels of two-dimensional dot plot SSC-A vs. side-scatter height (SSC-H) were set for gating singlets. BCECF fluorescence was detected with the filter for fluorescein isothiocyanate (FITC; 530/30) and used to exclude non-viable cells as previously described (Puga Molina et al., 2017). Positive cells for $DiSC_3(5)$ fluorescence was detected with the filter for allophycocyanin (APC; 585/40). Because $DiSC_3(5)$ is positively charged, cell hyperpolarization increases dye incorporation and intracellular fluorescence. Recordings were initiated after reaching steady-state fluorescence (1–3 min).

Mouse sperm samples were centrifuged at 200 × g for 10 min and resuspended in TYH media without BSA. Before recording, 5 nM $DiSC_3(5)$ and 900 nM Hoechst 33342 were added. Data were recorded as individual cellular events on a FACSCanto II TM cytometer (Becton Dickinson).

FSC-A and SSC-A data were collected from 20,000 events per recording. Threshold levels of two-dimensional dot plot SSC-A vs. SSC-H were set for gating singlets. Hoechst 33342 fluorescence was detected with the filter for pacific blue (Pacific Blue; 450/50) and used to exclude non-viable cells. $DiSC_3(5)$ fluorescence was detected with the filter for allophycocyanine (APC; 585/40).

In both mouse and human sperm experiments, membrane potential fluorescent signal was calibrated by adding 1 μM valinomycin and sequential adding KCl corresponding to 4.98, 7.48, 12.48, 22.48, and 42.48 mM K^+ for HTF and 5.90, 8.4, 13.4, 23.4, and 43.4 mM K^+ for TYH (Chávez et al., 2013). Theoretical values were obtained by using the Nernst equation, assuming an intracellular K^+ concentration of 120 mM (Linares-Hernández et al., 1998) and considering room temperature as 298.15°K. The final sperm membrane potential was obtained by linearly interpolating the median fluorescence of the unknown sample to the calibration curve of each trace.

Determination of Membrane Potential by Spectrophotometry

After swim-up incubation, human sperm samples were centrifuged at 400 × *g* for 5 min, resuspended in non-capacitating HTF media with 5 mg/ml of BSA A-2153 (Sigma), and 4 × 10^6 sperm were transferred to a gently stirred cuvette at 310.15°K. $DiSC_3(5)$ was added to a final concentration of 1 μM. Fluorescence was monitored with a Varian Cary Eclipse fluorescence spectrophotometer at 620 nm excitation and 670 nm emission as described before (Chávez et al., 2013). Calibration was performed by adding 1 μM valinomycin and sequential additions of KCl as described for flow cytometry experiments. The final sperm membrane potential was obtained by linearly interpolating the theoretical membrane potential values versus arbitrary units of fluorescence of each trace.

Acrosomal Status

To assess acrosomal status, 50 μl human sperm samples were treated with 10 μM of the calcium ionophore A23187 or DMSO (vehicle) for 30 min before the end of the capacitation incubation time. After incubation, sperm were fixed at 4°C by adding 50 μl of 12.5% w/v paraformaldehyde in 2.28 M Tris. Sperm were then spotted onto slides, dried, washed 3 times for 5 min and one time for 15 min with DPBS containing 0.1% v/v Tween 20 (t-DPBS), and stained with 100 μg/ml of FITC-labeled *Pisum sativum* agglutinin dissolved in t-DPBS. After washing, slides were observed under an EVOS® FL Cell Imaging System epifluorescence microscope at 40×. Sperm were scored as acrosome intact if a bright staining was observed in the acrosome, or as acrosome reacted when either fluorescent staining was restricted to the equatorial segment or no labeling was observed. The percentage of sperm that underwent induced acrosomal exocytosis was obtained by subtracting the percentage of acrosome reacted sperm incubated with DMSO from the percentage of acrosome reacted sperm incubated with A23187.

Computer-Assisted Sperm Analysis (CASA)

Aliquots (3 μl) of sperm suspension were placed into a 20 micron Leja standard count 4 chamber slide, pre-warmed at 37°C. CASA analysis was performed with a Hamilton–Thorne digital image analyzer (HTR-CEROS II v.1.7; Hamilton–Thorne Research, Beverly, MA, United States). Phase alignment was checked, and the settings used for the analysis were selected as follows: objective 1: Zeiss 10XNH; min total count: 200; frames acquired, 30; frame rate, 60 Hz; camera exposure: 8 ms; camera gain: 300; integrated time: 500 ms; elongation max%: 100; elongation min%: 1; head brightness min 170; head size max: 50 μm^2; head size min: 5 μm^2; static tail filter: false; tail brightness min: 70; tail brightness auto offset: 8; tail brightness mode: manual; progressive STR (%): 80; progressive VAP (μm/s): 25. The criteria used to define hyperactivated sperm were: curvilinear velocity (VCL) >150 μm/s, lateral head displacement (ALH) >7.0 μm, and linearity coefficient (LIN) <50% (Mortimer et al., 1998).

Calculations and Statistical Analyses

Data are expressed as mean ± standard error of the mean (SEM). Independent experiments were carried out with samples from different donors or patients. A probability (*p*) value $p < 0.05$ was considered statistically significant. A value of $p < 0.05$ was indicated with an *, $p < 0.01$ with **, and $p < 0.001$ with ***. Calculations were performed with Microsoft Office 365 ProPlus spreadsheet, and statistical analyses were performed with GraphPad Prism version 6.01, GraphPad Software (La Jolla, CA, United States). To test whether values were in a Gaussian distribution, D'Agostino-Pearson, Shapiro-Wilk, and Kolmogorov-Smirnov tests were run in parallel. Parametric or non-parametric comparisons were used as dictated by the data distribution. Spearman test was used for correlations. The differences between means from two groups were analyzed by paired or unpaired *t*-test, depending on the condition tested. The receiving operating characteristic (ROC) curve and the maximum Youden index were used to determine the optimal cut-off value for depolarized and hyperpolarized samples.

RESULTS

Flow Cytometry Can Be Used to Measure Absolute Values of Sperm Membrane Potential

Our method of calculating absolute sperm membrane potential values is based on the properties of the cationic voltage-sensitive dye $DiSC_3(5)$, which distributes across cellular membranes in response to electrochemical gradients. $DiSC_3(5)$ enters the sperm upon membrane hyperpolarization, increasing intracellular fluorescence. $DiSC_3(5)$ has been used to measure mammalian sperm membrane potential by spectrophotometry (Espinosa and Darszon, 1995; Muñoz-Garay et al., 2001; Demarco et al., 2003; Santi et al., 2010). Since flow-cytometry in association with $DiSC_3$-(5) was not previously used to determine absolute sperm membrane potential values, we first validated our method. To do so, we conducted DiSC$_3$(5) flow cytometry experiments with both wild type (WT) and *Slo3*$^{-/-}$ mouse sperm and compared our values to those previously measured by spectrophotometry (Santi et al., 2010). Forward scatter area (FSC-A) and side scatter area (SSC-A) light detection were used to identify sperm cells based on size and granularity (**Figure 1A**). To exclude non-single cells (doublets or debris), singlets were selected with SSC-A and side-scatter height (SSC-H) (**Figure 1B**; Escoffier et al., 2015). Hoechst 33342 dye was used to differentiate between live and dead sperm (**Figure 1C**), and DiSC$_3$(5) fluorescence was analyzed only in live sperm (see section Materials and Methods).

To calibrate the fluorescent signal, we constructed a calibration curve by using the K$^+$ ionophore valinomycin and sequential additions of known concentrations of KCl. Addition of valinomycin causes membrane hyperpolarization up to the value of the K$^+$ equilibrium potential, causing DiSC$_3$(5) to enter the

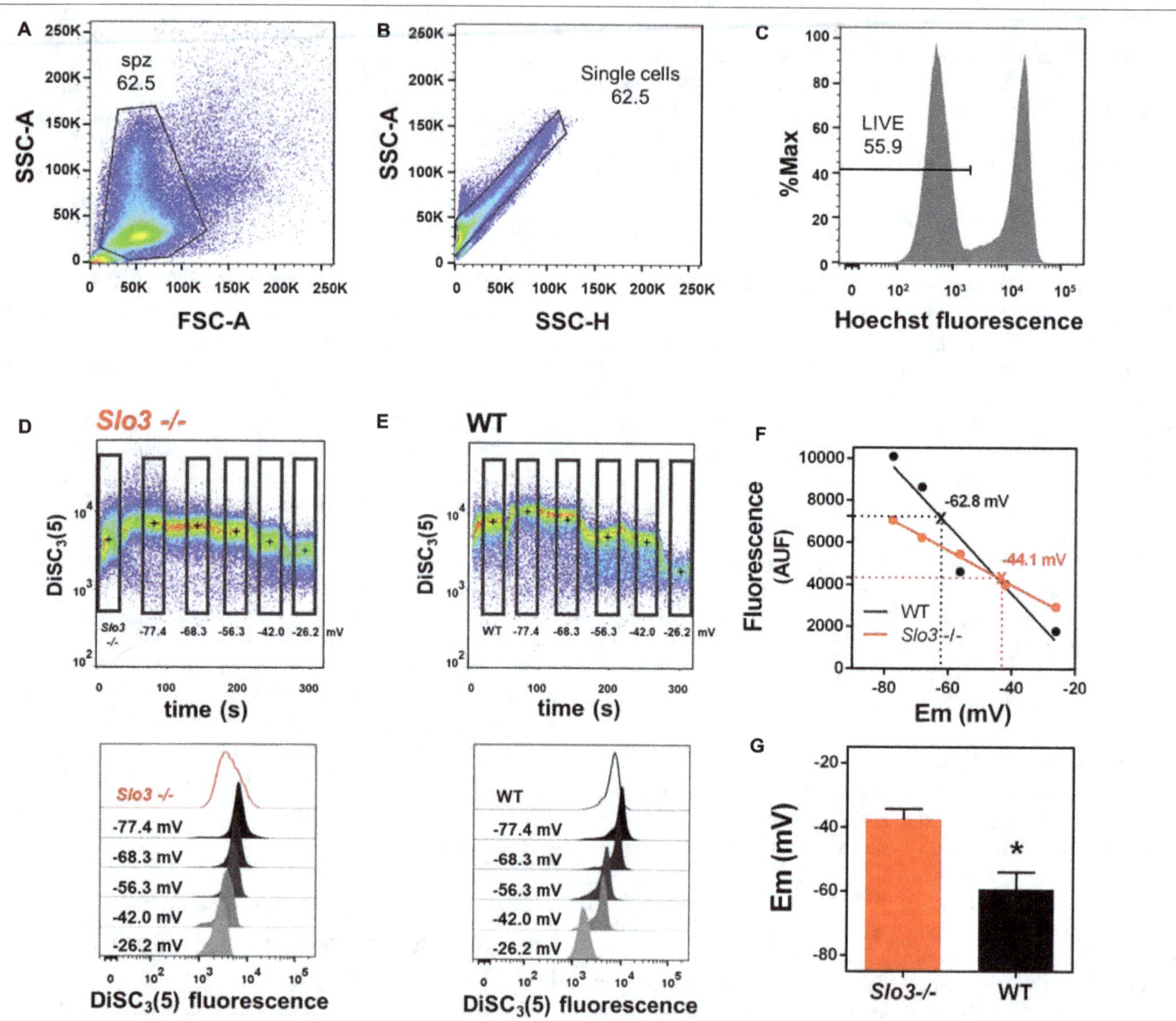

FIGURE 1 | Flow cytometry can be used to determine absolute values of membrane potential in wild type and *Slo3*$^{-/-}$ mouse sperm. **(A)** Forward-scatter (FSC) and side-scatter (SSC) light data were collected. Threshold levels for side-scatter area (SSC-A) and forward-scatter area (FSC-A) were set to exclude signals from cellular debris or cells with abnormal morphology. **(B)** Threshold levels of two-dimensional dot plot of SSC-A vs. side-scatter height (SSC-H) were set to include only single cells and exclude clumps. **(C)** Cells with bright Hoechst staining were excluded to measure DiSC$_3$(5) fluorescence only in live sperm. **(D,E)** Upper panel: Representative dot plot of DiSC$_3$(5) fluorescence from *Slo3*$^{-/-}$ **(D)** and WT **(E)** mouse sperm incubated in capacitated conditions. Calibration was performed by adding 1 μM valinomycin and sequentially adding KCl, corresponding to the theoretical plasma membrane potential values of −77.4, −68.3, −56.3, −42.0, and −26.2 mV ([K$^+$]$_i$ of 120 mM). Black crosses indicate the median DiSC$_3$(5) fluorescence of sperm within the gates (rectangles) defined for each addition. Lower panels: Histograms of DiSC$_3$(5) fluorescence from selected gates as indicated in flow cytometry dot plots. **(F)** Linear regression of the calibration curves constructed from the median DiSC$_3$(5) fluorescence from *Slo3*$^{-/-}$ and WT sperm obtained in D and E. Interpolated values for each curve are indicated with X and dotted lines. *Slo3*$^{-/-}$ r^2 = 0.9948; WT r^2 = 0.9311. **(G)** Membrane potential of *Slo3*$^{-/-}$ and WT capacitated sperm. *P = 0.0265 by unpaired t-test.

sperm, leading to increased intracellular fluorescence. Sequential KCl additions cause depolarization of the plasma membrane to the corresponding K^+ equilibrium potential values and decreased intracellular fluorescence. The membrane potential values after addition of valinomycin and KCl were calculated according to the Nernst equation, assuming a $[K^+]_i$ of 120 mM (**Figures 1D,E**). The absolute sperm membrane potential values were obtained by linearly interpolating the theoretical membrane potential values versus arbitrary units of fluorescence of each trace (**Figure 1F**). The membrane potential values obtained with this technique from WT (−59.4 ± 5.3 mV) and *Slo3*$^{-/-}$ (−37.5 ± 3.3 mV) sperm (**Figure 1G**) were similar to those reported by spectrophotometry by our group (−60 mV for WT and −40 mV for *Slo3*$^{-/-}$) (Santi et al., 2010). Thus, we concluded that our flow cytometric method of measuring absolute membrane potential values was valid for mouse sperm.

Human Sperm Incubated in Capacitation Conditions Are More Hyperpolarized Than Non-capacitated Sperm

Previous flow cytometry studies of human sperm membrane potential showed that non-capacitated sperm were more depolarized than sperm incubated in capacitating media (López-González et al., 2014; Brukman et al., 2019), but absolute membrane potential values were not reported. Here, we used our flow cytometric technique to measure the absolute membrane potential values in both capacitated and non-capacitated sperm from normozoospermic donors. The fluorescence probe BCECF-AM was used as an indicator of live sperm, and only BCECF-positive cells were analyzed (Puga Molina et al., 2017, 2018b; **Supplementary Figures S1A–C**). We conducted a calibration curve as we had done for mouse sperm (**Figures 2A–C**). We found that human sperm incubated in capacitation conditions were, on average, significantly more hyperpolarized than non-capacitated sperm (−45.2 ± 3.2 vs. −35.7 ± 2.8 mV, n = 13, respectively) (**Figure 2D**). However, some donor samples did not undergo hyperpolarization in capacitating media.

The spectrophotometry assay is widely used to measure absolute membrane potential values in sperm (Linares-Hernández et al., 1998; Patrat et al., 2002; Santi et al., 2010; Chávez et al., 2013). Therefore, we compared the membrane potential value obtained by spectrophotometry and flow cytometry in a donor sample. We obtained similar membrane potential values with the two techniques (**Supplementary Figure S1**). This result further indicates that our flow cytometric method could be used to determine human sperm membrane potential.

Human Sperm Membrane Potential Is a Good Indicator of the Ability of Sperm to Undergo Sapacitation

Mouse sperm that do not hyperpolarize, do not hyperactivate and do not undergo regulated acrosomal exocytosis, the two endpoints of sperm capacitation (Demott and Suarez, 1992; Yanagimachi, 1994; Buffone et al., 2009). To determine whether capacitated human sperm membrane potential correlated with the ability of sperm to undergo acrosomal exocytosis, we used our flow cytometry method to calculate membrane potential in 17 capacitated donor normozoospermic sperm samples. In parallel, we treated the sperm with the calcium ionophore A23187, which induces acrosomal exocytosis (Köhn et al., 1997; Moody et al., 2017; Puga Molina et al., 2017) and determined the percentage of sperm in each sample that underwent acrosomal exocytosis. A scatter plot comparing the two values revealed that the membrane potential values obtained by flow cytometry correlated significantly with the percentage of cells that underwent acrosomal exocytosis (**Figure 3A**).

To determine whether capacitated sperm membrane potential correlated with sperm hyperactivation (HA), we used computer-assisted sperm analysis to measure three parameters associated with HA: curvilinear velocity (VCL), amplitude of lateral head displacement (AHL), and linearity (LIN). Sperm with values of VCL>150 μm/s, AHL>7.0 μm and LIN <50% were considered hyperactivated (Mortimer et al., 1998). The percentage of sperm in each of 27 normozoospermic donor samples, correlated significantly with membrane potential values (**Figure 3B**). Specifically, VCL and ALH values (**Figures 3C,D**), but not LIN values (**Figure 3E**), correlated with sperm membrane potential. Together, these data indicate that human sperm membrane potential is a good indicator of the ability of sperm to undergo capacitation.

Membrane Potential of Capacitated Human Sperm Correlates With Fertilization Ratio in IVF Patients

Next, we wanted to determine whether the membrane potential could indicate the ability of sperm to fertilize an egg. To address this question, we performed our flow cytometric assay on excess samples from 49 normozoospermic men whose sperm was used for conventional IVF. We found that the percentage of fertilized oocytes (reported as fertilization ratio) from these patients significantly correlated with the absolute value of membrane potential of capacitated sperm. Those with more negative membrane potential had higher fertilization ratios than those with more positive membrane potential (**Figure 4**).

If IVF failure were caused by impaired sperm capacitation, this defect would be bypassed by ICSI. Thus, we reviewed the ICSI outcome of 14 patients who underwent this procedure and whose sperm resulted in an IVF ratio of less than 0.7. In three cases, the fertilization ratio was the same in ICSI and conventional IVF. However, for the other 11, the ICSI fertilization ratio was higher than the IVF ratio (mean values n = 14 0.8648 vs. 0.4208; Wilcoxon test, P = 0.0005) (**Supplementary Figure 2A**). This result suggests that the low IVF ratios were related to impaired sperm capacitation.

Fertile Sperm Are Hyperpolarized

Given the correlation we observed between sperm membrane potential values and fertilization ratios in IVF, we wondered whether we could detect a significant difference in sperm membrane potential values between patients with successful and non-successful IVF, which are defined as fertilization ratio

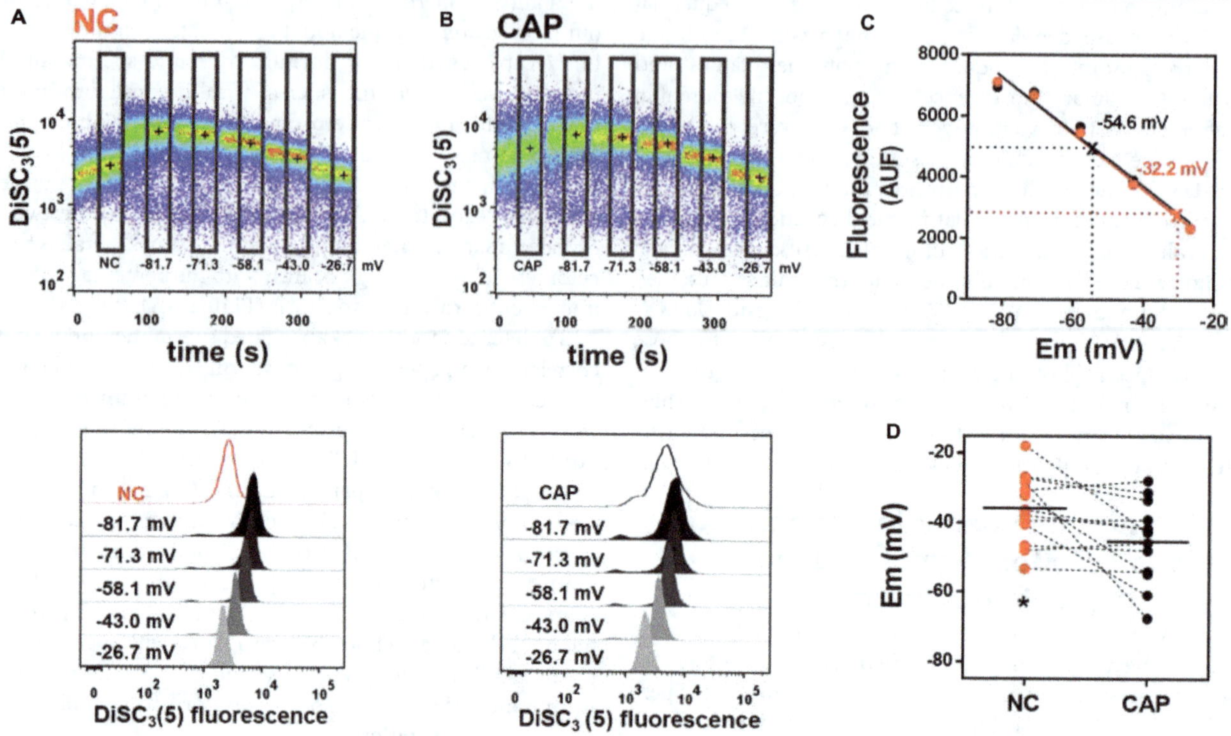

FIGURE 2 | Incubation in capacitating media hyperpolarizes human sperm. **(A,B)** Upper panel: Representative dot plot of $DiSC_3(5)$ fluorescence traces from human donor sperm incubated in non-capacitated (**A**, "NC") or capacitating (**B**, "CAP") HTF media. Black crosses indicate the median $DiSC_3(5)$ fluorescence of sperm within the gates (rectangles) defined for each addition. Calibration was performed as in **Figure 1** with 1 μM valinomycin and sequential additions of KCl, corresponding to the theoretical plasma membrane potential values of –81.7, –71.3, –58.1, –43.0, and –26.7 mV. Lower panels: Histograms of $DiSC_3(5)$ fluorescence from selected gates as indicated in flow cytometry dot plots above. **(C)** Linear regression of the calibration curves built from the median fluorescence from NC and CAP sperm obtained in panels **A,B**. Interpolated values for each curve are indicated. NC r^2 = 0.9670, CAP r^2 = 0.9860. **(D)** Sperm membrane potential values in both NC and CAP media were obtained by linearly interpolating the theoretical membrane potential values versus arbitrary units of fluorescence of each trace. Dashed lines connect the same samples incubated in NC and CAP media. *P = 0.0212 by paired t-test.

>0.7 or <0.7, respectively (Harris et al., 2019). This cut-off was determined by calculating the mean fertilization ratio in conventional IVF cases quarterly and yearly. Thus, we dichotomized the samples into those with fertilization ratio >0.7 (n = 27) and those with fertilization ratio <0.7 (n = 22) and compared their sperm membrane potential values. Whereas sperm samples with fertilization ratio >0.7 had an average membrane potential of −58.03 ± 3.00 mV, sperm samples with fertilization ratio <0.7 had an average membrane potential of −40.61 ± 2.60 mV (**Figure 5A**).

We next investigated whether sperm samples capable of fertilizing an egg, hyperpolarize during capacitation. These experiments require measuring the membrane potential before (time = 0 h) and after capacitation (time = 18 h). This kind of experiment was not possible to do using fresh sperm because these samples were obtained after finishing clinical procedures and were kept in capacitating media for 2–4 h. Therefore, we did not have a real 0 time point. For this reason, we decided to use and aliquot of frozen samples from anonymous donors that had resulted in pregnancies. We used flow cytometry in these frozen samples to measure membrane potential before (t = 0) and after capacitation (t = 18 h). We found that all these fertile sperm samples underwent hyperpolarization after capacitation, changing from −47.9 ± 4.4 to −62.5 ± 4.1 mV (**Figure 5B**). Although there could be many differences between frozen and fresh sperm samples, it is noteworthy that the mean membrane potential value of frozen sperm from fertile donors after capacitation was similar to the membrane potential value of fresh sperm samples from patients with successful IVF (fertilization ratio >0.7) (**Figure 5A**). In addition, the mean membrane potential values of the frozen sperm from fertile donors before capacitation, was similar to that of fresh sperm from patients with fertilization ratio <0.7. These findings suggest that infertile sperm fail to hyperpolarize in capacitating conditions: even though the samples with lower fertilization ratio were incubated in capacitated conditions, they apparently failed to undergo hyperpolarization and failed to capacitate and fertilize. The frozen samples hyperpolarized and all of them were capable of fertilizing an egg.

Membrane Potential May Be Used to Predict Fertility Success

Finally, we wanted to determine whether membrane potential values could be used to predict sperm capacitation state and fertilization success. To do this, we first determined a value of

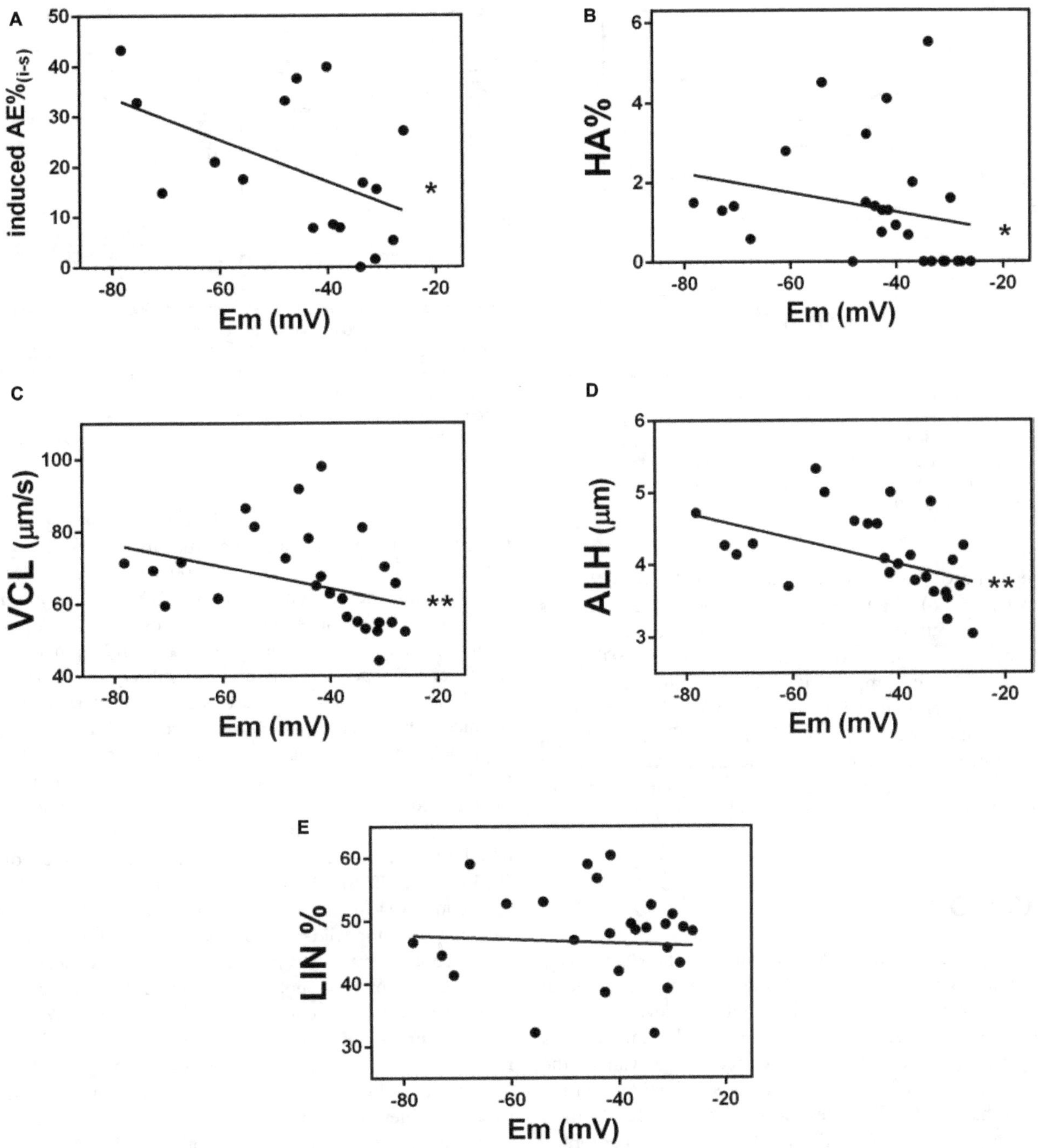

FIGURE 3 | Membrane potential correlates with events related to capacitation. Correlation between absolute values of membrane potential (Em) of donor sperm incubated in HTF non-commercial capacitating media and the following: **(A)** acrosomal exocytosis (AE) induced by 10 μM A23187 (*P = 0.0366); **(B)** hyperactivated motility (HA%) (r = −0.4865, *P = 0.0101); **(C)** curvilinear velocity (VCL) (r = −0.5000, **P = 0.0079); **(D)** lateral head displacement (ALH) (r = −0.5497, **P = 0.0030), and **(E)** linearity coefficient (LIN) (r = −0.0464, P = 0.8182).

membrane potential that allowed us to characterize a sample as either hyperpolarized or depolarized. We used the receiving operating characteristic curve and the maximum Youden index to determine the optimal cut-off value. We considered samples with fertilization ratio >0.7 as the reference for a positive outcome and <0.7 as a negative outcome. The optimal cut-off with 81.82% (59.72 to 84.81%) sensitivity and 88.89% (70.84 to 97.65%) specificity was −46 mV (**Figure 6A**). We then applied this cut-off value and found that those samples with a sperm membrane potential value more hyperpolarized than −46 mV had a significantly higher IVF fertilization ratio than those with a sperm membrane potential value

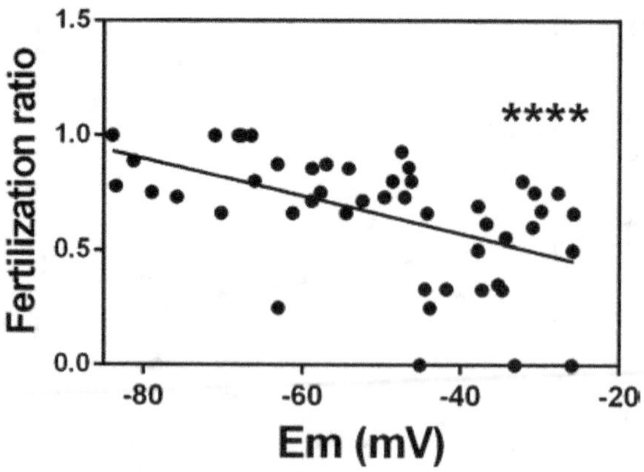

FIGURE 4 | *In vitro* fertilization ratio correlates with sperm membrane potential in patients with normozoospermic infertility. Spearman correlation between sperm membrane potential (Em) from normozoospermic patients undergoing conventional *in vitro* fertilization and fertilization ratio. Fertilization ratio was calculated as the number of normally fertilized mature oocytes with two pronuclei divided by total number of inseminated mature oocytes. $n = 49$, $r = -0.5855$, $^{****}P < 0.0001$.

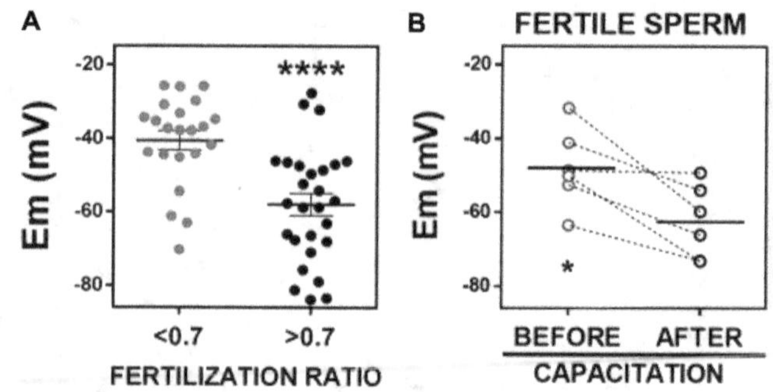

FIGURE 5 | Fertile sperm are hyperpolarized. **(A)** Sperm membrane potential (Em) values from patients with *in vitro* fertilization ratios <0.7 ($n = 22$; -40.61 ± 2.60 mV) or >0.7 ($n = 27$, -58.03 ± 3.00 mV). $^{****}P < 0.0001$ by unpaired *t*-test. **(B)** Membrane potential of fertile frozen sperm samples from patients that conceived a pregnancy, incubated in commercial capacitating media for 1 h (before capacitation, -47.92 ± 4.38 mV) or 18 h (after capacitation, -62.51 ± 4.05 mV). $n = 6$, $^{*}P = 0.0146$ by paired *t*-test.

more depolarized than −46 mV (0.46 ± 0.06, $n = 21$, vs. 0.80 ± 0.03, $n = 28$) (**Figure 6B**). Furthermore, the percentages of sperm that underwent induced acrosomal exocytosis (**Figure 6C**) and hyperactivated motility (**Figure 6D**) were significantly higher in samples with sperm membrane potential values more hyperpolarized than −46 mV. However, ICSI fertilization ratios were not significantly different between sperm samples with membrane potential values more positive and more negative than −46 mV (**Supplementary Figure S2**). This result is not surprisingly because ICSI bypasses sperm capacitation.

DISCUSSION

Here, we report a new method that combines flow-cytometry with the voltage sensitive dye $DiSC_3(5)$ to quantify human sperm membrane potential. This technique could be developed as a new tool to predict sperm fertility capacity. This method has several advantages over other available methods to evaluate the ability of human sperm to capacitate. It is less subjective and time consuming than the CapScore test, which assays the localization pattern of a ganglioside (GM1) within the plasma membrane as a marker of capacitation. This method requires staining, counting, and correctly identifying staining patterns in more than 150 individual sperm (Moody et al., 2017). Patch clamp can be used to measure sperm membrane potential, but the flow cytometry method is simpler and can evaluate membrane potential in higher number of sperm than this technique (Brown et al., 2016). Finally, our flow cytometry method excludes non-viable sperm and requires a smaller sperm sample than does spectrophotometry (0.25×10^6 sperm vs. 4×10^6 sperm).

We argue that quantification of human sperm membrane potential by flow cytometry is a valid method to predict human sperm fertility success for several reasons. First, hyperpolarization is a key event in sperm becoming competent to fertilize an egg in many mammalian species (Zeng et al., 1995; Hernández-González et al., 2007; López-González et al., 2014). In murine and bovine sperm, lack of hyperpolarization is associated with failure to undergo acrosomal exocytosis (Zeng et al., 1995; De La Vega-Beltran et al., 2012). An increase in membrane K^+ permeability and the subsequent sperm plasma membrane hyperpolarization are essential for sperm capacitation in mice (Chávez et al., 2013). Furthermore, human sperm also hyperpolarize under capacitating conditions (López-González et al., 2014). Brown et al. showed an association between depolarized membrane potential values and poor fertilization rate, as 2 of 19 IVF patients that they analyzed had highly depolarized membrane potential and a low fertilization ratio (Brown et al., 2016).

Second, we validated our method by showing that it produced similar values for wild-type and *Slo3*$^{-/-}$ mouse sperm as have been reported by other methods (Santi et al., 2010). Third, the mean membrane potential value of human sperm from donors capacitated in commercial IVF media (-57.7 ± 4.1 mV, $N = 22$, **Supplementary Figure S3**) is consistent with the value reported by Patrat et al. (2002) from spectrofluorimetric assays (-57.8 ± 2.20 mV, $n = 12$). In addition, we obtained similar values of human sperm membrane potential by spectrophotometry and flow cytometry. Fourth, the mean value of sperm membrane potential we calculated from patients with fertilization ratio <0.7 (-40.61 ± 2.60 mV) was similar to the value Calzada and Tellez (1997) obtained via a radioactivity assay of sperm from patients with idiopathic infertility (-35.00 ± 1.60 mV). Our value was also similar to the mean membrane potential value of non-capacitated sperm that Linares-Hernández et al. (1998) measured with spectrophotometry (-40.00 ± 6.00 mV). Conversely, we found that membrane potential values of capacitated sperm from patients with successful IVF (-58.03 ± 3.00 mV), from frozen fertile samples (-62.5 ± 4.1 mV), and from fertile donors included in this study (-64.1 ± 7.9 mV

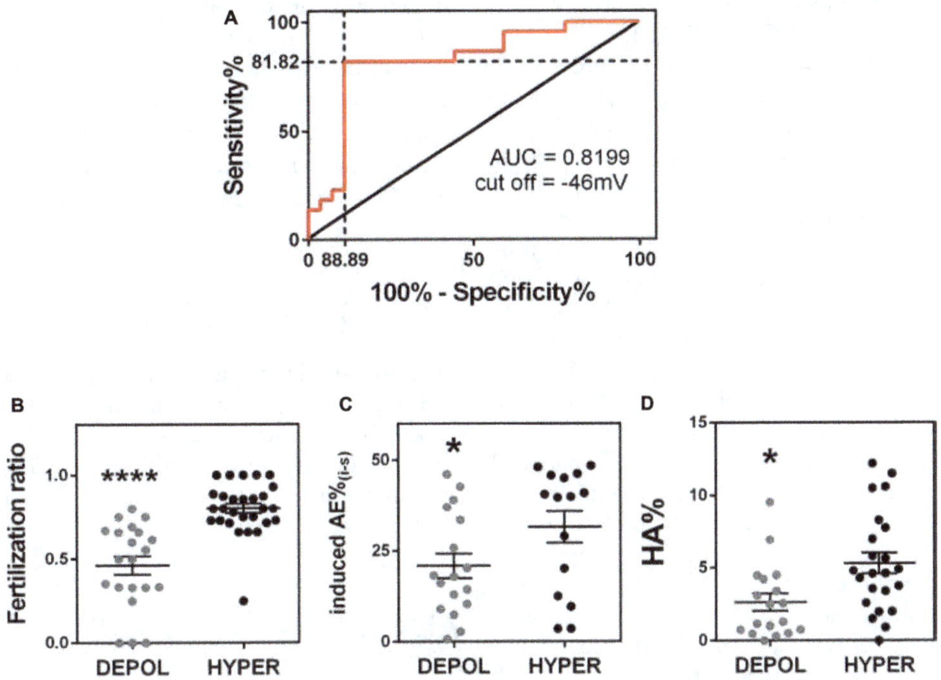

FIGURE 6 | Membrane potential predicts fertility success. **(A)** Receiver operating characteristic curve analysis of model including the sperm membrane potential from 49 normozoospermic infertile patients undergoing conventional *in vitro* fertilization. A fertilization ratio >0.7 was considered positive and <0.7 was considered negative. Area under the curve = 0.8199, $P = 0.0014$. The optimal cut-off value was –45.68 mV (81.82% sensitivity and 88.89% specificity). **(B–D)** Considering the cut off-value of –46 mV, sperm samples were classified as hyperpolarized (HYPER, membrane potential more negative than –46 mV) or depolarized (DEPOL, membrane potential values more positive than –46 mv) and compared to panel **(B)** fertilization ratio ($n = 49$, ****$P < 0.0001$); **(C)** induced acrosomal exocytosis ($n = 32$, *$P = 0.049$); and **(D)** hyperactivated motility ($n = 41$, *$P = 0.031$). All *P*-values were calculated by a Kolmogorov-Smirnov test.

$n = 4$, dark gray, **Supplementary Figure S3**) were similar to the reported values of sperm membrane potential from fertile donors, measured by a radioactivity assay (Calzada -75.0 ± 1.9 mV, $n = 10$).

Fifth, we argue that our method is valid because we found that human sperm, like mouse sperm, hyperpolarized when incubated in capacitating media. However, the extent of this hyperpolarization was smaller in human sperm (mean difference 9.24 mV) than in mouse sperm (mean difference ~15–30 mV) (Espinosa and Darszon, 1995; Zeng et al., 1995; Muñoz-Garay et al., 2001; Demarco et al., 2003; Hernández-González et al., 2006; Santi et al., 2010; De La Vega-Beltran et al., 2012). This difference in membrane potential between capacitated and non-capacitated human sperm is similar to the 5 mV difference reported by using the patch clamp technique (Brown et al., 2016). It is also noteworthy that human capacitated sperm membrane potential values were more heterogeneous than were mouse capacitated sperm values (coefficients of variation 25.7% vs. 0.29%, respectively), even though all the samples analyzed were normozoospermic (≥32% progressive motility; ≥40% total motility; $\geq 15 \times 10^6$ cells/ml). This variability, along with the small difference in membrane potential values between capacitated and non-capacitated sperm, could explain why changes in membrane potential of human sperm during capacitation are difficult to detect by other methods (Puga Molina et al., 2018a).

Sixth, by using this methodology, we found that membrane hyperpolarization positively correlated with the two endpoints of sperm capacitation: hyperactivated motility and acrosomal exocytosis. Hyperpolarization of the plasma membrane is necessary and sufficient for acrosomal exocytosis of mouse sperm (De La Vega-Beltran et al., 2012), but this is the first report that correlates membrane potential with both hyperactivation and the acrosomal exocytosis and highlights the importance of membrane potential in human sperm capacitation.

Finally, we reported here that hyperpolarization measured by our method correlates with IVF success. Only two previous studies attempted to find an association between membrane potential values and human fertility, but the techniques used to measure sperm membrane potential (patch clamp or radioactivity assays) are extremely challenging and not suitable to clinical implementation (Calzada and Tellez, 1997; Brown et al., 2016). Brown et al. showed that sperm plasma membrane depolarization, measured with the patch clamp technique, was associated with low IVF rates. However, these authors did not report a correlation between the values of membrane potential and fertilization ratio. Additionally, they did not address whether the mean values of sperm membrane potential from successful and unsuccessful IVF significantly differed (Brown et al., 2016). Interestingly our results agree with the results also reported in this issue which were independently obtained by Dr. Krapf's group showing that IVF rates correlate to human sperm membrane potential values measured by the spectrophotometry technique (Baro Graf et al., 2020).

Until now, the fluorescent probes DiSC3(5) or DiSBAC2(3) have only been used in combination with flow cytometry to report relative changes in sperm membrane potential (López-González et al., 2014; Escoffier et al., 2015; Puga Molina et al., 2017, 2018b; Brukman et al., 2019) and not absolute values. However, we were able to build upon spectrofluorimetric assays in which $DiSC_3(5)$ fluorescence was conveniently calibrated by using valinomycin and different KCl concentrations, permitting measurement of sperm membrane potential values (Zeng et al., 1995; Demarco et al., 2003; Chávez et al., 2013). Importantly, $DiSC_3(5)$ has no toxic effects on sperm function at the concentrations used (López-González et al., 2014). When constant concentrations of sperm and dye are used, $DiSC_3$ provides reproducible estimates of plasma membrane potential and good signal-to-noise ratio. One potential challenge with using $DiSC_3(5)$ is that it binds to mitochondria in their normal energized state, and the resulting mitochondrial fluorescence could contribute to the fluorescence signal (Rink et al., 1980). However, we previously measured $DiSC_3(5)$ fluorescence in the presence and absence of several mitochondrial uncouplers (CCCP, antimycin, and oligomycin) and showed that, in all conditions, the plasma membrane potential of valinomycin-treated mouse sperm responds to the external K^+ concentration in accordance with the Nernst equation (Chávez et al., 2013). In addition, Baro Graf et al. (2019) showed that the mitochondrial electron transport inhibitor rotenone does not affect $DiSC_3(5)$ membrane potential measurements in human sperm.

In summary, our data indicate that the absolute value of sperm membrane potential is a good indicator of human sperm fertilizing ability. We found that a membrane potential value of −46 mV could be used to classify the sperm samples as depolarized or hyperpolarized and predict their fertilization success. However, a larger cohort of patients is needed to determine a more accurate cut-off value of membrane potential for use in a clinical setting. Our findings also suggest the possibility of using capacitated sperm membrane potential values as a novel tool to diagnose idiopathic normozoospermic male infertility. In addition, this method could be developed as a fast, simple, clinically feasible assay to personalize fertility treatment plans for normozoospermic infertile men (Oehninger et al., 2014; Palermo et al., 2015). For example, normozoospermic men whose sperm have hyperpolarized values of membrane potential could be guided by clinicians to approaches such as intrauterine insemination or conventional IVF. Conversely, men with sperm with depolarized values of membrane potential might be able to avoid the emotional, physical, and financial costs associated with repeated intrauterine or IVF cycles by being guided to ICSI. Given that few IVF clinics are likely to have a flow cytometer, future work will be aimed at developing a more automated method to measure sperm membrane potential.

ETHICS STATEMENT

The studies involving human participants were reviewed and approved by Washington University Institutional Review Board. The patients/participants provided their written informed consent to participate in this study. The animal study was reviewed and approved by Animal Care and Use Committee at Washington University.

AUTHOR CONTRIBUTIONS

LP, CS, SG, and PL conceived and planned the experiments. LP and SG performed the experiments, analyzed the data, and obtained consent from patients. LP and CS discussed the results and wrote the manuscript. AB-A performed spectrophotometry assays and helped with mouse experiments. All authors contributed to revising the manuscript and read and approved the submitted version.

FUNDING

This work was supported by NIH grants R01HD069631 and R01HD095628 to CS.

ACKNOWLEDGMENTS

We thank Yang-Yang Yuan for helping with mice and sperm samples, the Fertility and Reproductive Medicine Center for providing human sperm samples, Paul Schlesinger for the use of Spectrophotometer, Jeremias Incicco for their help with statistical analysis, and Deborah Frank for editorial help.

REFERENCES

Austin, C. R. (1951). Observations on the penetration of the sperm in the mammalian egg. *Aust. J. Sci. Res. Ser. B Biologic. Sci.* 4, 581–596. doi: 10.1071/BI9510581

Baro Graf, C., Ritagliati, C., Stival, C., Balestrini, P. A., Buffone, M. G., and Krapf, D. (2019). Determination of a robust assay for human sperm membrane potential analysis. *Front. Cell Dev. Biol.* 7:101. doi: 10.3389/fcell.2019.00101

Baro Graf, C., Ritagliati, C., Torres-Monserrat, V., Stival, C., Carizza, C., Buffone, M. G., et al. (2020). Membrane potential assessment by fluorimetry as a predictor tool of human sperm fertilizing capacity. *Front. Cell Dev. Biol.* 7:383. doi: 10.3389/fcell.2019.00383

Bracke, A., Peeters, K., Punjabi, U., Hoogewijs, D., and Dewilde, S. A. O. (2018). A search for molecular mechanisms underlying male idiopathic infertility. *Reprod. Biomed. Online* 36, 327–339. doi: 10.1016/j.rbmo.2017.12.005

Brown, S. G., Publicover, S. J., Mansell, S. A., Lishko, P. V., Williams, H. L., Ramalingam, M., et al. (2016). Depolarization of sperm membrane potential is a common feature of men with subfertility and is associated with low fertilization rate at IVF. *Hum. Reprod* 31, 1147–1157. doi: 10.1093/humrep/dew056

Brukman, N. G., Nuñez, S. Y., Puga Molina, L., del, C., Buffone, M. G., Darszon, A., et al. (2019). Tyrosine phosphorylation signaling regulates Ca 2+ entry by affecting intracellular pH during human sperm capacitation. *J. Cellular Physiol.* 234, 5276–5288. doi: 10.1002/jcp.27337

Buffone, M. G., Rodriguez-Miranda, E., Storey, B. T., and Gerton, G. L. (2009). Acrosomal exocytosis of mouse sperm progresses in a consistent direction in response to zona pellucida. *J. Cellular Physiol.* 220, 611–620. doi: 10.1002/jcp.21781

Calzada, L., and Tellez, J. (1997). Defective function of membrane potential (Ψ) on sperm of infertile men. *Arch. Androl.* 38, 151–155. doi: 10.3109/01485019708987892

Chang, M. C. (1951). Fertilizing capacity of spermatozoa deposited into the fallopian tubes. *Nature* 168, 697–698. doi: 10.1038/168697b0

Chávez, J. C., De La Vega-Beltrá, N. J. L., Escoffier, J., Visconti, P. E., Treviñ, O. C. L., Darszon, A., et al. (2013). Ion permeabilities in mouse sperm reveal an external trigger for SLO3-dependent hyperpolarization. *PLoS ONE* 8:e60578. doi: 10.1371/journal.pone.0060578

De La Vega-Beltran, J. L., Sánchez-Cárdenas, C., Krapf, D., Hernandez-González, E. O., Wertheimer, E., Treviño, C. L., et al. (2012). Mouse sperm membrane potential hyperpolarization is necessary and sufficient to prepare sperm for the acrosome reaction. *J. Biologic. Chem.* 287, 44384–44393. doi: 10.1074/jbc.M112.393488

Demarco, I. A., Espinosa, F., Edwards, J., Sosnik, J., La Vega-Beltran, J. L., Hockensmith, J. W., et al. (2003). Involvement of a Na+/HCO Cotransporter in Mouse Sperm Capacitation. *J. Biologic. Chem.* 278, 7001–7009. doi: 10.1074/jbc.m206284200

Demott, R. P., and Suarez, S. S. (1992). Hyperactivated sperm progress in the mouse oviduct. *Biol. reprod.* 46, 779–785. doi: 10.1095/biolreprod46.5.779

Escoffier, J., Navarrete, F., Haddad, D., Santi, C. M., Darszon, A., and Visconti, P. E. (2015). Flow Cytometry Analysis Reveals That Only a Subpopulation of Mouse Sperm Undergoes Hyperpolarization During Capacitation. *Biol. Reprod.* 92, 1–11. doi: 10.1095/biolreprod.114.127266

Espinosa, F., and Darszon, A. (1995). Mouse sperm membrane potential: changes induced by Ca 2+. *FEBS Lett.* 372, 119–125. doi: 10.1016/0014-5793(95)00962-9

Harris, A. L., Vanegas, J. C., Hariton, E., Bortoletto, P., Palmor, M., Humphries, L. A., et al. (2019). Semen parameters on the day of oocyte retrieval predict low fertilization during conventional insemination IVF cycles. *J. Assist. Reprod. Genet.* 36, 291–298. doi: 10.1007/s10815-018-1336-1339

Hernández-González, E. O., Sosnik, J., Edwards, J., Acevedo, J. J., Mendoza-Lujambio, I., López-González, I., et al. (2006). Sodium and epithelial sodium channels participate in the regulation of the capacitation-associated hyperpolarization in mouse sperm. *J. Biologic. Chem.* 281, 5623–5633. doi: 10.1074/jbc.M508172200

Hernández-González, E. O., Treviño, C. L., Castellano, L. E., De La Vega-Beltrán, J. L., Ocampo, A. Y., Wertheimer, E., et al. (2007). Involvement of cystic fibrosis transmembrane conductance regulator in mouse sperm capacitation. *J. Biologic. Chem.* 282, 24397–24406. doi: 10.1074/jbc.M701603200

Köhn, F. M., Mack, S. R., Schill, W. B., and Zaneveld, L. J. (1997). Detection of human sperm acrosome reaction: comparison between methods using double staining. Pisum sativum agglutinin, concanavalin A and transmission electron microscopy. *Hum. Reprod.* 12, 714–721. doi: 10.1093/humrep/12.4.714

Kumar, N., and Singh, A. (2015). Trends of male factor infertility, an important cause of infertility: a review of literature. *J. Hum. Reprod. Sci.* 8, 191–196. doi: 10.4103/0974-1208.170370

Linares-Hernández, L., Guzmán-Grenfell, A. M., Hicks-Gomez, J. J., and González-Martínez, M. T. (1998). Voltage-dependent calcium influx in human sperm assessed by simultaneous optical detection of intracellular calcium and membrane potential. *Biochim. Biophys. Acta Biomembr.* 1372, 1–12. doi: 10.1016/S0005-2736(98)00035-32

López-González, I., Torres-Rodríguez, P., Sánchez-Carranza, O., Solís-López, A., Santi, C. M., Darszon, A., et al. (2014). Membrane hyperpolarization during human sperm capacitation. *Mol. Hum. Reprod.* 20, 619–629. doi: 10.1093/molehr/gau029

Moody, M. A., Cardona, C., Simpson, A. J., Smith, T. T., Travis, A. J., and Ostermeier, G. C. (2017). Validation of a laboratory-developed test of human sperm capacitation. *Mol. Reprod. Dev.* 84, 408–422. doi: 10.1002/mrd.22801

Mortimer, S. T., Swan, M. A., and Mortimer, D. (1998). Effect of seminal plasma on capacitation and hyperactivation in human spermatozoa. *Hum. Reprod.* 13, 2139–2146. doi: 10.1093/humrep/13.8.2139

Muñoz-Garay, C., José, L., Delgado, R., Labarca, P., Felix, R., and Darszon, A. (2001). Inwardly rectifying K+ channels in spermatogenic cells: functional expression and implication in sperm capacitation. *Dev. biol.* 234, 261–274. doi: 10.1006/dbio.2001.0196

Oehninger, S., Franken, D. R., and Ombelet, W. (2014). Sperm functional tests. *Fertil. Steril.* 102, 1528–1533. doi: 10.1016/j.fertnstert.2014.09.044

Palermo, G. D., Neri, Q. V., and Rosenwaks, Z. (2015). To ICSI or not to ICSI. *Semin. Reprod. Med.* 33, 92–102. doi: 10.1055/s-0035-1546825

Patrat, C., Serres, C., and Jouannet, P. (2002). Progesterone induces hyperpolarization after a transient depolarization phase in human spermatozoa. *Biol. Reprod.* 66, 1775–1780. doi: 10.1095/biolreprod66.6.1775

Puga Molina, L. C., Luque, G. M., Balestrini, P. A., Marín-Briggiler, C. I., Romarowski, A., and Buffone, M. G. (2018a). Molecular Basis of Human Sperm Capacitation. *Front. Cell Dev. Biol.* 6:72. doi: 10.3389/fcell.2018.00072

Puga Molina, L. C., Pinto, N. A., Torres, N. I., González-Cota, A. L., Luque, G. M., Balestrini, P. A., et al. (2018b). CFTR/ENaC dependent regulation of membrane potential during human sperm capacitation is initiated by bicarbonate uptake through NBC. *J. Biologic. Chem.* 293, 9924–9936. doi: 10.1074/jbc.RA118.003166

Puga Molina, L. C., Pinto, N. A., Torres Rodríguez, P., Romarowski, A., Vicens Sanchez, A., Visconti, P. E., et al. (2017). Essential Role of CFTR in PKA-Dependent Phosphorylation. Alkalinization, and Hyperpolarization During Human Sperm Capacitation. *.J. Cell. Physiol.* 232, 1404–1414. doi: 10.1002/jcp.25634

Rink, T. J., Montecucco, C., Hesketh, T. R., and Tsien, R. Y. (1980). Lymphocyte membrane potential assessed with fluorescent probes. *BBA Biomembr.* 595, 15–30. doi: 10.1016/0005-2736(80)90243-90246

Santi, C. M., Martínez-López, P., de la Vega-Beltrán, J. L., Butler, A., Alisio, A., Darszon, A., et al. (2010). The SLO3 sperm-specific potassium channel plays a vital role in male fertility. *FEBS lett.* 584, 1041–1046. doi: 10.1016/j.febslet.2010.02.005

Sharma, R., Biedenharn, K. R., Fedor, J. M., and Agarwal, A. (2013). Lifestyle factors and reproductive health: taking control of your fertility. *Reprod. Biol. Endocrinol.* 11:66. doi: 10.1186/1477-7827-11-66

World Health Organization [WHO] (2010). *WHO Laboratory Manual for the Examination and Processing of Human Semen*, 2nd Edn, 286. doi: 10.1038/aja.2008.57

Yanagimachi, R. (1994). *Mammalian fertilization*. E. Knobil. New York, NY: Raven Press.

Zeng, X.-H., Yang, C., Kim, S. T., Lingle, C. J., and Xia, X.-M. (2011). Deletion of the Slo3 gene abolishes alkalization-activated K+ current in mouse spermatozoa. *Proc. Nat. Acad. Sci.* 108, 5879–5884. doi: 10.1073/pnas.1100240108

Zeng, Y., Clark, E. N., and Florman, H. M. (1995). Sperm membrane potential: hyperpolarization during capacitation regulates zona pellucida-dependent acrosomal secretion. *Dev. biol.* 171, 554–563. doi: 10.1006/dbio.1995.1304

12

Proteomic Changes in Human Sperm During Sequential *in vitro* Capacitation and Acrosome Reaction

Judit Castillo[1]*, Orleigh Adeleccia Bogle[1], Meritxell Jodar[1], Forough Torabi[2], David Delgado-Dueñas[1], Josep Maria Estanyol[3], Josep Lluís Ballescà[4], David Miller[2] and Rafael Oliva[1,5]*

[1] Molecular Biology of Reproduction and Development Research Group, Institut d'Investigacions Biomèdiques August Pi i Sunyer (IDIBAPS), Fundació Clínic per a la Recerca Biomèdica, Department of Biomedical Sciences, Faculty of Medicine and Health Sciences, Universitat de Barcelona, Barcelona, Spain, [2] LIGHT Laboratories, Leeds Institute of Cardiovascular and Metabolic Medicine, University of Leeds, Leeds, United Kingdom, [3] Proteomics Unit, Scientific and Technical Services, Universitat de Barcelona, Barcelona, Spain, [4] Clinic Institute of Gynaecology, Obstetrics and Neonatology, Hospital Clínic, Barcelona, Spain, [5] Biochemistry and Molecular Genetics Service, Hospital Clínic, Barcelona, Spain

***Correspondence:**
Judit Castillo
juditcastillo@ub.edu
Rafael Oliva
roliva@ub.edu

The male gamete is not completely mature after ejaculation and requires further events in the female genital tract to acquire fertilizing ability, including the processes of capacitation and acrosome reaction. In order to shed light on protein changes experienced by the sperm cell in preparation for fertilization, a comprehensive quantitative proteomic profiling based on isotopic peptide labeling and liquid chromatography followed by tandem mass spectrometry was performed on spermatozoa from three donors of proven fertility under three sequential conditions: purification with density gradient centrifugation, incubation with capacitation medium, and induction of acrosome reaction by exposure to the calcium ionophore A23187. After applying strict selection criteria for peptide quantification and for statistical analyses, 36 proteins with significant changes in their relative abundance within sperm protein extracts were detected. Moreover, the presence of peptide residues potentially harboring sites for post-translational modification was revealed, suggesting that protein modification may be an important mechanism in sperm maturation. In this regard, increased levels of proteins mainly involved in motility and signaling, both regulated by protein modifiers, were detected in sperm lysates following incubation with capacitation medium. In contrast, less abundant proteins in acrosome-reacted cell lysates did not contain potentially modifiable residues, suggesting the possibility that all those proteins might be relocated or released during the process. Protein-protein interaction analysis revealed a subset of proteins potentially involved in sperm maturation, including the proteins Erlin-2 (ERLIN2), Gamma-glutamyl hydrolase (GGH) and Transmembrane emp24 domain-containing protein 10 (TMED10). These results contribute to the current knowledge of the molecular basis of human fertilization. It should now be possible to further validate the potential role of the detected altered proteins as modulators of male infertility.

Keywords: sperm, spermatozoa, capacitation, acrosome reaction, proteomics, mass spectrometry, TMT labeling

INTRODUCTION

Mammalian fertilization relies on the ability of spermatozoa to penetrate through the zona pellucida (ZP) and fuse with the oolemma. Testicular spermatozoa, however, although morphologically mature, lack this essential capacity and additional post-gonadal stages of maturation are required in both the male and the female reproductive tracts. After being released into the lumen of the seminiferous tubules, testicular spermatozoa are sequentially modified throughout their transit in the epididymis, acquiring forward progressive motility (Dacheux and Dacheux, 2014). However, maturation is not completed until spermatozoa undergo capacitation during their journey through the female genital tract (Visconti et al., 1998; Stival et al., 2016; Puga Molina et al., 2018a). Sperm are only capable of successfully fertilizing the oocyte after completing this essential post-ejaculatory step, which is a prerequisite to the acrosome reaction (Barros, 1967; Gaddum and Blandau, 1970; Visconti and Kopf, 1998; Visconti et al., 1998, 2011; De Jonge, 2005; Liu et al., 2007).

Sperm capacitation is a recognized phenomenon associated with acquisition of hyperactive motility comprising a complex set of highly regulated molecular and physiological events. As mature spermatozoa are no longer engaged in nuclear gene expression (Oliva, 2006; Jodar et al., 2013), understanding the role of protein modifiers, cell-cell communication and signaling pathways is essential (Baldi et al., 1996; Halet et al., 2003; De Jonge, 2005; Visconti et al., 2011; Buffone et al., 2012; Signorelli et al., 2012; Cuasnicú et al., 2016; Barrachina et al., 2018; Torabi et al., 2017b). For instance, many studies have correlated capacitation with an increase in cholesterol efflux from the sperm membrane (Visconti et al., 2002; Gadella et al., 2008) that modulates intracellular levels of calcium and bicarbonate ions (Visconti et al., 2011; Battistone et al., 2013; Li et al., 2014; Puga Molina et al., 2018a). As a consequence, other changes during capacitation include the hyperpolarization of the sperm plasma membrane (Puga Molina et al., 2017, 2018b), and the enhanced activity of protein kinases, phosphatases and acetylases (Ficarro et al., 2003; Ickowicz et al., 2012; Battistone et al., 2014; Sati et al., 2014; Wang J. et al., 2015; Puga Molina et al., 2017; Ritagliati et al., 2018). In addition, protein regulation through redox signaling has been proposed as one of the critical properties of sperm capacitation (O'Flaherty, 2015). All these changes occur prior to the acrosome reaction, a calcium-dependent process leading to a sequential release of the acrosomal contents (Buffone et al., 2008), which includes hydrolytic enzymes, such as acrosin and hyaluronidase, that allow sperm penetration through the ZP and subsequent fusion with the oocyte membrane (Brucker and Lipford, 1995; Patrat et al., 2000; Ickowicz et al., 2012; De Jonge and Barratt, 2013; Petit et al., 2013; Sánchez-Cárdenas et al., 2014; Singh and Rajender, 2015; Ito and Toshimori, 2016; Torabi et al., 2017a). The role of kinases and tyrosine phosphorylation has been also established as essential for sperm to correctly undergo acrosome reaction (Ickowicz et al., 2012; Breitbart and Finkelstein, 2015).

The analysis of protein profiles of lysates obtained from human sperm cell has revealed a complex set of proteins involved in processes culminating in oocyte fertilization, including capacitation, the acrosome reaction, oocyte penetration and sperm-oocyte fusion (Castillo et al., 2018). Indeed, capacitation is the event most studied by the application of quantitative proteomic strategies in human (Ficarro et al., 2003; Secciani et al., 2009; Wang J. et al., 2015; Yu et al., 2015; Hernández-Silva et al., 2019) as well as in model species, such as mice (Baker et al., 2010), boars (Bailey et al., 2005; Kwon et al., 2014), bulls (Park et al., 2012) and buffalo (Jagan Mohanarao and Atreja, 2011; Hou et al., 2019). Recently, Hernández-Silva et al. (2019) approached the proteomic study of human sperm capacitation from the alternative perspective of the seminal fluid components bathing sperm during and following ejaculation. Interestingly, they found a group of seminal fluid derived proteins attached to the sperm surface which inhibits the progress of capacitation by negatively affecting sperm hyperactivation and protein tyrosine phosphorylation (Hernández-Silva et al., 2019).

The study of the sperm protein composition is contributing not only to increase the knowledge of the male gamete structure and cargo, but also of past and future events related to sperm development and oocyte fertilization, respectively (Amaral et al., 2014a; Codina et al., 2015; Castillo et al., 2018). Mass spectrometry (MS) strategies are rapidly evolving, and novel approaches are currently available that could provide further insights into the maturation of the ejaculated sperm (Codina et al., 2015). Also, identifying protein changes in abundance and post-translational modifications during the different steps of sperm maturation is a good strategy to find candidates that could act as male infertility biomarkers with predictive, diagnostic and prognostic potentials (Rahman et al., 2013; Amaral et al., 2014a; Jodar et al., 2017). However, while the involvement of sperm proteins in ZP binding has been explored by proteomics (Redgrove et al., 2011; Petit et al., 2013), the sperm protein profile after the acrosomal exocytosis has not yet been addressed by MS. In the current study we employed a quantitative proteomics strategy based on isotopic peptide labeling using tandem mass tags (TMT), protein identification by liquid chromatography followed by tandem MS (LC-MS/MS), and strict and robust quantification and statistical analysis to evaluate changes in ejaculated spermatozoa after incubation in capacitation medium and calcium ionofore-induced acrosome reaction, aiming to improve the knowledge of the molecular mechanisms leading to post-ejaculation sperm maturation from a proteomic perspective.

MATERIALS AND METHODS

Biological Material and Sample Collection

Human semen samples were obtained from 3 donors of proven fertility attending the Assisted Reproduction Unit (FIVclinic) at the Clinic Institute of Gynaecology, Obstetrics and Neonatology, from the Hospital Clínic, Barcelona, Spain. The sample size was calculated by considering a balance between (1) a sufficient number of samples to statistically evaluate the significance of the resulting data, and (2) the maximum amount of analytical samples that can be analyzed by quantitative proteomics using

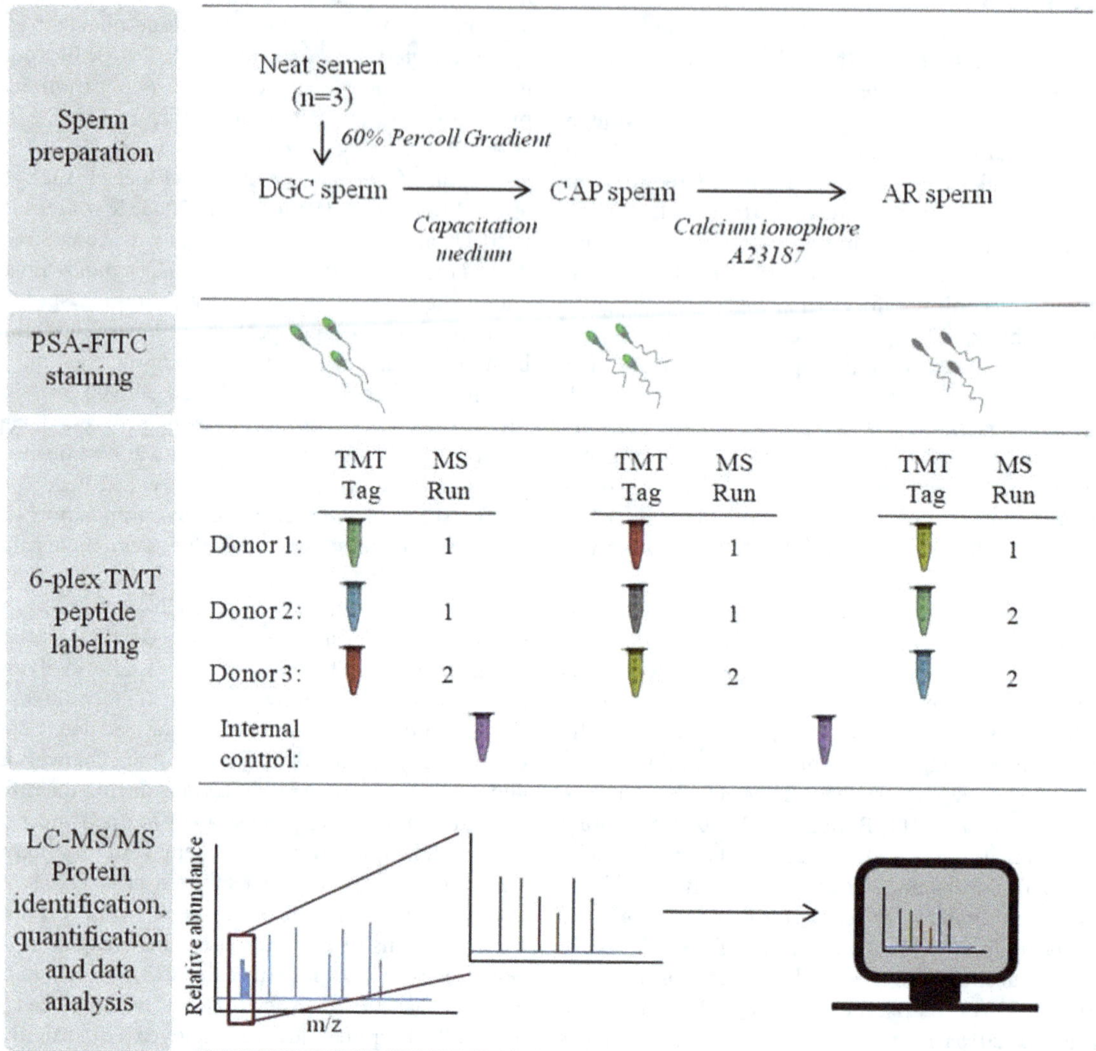

FIGURE 1 | Overall workflow of the experimental procedures. Steps followed for the identification of sperm protein alterations with TMT-LC-MS/MS after consecutive *in vitro* incubation with capacitation medium followed by induction of the acrosome reaction.

a unique set of Tandem Mass Tag^{TM} 6-plex (TMTsixplex^{TM}) Reagents. The ejaculates were collected by masturbation into sterile containers following a minimum of 3 days abstinence. Semen was allowed to liquefy at room temperature and an initial evaluation of the seminal parameters was taken for concentration and motility assessment using the automatic semen analysis system CASA (Computer Assisted Semen Analysis; Proiser, Paterna, Spain). Additional parameters such as sperm variability and morphology were also assessed, using 0.5% (w/v) Eosyn Y and Diff-quick^{TM} staining, respectively. All three ejaculates showed normal parameters according to the limits established by the World of Health Organization (WHO) (World Health Organization, 2010) and were classified as normozoospermic semen samples (**Supplementary Table S1**).

All samples were used in accordance with the appropriate ethical guidelines and Internal Review Board, and the biological material storing and processing was approved by the Clinical Research Ethics Committee of the Hospital Clínic of Barcelona. Written informed consents were obtained from all donors in accordance with the Declaration of Helsinki.

Sperm Preparation

Each ejaculate was processed under three sequential conditions (**Figure 1**): density-gradient centrifugation (DGC sperm), incubation in capacitation medium (CAP sperm) and incubation with the calcium ionophore A23187 to *in vitro* induce the acrosome reaction (AR sperm), following well-established protocols described elsewhere (World Health Organization, 2010; De Jonge and Barratt, 2013) with some minor modifications.

Density-Gradient Centrifugation

Spermatozoa were purified using a 60% Percoll® (Sigma-Aldrich, St Louis, MO, United States) gradient equilibrated with

Hepes-buffered Ham's F10 medium (Gibco, Life Technologies, United Kingdom) supplemented with sodium bicarbonate (0.2% NaHCO3; w/v; Merck, Darmstadt, Germany), sodium pyruvate (0.003% $C_3H_3NaO_3$; w/v; Sigma-Aldrich) and sodium DL lactate solution (0.36% v/v, Sigma-Aldrich). In order to ensure the complete elimination of the gradient material, the recovered sperm cells were washed twice with supplemented Hepes medium and centrifuged at 400 *g* for 10 min. This procedure allowed the purification of the samples from cells other than sperm while maintaining proportions of sperm subpopulations similar to the native semen sample (Mengual et al., 2003; Zhao et al., 2007; Wang G. et al., 2013). The sperm purification efficiency was checked using phase-contrast microscopy. All purified sperm samples contained <1% of potential contaminating cells. For each sample, an aliquot of 20 million of DGC sperm was taken for subsequent procedures of protein solubilization, while the remaining material was subjected to incubation with capacitation medium.

Sperm Incubation With Capacitation Medium

Capacitation medium consisted of Hepes-buffered Ham's F10 medium supplemented with 3.5% of bovine serum albumin (BSA; Sigma-Aldrich). DGC sperm were incubated in 1 ml of capacitation medium for each 10 million of sperm, for 3 h at 37°C with constant rotation. Aliquots of 20 million of CAP sperm from each biological replicates were taken for protein solubilization and the remaining material were used for the incubation with the calcium ionophore A23187.

Sperm Incubation With the Calcium Ionophore A23187 to Induce the Acrosome Reaction

To induce the acrosome reaction, 10 μL of the calcium ionophore A23187 (Sigma-Aldrich, stock solution 1.0 mM in DMSO) was added to approximately 10 million CAP sperm to get a final concentration of 10 μM, following WHO recommendations (World Health Organization, 2010). Spermatozoa were then incubated for 15 min at 37°C. Negative control aliquots were incubated with DMSO (vehicle control) for an equal amount of time (De Jonge and Barratt, 2013). Subsequently, 70% ethanol was added to stop the reaction and the spermatozoa were recovered by centrifugation at 400 *g* for 20 min (World Health Organization, 2010). The viability of the cells was monitored by eosin staining (World Health Organization, 2010). For each replicate, an aliquot of 20 million of AR sperm was used for protein solubilization.

Pisum sativum Agglutinin – Fluorescein Isothiocyanate (PSA-FITC) Labeling

The acrosome reaction was monitored by assessing the integrity of the sperm acrosome vesicle by the PSA-FITC labeling method (World Health Organization, 2010) (**Figure 1**). This fluorescent probe binds to the alpha-methyl mannose and labels the acrosomal content of sperm (Benoff et al., 1993). Briefly, 10 μl of each DGC, CAP, AR sperm and DMSO negative control (3 donors) were smeared on microscope slides in duplicates and were allowed to air dry. The slides were then fixed in 95% (v/v) ethanol for 30 min, and subsequently immersed in 25 μg/ml PSA-FITC staining solution, for 2 h at 4°C. The slides were washed in distilled water, air-dried and covered with mounting medium containing DAPI (Vectashield®, Vector Laboratories, Burlingame, CA, United States). The slides were visualized using a BX50 microscope (Olympus, Hamburg, Germany) equipped with a triple band pass filter, and images were acquired with an Olympus DP71 camera. The sperm acrosome status was categorized as: (1) intact acrosome (more than half of the sperm head with bright and uniform fluorescence); (2) reacted acrosome (a band of fluorescence localized to the equatorial segment or no fluorescing stain at all in the acrosome region); and (3) partially intact acrosome (all other sperm cells) (World Health Organization, 2010; De Jonge and Barratt, 2013). A minimum of 200 sperm were counted per slide and the mean of the two slides per sample represented the final value. Differences between the sperm treatments were evaluated by repeated measures ANOVA with Holm–Sidak correction. P-values < 0.05 were considered significant. Determination of the efficiency of the induction of acrosome reaction was also used as an indirect measure of efficiency on sperm capacitation (Torabi et al., 2017a).

Protein Solubilization and Quantification

From each sperm preparation (DGC, CAP and AR sperm; 3 donors), proteins were solubilized by incubating 20 million spermatozoa with 50 μL of lysis buffer containing 2% SDS and 1 mM Phenylmethylsulfonyl fluoride (PMSF), for 30 min at room temperature with constant gentle shaking. Lysates were centrifuged at 16,000 *g* for 10 min at 4°C. Proteins in the soluble fraction were quantified using the BCA method (Thermo Fisher Scientific, Rockford, IL, United States), following manufacturer's recommendations.

Sperm Peptide Isotopic Labeling (TMT 6-Plex)

A total of 9 protein extracts were used for the proteomic study, corresponding to the DGC, CAP and AR sperm preparations from three different semen donors (**Figure 1**). Differential peptide labeling was performed using Tandem Mass Tag^{TM} 6-plex (TMTsixplex^{TM}) Reagents (Thermo Fisher Scientific). The labeling procedure was adapted from the manufacturer's instructions after several studies conducted in our laboratory (Amaral et al., 2014b; Azpiazu et al., 2014; Bogle et al., 2017; Barrachina et al., 2018). Briefly, proteins were reduced in 9.5 mM tris (2-carboxyethyl) phosphine (TCEP) for 1 h at 55°C, and alkylated with 17 mM iodoacetamide (IAA) for 30 min in the dark. Six-volumes of cold acetone (−20°C) were added and proteins were allowed to precipitate overnight at −20°C. Samples were centrifuged at 17,500 *g* for 10 min, and resuspended in 100 mM triethylammonium bicarbonate (TEAB, Thermo Fisher Scientific) in order to reach a protein concentration of 1 μg/μl. Trypsin was then added at a 1:20 protease-to-protein ratio and the mixture was incubated overnight at 37°C with constant and gentle shaking. Prior to peptide labeling, aliquots were taken from each of the 9 samples and combined in equal amounts to represent the internal control sample. Subsequently, equal amounts of peptides from each sample and the internal control were labeled with TMT isobaric tags. After 1 h of incubation at room temperature, the reaction was quenched with 4 μl of 5% hydroxylamine for 15 min. Labeled peptides from each sample were then combined constituting two different multiplex pools, as indicated in **Figure 1**: Run 1 with 5 samples (TMT tags 127, 128, 129, 130, and 131) and 1 internal control (TMT tag 126), and Run 2 with 4 samples (TMT tags 127, 128, 129, and 130) and 1 internal control (TMT tag 126). The two multiplex pools containing labeled peptides were dried in a vacuum centrifuge to near dryness and resuspended in 20 μL of 0.5% trifluoracetic acid (TFA) in 5% acetonitrile. Subsequently, peptide purification was conducted by using Pierce C18 Spin Columns (Thermo Fisher Scientific) following manufacturer's indications.

Peptide Analysis by LC-MS/MS

Labeled peptides were analyzed via LC-MS/MS with an LTQ-Orbitrap Velos (Thermo-Fisher Scientific) interfaced with an Eksigent nanoLC ultra 2D plus system (AB Sciex, Switzerland). Peptides were injected onto a Pepmap 100 trap column (300 μm × 5 mm, 5 μm, 100 Å) at a flow rate of 400 nL/min. For analytical separation, the trap was switched inline to an Acclaim Pepmap C18 column (75 μm × 15 cm, 3 μm, 100 Å) using a 240 min linear gradient from 5 to 30% acetonitrile in 0.1% formic acid at a flow rate of 400 nL/min. MS/MS analyses were performed using an LTQ Orbitrap Velos (Thermo Fisher Scientific) with a nanoelectrospray ion source. The LTQ-Orbitrap Velos settings included one 30,000 resolution scan for precursor ions followed by MS2 scans of the 20 most intense precursor ions in positive ion mode. MS/MS data acquisition was completed using Xcalibur 2.1 (Thermo Fisher Scientific). The fragmentation method used for identification of TMT labeled peptides was based on higher energy collisional dissociation (HCD) with 40% fixed collision energy (CE).

LC-MS/MS Raw Data Analysis for Protein Identification and Quantification

LC-MS/MS data were analyzed by Proteome Discoverer 1.4.1.14 (Thermo Fisher Scientific). For database searching, raw MS files were submitted to an in-house *Homo sapiens* UniProtKB/Swiss-Prot 2018 database including *Sus scrofa* trypsin (HUMAN_PIG_Uniprot_Release_2018_03.fasta). SEQUEST HT version 28.0 was used (Thermo Fisher Scientific). Searches were performed using the following settings: 2 maximum miss cleavage sites for trypsin, TMT as a N-Terminal modification, lysine-TMT (+229.163 Da) and methionine-oxidation (+15.995 Da) as dynamic modifications, cysteine-carbamidomethylation (+57.021 Da) as static modification, 20 ppm precursor mass tolerance, 0.6 Da fragment mass tolerance, and 5 ppm peak integration tolerance. The criteria used for protein identification was set as 1% FDR and a minimum of one peptide match per protein. The mass spectrometry proteomics data have been deposited to the ProteomeXchange Consortium via the PRIDE (Perez-Riverol et al., 2019) partner repository with the dataset identifier PXD014871.

Quantitative analysis were performed simultaneously with protein identification using Proteome Discoverer software. For quantification, only unambiguous and unique peptides were considered. For that, the 'ungrouping' of proteins from their respective families was used during the quantification process. This avoids the possible ambiguity associated with different isoforms of the same protein (Amaral et al., 2014b; Bogle et al., 2017; Barrachina et al., 2018). The normalized TMT quantification values for each identified spectrum were extracted from the ratio between the reported ion intensities corresponding to each individual sample (TMT-127 to TMT-131) and the reporter ion intensity from the internal control (TMT-126). Quantification values were corrected according to the isotopic purities of the reporter ions provided by the manufacturer.

Statistical Analysis of Proteomic Data Under Strict Quality Criteria

In order to avoid any chance of false positive findings, robust statistics were performed by applying strict selection criteria on the proteomic data. Specifically, only those proteins with at least 1 unique peptide quantified by ≥2 peptide-to-spectrum matches (PSMs) in all the samples, and with a coefficient of variation < 50% in at least 75% of the samples, were considered for further statistical analyses. This pipeline was set by our group in a previous publication (Barrachina et al., 2018). Statistical analysis were conducted in R (R Development Core Team, 2016) with the package "car" (Fox and Weisberg, 2011). Significant differences among the different sperm lysates in the three donors were evaluated using repeated-measures ANOVA test on log-transformed proteomic quantification values. P-values < 0.05 were considered significant if the assumption of sphericity assessed by Mauchly's test had not been violated. In contrast, Greenhouse–Geisser and Huynh–Feldt corrections were applied when data violated the sphericity assumption. Subsequently, the pairwise t-test combined with Holm–Sidak adjustment was applied to identify significant differences between pairs of sample preparations (DGC-CAP, CAP-AR, and DGC-AR). P-values < 0.05 after Holm–Sidak adjustment were considered significant. These results were further filtered by applying similar statistical analysis at peptide level, in order to discard those significant proteins whose corresponding individual peptides do not show statistically significant differences between sperm preparations. Protein abundance alterations were considered significant only when corrected p-values < 0.05 were found at both protein and peptide levels. GraphPad Prism 7 (GraphPad Software Inc., San Diego, CA, United States) was used for visualizing the results.

Functional Prediction of the Proteins Detected With Altered Abundance Using Public Databases

In order to predict the functional involvement of the proteins detected with abundance alterations after each sperm preparation

(DGC, CAP, and AR), different data were retrieved from the UniProt Knowledgebase[1] and Pubmed[2]. Gene Ontology (GO) enrichment analyses on terms related to biological processes and cellular components were performed with the Gene Ontology Consortium database[3] supported by PANTHER v13.1. The significance of the enrichment analyses was calculated by a Fisher's exact test. *P*-values < 0.05 after FDR adjustment were considered statistically significant.

Gene Ontology Consortium database was also used to retrieve a list of proteins associated to GO terms related to capacitation and acrosome reaction processes. Specifically, the selected GO terms were "capacitation," "acrosome reaction," "regulation of acrosome reaction," "acrosome assembly," "acrosome matrix dispersal," "positive regulation of acrosome reaction" and "negative regulation of acrosome reaction," setting *Homo sapiens* as organism. This list of proteins was submitted, together with the list of altered proteins found in this study, to the String database[4], in order to explore potential protein-protein interactions and functional association networks between altered proteins and proteins already known to have a role in ejaculated sperm maturation. For String analysis, the confidence threshold was set at 0.7 (high confidence).

Theoretical post-translational modifications (PTMs) in the differentially abundant peptides were predicted using data contained at the PhosphoSitePlus® database[5].

RESULTS

Induction of the Acrosome Reaction With the Calcium Ionophore A23187

Before initiating the proteomic analysis, PSA-FITC labeling was performed to assess the integrity of the sperm acrosome in DGC, CAP and AR sperm, as well as to indirectly measure the level of capacitation of the sperm cells (Torabi et al., 2017a). As seen in **Figure 2**, the absence of signals in the majority of AR sperm (>74%) after exposure to the calcium ionophore A23187 demonstrates that they had mostly undergone acrosomal exocytosis ($p < 0.01$ one-way ANOVA, Holm–Sidak correction). The significant increase in the number of cells with reacted acrosome also indirectly confirmed the efficiency of sperm capacitation. The three samples showed >85% live cells after incubation with calcium ionophore. PSA-FITC staining revealed between 22 and 30% of the cells with a spontaneously reacted acrosome in the DMSO control, which could be considered higher than expected. However, no remarkable changes were found when DMSO cells were compared to DGC or CAP sperm. Taking into account that these levels were equivalent between the three semen samples, no bias on proteomic data was expected.

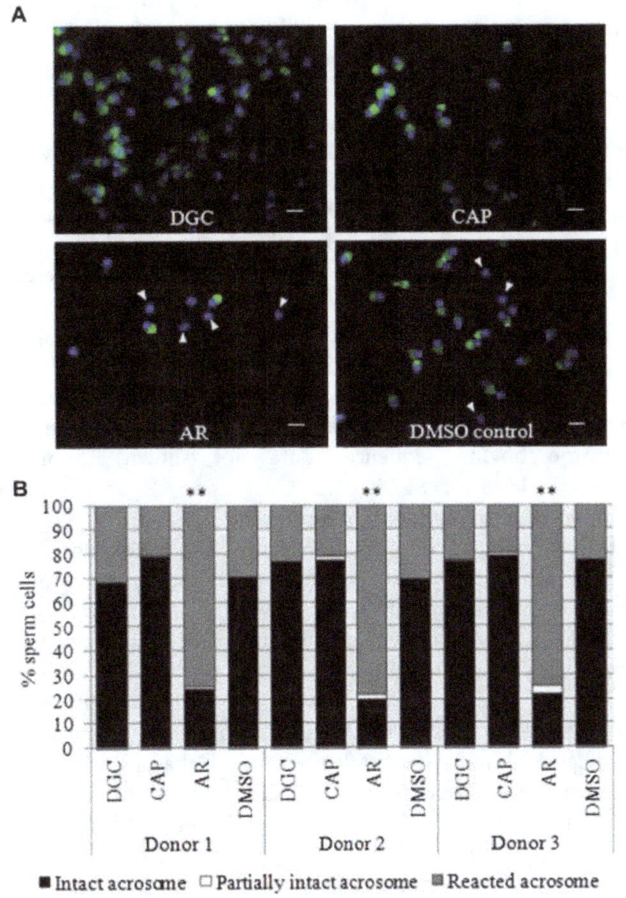

FIGURE 2 | PSA-FITC labeling for the assessment of acrosomal integrity. **(A)** Representative sperm PSA-FITC labeling of one donor sample. PSA-FITC labeling was conducted in purified sperm by density gradient centrifugation (DGC; upper left), sperm incubated with capacitation medium (CAP; upper right) and sperm in which the acrosome reaction was induced by incubation with a calcium ionophore A23187 (AR; lower left). Vehicle control is also shown (DMSO control; lower right). Acrosomal vesicles are shown in green and the sperm cells with reacted acrosomal vesicles are indicated by an arrowhead. Sperm nuclei are stained with DAPI (blue). Scale bar = 5 μM **(B)** Quantification of the number of sperm with an intact acrosome, partially intact acrosome and reacted acrosome in the three fertile donors used for this study. The number of spermatozoa was counted after PSA-FITC labeling on DGC, CAP, AR, and DMSO sperm. Significant differences in the percentage of sperm cells with reacted acrosomes are indicated with stars (*p*-value < 0.01; one-way ANOVA with Holm–Sidak correction).

Alterations in the Relative Abundance of Proteins After Differential Density Gradient Centrifugation, Incubation in Capacitation Medium and Induction of the Acrosome Reaction

A total of 3658 peptides corresponding to 781 proteins were identified by LC-MS/MS in the lysates from DGC, CAP and AR sperm from the three donor samples (**Supplementary Table S2**). TMT quantification values were determined for all samples in 1901 peptides from 484 proteins (**Supplementary Tables S2, S3**),

[1] https://www.uniprot.org/
[2] https://www.ncbi.nlm.nih.gov/pubmed
[3] http://geneontology.org/
[4] https://string-db.org/
[5] https://www.phosphosite.org

of which 860 peptides derived from 240 proteins met our strict quantification criteria (>1 PSM with <50% variability in >75% of the samples; **Supplementary Tables S2, S3**). Repeated-measures ANOVA test combined with *post hoc* pairwise *t*-test and Holm–Sidak correction revealed changes in the relative abundance of 48 sperm proteins. However, changes in the levels of albumin (ALB) and semenogelin 2 (SEMG2) were disregarded as they were most likely altered due to technical issues. Certainly, the marked increase of ALB seen in CAP sperm may have been due to the presence of bovine serum albumin in the capacitation medium. In fact, from the three peptides quantified for ALB, the only one not showing significant changes in abundance after incubation with capacitation medium was unique for *Homo sapiens,* while the other two were in common with the bovine sequence (data not shown). Similarly, the lower level of SEMG2 in CAP and AR sperm could be attributed to seminal plasma remnants in DGC sperm that were reduced or even eliminated after the consecutive sperm incubation conditions. Of note, no more proteins were found showing differences with a magnitude similar to SEMG2, which would discard additional artifactual extraneous contamination.

Relative inter-lysate changes in protein abundance were further validated by conducting quantitative analysis at the peptide level. This strategy revealed that peptides from some of the 48 proteins did not show significant differences following sequential incubation conditions. After *p*-value correction at both the peptide and protein levels, only 36 proteins showed significant inter-lysate differences and were considered for further analyses (**Table 1** and **Supplementary Table S4**). Of note, all these proteins have been identified in the human sperm cell by previous proteomic studies (Castillo et al., 2018). GO enrichment terms showed that this subset of 36 proteins was mainly involved in fertilization-related processes, including "fertilization," "sperm-egg recognition," and "acrosome reaction," and energy production-related processes, such as "ATP metabolic process" and "glycolytic process," among others ($p < 0.05$ after FDR correction; **Table 2**). Regarding localization in the sperm cell itself, the 5 most enriched cellular components were "sperm flagellum," "acrosomal vesicle," "mitochondrial proton-transporting ATP synthase," "acrosomal membrane," and "outer dense fiber" ($p < 0.05$ after FDR correction; **Table 2**).

Looking more closely at the 36 proteins with altered inter-lysate concentrations, 13 differed significantly between DGC and CAP sperm (9 with decreased and 4 with increased protein levels in CAP sperm lysates; **Figures 3A–D** and **Supplementary Figure S1**), and 13 differed significantly between DGC and AR sperm (8 with reduced abundance and 5 with increased abundance in AR sperm lysates; **Figures 3C–F** and **Supplementary Figure S2**). Interestingly, the relative abundance of 14 proteins was only altered after induction of the acrosome reaction (AR sperm; **Figures 3B–E**). Of those, 9 proteins showed lower and 5 higher levels of abundance in AR lysates (**Figure 3E** and **Supplementary Figure S3**).

Functional Roles of Sperm Proteins Differentially Solubilized After Consecutive Incubation in Capacitation Medium and Following Induction of the Acrosome Reaction

The small number of proteins with altered levels of abundance identified for each of the sperm preparation groups limited the usefulness of GO enrichment analysis for identifying potential functional roles of these proteins. Instead, this was evaluated by searching in public databases and close examination of the available literature. Eleven functional categories were identified in this way, including "sperm motility," "fertilization," "energy production," "signaling," "detoxification/antioxidant response," "protein degradation," "protein folding," "vesicular trafficking," "metabolism of folic acid," "RNA biogenesis" and "unknown." **Figure 4** shows the distribution of proteins in each of the functional groups according to the stage of post-ejaculatory sperm processing. The specific category for each protein is indicated in **Table 1**.

Following incubation of the DGC sperm in capacitation medium, differences in their relative abundance were detected in proteins involved in sperm motility, fertilization, energy production and signaling (**Figure 4**). Induction of the acrosome reaction resulted in the reduction of the abundance of proteins involved mainly in fertilization, which includes sperm-oocyte recognition, binding and fusion (**Figure 4**). In addition, reduced levels of proteins with known roles in sperm motility, energy production and metabolism of folic acid were also identified in AR lysates (**Figure 4** and **Table 1**). Interestingly, proteins with increased relative abundance following the acrosome reaction were related to energy production, signaling, protein degradation and vesicular trafficking (**Figure 4**). Regarding differences observed between DGC and AR groups, which tests for changes induced by the combination of both incubation in capacitation medium and the acrosome reaction on DGC sperm, proteins with altered abundance related to detoxification/antioxidant response, protein folding and RNA biogenesis were also revealed (**Figure 4**).

To further explore the potential functional roles of the lysate proteins with altered post-processing abundance or possible synergies between them, protein-protein interactions between these proteins and all proteins associated to GO terms related to capacitation or acrosome reaction were assessed using the STRING database. This analysis highlighted the interaction of altered proteins not previously related to these processes with other proteins known to play important roles in the maturation of ejaculated sperm (**Table 3** and **Supplementary Figure S4**). For example, ERLIN2, which differed in abundance between DGC and AR conditions, is known to interact with CFTR, a protein associated with the GO term for capacitation. Likewise, STRING analysis revealed an interaction between ATP5F1A (also known as ATP5A), the relative abundance of which was altered following incubation in CAP medium, with DLD, a protein related with the GO of "capacitation" (**Table 3** and **Supplementary Figure S4**).

TABLE 1 | Quantified proteins with an altered abundance after the consecutive incubation with capacitation medium and *in vitro* induction of the acrosome reaction.

Gene name	# Peptides quantified under strict criteria	#Peptide differentially abundant	DGC-CAP/CAP-AR/ DGC-AR	Abundance alteration	Related function
ACR	10	4	DGC-CAP; CAP-AR	↓	Fertilization
ACRBP	17	8	CAP-AR	↓	Fertilization
ACRV1	3	3	DGC-CAP; CAP-AR	↓	Fertilization
AKAP3	16	12	DGC-CAP	↓	Sperm motility
AKAP4	22	16	DGC-CAP	↓	Sperm motility
ATP5F1A	15	1	DGC-CAP	↑	Energy production
ATP5F1D	2	2	CAP-AR	↑	Energy production
ATP5IF1	3	1	DGC-AR	↑	Energy production
ATP5O	1	1	DGC-AR	↑	Energy production
CCT2	2	1	DGC-AR	↓	Protein folding
ENO1	11	1	DGC-AR	↓	Energy production
ERLIN2	1	1	DGC-AR	↑	Signaling
FAM209A	2	1	DGC-CAP	↑	Unknown
FAM71B	2	1	DGC-AR	↓	RNA biogenesis
GGH	5	2	CAP-AR	↓	Metabolism of folic acid
GLUL	3	1	DGC-CAP	↓	Signaling
GSTM3	9	3	DGC-AR	↓	Detoxification
HK1	19	2	CAP-AR	↓	Energy production
HSPA2	18	3	DGC-AR	↓	Protein folding
LYZL4	3	1	DGC-AR	↓	Fertilization
LYZL6	1	1	DGC-CAP	↓	Fertilization
ODF2	12	5	DGC-CAP	↓	Sperm motility
PGAM2	6	1	CAP-AR	↓	Sperm motility
PGK2	14	5	DGC-CAP	↓	Sperm motility
PHB2	1	1	DGC-CAP; CAP-AR	↑	Signaling
PSMA4	1	1	CAP-AR	↑	Protein degradation
REEP5	1	1	CAP-AR	↑	Signaling
ROPN1B	1	1	DGC-AR	↓	Sperm motility
RSPH1	1	1	DGC-AR	↑	Sperm motility
SLC2A14	1	1	DGC-AR	↓	Detoxification
SOD2	1	1	DGC-AR	↑	Detoxification
SPACA3	5	2	DGC-CAP	↓	Fertilization
SPACA7	1	1	CAP-AR	↓	Fertilization
TMED10	3	1	CAP-AR	↑	Vesicular trafficking
TUBA1A	1	1	DGC-CAP	↑	Sperm motility
ZPBP	10	2	CAP-AR	↓	Fertilization

DGC-CAP: proteins differentially detected after incubation with capacitation medium; CAP-AR: proteins differentially detected after induction of the acrosome reaction; DGC-AR: proteins differentially detected after incubation of capacitation medium followed by the induction of the acrosome reaction; ↑: increased abundance; ↓: decreased abundance; Related function: according to public databases.

Role of PTMs and Isoforms in Protein Abundance Alterations Detected After Incubation in Capacitation Medium and Following Induction of the Acrosome Reaction

To identify a possible mechanism behind the relative changes in protein abundance following the consecutive incubation of sperm with capacitation medium and the induction of the acrosome reaction, the presence of PTMs in residues from peptides with significant inter-lysate differences in relative abundance was explored by using data from the PhosphoSitePlus® database. Potentially phosphorylated, acetylated, ubiquitinated, succinylated and sumoylated residues were identified (**Figure 5** and **Supplementary Table S4**). Interestingly, no PTMs were described for the differential peptides identified for proteins with reduced abundance following induction of the acrosome reaction (**Figure 5B**). However, retrieved data revealed modified residues for all the significantly altered peptides corresponding to proteins with an increased relative abundance in AR lysates (**Figure 5B**). Described PTMs were also attributed to peptides corresponding to altered proteins after sperm incubation in capacitation medium, or after consecutive incubation with capacitation medium and following induction of the acrosome reaction (**Figures 5A–C**).

TABLE 2 | Gene Ontology (GO) terms enrichment analysis.

GO term	Genes	FDR
GO biological process		
Fertilization	11	1.34E-10
ATP metabolic process	7	1.42E-04
Glycolytic process	4	1.62E-03
Sperm-egg recognition	4	2.37E-03
Acrosome reaction	3	5.30E-03
Spermatogenesis	7	1.15E-02
Gluconeogenesis	3	2.18E-02
Inner mitochondrial membrane organization	3	2.74E-02
GO cellular component		
Sperm flagellum	8	5.84E-09
Acrosomal vesicle	8	8.16E-09
Mitochondrial proton-transporting ATP synthase complex	3	1.21E-03
Acrosomal membrane	3	1.28E-03
Extracellular vesicle	13	1.85E-03
Outer dense fiber	2	6.75E-03
Meiotic spindle	2	1.62E-02
Nucleus	23	1.71E-02
Sperm principal piece	2	3.91E-02

GO terms corresponding to biological processes and cellular components that are significantly enriched in the set of sperm proteins with altered abundance after incubation with capacitation medium and induction of the acrosome reaction. P-value < 0.05 after FDR correction.

In addition to the above observations, assignment of the peptides with altered abundance to specific protein isoforms was also undertaken. Three peptides were quantified for protein ATP5IF1, which showed increased protein levels only in comparison between DGC and AR sperm lysates. Following statistical analysis, the only peptide shown to differ significantly was exclusive for the ATP5IF1 isoform 1 (**Table 1** and **Supplementary Table S4**).

DISCUSSION

Studying the molecular processes that govern how ejaculated spermatozoa mature in the female genital tract and become competent to fertilize the oocyte is now a key component of basic research in the field of Andrology. The fundamental cellular and molecular mechanisms and their components driving capacitation and acrosome reaction processes, however, are not yet completely understood. Identifying sperm components displaying alterations in abundance during *in vitro* post-ejaculated sperm maturation could aid to unravel hidden molecular aspects which can impact on male fertility, and the use of novel high-throughput molecular approaches is a good strategy to help achieve this goal.

There are published reports that made use of MS to help identify protein differences before and after the induction of sperm capacitation in human and model species (Ficarro et al., 2003; Bailey et al., 2005; Sleight et al., 2005; Secciani et al., 2009; Baker et al., 2010; Zigo et al., 2013; Kwon et al., 2014; Wang J. et al., 2015; Hernández-Silva et al., 2019; Hou et al., 2019). However, the number of studies focusing on human sperm and using the most advanced techniques is limited. In addition, to the best of our knowledge, acrosomal exocytosis has not yet been evaluated from a proteomic perspective. In the present study, we applied, for the first time, a high-throughput proteomic procedure combined with isotopic peptide labeling to help characterize not only changes in the proteomic profile of healthy spermatozoa after *in vitro* incubation with capacitation medium, but also after the release of the acrosomal contents. It is important, however, to be mindful of the fact that human semen samples are biologically very heterogeneous and that among the sperm population, only a few sperm will be capable of becoming competent to fertilize the oocyte. Both intra- and inter-individual sample variance might influence the results of 'omics- based research and, therefore, setting strict criteria for data analysis becomes essential to improve the impact of these data (Lualdi and Fasano, 2019). In the current study, we applied robust statistics at both the protein and peptide levels and considered potential technical bias. This workflow led us to identify 36 sperm proteins with a remarkably altered abundance in sperm lysates as a consequence of the incubation with capacitation medium, the calcium ionophore-induced acrosome reaction or both joint processes.

In order to understand whether the apparent differences in protein abundance are truly reflective of novel factors that may be critical during the acquisition of sperm fertilization capacity, it is necessary to consider their potential causes and effects. This is highly relevant since spermatozoa are inactive at both the transcriptional and the translational levels, excluding the possibility of increased gene expression accounting for rises in the relative abundance of some proteins in sperm lysates and placing more emphasis on dynamic molecular changes due, perhaps, to protein modification, degradation or translocation (Signorelli et al., 2012; Jodar et al., 2013; Amaral et al., 2014a; Castillo et al., 2018). We found that incubation with capacitation medium induced quantitative changes in proteins involved mainly in sperm motility and signaling, which are processes regulated by PTMs. Indeed, it is widely thought that important cellular changes facilitating sperm motility during capacitation is mediated by tyrosine phosphorylation through protein kinase A (PKA) activation and the down-regulation of Ser/Thr phosphatases by Src family kinases (Ficarro et al., 2003; Visconti et al., 2011; Battistone et al., 2013; Signorelli et al., 2013; Wang J. et al., 2015). The A kinase anchoring proteins (AKAPS) are actively involved in PKA-dependent protein tyrosine phosphorylation, and a decrease in the relative inter-lysate abundance of AKAP3 and AKAP4 was found in the current study after incubation with capacitation medium. A requirement for AKAP3 degradation in sperm capacitation has been reported (Hillman et al., 2013; Vizel et al., 2015), which supports our results. Likewise, we found relative alterations in other proteins known to be involved in PKA-dependent signaling processes, including ROPN1B (Carr et al., 2001; Fiedler et al., 2013) and the acquisition of sperm motility, including PGK2 (Danshina et al., 2010; Shen et al., 2013; Liu et al., 2016; Huang et al., 2017), ODF2 (Huang et al., 2015; Wang X. et al., 2015; Zhao et al., 2018), and RSPH1 (also known as TSGA2) (Hui et al., 2006; Shetty et al., 2007; Onoufriadis et al., 2014).

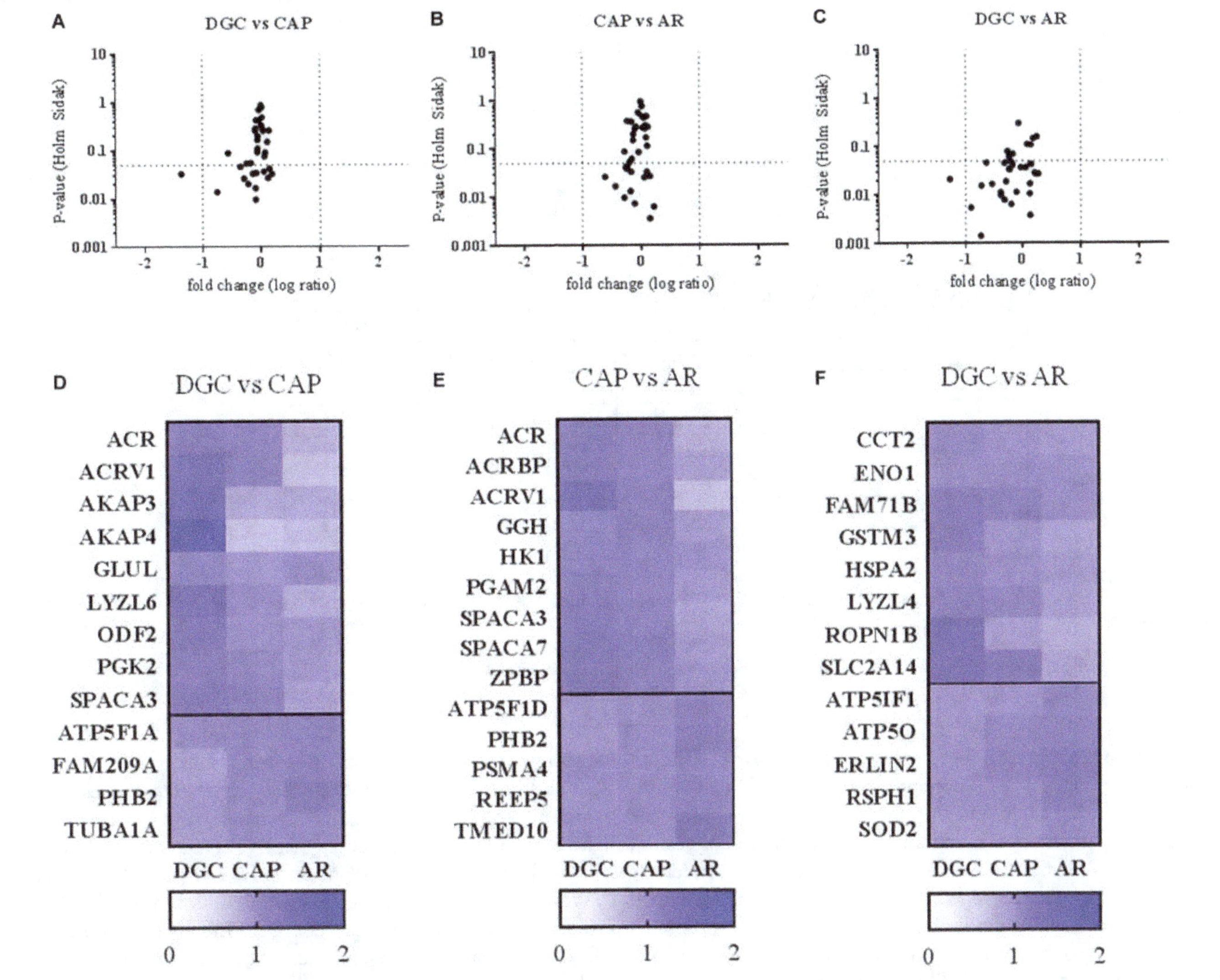

FIGURE 3 | Differences in the abundance of sperm proteins after incubation with capacitation medium and *in vitro* induction of the acrosome reaction. **(A–C)** *p*-value (repeated-measures ANOVA with Holm–Sidak correction) and fold changes (log ratio of TMT intensities of each sample with the internal control) for all quantified proteins (under strict criteria) after incubation with sperm capacitation medium (DGC vs. CAP), induction of the acrosome reaction (CAP vs. AR) and the combination of both treatments (DGC vs. AR). Fold change of −1 represents reduction to half, and +1 increasing to double (vertical dot lines). Horizontal dotted lines are set at *p*-value = 0.05. **(D–F)** heatmaps showing the ratio of TMT intensities from each sample with the internal control corresponding to proteins with statistically significant differences in their abundance after the different sperm treatments (DGC, CAP, and AR). Proteins with altered abundance were grouped depending on the treatment leading to the significant differences (DGC vs. CAP, CAP vs. AR, DGC vs. AR). Horizontal thick line separates proteins decreasing in abundance after the treatment (top) from those detected with higher protein levels (bottom).

While several proteomic reports can be found focused on sperm capacitation, this is the first study applying advanced proteomic strategies to analyze protein changes following the release of the acrosomal content. It is important to take into consideration that, although calcium influx is required to initiate the process, the use of a calcium ionophore does not mimic the natural trigger of the acrosome reaction, which requires binding to the zona pellucida (Liu and Baker, 1996a,b). However, tests simulating a zona-mediated physiological acrosome reaction are restricted by the limited availability of enough biological material for proteomic studies. Calcium ionophore A23187 is therefore an acceptable alternative when aiming to describe protein changes, since the results in terms of the quantitative loss of acrosomal contents should be equivalent. We found 9 proteins with a lower abundance after the acrosome reaction compared with lysates from CAP sperm, while 5 proteins seemed to increase their relative protein levels. Of note, none of the peptides from proteins with a lower abundance after the acrosome reaction contained residues with potential PTMs in their sequence. In contrast, all proteins with relatively higher abundance in AR lysates could be targets of protein modifiers. These results suggest that all proteins with apparently lower abundance in AR lysates may be released or relocated during the acrosome reaction, while those with relative increases in abundance may represent modified proteins

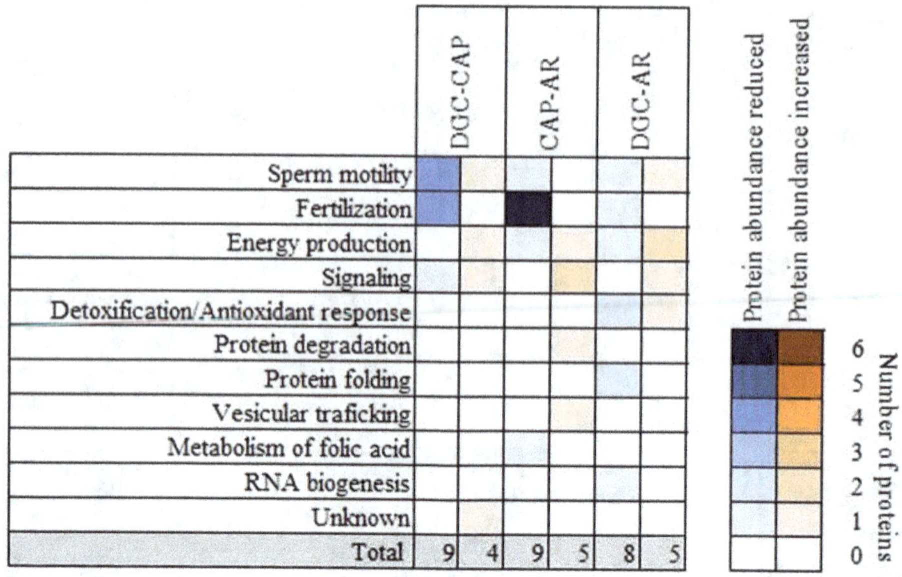

FIGURE 4 | Functional involvement of proteins detected with an altered abundance after incubation with capacitation medium and *in vitro* induction of the acrosome reaction. The results are based on the data contained in the public databases Uniprot KB and Pubmed. Proteins present at reduced abundance are shown in blue and proteins detected with increased abundance in orange. The intensity of the color increases according to the number of proteins related to each functional category. DGC-CAP: changes after incubation with capacitation medium. CAP-AR: changes after induction of the acrosome reaction; DGC-AR: changes after synergic effect of incubation with capacitation medium followed by induction of the acrosome reaction.

involved in signaling processes that have lost the corresponding PTM. In support of this hypothesis, many of the proteins with diminished protein levels after induction of the acrosome reaction are known to be components of the acrosomal vesicle, including ACR, ACRBP, ARV1, and SPACA7 and, therefore, those might be released together with the acrosomal content. However, potential changes in the distribution of sperm proteins should also be considered, as it has been observed in previous studies using a number of different methods (Torabi et al., 2017a). The lysis buffer used in this study to solubilize sperm proteins most likely gained access to compartments of the sperm during and following capacitation that were hidden beforehand. A similar effect would lead to the release of proteins following the acrosome reaction where the acrosomal vesicle is lost. This does not imply that our data is a technical artifact (notwithstanding the status of albumin and semenogelin, both disregarded); instead, we propose that it is mainly the dynamic changes in cellular and structural aspects of the sperm occurring during capacitation and the acrosome reaction that is the main driver of these results, although active enzymatic destruction of sperm proteins during these processes may also contribute. It should also be recognised that successive transitional stages take place before the complete release of the acrosome contents (Buffone et al., 2008). Therefore, further studies considering different time points during the acrosome reaction would shed light into the functional involvement of these proteins.

The finding of alterations in the abundance of sperm proteins already known to be involved in sperm capacitation and the acrosome reaction supports the reliability of the strategy followed by this study. Moreover, it also increases the interest in those (altered) proteins never associated previously with sperm functionality. For example, our results suggest that, in our *in vitro* conditions, sperm maturation induced changes in the ER lipid raft-associated 2 (ERLIN2) protein, which is known to mediate degradation of inositol 1,4,5-triphosphate receptors (Wang Y. et al., 2009; Wright et al., 2018). Interestingly, STRING analysis revealed the interaction of ERLIN2 with the cystic fibrosis transmembrane conductance regulator protein (CFTR), which is essential during sperm capacitation through PKA-dependent phosphorylation, alkalization and hyperpolarization (Puga Molina et al., 2017, 2018b). The reduction in the abundance of gamma-glytamyl hydrolase (GGH) in AR sperm is also noteworthy. The interaction analysis revealed the association of GGH with the T-complex protein 1 subunit beta (CCT2), which is a chaperone involved in sperm-ZP binding (Redgrove et al., 2011). Only an involvement of GGH in the metabolism of folic acid is reported in the literature (DeVos et al., 2008). However, since both GGH and CCT2 showed significant alterations in protein abundance after the process of acrosome reaction, GGH is suggested as a potential candidate for further study. In addition, GGH might also interact with Glutathione S-transferase Mu 3 protein (GSTM3), which has been previously related to capacitation and ZP binding using MS (Ficarro et al., 2003; Petit et al., 2013). Another novel protein thought to be involved in the process of the acrosome reaction is the Transmembrane em24 domain-containing protein 10 (TMED10), which, although not previously associated with sperm function, may be involved in vesicular trafficking in other cellular systems (Nakano et al., 2017; Luteijn et al., 2019).

TABLE 3 | Protein–protein interactions between altered proteins detected in this study and proteins associated to GO terms of capacitation and acrosome reaction.

Node1	Node2	Combined_score
ACRBP	ACR	0.776
ACRV1	SPACA1	0.827
AKAP3	ROPN1	0.943
AKAP4	PRKACA	0.901
ATP5F1A	ATP5F1D	0.999
ATP5F1A	ATP5O	0.999
ATP5F1A	DLD	0.893
ATP5F1A	ATPIF1	0.852
ATP5O	ATP5F1D	0.999
ATPIF1	ATP5F1D	0.837
CABYR	AKAP3	0.894
CABYR	AKAP4	0.736
CATSPER4	HSPA2	0.724
CCT2	GGH	0.907
CCT2	PSMA4	0.867
ENO1	DLD	0.713
ERLIN2	CFTR	0.906
GGH	GSTM3	0.902
GLUL	DLD	0.858
HSPA2	CATSPERD	0.758
HSPA2	CACNA1H	0.744
HSPA2	CATSPER2	0.730
HSPA2	CATSPER3	0.724
ODF2	PAFAH1B1	0.916
ODF2	PRKACA	0.901
ODF2	TUBA1A	0.900
PAFAH1B1	TUBA1A	0.982
PGAM2	ENO1	0.978
PGK2	PGAM2	0.980
PGK2	ENO1	0.935
PRKACA	TUBA1A	0.903
PSMA4	CFTR	0.907
ROPN1B	ROPN1	0.719
ROPN1L	AKAP3	0.946
SLC2A14	HK1	0.722
SOD2	ATP5O	0.771
TEX40	HSPA2	0.720
TUBA1A	CCT2	0.914
ZP2	ACR	0.766
ZP3	ACR	0.737

Proteins found with altered abundance in this study are highlighted in gray. Confidence score > 0.7 is set as high by STRING database.

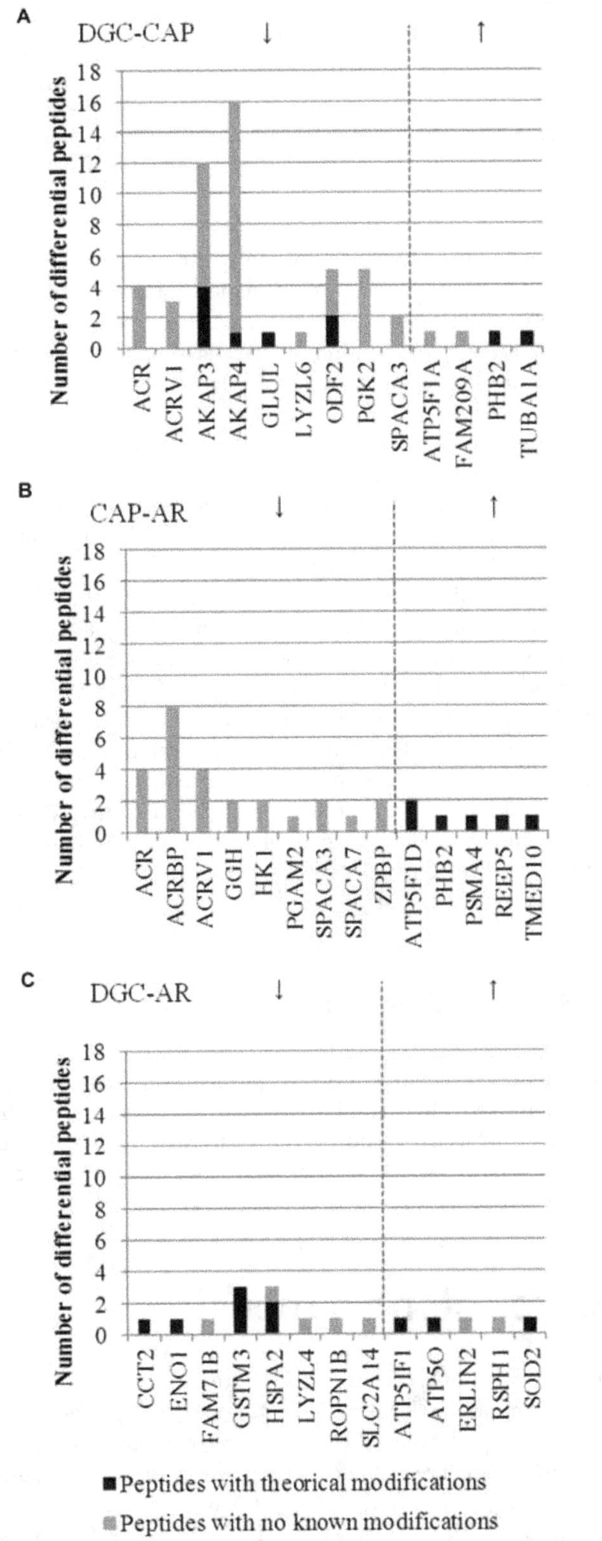

FIGURE 5 | Altered peptides with potential post-translational modifications corresponding to proteins identified with significantly different abundance after incubation with capacitation medium and *in vitro* induction of the acrosome reaction. **(A)** proteins found with altered abundance after incubation with *(Continued)*

Sperm capacitation and the acrosome reaction are complex processes involving many proteins and signaling pathways. Indeed, the sheer complexity precludes our obtaining a complete proteomic picture of these processes in just one MS-based study. A combination of data from high-throughput studies applying different approaches, such as enrichment in peptides with specific PTMs, the conduction of cell fractionation or the use of isobaric tags for protein quantification, among others, is required (Amaral et al., 2014a; Codina et al., 2015). In this study, we have applied

FIGURE 5 | Continued
capacitation medium. **(B)** proteins found with altered abundance after induction of the acrosome reaction. **(C)** proteins found with altered abundance after the synergic effect of incubation in capacitation medium followed by induction of the acrosome reaction. Arrows indicate whether the abundance of the proteins was increased or decreased after incubation with capacitation medium and *in vitro* induction of the acrosome reaction.

TMT labeling to quantify changes in sperm proteins in response to stimuli leading to an *in vitro* simulation of post-gonadal sperm maturation. We believe that our results increase the current knowledge about maturation of ejaculated sperm and suggest new players in the process. However, further experiments at peptide level are now required. By dissected the process of capacitation and the acrosome reaction at the peptide level, there is the possibility of understanding the roles of these proteins during the acquisition of competence to fertilize the oocyte and to confirm both the presence of modifications and alterations thereof in infertile patients. In addition, our results highlight the limitations of the currently available *in vitro* methods to mimic the *in vivo* situation. Capacitation and the acrosome reaction occur within the female reproductive system and thus, secretions from and components of the female tract may have an impact on sperm acquisition of fertilizing capacity. Therefore, the development of 3-D culture systems that mimic the oviduct and provide an *in vivo*-like environment to the sperm cell are desirable (Ferraz et al., 2017). A better understanding of the molecular mechanism mediating fertilization is essential in order to improve current infertility diagnosis and treatment.

ETHICS STATEMENT

The studies involving human participants were reviewed and approved by Clinical Research Ethics Committee of the Hospital Clínic of Barcelona. The donors provided their written informed consent to participate in this study.

AUTHOR CONTRIBUTIONS

OB, FT, and RO designed the study. JB was involved in donor samples collection. JC, OB, and FT performed the research. JE performed the proteomic technology. JC, MJ, FT, and DD-D analyzed the data. JC, MJ, and RO interpreted the data. JC, MJ, FT, DM, and RO drafted the manuscript. All authors critically reviewed and approved the final version of the manuscript.

FUNDING

This work was supported by grants to RO from the Spanish Ministry of Economy and Competitiveness (Ministerio de Economía y Competividad; fondos FEDER 'una manera de hacer Europa' PI13/00699, and PI16/00346), from Fundación Salud 2000 (SERONO 13-015), and from EU-FP7-PEOPLE-2011-ITN289880. JC is supported by the Sara Borrell Postdoctoral Fellowship from the Spanish Ministry of Economy and Competitiveness (Ministerio de Economía y Competitividad, Acción Estratégica en Salud, CD17/00109). MJ is granted by Government of Catalonia (Generalitat de Catalunya, pla estratègic de recerca i innovació en salut, PERIS 2016-2020, SLT002/1600337).

ACKNOWLEDGMENTS

We thank Raquel Ferreti and Alicia Diez for their assistance in the collection and routine analysis of semen samples.

SUPPLEMENTARY MATERIAL

FIGURE S1 | Proteins detected with altered abundance after incubation of the sperm cells with capacitation medium (DGC-CAP). The mean of the ratio between TMT intensities of the three donors and the internal control are shown for each protein at each sperm condition.

FIGURE S2 | Proteins detected with altered abundance after the combination of sperm incubation with capacitation medium and induction of the acrosome reaction (DGC-AR). The mean of the ratio between TMT intensities of the three donors and the internal control are shown for each protein at each sperm condition.

FIGURE S3 | Proteins detected with altered abundance after the induction of the acrosome reaction (CAP-AR). The mean of the ratio between TMT intensities of the three donors and the internal control are shown for each protein at each sperm condition.

FIGURE S4 | Protein–protein interaction networks between proteins found with altered abundance in this study and all those proteins associated with Gene Ontology terms related to capacitation and acrosome reaction. Proteins known to be functionally associated to the processes of capacitation and acrosome reaction were retrieved from the Gene Ontology Consortium database and submitted to STRING database together with the list of proteins found in this study with statistical significant differences in abundance. Only those protein-protein interactions with a high confidential score (>0.7) are shown.

TABLE S1 | Seminal parameters of the semen samples included in the study and obtained from 3 fertile donors.

TABLE S2 | Proteins identified in the three sperm donors and three sperm conditions by LC-MS/MS. The number of identified peptides, PSMs at both TMT runs, quantified peptides in all samples and quantified peptides that fit the strict selection criteria for statistics are indicated.

TABLE S3 | Peptides identified by LC-MS/MS containing quantification values.

TABLE S4 | Proteins identified with altered abundance. *P*-values after one way ANOVA for repeated measures and *t*-test with Holm–Sidak adjustment are provided for both proteins and peptides. *P*-values <0.05 are highlighted in green.

REFERENCES

Amaral, A., Castillo, J., Ramalho-Santos, J., and Oliva, R. (2014a). The combined human sperm proteome: cellular pathways and implications for basic and clinical science. *Hum. Reprod. Update* 20, 40–62. doi: 10.1093/humupd/dmt046

Amaral, A., Paiva, C., Attardo Parrinello, C., Estanyol, J. M., Ballescà, J. L., Ramalho-Santos, J., et al. (2014b). Identification of proteins involved in human sperm motility using high-throughput differential proteomics. *J. Proteome Res.* 13, 5670–5684. doi: 10.1021/pr500652y

Azpiazu, R., Amaral, A., Castillo, J., Estanyol, J. M., Guimerà, M., Ballescà, J. L., et al. (2014). High-throughput sperm differential proteomics suggests that epigenetic alterations contribute to failed assisted reproduction. *Hum. Reprod.* 29, 1225–1237. doi: 10.1093/humrep/deu073

Bailey, J. L., Tardif, S., Dubé, C., Beaulieu, M., Reyes-Moreno, C., Lefièvre, L., et al. (2005). Use of phosphoproteomics to study tyrosine kinase activity in capacitating boar sperm. *Theriogenology* 63, 599–614. doi: 10.1016/j.theriogenology.2004.09.034

Baker, M. A., Reeves, G., Hetherington, L., and Aitken, R. J. (2010). Analysis of proteomic changes associated with sperm capacitation through the combined use of IPG-strip prefractionation followed by RP chromatography LC-MS/ MS analysis. *Proteomics* 10, 482–495. doi: 10.1002/pmic.200900574

Baldi, E., Luconi, M., Bonaccorsi, L., Krausz, C., and Forti, G. (1996). Human sperm activation during capacitation and acrosome reaction: role of calcium, protein phosphorylation and lipid remodelling pathways. *Front. Biosci.* 1:d189–d205. doi: 10.2741/a125

Barrachina, F., Jodar, M., Delgado-Dueñas, D., Soler-Ventura, A., Estanyol, J. M., Mallofré, C., et al. (2018). Novel and conventional approaches for the analysis of quantitative proteomic data are complementary towards the identification of seminal plasma alterations in infertile patients. *Mol. Cell. Proteomics* 18:mcRA118.001248. doi: 10.1074/mcp.RA118.001248

Barros, C. (1967). Membrane vesiculation as a feature of the mammalian acrosome reaction. *J. Cell Biol.* 34, C1–C5. doi: 10.1083/jcb.34.3.C1

Battistone, M. A., Alvau, A., Salicioni, A. M., Visconti, P. E., Da Ros, V. G., and Cuasnicú, P. S. (2014). Evidence for the involvement of proline-rich tyrosine kinase 2 in tyrosine phosphorylation downstream of protein kinase a activation during human sperm capacitation. *Mol. Hum. Reprod.* 20, 1054–1066. doi: 10.1093/molehr/gau073

Battistone, M. A., Da Ros, V. G., Salicioni, A. M., Navarrete, F. A., Krapf, D., Visconti, P. E., et al. (2013). Functional human sperm capacitation requires both bicarbonate-dependent PKA activation and down-regulation of Ser/Thr phosphatases by Src family kinases. *Mol. Hum. Reprod.* 19, 570–580. doi: 10.1093/molehr/gat033

Benoff, S., Hurley, I., Cooper, G. W., Mandel, F. S., Hershlag, A., Scholl, G. M., et al. (1993). Fertilization potential in vitro is correlated with head-specific mannose-ligand receptor expression, acrosome status and membrane cholesterol content. *Hum. Reprod.* 8, 2155–2166. doi: 10.1093/oxfordjournals.humrep.a137997

Bogle, O. A., Kumar, K., Attardo-Parrinello, C., Lewis, S. E. M., Estanyol, J. M., Ballescà, J. L., et al. (2017). Identification of protein changes in human spermatozoa throughout the cryopreservation process. *Andrology* 5, 10–22. doi: 10.1111/andr.12279

Breitbart, H., and Finkelstein, M. (2015). Regulation of sperm capacitation and the acrosome reaction by PIP 2 and actin modulation. *Asian J. Androl.* 17, 597–600. doi: 10.4103/1008-682X.154305

Brucker, C., and Lipford, G. B. (1995). The human sperm acrosome reaction: physiology and regulatory mechanisms. An update. *Hum. Reprod. Update* 1, 51–62. doi: 10.1093/humupd/1.1.51

Buffone, M. G., Foster, J. A., and Gerton, G. L. (2008). The role of the acrosomal matrix in fertilization. *Int. J. Dev. Biol.* 52, 511–522. doi: 10.1387/ijdb.072532mb

Buffone, M. G., Ijiri, T. W., Cao, W., Merdiushev, T., Aghajanian, H. K., and Gerton, G. L. (2012). Heads or tails? Structural events and molecular mechanisms that promote mammalian sperm acrosomal exocytosis and motility. *Mol. Reprod. Dev.* 79, 4–18. doi: 10.1002/mrd.21393

Carr, D. W., Fujita, A., Stentz, C. L., Liberty, G. A., Olson, G. E., and Narumiya, S. (2001). Identification of sperm-specific proteins that interact with A-kinase anchoring proteins in a manner similar to the Type II regulatory subunit of PKA. *J. Biol. Chem.* 276, 17332–17338. doi: 10.1074/jbc.M011252200

Castillo, J., Jodar, M., and Oliva, R. (2018). The contribution of human sperm proteins to the development and epigenome of the preimplantation embryo. *Hum. Reprod. Update* 24, 535–555. doi: 10.1093/humupd/dmy017

Codina, M., Estanyol, J. M., Fidalgo, M. J., Ballescà, J. L., and Oliva, R. (2015). Advances in sperm proteomics: best-practise methodology and clinical potential. *Expert Rev. Proteomics* 12, 255–277. doi: 10.1586/14789450.2015.1040769

Cuasnicú, P. S., Da Ros, V. G., Weigel Muñoz, M., and Cohen, D. J. (2016). Acrosome reaction as a preparation for gamete fusion. *Adv. Anat. Embryol. Cell Biol.* 220, 159–172. doi: 10.1007/978-3-319-30567-7_9

Dacheux, J.-L., and Dacheux, F. (2014). New insights into epididymal function in relation to sperm maturation. *Reproduction* 147, R27–R42. doi: 10.1530/REP-13-0420

Danshina, P. V., Geyer, C. B., Dai, Q., Goulding, E. H., Willis, W. D., Kitto, G. B., et al. (2010). Phosphoglycerate Kinase 2 (PGK2) is essential for sperm function and male fertility in Micel. *Biol. Reprod.* 82, 136–145. doi: 10.1095/biolreprod.109.079699

De Jonge, C. (2005). Biological basis for human capacitation. *Hum. Reprod. Update* 11, 205–214. doi: 10.1093/humupd/dmi010

De Jonge, C. J., and Barratt, C. L. R. (2013). Methods for the assessment of sperm capacitation and acrosome reaction excluding the sperm penetration assay. *Methods Mol. Biol.* 927, 113–118. doi: 10.1007/978-1-62703-038-0_11

DeVos, L., Chanson, A., Liu, Z., Ciappio, E. D., Parnell, L. D., Mason, J. B., et al. (2008). Associations between single nucleotide polymorphisms in folate uptake and metabolizing genes with blood folate, homocysteine, and DNA uracil concentrations. *Am. J. Clin. Nutr.* 88, 1149–1158. doi: 10.1093/ajcn/88.4.1149

Ferraz, M. A. M. M., Henning, H. H. W., Stout, T. A. E., Vos, P. L. A. M., and Gadella, B. M. (2017). Designing 3-Dimensional *in vitro* oviduct culture systems to study mammalian fertilization and embryo production. *Ann. Biomed. Eng.* 45, 1731–1744. doi: 10.1007/s10439-016-1760-x

Ficarro, S., Chertihin, O., Westbrook, V. A., White, F., Jayes, F., Kalab, P., et al. (2003). Phosphoproteome analysis of capacitated human sperm: evidence of tyrosine phosphorylation of a kinase-anchoring protein 3 and valosin-containing protein/p97 during capacitation. *J. Biol. Chem.* 278, 11579–11589. doi: 10.1074/jbc.M202325200

Fiedler, S. E., Dudiki, T., Vijayaraghavan, S., and Carr, D. W. (2013). Loss of R2D2 Proteins ROPN1 and ROPN1L causes defects in murine sperm motility, phosphorylation, and fibrous sheath integrity1. *Biol. Reprod.* 88:41. doi: 10.1095/biolreprod.112.105262

Fox, J., and Weisberg, S. (2011). *An {R} Companion to Applied Regression, Second Edition*. Thousand Oaks, CA: Sage.

Gaddum, P., and Blandau, R. J. (1970). Proteolytic reaction of mammalian spermatozoa on gelatin membranes. *Science* 170, 749–751. doi: 10.1126/science.170.3959.749

Gadella, B. M., Tsai, P., Boerke, A., and Brewis, I. A. (2008). Sperm head membrane reorganisation during capacitation. *Int. J. Dev. Biol.* 52, 473–480. doi: 10.1387/ijdb.082583bg

Halet, G., Marangos, P., Fitzharris, G., and Carroll, J. (2003). Ca2+ oscillations at fertilization in mammals. *Biochem. Soc. Trans.* 31, 907–911. doi: 10.1042/bst0310907

Hernández-Silva, G., Fabián López-Araiza, J. E., López-Torres, A. S., Larrea, F., Torres-Flores, V., and Chirinos, M. (2019). Proteomic characterization of human sperm plasma membrane-associated proteins and their role in capacitation. *Andrology*. doi: 10.1111/andr.12627 [Epub ahead of print].

Hillman, P., Ickowicz, D., Vizel, R., and Breitbart, H. (2013). Dissociation between AKAP3 and PKARII promotes AKAP3 degradation in sperm capacitation. *PLoS One* 8:e68873. doi: 10.1371/journal.pone.0068873

Hou, Z., Fu, Q., Huang, Y., Zhang, P., Chen, F., Li, M., et al. (2019). Comparative proteomic identification buffalo spermatozoa during in vitro capacitation. *Theriogenology* 126, 303–309. doi: 10.1016/j.theriogenology.2018.12.025

Huang, Y.-L., Fu, Q., Yang, L., Guan, J.-L., Pan, H., Chen, F.-M., et al. (2015). Differences between high- and low-motility buffalo sperm identified by comparative proteomics. *Reprod. Domest. Anim.* 50, 443–451. doi: 10.1111/rda.12511

Huang, Z., Danshina, P. V., Mohr, K., Qu, W., Goodson, S. G., O'Connell, T. M., et al. (2017). Sperm function, protein phosphorylation, and metabolism differ in mice lacking successive sperm-specific glycolytic enzymes. *Biol. Reprod.* 97, 586–597. doi: 10.1093/biolre/iox103

Hui, L., Lu, J., Han, Y., and Pilder, S. H. (2006). The mouse t complex gene Tsga2, encoding polypeptides located in the sperm tail and anterior acrosome, maps to a locus associated with sperm motility and sperm-egg interaction Abnormalities1. *Biol. Reprod.* 74, 633–643. doi: 10.1095/biolreprod.105.045963

Ickowicz, D., Finkelstein, M., and Breitbart, H. (2012). Mechanism of sperm capacitation and the acrosome reaction: role of protein kinases. *Asian J. Androl.* 14, 816–821. doi: 10.1038/aja.2012.81

Ito, C., and Toshimori, K. (2016). Acrosome markers of human sperm. *Anat. Sci. Int.* 91, 128–142. doi: 10.1007/s12565-015-0323-9

Jagan Mohanarao, G., and Atreja, S. K. (2011). Identification of capacitation associated tyrosine phosphoproteins in buffalo (Bubalus bubalis) and cattle spermatozoa. *Anim. Reprod. Sci.* 123, 40–47. doi: 10.1016/j.anireprosci.2010.11.013

Jodar, M., Selvaraju, S., Sendler, E., Diamond, M. P., and Krawetz, S. A. (2013). The presence, role and clinical use of spermatozoal RNAs. *Hum. Reprod. Update* 19, 604–624. doi: 10.1093/humupd/dmt031

Jodar, M., Soler-Ventura, A., and Oliva, R. (2017). Semen proteomics and male infertility. *J. Proteomics* 162, 125–134. doi: 10.1016/j.jprot.2016.08.018

Kwon, W.-S., Rahman, M., Lee, J.-S., Kim, J., Yoon, S.-J., Park, Y.-J., et al. (2014). A comprehensive proteomic approach to identifying capacitation related proteins in boar spermatozoa. *BMC Genomics* 15:897. doi: 10.1186/1471-2164-15-897

Li, K., Xue, Y., Chen, A., Jiang, Y., Xie, H., Shi, Q., et al. (2014). Heat shock protein 90 has roles in intracellular calcium homeostasis, protein tyrosine phosphorylation regulation, and progesterone-responsive sperm function in human sperm. *PLoS One* 9:e115841. doi: 10.1371/journal.pone.0115841

Liu, D. Y., and Baker, H. W. (1996a). A simple method for assessment of the human acrosome reaction of spermatozoa bound to the zona pellucida: lack of relationship with ionophore A23187-induced acrosome reaction. *Hum. Reprod.* 11, 551–557. doi: 10.1093/humrep/11.3.551

Liu, D. Y., and Baker, H. W. (1996b). Relationship between the zona pellucida (ZP) and ionophore A23187-induced acrosome reaction and the ability of sperm to penetrate the ZP in men with normal sperm-ZP binding. *Fertil. Steril.* 66, 312–315. doi: 10.1016/s0015-0282(16)58459-3

Liu, D. Y., Liu, M. L., Clarke, G. N., and Baker, H. W. G. (2007). Hyperactivation of capacitated human sperm correlates with the zona pellucida-induced acrosome reaction of zona pellucida-bound sperm. *Hum. Reprod.* 22, 2632–2638. doi: 10.1093/humrep/dem245

Liu, X. X., Zhang, H., Shen, X. F., Liu, F. J., Liu, J., and Wang, W. J. (2016). Characteristics of testis-specific phosphoglycerate kinase 2 and its association with human sperm quality. *Hum. Reprod.* 31, 273–279. doi: 10.1093/humrep/dev301

Lualdi, M., and Fasano, M. (2019). Statistical analysis of proteomics data: a review on feature selection. *J. Proteomics* 198, 18–26. doi: 10.1016/j.jprot.2018.12.004

Luteijn, R. D., van Diemen, F., Blomen, V. A., Boer, I. G. J., Manikam Sadasivam, S., van Kuppevelt, T. H., et al. (2019). A genome-wide haploid genetic screen identifies heparan sulfate-associated genes and the macropinocytosis modulator TMED10 as factors supporting vaccinia virus infection. *J. Virol.* 93:e02160-18. doi: 10.1128/JVI.02160-18

Mengual, L., Ballescà, J. L., Ascaso, C., and Oliva, R. (2003). Marked differences in protamine content and P1 / P2 Ratios. *J. Androl.* 24, 438–447. doi: 10.1002/j.1939-4640.2003.tb02692.x

Nakano, N., Tsuchiya, Y., Kako, K., Umezaki, K., Sano, K., Ikeno, S., et al. (2017). TMED10 protein interferes with transforming growth factor (TGF)-β signaling by disrupting TGF-β receptor complex formation. *J. Biol. Chem.* 292, 4099–4112. doi: 10.1074/jbc.M116.769109

O'Flaherty, C. (2015). Redox regulation of mammalian sperm capacitation. *Asian J. Androl.* 17, 583–590. doi: 10.4103/1008-682x.153303

Oliva, R. (2006). Protamines and male infertility. *Hum. Reprod. Update* 12, 417–435. doi: 10.1093/humupd/dml009

Onoufriadis, A., Shoemark, A., Schmidts, M., Patel, M., Jimenez, G., Liu, H., et al. (2014). Targeted NGS gene panel identifies mutations in RSPH1 causing primary ciliary dyskinesia and a common mechanism for ciliary central pair agenesis due to radial spoke defects. *Hum. Mol. Genet.* 23, 3362–3374. doi: 10.1093/hmg/ddu046

Park, Y.-J., Kwon, W.-S., Oh, S.-A., and Pang, M.-G. (2012). Fertility-Related proteomic profiling bull spermatozoa separated by Percoll. *J. Proteome Res.* 11, 4162–4168. doi: 10.1021/pr300248s

Patrat, C., Serres, C., and Jouannet, P. (2000). The acrosome reaction in human spermatozoa. *Biol. Cell* 92, 255–266. doi: 10.1016/s0248-4900(00)01072-8

Perez-Riverol, Y., Csordas, A., Bai, J., Bernal-Llinares, M., Hewapathirana, S., Kundu, D. J., et al. (2019). The PRIDE database and related tools and resources in 2019: improving support for quantification data. *Nucleic Acids Res.* 47, D442–D450. doi: 10.1093/nar/gky1106

Petit, F. M., Serres, C., Bourgeon, F., Pineau, C., and Auer, J. (2013). Identification of sperm head proteins involved in zona pellucida binding. *Hum. Reprod.* 28, 852–865. doi: 10.1093/humrep/des452

Puga Molina, L. C., Luque, G. M., Balestrini, P. A., Marín-Briggiler, C. I., Romarowski, A., and Buffone, M. G. (2018a). Molecular basis of human sperm capacitation. *Front. Cell Dev. Biol.* 6:72. doi: 10.3389/fcell.2018.00072

Puga Molina, L. C., Pinto, N. A., Torres, N. I., Ana, L. G. C., Luque, G. M., Balestrini, P. A., et al. (2018b). CFTR/ENaC-dependent regulation of membrane potential during human sperm capacitation is initiated by bicarbonate uptake through NBC. *J. Biol. Chem.* 293, 9924–9936. doi: 10.1074/jbc.RA118.003166

Puga Molina, L. C., Pinto, N. A., Torres Rodríguez, P., Romarowski, A., Vicens Sanchez, A., Visconti, P. E., et al. (2017). Essential role of CFTR in PKA-Dependent phosphorylation, alkalinization, and hyperpolarization during human sperm capacitation. *J. Cell. Physiol.* 232, 1404–1414. doi: 10.1002/jcp.25634

R Development Core Team, (2016). *R: A Language and Environment for Statistical Computing.* Vienna: R Foundation for Statistical Computing, doi: 10.1007/978-3-540-74686-7

Rahman, M. S., Lee, J.-S., Kwon, W.-S., and Pang, M.-G. (2013). Sperm proteomics: road to male fertility and contraception. *Int. J. Endocrinol.* 2013:360986. doi: 10.1155/2013/360986

Redgrove, K. A., Anderson, A. L., Dun, M. D., McLaughlin, E. A., O'Bryan, M. K., Aitken, R. J., et al. (2011). Involvement of multimeric protein complexes in mediating the capacitation-dependent binding of human spermatozoa to homologous zonae pellucidae. *Dev. Biol.* 356, 460–474. doi: 10.1016/j.ydbio.2011.05.674

Ritagliati, C., Luque, G. M., Stival, C., Baro Graf, C., Buffone, M. G., and Krapf, D. (2018). Lysine acetylation modulates mouse sperm capacitation. *Sci. Rep.* 8:13334. doi: 10.1038/s41598-018-31557-5

Sánchez-Cárdenas, C., Servín-Vences, M. R., José, O., Treviño, C. L., Hernández-Cruz, A., and Darszon, A. (2014). Acrosome reaction and Ca2+ imaging in single human spermatozoa: new regulatory roles of [Ca2+]i1. *Biol. Reprod.* 91:67. doi: 10.1095/biolreprod.114.119768

Sati, L., Cayli, S., Delpiano, E., Sakkas, D., and Huszar, G. (2014). The pattern of tyrosine phosphorylation in human sperm in response to binding to zona pellucida or hyaluronic acid. *Reprod. Sci.* 21, 573–581. doi: 10.1177/1933719113504467

Secciani, F., Bianchi, L., Ermini, L., Cianti, R., Armini, A., La Sala, G. B., et al. (2009). Protein profile of capacitated versus ejaculated human sperm. *J. Proteome Res.* 8, 3377–3389. doi: 10.1021/pr900031r

Shen, S., Wang, J., Liang, J., and He, D. (2013). Comparative proteomic study between human normal motility sperm and idiopathic asthenozoospermia. *World J. Urol.* 31, 1395–1401. doi: 10.1007/s00345-013-1023-1025

Shetty, J., Klotz, K. L., Wolkowicz, M. J., Flickinger, C. J., and Herr, J. C. (2007). Radial spoke protein 44 (human meichroacidin) is an axonemal alloantigen of sperm and cilia. *Gene* 396, 93–107. doi: 10.1016/j.gene.2007.02.031

Signorelli, J., Diaz, E. S., and Morales, P. (2012). Kinases, phosphatases and proteases during sperm capacitation. *Cell Tissue Res.* 349, 765–782. doi: 10.1007/s00441-012-1370-3

Signorelli, J. R., Díaz, E. S., Fara, K., Barón, L., and Morales, P. (2013). Protein phosphatases decrease their activity during capacitation: a new requirement for this event. *PLoS One* 8:e81286. doi: 10.1371/journal.pone.0081286

Singh, A. P., and Rajender, S. (2015). CatSper channel, sperm function and male fertility. *Reprod. Biomed. Online* 30, 28–38. doi: 10.1016/j.rbmo.2014.09.014

Sleight, S. B., Miranda, P. V., Plaskett, N.-W., Maier, B., Lysiak, J., Scrable, H., et al. (2005). Isolation and proteomic analysis of mouse sperm detergent-resistant membrane fractions: evidence for dissociation of lipid rafts during capacitation. *Biol. Reprod.* 73, 721–729. doi: 10.1095/biolreprod.105.041533

Stival, C., Puga Molina, L., del, C., Paudel, B., Buffone, M. G., Visconti, P. E., et al. (2016). Sperm capacitation and acrosome reaction in mammalian sperm. *Adv. Anat. Embryol. Cell Biol.* 220, 93–106. doi: 10.1007/978-3-319-30567-7_5

Torabi, F., Binduraihem, A., and Miller, D. (2017a). Sedimentation properties in density gradients correspond with levels of sperm DNA fragmentation, chromatin compaction and binding affinity to hyaluronic acid. *Reprod. Biomed. Online* 34, 298–311. doi: 10.1016/j.rbmo.2016.11.011

Torabi, F., Bogle, O. A., Estanyol, J. M., Oliva, R., and Miller, D. (2017b). Zona pellucida-binding protein 2 (ZPBP2) and several proteins containing BX7B motifs in human sperm may have hyaluronic acid binding or recognition properties. *Mol. Hum. Reprod.* 23, 803–816. doi: 10.1093/MOLEHR/GAX053

Visconti, P. E., Galantino-Homer, H., Moore, G. D., Bailey, J. L., Ning, X., Fornes, M., et al. (1998). The molecular basis of sperm capacitation. *J. Androl.* 19, 242–248. doi: 10.1002/j.1939-4640.1998.tb01994.x

Visconti, P. E., and Kopf, G. S. (1998). Regulation of protein phosphorylation during sperm capacitation. *Biol. Reprod.* 59, 1–6. doi: 10.1095/biolreprod59.1.1

Visconti, P. E., Krapf, D., De La Vega-Beltrán, J. L., Acevedo, J. J., and Darszon, A. (2011). Ion channels, phosphorylation and mammalian sperm capacitation. *Asian J. Androl.* 13, 395–405. doi: 10.1038/aja.2010.69

Visconti, P. E., Westbrook, V. A., Chertihin, O., Demarco, I., Sleight, S., and Diekman, A. B. (2002). Novel signaling pathways involved in sperm acquisition of fertilizing capacity. *J. Reprod. Immunol.* 53, 133–150. doi: 10.1016/s0165-0378(01)00103-6

Vizel, R., Hillman, P., Ickowicz, D., and Breitbart, H. (2015). AKAP3 degradation in sperm capacitation is regulated by its tyrosine phosphorylation. *Biochim. Biophys. Acta* 1850, 1912–1920. doi: 10.1016/j.bbagen.2015.06.005

Wang, G., Guo, Y., Zhou, T., Shi, X., Yu, J., Yang, Y., et al. (2013). In-depth proteomic analysis of the human sperm reveals complex protein compositions. *J. Proteomics* 79, 114–122. doi: 10.1016/j.jprot.2012.12.008

Wang, J., Qi, L., Huang, S., Zhou, T., Guo, Y., Wang, G., et al. (2015). Quantitative phosphoproteomics analysis reveals a key role of insulin growth factor 1 receptor (IGF1R) tyrosine kinase in human sperm capacitation. *Mol. Cell. Proteomics* 14, 1104–1112. doi: 10.1074/mcp.M114.045468

Wang, X., Wei, Y., Fu, G., Li, H., Saiyin, H., Lin, G., et al. (2015). Tssk4 is essential for maintaining the structural integrity of sperm flagellum. *MHR Basic Sci. Reprod. Med.* 21, 136–145. doi: 10.1093/molehr/gau097

Wang, Y., Pearce, M. M. P., Sliter, D. A., Olzmann, J. A., Christianson, J. C., Kopito, R. R., et al. (2009). SPFH1 and SPFH2 mediate the ubiquitination and degradation of inositol 1,4,5-trisphosphate receptors in muscarinic receptor-expressing HeLa cells. *Biochim. Biophys. Acta* 1793, 1710–1718. doi: 10.1016/j.bbamcr.2009.09.004

World Health Organization, (2010). *Who Laboratory Manual For The Examination And Processing Of Human Semen*. Geneva: WHO.

Wright, F. A., Bonzerato, C. G., Sliter, D. A., and Wojcikiewicz, R. J. H. (2018). The erlin2 T65I mutation inhibits erlin1/2 complex-mediated inositol 1,4,5-trisphosphate receptor ubiquitination and phosphatidylinositol 3-phosphate binding. *J. Biol. Chem.* 293, 15706–15714. doi: 10.1074/jbc.RA118.004547

Yu, H., Diao, H., Wang, C., Lin, Y., Yu, F., Lu, H., et al. (2015). Acetylproteomic analysis reveals functional implications of lysine acetylation in human spermatozoa (sperm). *Mol. Cell. Proteomics* 14, 1009–1023. doi: 10.1074/mcp.M114.041384

Zhao, C., Huo, R., Wang, F.-Q., Lin, M., Zhou, Z.-M., and Sha, J.-H. (2007). Identification of several proteins involved in regulation of sperm motility by proteomic analysis. *Fertil. Steril.* 87, 436–438. doi: 10.1016/j.fertnstert.2006.06.057

Zhao, W., Li, Z., Ping, P., Wang, G., Yuan, X., and Sun, F. (2018). Outer dense fibers stabilize the axoneme to maintain sperm motility. *J. Cell. Mol. Med.* 22, 1755–1768. doi: 10.1111/jcmm.13457

Zigo, M., Jonáková, V., Šulc, M., and Maňásková-Postlerová, P. (2013). Characterization of sperm surface protein patterns of ejaculated and capacitated boar sperm, with the detection of ZP binding candidates. *Int. J. Biol. Macromol.* 61, 322–328. doi: 10.1016/j.ijbiomac.2013.07.014

13

Amino Acids of Seminal Plasma Associated With Freezability of Bull Sperm

Muhammet Rasit Ugur[1], Thu Dinh[1], Mustafa Hitit[1,2], Abdullah Kaya[3], Einko Topper[4], Bradley Didion[4] and Erdogan Memili[1*]

[1] Department of Animal and Dairy Sciences, Mississippi State University, Starkville, MS, United States, [2] Department of Animal Genetics, Kastamonu University, Kastamonu, Turkey, [3] Department of Reproduction and Artificial Insemination, Selçuk University, Konya, Turkey, [4] Alta Genetics, Inc., Watertown, WI, United States

*Correspondence:
Erdogan Memili
em149@ads.msstate.edu;
em149@msstate.edu

Sperm cryopreservation is an important technique for fertility management, but post-thaw viability of sperm differs among breeding bulls. With metabolites being the end products of various metabolic pathways, the contributions of seminal plasma metabolites to sperm cryopreservation are still unknown. These gaps in the knowledge base are concerning because they prevent advances in the fundamental science of cryobiology and improvement of bull fertility. The objective of this study was to test the hypothesis that seminal plasma amino acids are associated with freezability of bull sperm. To accomplish this objective, amino acid concentrations in seminal plasma from seven bulls of good freezability (GF) and six bulls of poor freezability (PF) were quantified using gas chromatography–mass spectrometry (GC–MS). Multivariate and univariate analyses were performed to identify potential freezability biomarkers. Pathways and networks analyses of identified amino acids were performed using bioinformatic tools. By analyzing and interpreting the results we demonstrated that glutamic acid was the most abundant amino acid in bull seminal plasma with average concentration of 3,366 ± 547.3 nM, which accounts for about 53% of total amino acids. The other most predominant amino acids were alanine, glycine, and aspartic acid with the mean concentrations of 1,053 ± 187.9, 429.8 ± 57.94, and 427 ± 101.3 nM. Pearson's correlation analysis suggested that phenylalanine concentration was significantly associated with post-thaw viability (r = 0.57, P-value = 0.043). Significant correlations were also found among other amino acids. In addition, partial least squares-discriminant analysis (PLS-DA) bi-plot indicated a distinct separation between GF and PF groups. Phenylalanine had the highest VIP score and was more abundant in the GF groups than in the PF groups. Moreover, pathway and network analysis indicated that phenylalanine contributes to oxidoreductase and antioxidant reactions. Although univariate analysis did not yield significant differences in amino acid concentration between the two groups, these findings are significant that they indicate the potentially important roles of amino acids in seminal plasma, thereby building a foundation for the fundamental science of cryobiology and reproductive biotechnology.

Keywords: amino acids, seminal plasma, freezability, bull sperm, metabolomics

INTRODUCTION

There is an urgent need for more efficient, sustainable, and profitable cattle farming to feed the ever-increasing world population. Artificial insemination (AI) using cryopreserved sperm is a significant tool for the agri-food industry to improve modern animal production. The first attempt on sperm cryopreservation was made in 1776 (Royere et al., 1996); since then significant progress has been made using various cryoprotective agents and protocols during the last two centuries. Such progress, however, has not yet achieved the desired level of success because post-thaw survivability of sperm cells is disappointingly low, <50%, despite the best effort put forward in developing preservation techniques (Nijs et al., 2009). During cryopreservation, sperm cells undergo cellular and molecular changes, among which are membrane damage, oxidative stress, DNA fragmentation, reduced mRNA–protein interactions, as well as epigenetic modifications (O'Connell et al., 2002; Flores et al., 2011; Valcarce et al., 2013). Such modifications have detrimental effects on sperm physiology and thus on fertility.

Bovine seminal plasma is composed of secretions from testis, epididymis, and accessory sex glands. Such mixture contains proteins, ions, and metabolites including amino acids, lipids, monosaccharides, nucleosides, minerals, electrolytes, and steroid hormones (Egea et al., 2014; Cheng et al., 2015). As metabolites are the end-products of metabolic pathways, they play significant roles in sperm physiology such as energy metabolism, motility, and regulation of metabolic activities (Bieniek et al., 2016). While some components of seminal plasma have positive influences on sperm cryotolerance, others have detrimental effects (Yeste, 2016; Recuero et al., 2019). Regardless, metabolites in seminal plasma can be used to estimate bull fertility and sperm freezability. Hamamah et al. (1993) analyzed seminal plasma from fertile and infertile men using ^{1}H nuclear magnetic resonance (NMR) spectra, and found significant differences in concentrations of glycerylphosphorylcholine citrate (GPC), and lactate between azoospermic and oligoasthenozoospermic patients. Lin et al. (2009) characterized the metabolite profiles of primate sperm to investigate the association between metabolism and energy supply. The association between glycolytic substrates and energy production, which is essential for motility, was determined using metabolomics approach in mouse spermatozoa (Goodson et al., 2012). More recently, using both NMR and gas chromatography–mass spectrometry (GC–MS), total of 96 metabolites and more than 10 biological pathways were identified in human sperm (Paiva et al., 2015).

Free amino acids of seminal plasma have various functions including reducing free radicals, protecting cells against denaturation, and providing oxidizable substrate to spermatozoa (Mann and Lutwak-Mann, 1981). However, identities and roles of seminal plasma amino acids during cryopreservation are not fully understood. Alanine, glycine, glutamine, histidine, and proline have been used as cryoprotectant agents for various species as they either inhibit lipid peroxidation or modulate osmotic mechanism (Heber et al., 1971; Renard et al., 1996; Trimeche et al., 1999; Jaiswal and Eisenbach, 2002; Dvořáková et al., 2005; Sangeeta et al., 2015). In addition to stabilizing proteins, amino acids also possess antioxidant properties to protect sperm cells from cold shock (Atessahin et al., 2008). For example, proline improves motility and protects sperm cells against damages caused by free radicals by stabilizing the membrane structure and function during the freezing (Rudolph et al., 1986; Smirnoff and Cumbes, 1989). Additionally, alanine and glutamine also affect the motility and viability of the sperm (Koskinen et al., 1989; Khlifaoui et al., 2005; Amirat-Briand et al., 2009) by to some extent improving the cryoprotective effects of glycerol.

Recently, we have identified 63 seminal plasma metabolites of which 21 were amino acids from bulls with different field fertility scores (Velho et al., 2018) demonstrating the importance of metabolite profiles between low and high fertility bulls. Seminal plasma addition before freezing also influenced on post-thaw bull sperm kinematics (Nongbua et al., 2018). To investigate further the impacts of seminal plasma composition on sperm cells, in this study we ascertained the relationship between freezability and amino acids in bull seminal plasma.

MATERIALS AND METHODS

Semen Collection and Determination of Bull Semen Freezability

Seminal plasma samples from 13 bulls with various freezability and semen freezability data were provided by a commercial breeding company (Alta Genetics Inc., Watertown, WI, United States). The bulls were housed in the same nutrition and management environment to prevent sample variation. Semen was collected using artificial vagina and protease inhibitor was added immediately. Semen was then centrifuged at 800 × *g* for 15 min to separate the seminal plasma and sperm. This seminal plasma was transferred into sterile microcentrifuge tubes and centrifuged again at 800 × *g* for 15 min to completely eliminate sperm in the sample. Following this second centrifugation, seminal plasma was transferred into new tubes and shipped to Mississippi State University (MSU) in a liquid nitrogen tank.

Bull semen was extended with commercial egg-yolk–tris-based extender, and then frozen at Alta Genetics using standard protocols (Pace et al., 1981). Briefly, fresh semen was collected from bulls via artificial vagina, and semen was evaluated for concentration, volume, color, and motility. Then, semen was extended with one-step egg-yolk–tris–glycerol extender. The extender included 20% egg-yolk and 6% glycerol. This is called initial extension which includes fourfold dilution with extender at 32°C. The extended semen was cooled down to 5°C within 90 min. Then, the remaining extender was added at 5°C to complete extension, and packaged into quarter cc straws (250 μl) and let semen equilibrate for 3–4 h. Following the equilibration process, straws were frozen using automated freezer machine. The freezing was completed within 14 min (temperature from 5°C to −196°C), and stored in a liquid nitrogen tank.

Post-thaw sperm viability was assessed using flow cytometry (CyFlow SL, Partec, Germany). Fluorescent stain combinations of SYBR-14 with propidium iodide (SYBR-14/PI, Live/Dead Sperm Viability Kit L-7011, Thermo Fisher Scientific) were used as described previously (Garner et al., 1994; Nagy et al., 2004). Membrane integrity of 10,000 sperm cells from each collection was measured with the highest accuracy and objectivity. We verified that biological sample preparations, instrument configurations, and data analysis were compliant with the recommendations set by the International Society for Advancement of Cytometry on the minimum information necessary. The CyFlow SL (Partec, Münster, Germany) instrument equipped with 488 nm blue state laser allowed excitation of SYBR14 and PI to measure sperm viability. It was also fully equipped with five parameters: FSC, SSC, red, green, and orange/yellow colors. With the Partec FloMax software, the instrument allowed a real-time data acquisition, data display, and data evaluation.

The quality control measures and repeatability of flow cytometric sperm viability analysis were routinely verified by control samples which consisted of positive (100% dead sperm) and negative control (100% live sperm) of standard biological samples and their mixture of different ratios (100/100, 75/25/50/50, 25/75, and 100/100% dead and live sperm combinations). Another quality measure we used was the control of reagents (SYBR-14 and PI). The reagents and biological standards were used to calibrate the instrument settings and data processing. In the calibration, non-sperm particles were gated out and not included in the calculations. Partially stained (green and red) moribund sperm were considered as dead in the analysis. The percentage of live (green) sperm is used as a measure of sperm freezability parameter, the percentage of sperm that maintained membrane integrity during freeze–thawing process. The following formula was used to count the percentage of viable sperm: The% Viable sperm = The number of viable sperm/Total sperm (viable + dead + moribund) × 100.

Collectively, a unique freezability phenotype was generated to characterize variation among bulls for their lifetime post-thaw viability of sperm. For this particular research, we used post-thaw viability data generated over 8 years period (between 2008 and 2016). The database included 100,448 ejaculates from 860 Holstein bulls that were collected at least 20 different times in approximately 3 months period. The average and standard deviation of post-thaw viability for individual bulls were calculated, and then bulls were ranked based on average post-thaw semen viability. The threshold was the population average which consisted of the 100,448 ejaculates from 860 Holstein bulls. The average post-thaw viabilities of all bulls ranged from 33.03 to 67.3% (population average 54.7 ± 5.4%). The bulls were then classified as GF and PF based on average post-thaw viability score and the differences from the population average. The population average was our threshold to classify GF and PF groups. Bulls with greater sperm post-thaw viability than population average grouped as GF while those lower than average were considered as PF. Total of 13 bulls were selected with high confidence among 860 bulls for the presented study (**Table 1**).

TABLE 1 | Semen freezability phenotypes of the Holstein bulls used for GC–MS analysis: **(A)** Bulls 1–7 were defined as good freezability (GF) and Bulls 8–13 were grouped as poor freezability (PF) and **(B)** Percent differences of good and poor freezing phenotypes from the population average.

(A)

Bull No.	Freezability status	Average post-thaw viability (%)	Difference from population average (%)
1	Good freezability	66.19	11.50
2		64.40	9.71
3		64.28	9.59
4		62.34	7.65
5		61.95	7.26
6		59.92	5.23
7		58.37	3.68
8	Poor freezability	55.03	0.34
9		54.92	0.23
10		54.77	−0.08
11		52.68	−2.01
12		49.23	−5.46
13		48.93	−5.76

(B)

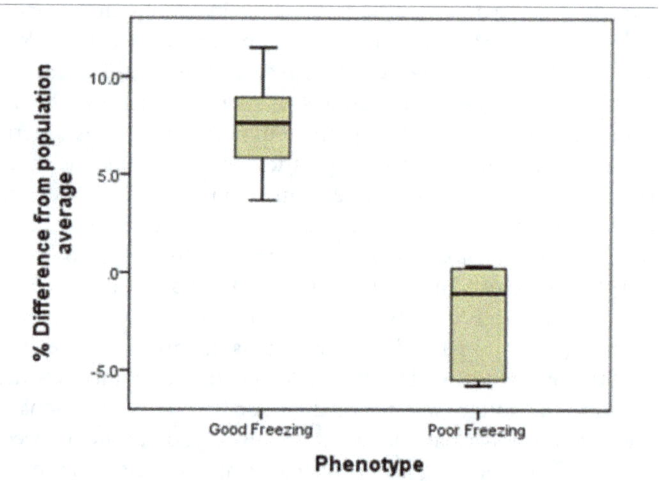

Bulls were classified as good freezability and poor freezability based on average post-thaw viability scores and the percent differences from the population average ($P < 0.001$).

Sample Preparation for Gas Chromatography–Mass Spectrometry Analysis

The amino acid analyses of seminal plasma from 13 bulls with various freezability were performed using EZfaast Amino Acid kit (©Phenomenex Inc., Torrance, CA, United States) as previously described by Kaspar et al. (2008). All samples were prepared and analyzed according to protocol that provided by Phenomenex Inc., Torrance, CA, United States. Briefly, 10 μl of seminal plasma and 25 μl of internal standard solution (norvaline 0.02 nM and *N*-propanol 10%) were pipetted into glass sample preparation vials. Solution in the sample preparation vial was passed through the sorbent tip using a syringe. Then, 200 μl of *N*-propanol was pipetted into the same vial and passed through the sorbent tip and into syringe barrel. Drained liquid from sorbent tip was discarded. One hundred and twenty microliters of sodium hydroxide and 80 μl of *N*-propanol were pipetted into same glass vial, and the particles inside the sorbent tip were ejected into solution. A volume of 50 μl of chloroform–propyl chloroformate, and 100 μl of iso-octane were transferred to the tube and the resulted mixture was vortexed for 1 min after each adding. Transparent part of the (upper) organic layer transferred into autosampler vial, and evaporation of the solvent was achieved using a TurboVap® LV evaporator (Biotage, Charlotte, NC, United States) with a gentle stream of nitrogen at 30°C. The extract was then suspended in 50 μl of solution containing iso-octane (80%) and chloroform (20%) and transferred to an amber glass vial having a fixed insert (Agilent Technologies, Santa Clara, CA, United States) for the analysis using GC–MS.

Amino Acid Analysis Using Gas Chromatography–Mass Spectrometry

We used recommended GC-MS parameters to analyze the seminal plasma amino acids and the reference standards in an Agilent 7890A GC System that was coupled to an Agilent 5975C inert XL MSD with triple-axis mass detector, an Agilent 7693 Series Autosampler, and a capillary column (Zebron™ EZ-AAA 10 m × 0.25 mm; ©Phenomenex, Santa Clara, CA, United States). The derivatized mixture (1.5 μl) was injected into the inlet that was heated at 250°C with 1:15 split ratio. Following the injection of the sample at 3 ml/min, standard septum purge was performed using helium carrier gas at 1 ml/min constant flow rate. Auxiliary, ion source, and quadrupole were heated at 310, 240, and 180°C, respectively. The oven was programmed initially at 110°C, and ramped up to 320°C within 11 min. The solvent delay time was at 1.30 min. The MS was operated in selected ion monitoring (SIM) mode and appropriate ion sets were selected. All amino acids were identified based on retention times, target and qualifier ions in comparison with authentic standards supplied by ©Phenomenex Inc., Torrance, CA, United States (**Table 2**). For calibration, increasing volumes of the diluted standards (0, 5, 10, 40, 80, 160, and 200 nmol/ml) were as described above. Abundances of the target ions of amino acids were divided by abundance of target ion of the internal standard (norvaline) and the unitless ratios were used to calculate amino acid concentrations using internal standard calibration.

Statistical Analysis

The associations between freezability of sperm and concentration of seminal plasma amino acids were assessed using both univariate and multivariate approaches. For univariate approach, a generalized linear mixed model was used to determine the statistical significance between GF and PF groups. The variance was estimated by the GLIMMIX procedure of SAS 9.4 (SAS Institute Inc., Cary, NC, United States). The Kenward–Roger approximation was used to calculate the degree of freedom in case of heterogeneous variances. In addition, correlations among seminal plasma amino acids and correlations between seminal plasma amino acid concentrations and freezability scores were determined using Pearson's correlation (Xia and Wishart, 2011). For multivariate analyses, MetaboAnalyst 3.0[1] (Xia et al., 2015) was used. For each variable, an observation was subtracted from the overall mean and the difference was divided by the standard deviation. This scaling or normalization of the data allowed us to bring the variances of all variables to the value of 1 while preserving the relative variability among observations within a variable. Following the normalization of data, partial least squares regression-discriminant analysis (PLS-DA) was performed and the bi-plot was constructed. The VIP scores in PLS-DA were calculated to identify significance of variables on phenotype. A VIP score >1.5 was considered as significant for group separation, and the significance level of 0.05 was used to determine statistical significance for other analyses. GraphPad Prism 8 was used (GraphPad Software, Inc., La Jolla, CA, United States) to generate some of the figures.

TABLE 2 | Selected ions and retention times for the SIM analysis of 22 amino acids, dipeptides and internal standard (norvaline).

Amino acid	Abbreviation	Retention time	Target ion (*m/z*)	Qualifier ion (*m/z*)
Alanine	ALA	1.42	130	88
Glycine	GLY	1.53	116	207
Alpha-aminobutyric acid	ABA	1.64	144	102
Valine	VAL	1.74	158	116
Beta-aminobutyric acid	Beta-AiB	1.83	158	116
Norvaline	NOR	1.88	158	72
Leucine	LEU	1.97	172	76
Allo-isoleucine	aILE	2.00	172	130
Isoleucine	ILE	2.03	172	130
Threonine	THR	2.25	160	101
Serine	SER	2.29	146	203
Proline	PRO	2.37	156	243
Asparagine	ASN	2.47	155	69
Aspartic acid	ASP	3.04	216	130
Methionine	MET	3.08	203	277
4-Hydroxyproline	4HYP	3.22	172	86
Glutamic acid	GLU	3.42	230	170
Phenylalanine	PHE	3.45	206	190
Alpha-aminoadipic acid	AAA	3.73	244	98
Ornithine	ORN	4.48	156	70
Lysine	LYS	4.75	170	128
Tyrosine	TYR	5.24	206	107
Tryptophan	TRP	5.54	130	

All amino acids were identified based on retention time, target and qualifier ions.

Pathway and Network Analysis

Pathways and network analyses of amino acids were performed using bioinformatic tools. The pathway-based compound-reaction-enzyme-gene networks were identified using MetScape 3.1 (Karnovsky et al., 2012) which was plug in Cytoscape 3.7.1[2]. Interactomes of gene products defined by MetScape 3.1

[1] http://www.metaboanalyst.ca
[2] https://cytoscape.org/

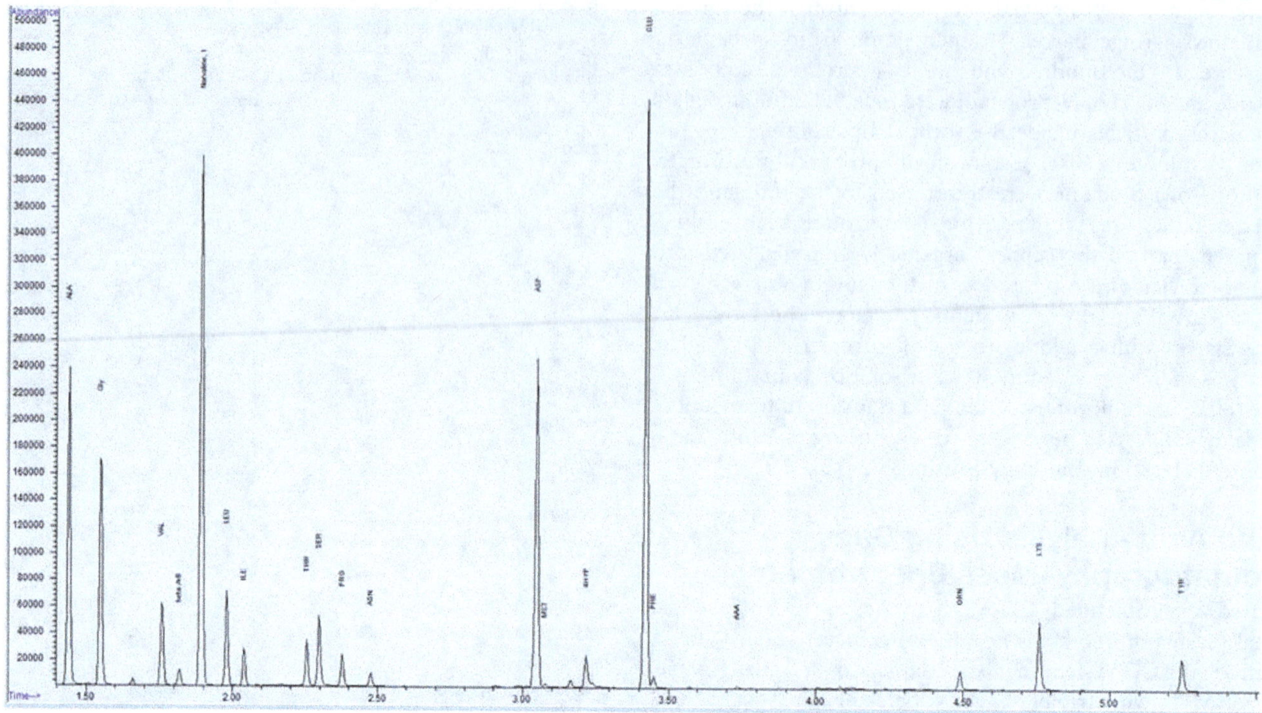

FIGURE 1 | Representative GC–MS chromatogram of bull seminal plasma. Total of 21 amino acids were identified using SIM (selected ion monitoring), Norvaline used as an internal standard with a concentration of 200 nM.

were identified using the biological networks gene ontology tool (BiNGO) within Cystoscope 3.7.1. A merged network was created in Cystoscope by entering subjected genes to analyze the interactome of genes for Bos Taurus, and significance level was set as 0.05.

TABLE 3 | Average amino acid concentrations (nM) of seminal plasma from good and poor freezability semen (mean ± SD).

Amino acid	Good freezability	Poor freezability	Both
Alanine	943.4 ± 232.9	1180.00 ± 318.6	1053 ± 187.9
Glycine	464.7 ± 90.62	389.10 ± 73.09	429.8 ± 57.94
α-Aminobutyric acid	6.349 ± 3.17	9.65 ± 4.258	7.874 ± 2.53
Valine	145.3 ± 13.89	134.80 ± 33.49	140.5 ± 16.43
β-Aminobutyric acid	92.77 ± 13.81	94.03 ± 25.50	93.35 ± 13.28
Leucine	140.7 ± 15.73	141.00 ± 26.44	140.8 ± 14.18
Allo-isoleucine	4.70 ± 1.67	7.32 ± 4.348	5.912 ± 2.13
Isoleucine	54.06 ± 5.93	45.66 ± 13.38	50.19 ± 6.73
Threonine	104.3 ± 19.67	149.10 ± 36.93	125 ± 20.20
Serine	250.2 ± 52.74	310.90 ± 63.93	278.2 ± 40.14
Proline	35.56 ± 9.34	46.87 ± 17.39	40.78 ± 9.18
Asparagine	1.98 ± 1.90	4.02 ± 1.63	2.92 ± 1.25
Aspartic acid	412.0 ± 120.3	444.40 ± 181.7	427 ± 101.3
Methionine	7.851 ± 1.99	10.27 ± 3.16	8.97 ± 1.76
4-Hydroxyproline	49.50 ± 9.74	44.45 ± 5.21	47.17 ± 5.59
Glutamic acid	3567 ± 899.8	3131.00 ± 635.6	3366 ± 547.3
Phenylalanine	25.53 ± 2.06	18.72 ± 1.28	22.38 ± 1.56
α-Aminoadipic acid	18.21 ± 3.23	16.23 ± 1.53	17.29 ± 1.83
Ornithine	33.39 ± 4.83	27.27 ± 3.98	30.56 ± 3.18
Lysine	77.43 ± 13.63	58.42 ± 12.76	68.65 ± 9.42
Tyrosine	14.25 ± 2.71	11.26 ± 2.78	12.87 ± 1.91

RESULTS

Amino Acid Concentration in Bull Seminal Plasma

Twenty-one amino acids were detected in bull seminal plasma (**Figure 1**). Free amino acid concentrations of bull seminal

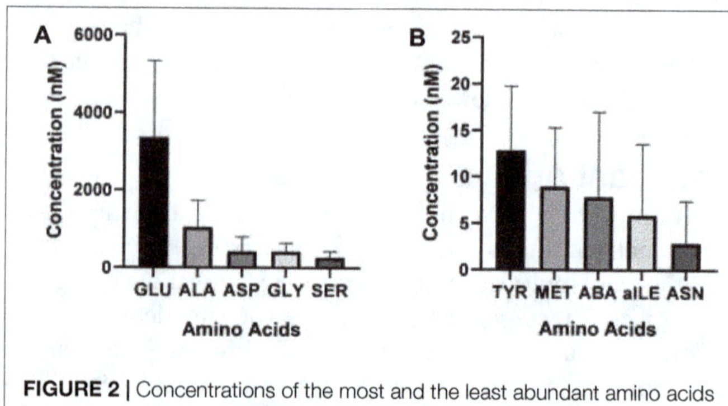

FIGURE 2 | Concentrations of the most and the least abundant amino acids in bull seminal plasma. **(A)** The most abundant amino acids in bull seminal plasma was glutamic acid. Alanine, glycine, aspartic acid, and serine were the other predominant amino acids in bull seminal plasma. **(B)** The least predominant amino acids were tyrosine, methionine, alpha aminobutyric acid, allo-isoleucine, and asparagine.

A

	PTV	ALA	GLY	ABA	VAL	betaAIB	LEU	aILE	ILE	THR	SER	PRO	ASN	ASP	MET	HYP	GLU	PHE	AAA	ORN	LYS	TYR
PTV	1.000	-0.230	0.196	-0.200	0.027	-0.050	-0.047	-0.219	0.106	-0.326	-0.115	-0.228	-0.217	-0.063	-0.238	0.112	0.322	0.565	0.365	0.176	0.085	-0.025
		0.450	0.520	0.513	0.931	0.870	0.878	0.472	0.730	0.277	0.708	0.455	0.477	0.838	0.435	0.715	0.284	0.044	0.221	0.565	0.781	0.936
ALA		1.000	0.389	0.910	0.860	0.653	0.636	0.673	0.774	0.945	0.611	0.645	0.511	0.437	0.559	0.151	0.006	-0.083	-0.147	-0.145	-0.150	-0.200
			0.188	<.0001	0.001	0.016	0.020	0.012	0.002	<.0001	0.026	0.017	0.074	0.135	0.047	0.623	0.984	0.787	0.631	0.637	0.625	0.513
GLY			1.000	0.504	0.544	0.811	0.812	0.741	0.695	0.331	0.238	0.774	0.716	0.651	0.754	0.268	0.606	0.340	0.190	-0.479	-0.583	-0.596
				0.079	0.055	0.002	0.002	0.004	0.008	0.270	0.434	0.002	0.006	0.016	0.003	0.375	0.028	0.256	0.535	0.098	0.036	0.032
ABA				1.000	0.873	0.690	0.697	0.742	0.735	0.805	0.465	0.811	0.498	0.635	0.614	0.240	0.048	-0.140	0.004	-0.366	-0.343	-0.356
					<.0001	0.009	0.008	0.004	0.004	0.002	0.110	0.002	0.084	0.020	0.026	0.430	0.876	0.647	0.989	0.219	0.252	0.233
VAL					1.000	0.744	0.781	0.801	0.917	0.741	0.270	0.771	0.391	0.713	0.618	-0.041	-0.037	-0.014	0.036	-0.278	-0.288	-0.316
						0.004	0.002	0.001	<.0001	0.004	0.372	0.002	0.186	0.006	0.024	0.894	0.904	0.964	0.908	0.358	0.339	0.293
betaAIB						1.000	0.943	0.935	0.804	0.562	0.202	0.860	0.739	0.769	0.835	0.031	0.444	0.148	0.240	-0.520	-0.556	-0.598
							<.0001	<.0001	0.002	0.045	0.509	0.001	0.004	0.002	0.001	0.921	0.129	0.628	0.430	0.068	0.049	0.031
LEU							1.000	0.953	0.883	0.570	0.185	0.896	0.727	0.787	0.859	0.086	0.303	0.127	0.246	-0.514	-0.505	-0.507
								<.0001	<.0001	0.042	0.544	<.0001	0.005	0.001	0.001	0.780	0.314	0.679	0.419	0.072	0.079	0.077
aILE								1.000	0.822	0.621	0.169	0.941	0.696	0.818	0.881	-0.088	0.198	-0.015	0.099	-0.552	-0.567	-0.575
									0.002	0.024	0.580	<.0001	0.008	0.002	<.0001	0.776	0.518	0.962	0.747	0.051	0.043	0.040
ILE									1.000	0.689	0.267	0.756	0.559	0.671	0.708	0.034	0.119	0.176	0.081	-0.266	-0.277	-0.301
										0.009	0.378	0.003	0.047	0.012	0.007	0.912	0.699	0.565	0.793	0.379	0.359	0.318
THR										1.000	0.743	0.553	0.579	0.320	0.592	0.099	0.028	-0.147	-0.217	-0.147	-0.173	-0.231
											0.004	0.050	0.038	0.286	0.033	0.748	0.927	0.632	0.476	0.632	0.572	0.447
SER											1.000	0.179	0.501	-0.185	0.231	0.496	0.261	0.083	-0.235	0.061	-0.038	-0.108
												0.558	0.081	0.545	0.447	0.084	0.389	0.787	0.439	0.843	0.903	0.725
PRO												1.000	0.681	0.801	0.801	0.127	0.159	0.032	0.062	-0.606	-0.586	-0.544
													0.010	0.001	0.001	0.679	0.604	0.918	0.841	0.028	0.035	0.055
ASN													1.000	0.368	0.728	0.293	0.519	0.335	0.078	-0.603	-0.576	-0.570
														0.216	0.005	0.331	0.069	0.263	0.800	0.029	0.040	0.042
ASP														1.000	0.768	-0.211	0.239	-0.248	0.381	-0.634	-0.645	-0.630
															0.002	0.488	0.432	0.413	0.199	0.020	0.017	0.021
MET															1.000	-0.069	0.367	-0.133	0.051	-0.498	-0.525	-0.569
																0.824	0.217	0.666	0.868	0.083	0.065	0.043
HYP																1.000	0.254	0.363	0.078	0.030	0.120	0.187
																	0.402	0.223	0.800	0.922	0.696	0.541
GLU																	1.000	0.250	0.532	-0.399	-0.562	-0.655
																		0.409	0.061	0.177	0.046	0.015
PHE																		1.000	0.007	-0.024	0.031	0.027
																			0.981	0.937	0.920	0.930
AAA																			1.000	-0.513	-0.498	-0.483
																				0.073	0.083	0.094
ORN																				1.000	0.919	0.826
																					<.0001	0.002
LYS																					1.000	0.962
																						<.0001
TYR																						1

B

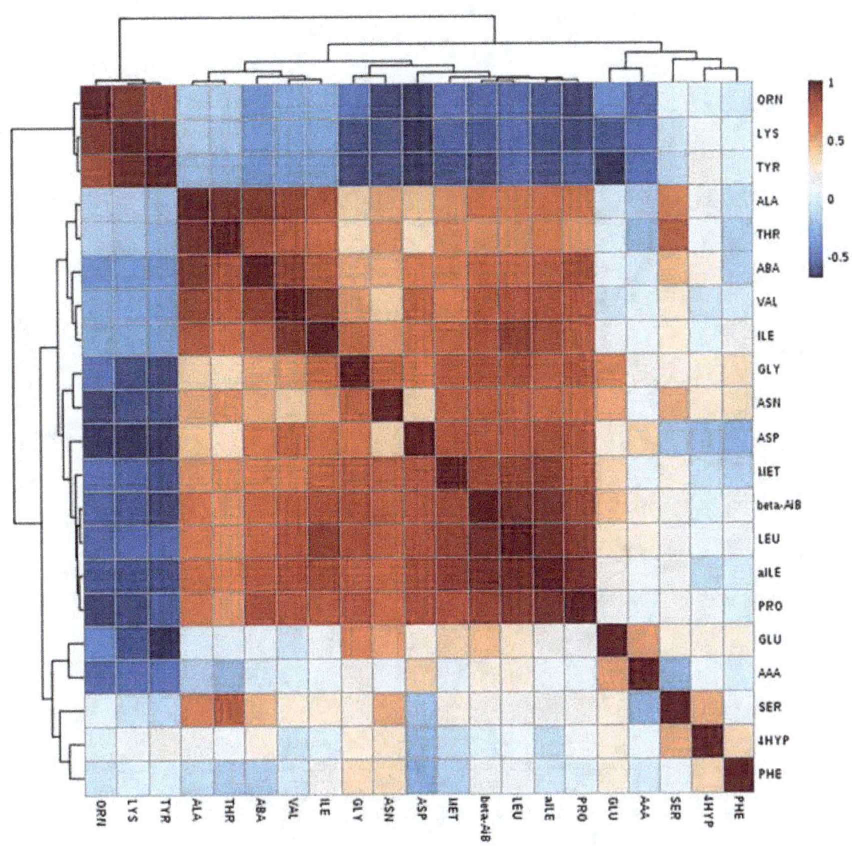

FIGURE 3 | Pearson's correlations among amino acids identified in bull seminal plasma. **(A)** Correlation matrix of amino acid concentrations in seminal plasma [shaded lines: Pearson correlation coefficients (*r*); white boxes: *P*-value; highlighted boxes: $P < 0.05$). **(B)** Heatmap of Pearson's correlations among amino acids identified in bull seminal plasma.

plasma are depicted in **Table 3**. Among these, glutamic acid was the most abundant amino acid in seminal plasma with an average concentration of 3366 ± 547.3 (mean ± SD) nM, which accounts for approximately 53% of all the amino acids. The other most predominant amino acids were alanine, glycine, aspartic acid, and serine with mean concentrations of 1053 ± 187.9, 429.8 ± 57.94, 427 ± 101.3, and 278.2 ± 40.14 nM, respectively (**Figure 2A**). The least abundant were tyrosine, methionine, alpha-aminobutyric acid, allo-isoleucine, and asparagine with mean concentrations of 12.87 ± 1.91, 8.97 ± 1.76, 7.87 ± 2.53, 5.91 ± 2.13, and 2.92 ± 1.25 nM, respectively (**Figure 2B**).

Identification of Potential Freezability Biomarkers

There was no significant difference in amino acid concentrations between GF and PF groups ($P > 0.05$). However, phenylalanine concentration was significantly correlated with average post-thaw viability ($r = 0.57$, P-value = 0.044). Additionally, there were significant correlations among individual amino acids (**Figure 3**), such as the concentration of proline was positively correlated with leucine ($r = 0.90$, P-value < 0.0001), iso-leucine positively correlated with valine ($r = 0.92$, P-value < 0001), and the concentration of threonine was positively correlated with alanine ($r = 0.95$, P-value < 0001).

The multivariate analysis, PLS-DA, of seminal plasma amino acids showed a distinct separation between GF and PF bulls (**Figure 4**). PLS-DA was used for the classification. A variable importance in projection (VIP) score, which is widely used in PLS-DA, rank the amino acids considering their significance in discrimination between the GF and PF bulls. VIP score is referred as a weighted sum of squares of the PLS loadings. The X-axis specifies the VIP scores to each variable on the Y-axis. Therefore, amino acids with VIP score >1.5 was identified as phenylalanine, and VIP score in the corresponding heat map demonstrated that phenylalanine is more abundant in seminal plasma of the GF bulls than in that of PF bulls (**Figure 5**).

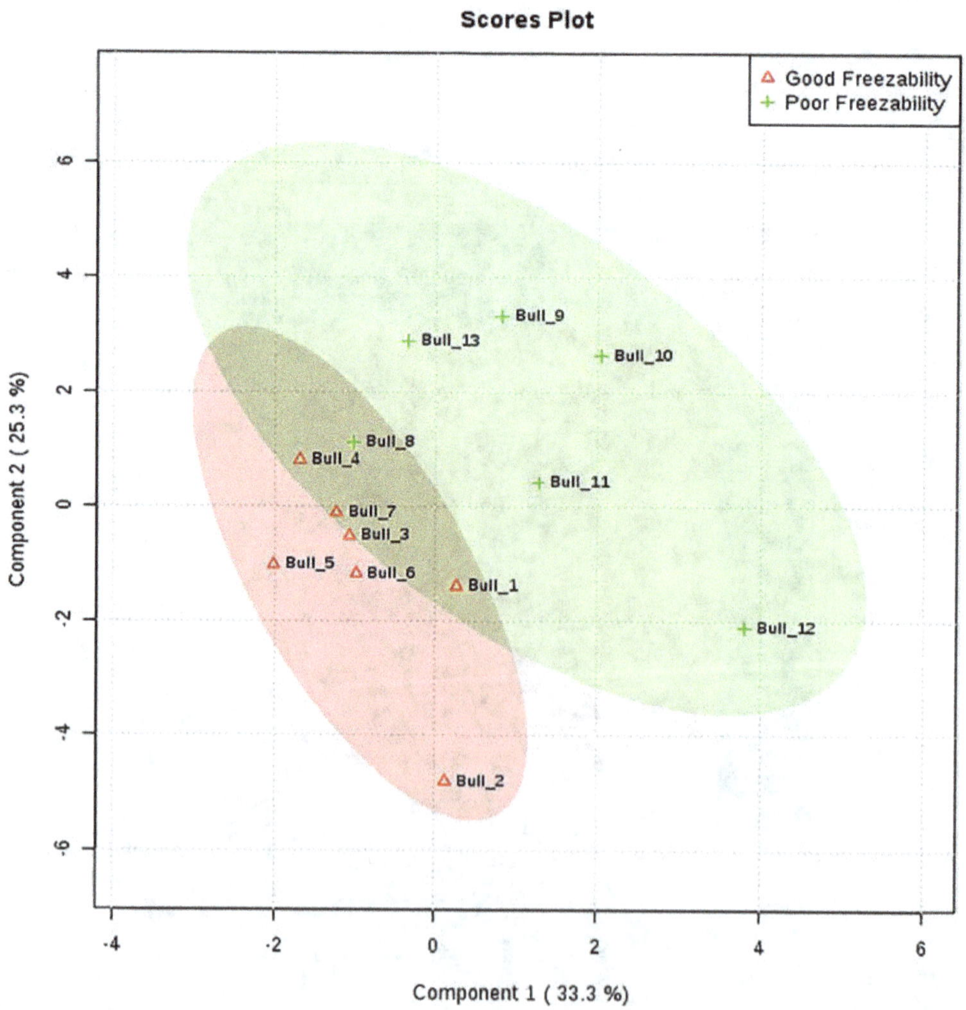

FIGURE 4 | Partial least squares discriminant analysis (2D PLS-DA) of the seminal plasma amino acids from good freezability (GF) and poor freezability (PF) bulls. The plots indicate a separation between GF and PF bulls. PLS-DA was obtained with two components.

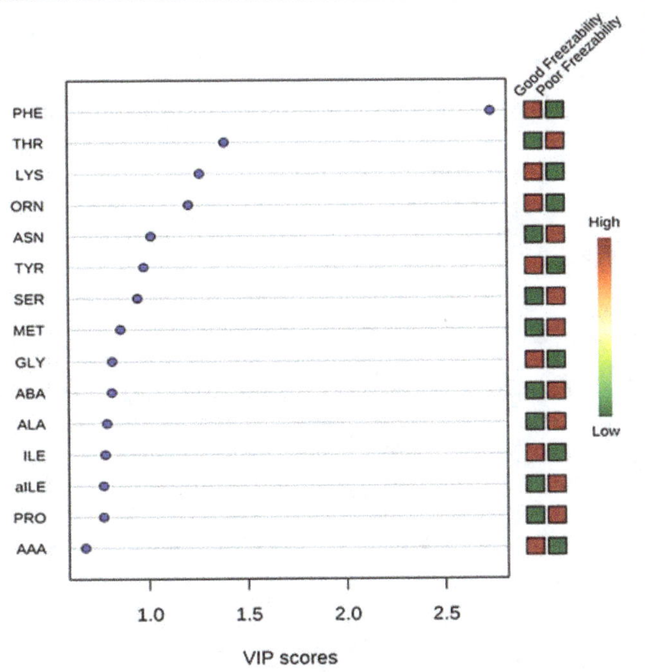

FIGURE 5 | Variable importance in projection (VIP) plot displays the top 15 most important amino acid features identified by PLS-DA. Colored boxes on right indicate concentration of corresponding amino acid from GF and PF samples. VIP score is a weighted based on PLS-DA model.

Pathways and Networks of Seminal Plasma Amino Acids

Pathway and network analyses of the amino acids with highest VIP scores (phenylalanine and threonine) and the most abundant amino acids (glutamic acid, alanine, and glycine) were performed using MetScape (3.1.3) (Karnovsky et al., 2012). By analyzing the results, we showed that phenylalanine was involved in tyrosine metabolism, and interacted with several compounds and genes (**Figure 6A**). The interactome of phenylalanine showed that this amino acid contributes to a number of cellular and biological processes, such as antioxidant detoxification, metabolic processes of reactive oxygen species, and oxidoreductase activity (**Table 4**). Threonine was involved in glycine, serine, alanine, and threonine metabolism and it shows significant gene ontology in terms of cellular amino acids and derivative metabolic processes (**Figure 6B**). Glutamic acid was correlated with many genes, enzymes, and other reactions (**Figure 6C**), most of which occur in mitochondria. It has a significant interactome regarding oxidoreductase activity, regulation of cell death, and the oxoacid metabolic process. It also contributes to histidine metabolism, the urea cycle, and the metabolism of arginine, proline, glutamate, aspartate, and asparagine, and Vitamin B9 (folate) metabolism. Alanine created a significant gene ontology in terms of ligase activity and forming carbon–oxygen bonds, and is also involved in pathways of glycine, serine, alanine, and threonine metabolism (**Figure 6D**). Finally, glycine is involved in seven different biological and cellular pathways, and has generated significant gene ontology in terms of oxidoreductase activity (acting on the CH-NH_2 group of donors), sarcosine oxidase activity, and D-amino-acid oxidase activity. All findings are summarized in **Table 4**.

DISCUSSION

Successful sperm cryopreservation is an imperative element of fertility management and assisted reproductive studies (ART). The contributions that seminal plasma metabolites have on sperm cryopreservation are still largely unknown. In this present study, we performed GC–MS analyses to investigate the amino acid profiles of bull seminal plasma and classify potential biomolecular markers of freezability. Consecutively, bioinformatic tools were used to identify network and biological pathways of seminal plasma amino acids. To the extent of our knowledge, our study is the first to conduct an extensive assessment of amino acids in bull seminal plasma considering association of specific seminal plasma amino acids with freezability phenotypes.

Seminal plasma is a complex fluid composed of a broad range of metabolites such as organic compounds and energy substrates. Biochemical compositions of seminal plasma differ among species and even among individual males (Killian et al., 1993). This may be due to different management and feeding variations as well as metabolic activity of sperm. These metabolites in seminal plasma have functional roles in sperm preservation, motility, and control of metabolic activity (Bieniek et al., 2016). Amino acids and peptides are the major biochemical compounds found in bovine sperm and its seminal plasma. There is a wide range of amino acids in seminal plasma of which concentrations of many rise after ejaculation due to the massive proteolytic activities occurring in semen (Mann, 1964). Amino acids function as oxidizable substrates for the energy supply, causing reactions in semen (Neumark and Schındler, 2007).

The most abundant amino acid present in seminal plasma is glutamic acid accompanied by a considerable level of glutamic oxaloacetic transaminase (GOT) activity (Flipse, 1960). As in earlier bull semen studies, the abundance of glycine, alanine, serine, aspartic acid, and glutamic acid is found to be high and high levels of amino acids in seminal plasma are higher than in sperm (Roussel and Stallcup, 1967). In a recent study aimed at analyzing metabolomes of seminal plasma from bulls with somewhat higher vs. lower fertility, researchers have identified 63 metabolites, in seminal plasma, of which 21 are amino acids that can be potential biomarker of fertility. Abundances of L-leucine and ornithine differed between the fertility groups, and the levels of fructose were correlated with those of glutamic acid and amino-butyrolactone (Velho et al., 2018). In other studies, researchers have determined different numbers of amino acids and peptides, in seminal plasma of bull, where glutamic and aspartic acid were the most abundant, and were associated with fertility and pregnancy rates (al-Hakim et al., 1970; Holden et al., 2017). Also, seminal plasma of human and other species were found to contain large numbers of amino acids (Engel et al., 2019; Santiago-Moreno et al., 2019). Fertility and sperm freezability are not always related. This current study was aimed at ascertaining

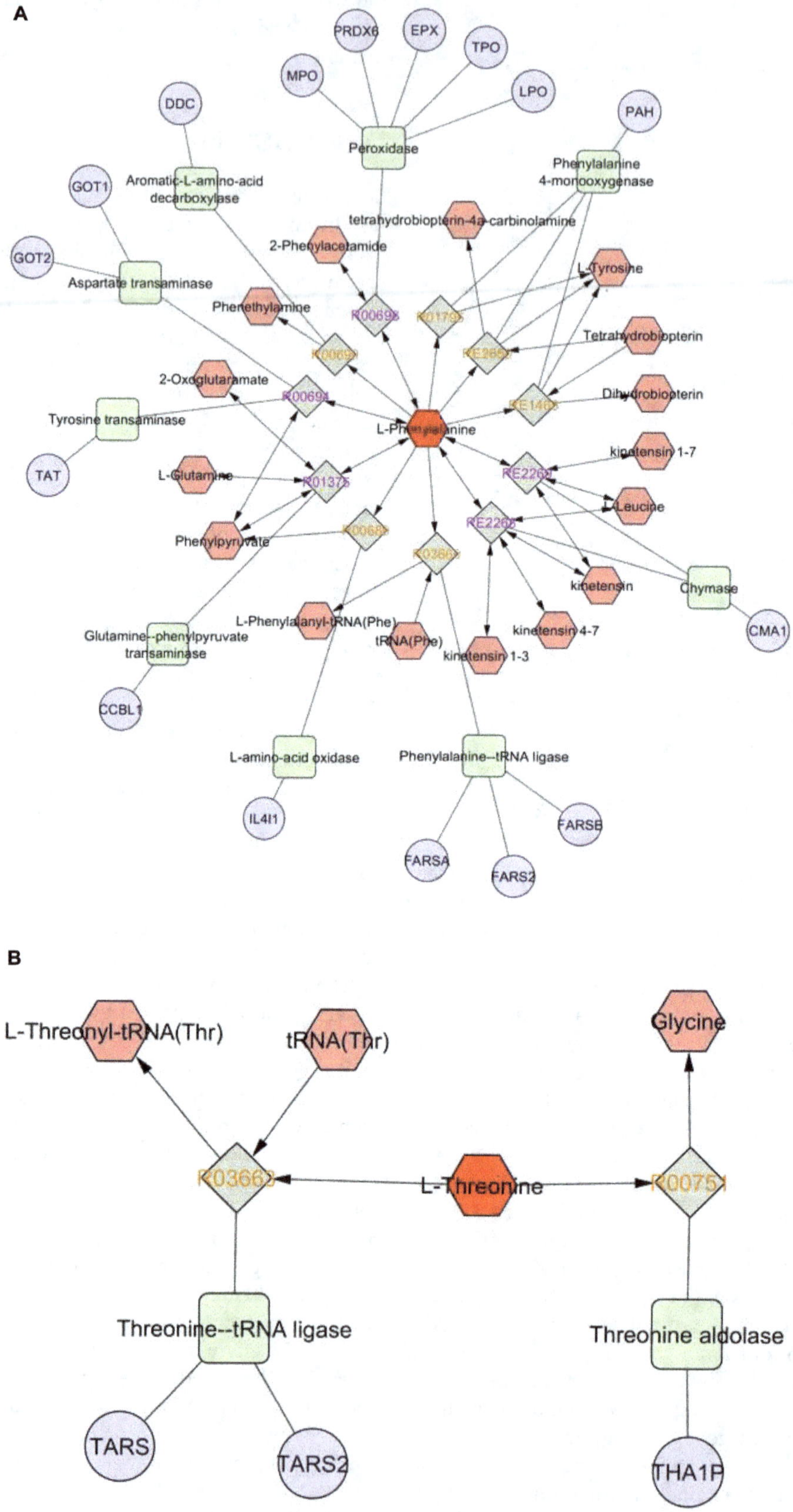

FIGURE 6 | Continued

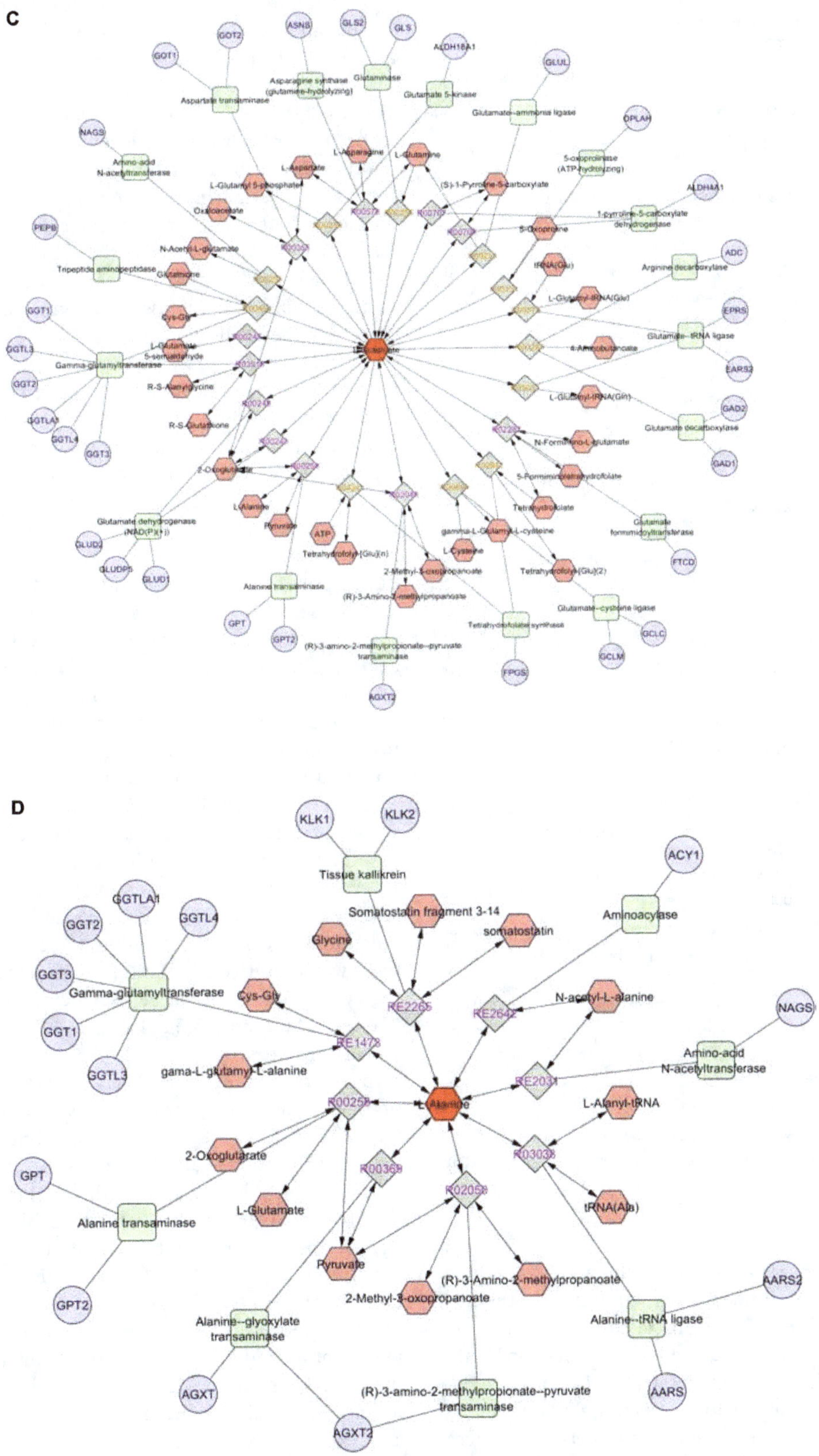

FIGURE 6 | Pathway and network analyses of the amino acids with highest VIP scores (phenylalanine, threonine) and the most abundant amino acids (glutamic acid, alanine) were performed using MetScape. **(A)** Phenylalanine, **(B)** threonine, **(C)** glutamate, and **(D)** alanine. Amino acids are shown in red hexagons. Gray square: Reaction node with reaction ID; Pale red hexagon: Compound node; Green square: Enzyme node; Blue circle: Gene node.

TABLE 4 | The interactome of amino acid shows that amino acid contributes to a great number of cellular and biological processes, such as antioxidant detoxification, reactive oxygen species metabolic processes, and oxidoreductase activity.

Amino acid	GO ID	Description	*P*-value
Phenylalanine	10602	Oxidoreductase activity, acting on paired donors, with incorporation or reduction of molecular oxygen, reduced pteridine as one donor, and incorporation of one atom of oxygen	0.003
	10636	Cellular biosynthetic process	0.007
	10652	Oxygen and reactive oxygen species metabolic process	0.025
	10677	Response to stress	0.016
	10678	Response to oxidative stress	<0.0001
	10680	Tyrosine metabolic process	0.004
	10733	Oxidoreductase activity, acting on peroxide as acceptor	<0.0001
	10735	Response to reactive oxygen species	<0.0001
	10738	Antioxidant activity	<0.0001
	10788	Hydrogen peroxide metabolic process	0.012
	10789	Hydrogen peroxide catabolic process	0.007
	10865	Vitamin binding	<0.0001
	10879	Peroxiredoxin activity	0.007
	10894	Oxidation reduction	0.001
	10913	Cellular response to reactive oxygen species	0.013
	11069	Fatty acid transport	0.008
Threonine	11913	Cellular amino acid and derivative metabolic process	0.017
Glutamic acid	8483	Transaminase activity	<0.0001
	16639	Oxidoreductase activity, acting on the CH-NH_2 group of donors, NAD or NADP as acceptor	0.001
	12782	Regulation of cell death	0.047
	43436	Oxoacid metabolic process	<0.0001
Alanine	15707	Ligase activity, forming carbon–oxygen bonds	0.017
	15722	Small molecule metabolic process	0.008
Glycine	16641	Oxidoreductase activity, acting on the CH-NH group of donors, oxygen as acceptor	0.001
	8115	Sarcosine oxidase activity	0.001
	3884	D-Amino-acid oxidase activity	0.003
	17834	Oxidoreductase activity, acting on the CH-NH_2 group of donors	0.016

seminal plasma amino acids associated with sperm freezability. In the current study, we identified the glutamic acid as the most abundant amino acid. We also demonstrated that glutamic acid was correlated with a number of genes, enzymes, and other reactions, most of which occur in mitochondria. This provides an important evidence of interactome regarding oxidoreductase activity, regulation of cell death, the oxoacid metabolic process, and significant possibility of influence on cell energy production.

The other most predominant amino acids revealed in our study were alanine, glycine, aspartic acid, and serine. When these amino acids in seminal plasma were compared to those found in human seminal plasma (Li et al., 2019), profiles of some seminal plasma amino acids were similar to those profiles we found such as serine, glycine, and glutamic acids. The least abundant in our study, on the other hand, are tyrosine, methionine, alpha-aminobutyric acid, allo-isoleucine, and asparagine, and are found to be similar with the low levels of amino acids of methionine and tyrosine in bull (Assumpção et al., 2005). Also, in domestic fowl, valine, serine, glycine, and alanine were the most abundant amino acids followed by glutamic acid (Santiago-Moreno et al., 2019). The alanine created a significant gene ontology in terms of its ligase activity and formed carbon–oxygen bonds, and is also involved in pathways of glycine, serine, alanine, and threonine metabolism.

During the cryopreservation process, sperm undergo critical cryo-injury based on membrane damage, oxidative stress, and DNA fragmentation which reduce post-thaw viability of sperm cells. Even though the exact cryo-protectant mechanisms of amino acids have not been clearly understood, it is presumed they may bind phospholipid membrane bilayers and stabilize the cell membranes (Bilodeau et al., 2001). In addition, osmo-regulative and antioxidative features may provide resilience during freezing–thawing (Kruuv and Glofcheski, 1992; Farshad and Hosseini, 2013). However, there are not a great number of studies that have investigated the protective influence of amino acids against cryo-injury. Previous studies have claimed that seminal plasma supplementation of amino acids into semen extenders improved sperm viability, acrosome integrity and membrane integrity of sperm (Ali Al Ahmad et al., 2008), and post-thaw semen quality (Saravia et al., 2009). More specifically, in human research, it was found that addition of glutamine to semen as a cryoprotectant agent increased post-thaw motility in human sperm (Atessahin et al., 2008). In animal studies, supplementation of extender solutions with glutamine, glycine, and cysteine enhanced acrosome and membrane integrity of buffalo bull semen (El-Sheshtawy et al., 2008). Additionally, there was a positive correlation between membrane integrity and the concentration of valine, isoleucine and leucine, and lysine (Santiago-Moreno et al., 2019).

One of the most common negative consequences of cryopreservation of sperm cell is DNA damage, and majority of DNA lesions in sperm cells is caused by oxidative stress (Zribi et al., 2010). Seminal plasma content plays a significant role in protection against oxidative stress. Aitken and Baker (2004) clarified that taurine and hypotaurine are the amino acids that reduce oxidative stress through binding to the oxidizing agents. In addition, supplementation of donkey semen with glutamine reduced DNA fragmentation index (Bottrel et al., 2018). Sangeeta et al. (2015) reported that supplementation of ram sperm with L-glutamine and L-proline reduced lipid peroxidation and increased acrosomal integrity. Glutamic acid is the key component of glutathione which has been demonstrated to inhibit cellular damage resulting from lipid peroxidation and reactive oxygen species (Arai et al., 1999). In the present study, we showed that phenylalanine is more abundant in seminal plasma of the GF bulls than in that of PF bulls. It has significant gene ontology terms for antioxidant activity, response to oxidative stress, and oxidoreductase activity through its actions on peroxide as acceptor, and metabolic processes of oxygen as well as reactive oxygen species. We postulate that phenylalanine could have an antioxidant effect, and increased concentrations of phenylalanine in seminal plasma may reduce DNA damage caused by oxidative stress. Moreover, PLS-DA results demonstrate a distinct separation between GF and PF groups. Thus, the abundance of glutamic acid may explain protective effects of seminal plasma during cryopreservation. Furthermore, glutamine may play an important role in gene expression redox-potential, and cell integrity (Curi et al., 2005). It has been assumed electrostatic interactions between plasma membrane phospholipids and amino acids help to generate a layer on the sperm surface, and which thus protects the sperm cell from cryo-injury (Anchordoguy et al., 1988; Kundu et al., 2001).

CONCLUSION

We have found that glutamic acid, alanine, and glycine are the predominant metabolites in bull seminal plasma. It is clear that there is a distinct separation of the amino acid profiles for the seminal plasmas of GF and PF bulls. According to our findings, phenylalanine could be considered as a freezability biomarker, and may be used as a cryoprotectant supplement. In addition, amino acid profiles of the seminal plasma could be used to determine the freezability phenotypes. These findings help us better understand the exact mechanisms of cryopreservation for sperm cells as well as other cell types.

AUTHOR CONTRIBUTIONS

MU, AK, TD, and EM conceptualized the study. MU, TD, and MH curated the data. MU, TD, MH, and EM carried out the investigations. AK, BD, and ET provided the essential samples and phenotypic data. MU, TD, MH, AK, and EM wrote the original draft, and reviewed and edited the manuscript.

FUNDING

This project was supported by the Agriculture and Food Research Initiative Competitive Grant No. 2017-67016-26507 from the USDA National Institute of Food and Agriculture. Partial funding was provided by the Mississippi Agricultural Forestry Experiment Station, and by Alta Genetics Inc., Watertown, WI, United States. MH was funded through a competitive international postdoctoral fellowship by the Scientific and Technological Research Council of Turkey (TUBITAK). MU was funded through a competitive graduate fellowship from the Turkish Ministry of National Education.

REFERENCES

Aitken, R. J., and Baker, M. A. (2004). Oxidative stress and male reproductive biology. *Reprod. Fertil. Dev.* 16, 581–588. doi: 10.1071/RD03089

al-Hakim, M. K., Graham, E. F., and Schmehl, M. L. (1970). Free amino acids and amino compounds in bovine seminal plasma. *J. Dairy Sci.* 53, 84–88. doi: 10.3168/jds.S0022-0302

Ali Al Ahmad, M., Chatagnon, G., Amirat-Briand, L., Moussa, M., Tainturier, D., Anton, M., et al. (2008). Use of glutamine and low density lipoproteins isolated from egg yolk to improve buck semen freezing. *Reprod. Domest. Anim.* 43, 429–436. doi: 10.1111/j.1439-0531.2007.00930.x

Amirat-Briand, L., Bencharif, D., Vera-Munoz, O., Bel Hadj Ali, H., Destrumelle, S., Desherces, S., et al. (2009). Effect of glutamine on post-thaw motility of bull spermatozoa after association with LDL (low density lipoproteins) extender: preliminary results. *Theriogenology* 71, 1209–1214. doi: 10.1016/j.theriogenology.2008.10.002

Anchordoguy, T., Carpenter, J. F., Loomis, S. H., and Crowe, J. H. (1988). Mechanisms of interaction of amino acids with phospholipid bilayers during freezing. *Biochim. Biophys. Acta Biomembr.* 946, 299–306. doi: 10.1016/0005-2736(88)90405-90401

Arai, M., Imai, H., Koumura, T., Yoshida, M., Emoto, K., Umeda, M., et al. (1999). Mitochondrial phospholipid hydroperoxide glutathione peroxidase plays a major role in preventing oxidative injury to cells. *J. Biol. Chem.* 274, 4924–4933. doi: 10.1074/jbc.274.8.4924

Assumpção, T. I., Torres, R. A. A., Sousa, M. V., and Ricart, C. A. O. (2005). Correlation between fertility and levels of protein, sugar and free amino acids in seminal plasma of Nelore bulls. *Arq. Bras. Med. Vet. Zootec.* 57, 55–61. doi: 10.1590/S0102-09352005000100008

Atessahin, A., Bucak, M. N., Tuncer, P. B., and Kizil, M. (2008). Effects of anti-oxidant additives on microscopic and oxidative parameters of angora goat semen following the freeze-thawing process. *Small Rumin. Res.* 77, 38–44. doi: 10.1016/j.smallrumres.2008.03.002

Bieniek, J. M., Drabovich, A. P., and Lo, K. C. (2016). Seminal biomarkers for the evaluation of male infertility. *Asian J. Androl.* 18, 426–433. doi: 10.4103/1008-682X.175781

Bilodeau, J.-F., Blanchette, S., Gagnon, C., and Sirard, M.-A. (2001). Thiols prevent H2O2-mediated loss of sperm motility in cryopreserved bull semen. *Theriogenology* 56, 275–286. doi: 10.1016/S0093-691X(01)00562-563

Bottrel, M., Acha, D., Ortiz, I., Hidalgo, M., Gósalvez, J., Camisão, J., et al. (2018). Cryoprotective effect of glutamine, taurine, and proline on post-thaw semen quality and DNA integrity of donkey spermatozoa. *Anim. Reprod. Sci.* 189, 128–135. doi: 10.1016/j.anireprosci.2017.12.021

Cheng, Y., Yang, X., Deng, X., Zhang, X., Li, P., Tao, J., et al. (2015). Metabolomics in bladder cancer: a systematic review. *Int. J. Clin. Exp. Med.* 8, 11052–11063.

Curi, R., Lagranha, C. J., Doi, S. Q., Sellitti, D. F., Procopio, J., Pithon-Curi, T. C., et al. (2005). Molecular mechanisms of glutamine action. *J. Cell. Physiol.* 204, 392–401. doi: 10.1002/jcp.20339

Dvořáková, K., Moore, H. D. M., Šebková, N., and Paleèek, J. (2005). Cytoskeleton localization in the sperm head prior to fertilization. *Reproduction* 130, 61–69. doi: 10.1530/rep.1.00549

Egea, R. R., Puchalt, N. G., Escrivá, M. M., and Varghese, A. C. (2014). OMICS: current and future perspectives in reproductive medicine and technology. *J. Hum. Reprod. Sci.* 7, 73–92. doi: 10.4103/0974-1208.138857

El-Sheshtawy, R. I., El-Sisy, G. A., and El-Nattat, W. S. (2008). Use of selected amino acids to improve buffalo bull semen cryopreservation. *Glob. Vet.* 2, 146–150.

Engel, K. M., Baumann, S., Rolle-Kampczyk, U., Schiller, J., von Bergen, M., and Grunewald, S. (2019). Metabolomic profiling reveals correlations between spermiogram parameters and the metabolites present in human spermatozoa and seminal plasma. *PLoS One* 14:e0211679. doi: 10.1371/journal.pone.0211679

Farshad, A., and Hosseini, Y. (2013). The cryoprotective effects of amino acids supplementation on cooled and post-thaw Markhoz bucks semen quality. *Small Rumin. Res.* 114, 258–263. doi: 10.1016/j.smallrumres.2013.07.007

Flipse, R. J. (1960). Metabolism of bovine semen. IX. Glutamic-oxaloacetic and glutamic-pyruvic transaminase activities. *J. Dairy Sci.* 43, 773–776. doi: 10.3168/jds.S0022-0302(60)90237-X

Flores, E., Ramió-Lluch, L., Bucci, D., Fernández-Novell, J. M., Peña, A., and Rodríguez-Gil, J. E. (2011). Freezing-thawing induces alterations in histone H1-DNA binding and the breaking of protein-DNA disulfide bonds in boar sperm. *Theriogenology* 76, 1450–1464. doi: 10.1016/j.theriogenology.2011.05.039

Garner, D. L., Johnson, L. A., Yue, S. T., Roth, B. L., and Haugland, R. P. (1994). Dual DNA staining assessment of bovine sperm viability using SYBR-14 and propidium iodide. *J. Androl.* 15, 620–629. doi: 10.1002/j.1939-4640.1994.tb00510.x

Goodson, S. G., Qiu, Y., Sutton, K. A., Xie, G., Jia, W., and O'Brien, D. A. (2012). Metabolic substrates exhibit differential effects on functional parameters of mouse sperm capacitation1. *Biol. Reprod.* 87:75. doi: 10.1095/biolreprod.112.102673

Hamamah, S., Seguin, F., Barthelemy, C., Akoka, S., Le Pape, A., Lansac, J., et al. (1993). 1H nuclear magnetic resonance studies of seminal plasma from fertile and infertile men. *J. Reprod. Fertil.* 97, 51–55. doi: 10.1530/JRF.0.0970051

Heber, U., Tyankova, L., and Santarius, K. A. (1971). Stabilization and inactivation of biological membranes during freezing in the presence of amino acids. *BBA Biomembr.* 241, 578–592. doi: 10.1016/0005-2736(71)90056-90053

Holden, S. A., Fernandez-Fuertes, B., Murphy, C., Whelan, H., O'Gorman, A., Brennan, L., et al. (2017). Relationship between in vitro sperm functional assessments, seminal plasma composition, and field fertility after AI with either non-sorted or sex-sorted bull semen. *Theriogenology* 87, 221–228. doi: 10.1016/j.theriogenology.2016.08.024

Jaiswal, B. S., and Eisenbach, M. (2002). "Capacitation," in *Fertilization*, ed. D. M. Hardy (San Diego: Academic Press), 57–117.

Karnovsky, A., Weymouth, T., Hull, T., Tarcea, V. G., Scardoni, G., Laudanna, C., et al. (2012). Metscape 2 bioinformatics tool for the analysis and visualization of metabolomics and gene expression data. *Bioinformatics* 28, 373–380. doi: 10.1093/bioinformatics/btr661

Kaspar, H., Dettmer, K., Gronwald, W., and Oefner, P. J. (2008). Automated GC-MS analysis of free amino acids in biological fluids. *J. Chromatogr. B Anal. Technol. Biomed. Life Sci.* 870, 222–232. doi: 10.1016/j.jchromb.2008.06.018

Khlifaoui, M., Battut, I., Bruyas, J. F., Chatagnon, G., Trimeche, A., and Tainturier, D. (2005). Effects of glutamine on post-thaw motility of stallion spermatozoa: an approach of the mechanism of action at spermatozoa level. *Theriogenology* 63, 138–149. doi: 10.1016/J.THERIOGENOLOGY.2004.04.012

Killian, G. J., Chapman, D. A., and Rogowski, L. A. (1993). Fertility-associated proteins in Holstein bull seminal plasma. *Biol. Reprod.* 49, 1202–1207. doi: 10.1095/biolreprod49.6.1202

Koskinen, E., Junnila, M., Katila, T., and Soini, H. (1989). A preliminary study on the use of betaine as a cryoprotective agent in deep freezing of stallion semen. *J. Vet. Med. Ser. A* 36, 110–114. doi: 10.1111/j.1439-0442.1989.tb00710.x

Kruuv, J., and Glofcheski, D. J. (1992). Protective effects of amino acids against freeze-thaw damage in mammalian cells. *Cryobiology* 29, 291–295. doi: 10.1016/0011-2240(92)90028-Z

Kundu, C. N., Das, K., and Majumder, G. C. (2001). Effect of amino acids on goat cauda epididymal sperm cryopreservation using a chemically defined model system. *Cryobiology* 42, 21–27. doi: 10.1006/cryo.2001.2296

Li, M. J., Zhang, Z. M., Fan, F., Ma, P., Wang, Y., and Lu, H. M. (2019). Exploring asthenozoospermia seminal plasma amino acid disorder based on GC-SIM-MS combined with chemometrics methods. *Anal. Methods* 11, 2895–2902. doi: 10.1039/c9ay00134d

Lin, C. Y., Hung, P. H., VandeVoort, C. A., and Miller, M. G. (2009). 1H NMR to investigate metabolism and energy supply in rhesus macaque sperm. *Reprod. Toxicol.* 28, 75–80. doi: 10.1016/j.reprotox.2009.03.005

Mann, T. (1964). *The Biochemistry of Semen and of the Male Reproductive Tract.* New York, NY: John Wiley & Sons.

Mann, T., and Lutwak-Mann, C. (eds). (1981). "Biochemistry of seminal plasma and male accessory fluids; application to andrological problems," in *Male Reproductive Function and Semen* (London: Springer), 269–336. doi: 10.1007/978-1-4471-1300-3_9

Nagy, S., Jansen, J., Topper, E. K., and Gadella, B. M. (2004). A triple-stain flow cytometric method to assess plasma- and Acrosome-membrane integrity of cryopreserved bovine sperm immediately after thawing in presence of egg-yolk particles1. *Biol. Reprod.* 68, 1828–1835. doi: 10.1095/biolreprod.102.011445

Neumark, H., and Schındler, H. (2007). Amino acids, amines and peptides of ram epididymal semen. *Reproduction* 14, 469–471. doi: 10.1530/jrf.0.0140469

Nijs, M., Creemers, E., Cox, A., Janssen, M., Vanheusden, E., Castro-Sanchez, Y., et al. (2009). Influence of freeze-thawing on hyaluronic acid binding of human spermatozoa. *Reprod. Biomed. Online* 19, 202–206. doi: 10.1016/S1472-6483(10)60073-9

Nongbua, T., Al-Essawe, E. M., Edman, A., Johannisson, A., and Morrell, J. M. (2018). Adding bovine seminal plasma prior to freezing improves post-thaw bull sperm kinematics but decreases mitochondrial activity. *Syst. Biol. Reprod. Med.* 64, 183–190. doi: 10.1080/19396368.2018.1455245

O'Connell, M., McClure, N., and Lewis, S. E. M. (2002). The effects of cryopreservation on sperm morphology, motility and mitochondrial function. *Hum. Reprod.* 17, 704–709. doi: 10.1093/humrep/17.3.704

Pace, M. M., Sullivan, J. J., Elliott, F. I., Graham, E. F., and Coulter, G. H. (1981). Effects of thawing temperature, number of spermatozoa and spermatozoal quality on fertility of bovine spermatozoa packaged in. 5-ml French straws. *J. Anim. Sci.* 53, 693–701. doi: 10.2527/jas1981.533693x

Paiva, C., Amaral, A., Rodriguez, M., Canyellas, N., Correig, X., Ballescà, J. L., et al. (2015). Identification of endogenous metabolites in human sperm cells using proton nuclear magnetic resonance (1H-NMR) spectroscopy and gas chromatography-mass spectrometry (GC-MS). *Andrology* 3, 496–505. doi: 10.1111/andr.12027

Recuero, S., Fernandez-Fuertes, B., Bonet, S., Barranco, I., and Yeste, M. (2019). Potential of seminal plasma to improve the fertility of frozen-thawed boar spermatozoa. *Theriogenology* 137, 36–42. doi: 10.1016/j.theriogenology.2019.05.035

Renard, P., Grizard, G., Griveau, J.-F., Sion, B., Boucher, D., and Le Lannou, D. (1996). Improvement of motility and fertilization potential of postthaw human sperm using glutamine. *Cryobiology* 33, 311–319. doi: 10.1006/CRYO.1996.0031

Roussel, J. D., and Stallcup, O. T. (1967). Some amino acid aspects of bovine semen. *Fertil. Steril.* 18, 331–341. doi: 10.1016/S0015-0282(16)36306-36303

Royere, D., Barthelemy, C., Hamamah, S., and Lansac, J. (1996). Cryopreservation of spermatozoa: a 1996 review. *Hum. Reprod. Update* 2, 553–559. doi: 10.1093/humupd/2.6.553

Rudolph, A. S., Crowe, J. H., and Crowe, L. M. (1986). Effects of three stabilizing agents—Proline, betaine, and trehalose—on membrane phospholipids. *Arch. Biochem. Biophys.* 245, 134–143. doi: 10.1016/0003-9861(86)90197-90199

Sangeeta, S., Arangasamy, A., Kulkarni, S., and Selvaraju, S. (2015). Role of amino acids as additives on sperm motility, plasma membrane integrity and lipid peroxidation levels at pre-freeze and post-thawed ram semen. *Anim. Reprod. Sci.* 161, 82–88. doi: 10.1016/j.anireprosci.2015.08.008

Santiago-Moreno, J., Bernal, B., Pérez-Cerezales, S., Castaño, C., Toledano-Díaz, A., Esteso, M. C., et al. (2019). Seminal plasma amino acid profile in different breeds of chicken: role of seminal plasma on sperm cryoresistance. *PLoS One* 14:e0209910. doi: 10.1371/journal.pone.0209910

Saravia, F., Wallgren, M., Johannisson, A., Calvete, J. J., Sanz, L., Peña, F. J., et al. (2009). Exposure to the seminal plasma of different portions of the boar ejaculate modulates the survival of spermatozoa cryopreserved in MiniFlatPacks. *Theriogenology* 71, 662–675. doi: 10.1016/j.theriogenology.2008.09.037

Smirnoff, N., and Cumbes, Q. J. (1989). Hydroxyl radical scavenging activity of compatible solutes. *Phytochemistry* 28, 1057–1060. doi: 10.1016/0031-9422(89)80182-80187

Trimeche, A., Yvon, J. M., Vidament, M., Palmer, E., and Magistrini, M. (1999). Effects of glutamine, proline, histidine and betaine on post-thaw motility of stallion spermatozoa. *Theriogenology* 52, 181–191. doi: 10.1016/s0093-691x(99)00120-x

Valcarce, D. G., Cartón-García, F., Herráez, M. P., and Robles, V. (2013). Effect of cryopreservation on human sperm messenger RNAs crucial for fertilization and early embryo development. *Cryobiology* 67, 84–90. doi: 10.1016/j.cryobiol.2013.05.007

Velho, A. L. C., Menezes, E., Dinh, T., Kaya, A., Topper, E., Moura, A. A., et al. (2018). Metabolomic markers of fertility in bull seminal plasma. *PLoS One* 13:e0195279. doi: 10.1371/journal.pone.0195279

Xia, J., Sinelnikov, I., Han, B., and Wishart, D. S. (2015). MetaboAnalyst 3.0–making metabolomics more meaningful. *Nucleic Acids* 43, W251–W257. doi: 10.1093/nar/gkv380

Xia, J., and Wishart, D. S. (2011). Web-based inference of biological patterns, functions and pathways from metabolomic data using metaboanalyst. *Nat Protoc.* 6, 743–760. doi: 10.1038/nprot.2011.319

Yeste, M. (2016). Sperm cryopreservation update: cryodamage, markers, and factors affecting the sperm freezability in pigs. *Theriogenology* 85, 47–64. doi: 10.1016/j.theriogenology.2015.09.047

Zribi, N., Feki Chakroun, N., El Euch, H., Gargouri, J., Bahloul, A., and Ammar Keskes, L. (2010). Effects of cryopreservation on human sperm deoxyribonucleic acid integrity. *Fertil. Steril.* 93, 159–166. doi: 10.1016/j.fertnstert.2008.09.038

14

A Kinase Anchor Protein 4 Is Vulnerable to Oxidative Adduction in Male Germ Cells

Brett Nixon[1,2]*, Ilana R. Bernstein[1,2], Shenae L. Cafe[1,2], Maryse Delehedde[3], Nicolas Sergeant[3,4], Amanda L. Anderson[1,2], Natalie A. Trigg[1,2], Andrew L. Eamens[1,2], Tessa Lord[1,2], Matthew D. Dun[5,6], Geoffry N. De Iuliis[1,2] and Elizabeth G. Bromfield[1,2,7]

[1] Priority Research Centre for Reproductive Science, School of Environmental and Life Sciences, Discipline of Biological Sciences, The University of Newcastle, Callaghan, NSW, Australia, [2] Pregnancy and Reproduction Program, Hunter Medical Research Institute, New Lambton Heights, NSW, Australia, [3] SPQI – 4BioDx-Breeding Section, Lille, France, [4] University of Lille, INSERM UMRS, Lille, France, [5] Cancer Signalling Research Group, School of Biomedical Sciences and Pharmacy, Faculty of Health and Medicine, University of Newcastle, Callaghan, NSW, Australia, [6] Priority Research Centre for Cancer Research Innovation and Translation, Hunter Medical Research Institute, New Lambton Heights, NSW, Australia, [7] Department of Biochemistry and Cell Biology, Faculty of Veterinary Medicine, Utrecht University, Utrecht, Netherlands

Correspondence:
Brett Nixon
brett.nixon@newcastle.edu.au

Oxidative stress is a leading causative agent in the defective sperm function associated with male infertility. Such stress commonly manifests via the accumulation of pathological levels of the electrophilic aldehyde, 4-hydroxynonenal (4HNE), generated as a result of lipid peroxidation. This highly reactive lipid aldehyde elicits a spectrum of cytotoxic lesions owing to its propensity to form stable adducts with biomolecules. Notably however, not all elements of the sperm proteome appear to display an equivalent vulnerability to 4HNE modification, with only a small number of putative targets having been identified to date. Here, we validate one such target of 4HNE adduction, A-Kinase Anchor Protein 4 (AKAP4); a major component of the sperm fibrous sheath responsible for regulating the signal transduction and metabolic pathways that support sperm motility and capacitation. Our data confirm that both the precursor (proAKAP4), and mature form of AKAP4, are conserved targets of 4HNE adduction in primary cultures of post-meiotic male germ cells (round spermatids) and in mature mouse and human spermatozoa. We further demonstrate that 4HNE treatment of round spermatids and mature spermatozoa results in a substantial reduction in the levels of both proAKAP4 and AKAP4 proteins. This response proved refractory to pharmacological inhibition of proteolysis, but coincided with an apparent increase in the degree of protein aggregation. Further, we demonstrate that 4HNE-mediated protein degradation and/or aggregation culminates in reduced levels of capacitation-associated phosphorylation in mature human spermatozoa, possibly due to dysregulation of the signaling framework assembled around the AKAP4 scaffold. Together, these findings suggest that AKAP4 plays an important role in the pathophysiological responses to 4HNE, thus strengthening the importance of AKAP4 as a biomarker of sperm quality, and providing the impetus for the design of an efficacious antioxidant-based intervention strategy to alleviate sperm dysfunction.

Keywords: 4-hydroxynonenal, A-kinase anchor protein 4, male germ cells, oxidative stress, spermatozoa, sperm capacitation, sperm motility

INTRODUCTION

A male factor is implicated in approximately half of all cases of infertility (Dohle et al., 2005), and in the majority of these individuals, the underlying etiology is attributed to dysregulation of sperm function (Aitken, 2018). Among the myriad of causative agents, oxidative stress has repeatedly been implicated as a key contributor to the loss of sperm developmental and functional competence (Tremellen, 2008; Aitken et al., 2010). Indeed, notwithstanding the important physiological role that reactive oxygen species (ROS) serve to drive the latter phases of sperm maturation (Aitken and Nixon, 2013), exposure to even modest levels of ROS has the potential to induce a state of oxidative stress that deleteriously affects the unique physiology of the male gamete (Aitken et al., 2016). Notably, the legion of pathologic impacts resulting from elevated ROS vary considerably depending on the timing of exposure, with recent evidence suggesting that the round spermatid stage of development is particularly sensitive to oxidative attack. Specifically, post-ROS exposure, round spermatids rapidly succumb to a novel form of regulated cell death, termed ferroptosis (Bromfield et al., 2019). By contrast, equivalent levels of ROS elicit functional lesions in the mature spermatozoon, which compromise their fertilization potential, but does not negatively impact their viability (Bromfield et al., 2015). Such differential pathogenesis may be attributed to the highly specialized architecture of the male germ cell, which depending on their stage of differentiation, features an abundance of substrates for free radical attack, minimal antioxidant defense enzymes, and limited capacity for self-repair when oxidative damage is sustained (Walters et al., 2018b).

Irrespective of the timing of oxidative stress exposure, a virtually ubiquitous response to this insult is lipid peroxidation, a process whereby hydroxyl radicals attack the unsaturated fatty acyl chains of membrane phospholipids (Hauck and Bernlohr, 2016). The ensuing peroxidation reactions generate appreciable levels of highly reactive short chain carbonyl compounds. Among the most abundant and cytotoxic of these secondary oxidation products is 4-hydroxynonenal (4HNE) (Petersen and Doorn, 2004); an aldehyde that has become a major focus in the field due to the pathophysiological impact it exerts on both male (Aitken et al., 2012; Baker et al., 2015; Bromfield et al., 2017b) and female germ cells (Lord et al., 2015; Mihalas et al., 2017, 2018). Under normal physiological conditions, aldehyde-metabolizing enzymes function to detoxify 4HNE, and to abrogate its cellular accumulation, thus limiting its ability to propagate oxidative cellular damage (Hauck and Bernlohr, 2016). However, when challenged with either chronic or acute oxidative stress, 4HNE can accrue within the cellular environment, and, owing to its inherent stability and rapid diffusion, direct the formation of Michael adducts with nucleophilic sites in DNA, lipids and proteins (LoPachin et al., 2009). Curiously, despite 4HNE being capable of disseminating across large functional boundaries, not all elements of the cellular proteome display equivalent susceptibility to 4HNE carbonylation, with only a relatively small number of putative targets identified in spermatozoa to date (Aitken et al., 2012).

In seeking to reconcile the mechanisms underpinning the pathophysiology of 4HNE accumulation, recent studies have reported the application of affinity-based isolation techniques coupled with mass spectrometry to identify 4HNE adducted proteins harbored by oxidatively stressed human spermatozoa (Baker et al., 2015). Among the dominant 4HNE targets identified was A-kinase anchoring protein 4 (AKAP4). AKAP4 is encoded by a single gene located on the X chromosome and synthesized as a precursor pro-polypeptide before undergoing cleavage of the first 188 amino acids to release the mature AKAP4 protein (Carrera et al., 1996; Turner et al., 1998). AKAP4 is subsequently incorporated into the fibrous sheath (Brown et al., 2003); a unique cytoskeletal structure surrounding the axoneme and outer dense fibers that extends throughout the principal-piece of the sperm flagellum (Eddy et al., 2003). Aside from structural contributions to the fibrous sheath, AKAP4 has been implicated as a subcellular scaffold responsible for the tethering of cyclic AMP-dependent protein kinase (PKA), thereby compartmentalizing PKA within the immediate proximity of its enzymatic substrates (Eddy, 2007). Via the targeted positioning of PKA, AKAP4 exerts influence over the specificity of the signal transduction and metabolic processes that support sperm motility and capacitation (Luconi et al., 2011; Sergeant et al., 2019). The importance of AKAP4 in the organization and integrity of the fibrous sheath has been elegantly highlighted by gene ablation studies in which male mice lacking AKAP4 are rendered infertile due to lesions in the progressive motility profiles of their spermatozoa (Miki et al., 2002; Fang et al., 2019). Indeed, while the number of spermatozoa produced by *Akap4* knockout animals remains unchanged, these cells display aberrant fibrous sheath development, a shortened flagella, and a substantially reduced abundance of signal transduction and glycolytic enzymes usually associated with the fibrous sheath (Miki et al., 2002).

These findings take on added significance in view of the dramatic under-representation of AKAP4 in the spermatozoa of infertile human patients (Moretti et al., 2007; Redgrove et al., 2012; Frapsauce et al., 2014). More recent work has also established positive correlations between the levels of AKAP4, and/or that of the proAKAP4 precursor molecule, with key sperm quality and fertility indicators in a number of livestock species (Peddinti et al., 2008; Blommaert et al., 2019; Sergeant et al., 2019). Taken together, these cross species analyses identify the potential use of proAKAP4 and AKAP4 as diagnostic biomarkers of overall semen quality (Sergeant et al., 2019). At present however, it remains uncertain what factor(s) contribute to the striking differences in proAKAP4 and AKAP4 levels documented in livestock (Blommaert et al., 2019) and human spermatozoa (Jumeau et al., 2018). Here, we sought to validate proAKAP4 and AKAP4 as targets for chemical alkylation by 4HNE, and to explore the consequences of 4HNE-mediated alkylation of proAKAP4 and AKAP4 during key phases of sperm development.

MATERIALS AND METHODS

Ethics Statement

All experimental procedures involving animals were conducted with the approval of the University of Newcastle's Animal Care and Ethics Committee (ACEC) (approval numbers: A-2013-322, A-2018-826). Experiments involving human spermatozoa were performed with semen samples obtained with informed written consent from a panel of healthy normozoospermic donors assembled for the Reproductive Science Group at the University of Newcastle. Volunteer involvement and all experimental procedures were performed in strict accordance with institutional ethics approvals granted by the University of Newcastle Human Research and Ethics Committee (approval number H-2013-0319).

Reagents

Unless specified, chemical reagents were obtained from Sigma-Aldrich (St. Louis, MO, United States) and were of research grade. Cell culture reagents were purchased from Sigma-Aldrich or Thermo Fisher Scientific (Waltham, MA, United States). The following primary antibodies were used to characterize proteins of interest: monoclonal anti-AKAP4 antibody clone 7E10 (4BDX-1602; 4BioDx, Lille, France), monoclonal anti-proAKAP4 antibody clone 6F12 (4BDX-1701; 4BioDx), rabbit polyclonal anti-4HNE (HNE11-S; Alpha Diagnostic International, San Antonio, TX, United States), rabbit polyclonal anti-androgen receptor (SAB4501575; Sigma-Aldrich), rabbit polyclonal anti-GAPDH antibodies (G9545; Sigma-Aldrich), monoclonal anti-phosphotyrosine (PT66) (P5872; Sigma-Aldrich), rabbit polyclonal anti-phospho (Ser/Thr) PKA substrate (9621; Cell Signaling, Danvers, MA, United States), and rabbit polyclonal anti-amyloid fibrils OC (ab2286; Merck Millipore, Kenilworth, NJ, United States). Appropriate horseradish peroxidase (HRP)-conjugated and Alexa Fluor-conjugated secondary antibodies were obtained from Sigma-Aldrich and Thermo Fisher Scientific, respectively. Bovine serum albumin (BSA) and 3-[(3-cholamidopropyl)dimethylammonio]-1-propanesulfonate (CHAPS) were obtained from Research Organics (Cleveland, OH, United States), Dulbecco's Modified Eagle Medium (DMEM) was purchased from Thermo Fisher Scientific, Tris was purchased from ICN Biochemicals (Castle Hill, NSW, Australia), nitrocellulose was purchased from GE Healthcare (Buckinghamshire, United Kingdom), Mowiol 4-88 was purchased from Calbiochem (La Jolla, CA, United States), and the paraformaldehyde used in this study was purchased from ProSciTech (Thuringowa, QLD, Australia).

Mouse Germ Cell Isolation

Swiss mice were obtained from a breeding colony held at the institutes' central animal house and maintained according to the recommendations prescribed by the ACEC. Mice were housed under a controlled lighting regimen (16L:8D) at 21–22°C and were supplied with food and water *ad libitum*. Prior to dissection, animals were euthanized via CO_2 inhalation. Enriched populations of spermatocytes and spermatids were isolated from dissected adult mouse testes using density sedimentation at unit gravity as described previously (Nixon et al., 2014; Bromfield et al., 2017b). Briefly, testes were disassociated and tubules were sequentially digested with 0.5 mg/ml collagenase/DMEM and 0.5% (v/v) trypsin/EDTA to remove extra-tubular contents and interstitial cells. The remaining cells were loaded atop a 2–4% (w/v) BSA/DMEM gradient to separate male germ cell types according to their density. Consistent with previous data (Bromfield et al., 2019), this method resulted in the isolation of pachytene spermatocytes (>90% purity) and round spermatids (>85% purity) with minimal somatic cell contamination. Unless stated otherwise, spermatocytes and spermatids were pooled from 2 to 4 mice to achieve adequate cell numbers for subsequent analyses. Experiments were conducted on three independently pooled samples.

Preparation of Mouse and Human Spermatozoa

Mature spermatozoa were isolated from the cauda epididymides of adult mice by retrograde perfusion and subsequently allowed to disperse into Biggers, Whitten and Whittingham medium (BWW) as previously described (Walsh et al., 2008; Dun et al., 2012). By contrast, corpus spermatozoa were recovered by placing each sampled corpus segment into a 500 μl droplet of modified BWW. After making multiple incisions with a razor blade, the spermatozoa were gently washed into the medium via mild agitation. The resulting suspensions were next placed atop a 27% Percoll density gradient and subjected to centrifugation at 400 × *g* for 15 min at room temperature (RT). The pellet, consisting of an enriched population of >95% corpus spermatozoa was resuspended in fresh BWW and then re-centrifuged at 400 × *g* for 2 min at RT to again pellet the cells and to allow for the removal of excess Percoll (Zhou et al., 2018). These cell preparations were then pooled with those of the cauda epididymis and assessed for viability and motility as previously described (Zhou et al., 2018), prior to being allocated to appropriate treatment groups in preparation for further analysis. In all samples, >80% of the mouse spermatozoa were deemed viable and motile prior to treatment.

Human semen samples were collected following sexual abstinence of at least 2 days. Following collection, all samples were maintained at 37°C and sample analysis was initiated after completion of liquefaction and within 1 h of ejaculation. Each sample was analyzed for total sperm count, motility, morphology and vitality as described previously (Walters et al., 2018a); with all samples used in this study exceeding WHO reference values of 58% live cells, 15 × 10^6 cells/ml, 1.5 ml ejaculate volume, 40% total motility and 4% normal morphology. After assessment, semen samples were fractionated over a discontinuous Percoll density gradient (comprising 40 and 80% Percoll suspensions) by centrifugation at 500 × *g* for 30 min at RT (Redgrove et al., 2011). This study was restricted to the use of good quality spermatozoa collected from the base of the 80% Percoll suspension as opposed to the poor quality cells partitioning at the 40/80% Percoll interface. After centrifugation, sperm pellets were resuspended in BWW and washed by centrifugation at

500 × *g* for 15 min at RT. Post-washing, the cells were again resuspended in fresh BWW prior to experimental use. A routine assessment of semen parameters was conducted for all donors in accordance with World Health Organization (WHO) criteria and corresponding to the checklist published by Bjorndahl et al. (2016). At least 100 cells were assessed for determination of cell motility, viability and morphology, with at least five microscope fields of view being examined for each count. Sperm morphology was assessed in accordance with WHO criteria using bright field microscopy (×400 magnification; Olympus CX40; Olympus Corporation, Tokyo, Japan). Sperm motility was assessed using phase contrast microscope optics (×400 magnification), with cells being classified as either motile (that is, sperm that displayed any form of motility, ranging from rapid progressive to non-progressive) or immotile.

4HNE Treatment

Oxidative stress was induced in germ cells and mature spermatozoa via direct 4HNE (Cayman chemicals, Ann Arbor, MI, United States) challenge, in accordance with our previously established protocols (Bromfield et al., 2015, 2017b; Walters et al., 2018a). For both germ cells and mature spermatozoa, 4HNE treatment regimens (consisting of 4HNE concentrations of either 50 or 100 μM and exposure periods of either 1 or 3 h at 37°C) were selected based on our prior *in vitro* experimentation, in which these conditions were shown to robustly promote the loss and/or dysregulation of alternative 4HNE targeted proteins in male germ cells (Bromfield et al., 2015, 2017a). We also note that the concentrations of 4HNE used herein fall within the range normally associated with low levels of oxidative stress *in vivo* (Uchida, 2003; Chen and Niki, 2006), but are considered sub-lethal such that they are below those required to elicit significant elevation of apoptotic hallmarks (i.e., caspase activation and annexin V binding) or DNA fragmentation (i.e., TUNEL positivity) under comparable *in vitro* incubation periods to those assessed in our study (Aitken et al., 2012). Post-incubation, residual 4HNE was removed via centrifugation at 500 × *g* for 3 min at RT, and resuspension in pre-warmed DMEM or BWW for germ cells and spermatozoa, respectively. Consistent with our previous studies (Bromfield et al., 2015, 2017a; Walters et al., 2018a), the use of these conditions resulted in the death of <20% of the cells under examination (**Supplementary Figure S1**). In accordance with previous studies (Aitken et al., 2012; Bromfield et al., 2017b, 2019), we also noted that these experimental treatments elicited robust levels of oxidative stress as measured by labeling of the target germ cell populations with MitoSOX Red (MSR) and dihydroethidium (DHE) probes (reference values: ~40–45% human spermatozoa stained positive for MSR and DHE following 50 μM 4HNE treatment for 3 h). By contrast, equivalent analysis of untreated germ cells confirmed relatively low basal levels of oxidative stress (reference values: <10% human spermatozoa stained positive for MSR and DHE following 50 μM 4HNE treatment for 3 h). Where indicated, an additional control group was incorporated in which male germ cells were pretreated with reduced glutathione (GSH; 4 mM) for 10 min prior to the addition of 4HNE (100 μM). The cells were then co-incubated with both GSH and 4HNE throughout the exposure period (i.e., 3 h for round spermatids and 1 h for spermatozoa). Alternatively, following the completion of 4HNE exposure, the cells were washed twice with BWW (via centrifugation at 500 × *g* for 3 min at RT) to remove residual 4HNE before being resuspended in either DMEM (round spermatids) or BWW (spermatozoa) supplemented with reduced GSH (4 mM) and incubated for an additional 30 min. At the completion of either treatment regimen, gametes were washed twice in BWW via centrifugation at 500 × *g* for 3 min at RT before being processed in accordance with the relevant protocols described below.

Sodium Dodecyl Sulfate (SDS) Polyacrylamide Gel Electrophoresis and Immunoblotting

Following 4HNE treatment, cells were centrifuged at 500 × *g* for 3 min at RT, and the resulting pellets resuspended in SDS-based protein extraction buffer as previously described (Reid et al., 2012). Protein extracts were then boiled in the presence of NuPAGE LDS sample buffer (Thermo Fisher Scientific) containing 8% β-mercaptoethanol, and subjected to SDS-polyacrylamide gel electrophoresis (SDS-PAGE) using 4–12% Bis–Tris pre-cast gels (Thermo Fisher Scientific). Post-electrophoresis, separated proteins were transferred to nitrocellulose membranes using standard Western blotting techniques (Towbin et al., 1979). To detect proteins of interest, membranes were blocked in 3% BSA (w/v) in Tris-buffered saline supplemented with 0.1% Tween-20 (v/v; TBST, pH 7.4), and then probed with either anti-proAKAP4, anti-AKAP4, anti-4HNE, anti-phospho-PKA substrate, or anti-phosphotyrosine antibodies, as appropriate. All primary antibodies were diluted 1:1000 in TBST supplemented with 1% BSA and probing reactions were conducted overnight at 4°C on a rotating platform. Membranes were next washed in three changes of TBST (10 min/wash) and thereafter, the appropriate secondary antibodies were applied to each membrane for 1 h at RT on a rotating platform. The membranes were again washed with three changes of TBST (10 min/wash), and labeled proteins were then visualized using an enhanced chemiluminescence detection kit according to the manufacturer's instructions (ECL plus, GE Healthcare). After visualization of the abundance of proteins of interest, all immunoblotted membranes were stripped prior to being re-incubated with anti-GAPDH antibodies (1:4000 dilution), and with the corresponding secondary antibody (washing was performed as outlined above), to demonstrate equivalent protein loading. Band density was quantified in each of three replicate blots using ImageJ software (version 1.48v; National Institute of Health, Bethesda, MD, United States) and the abundance of each protein of interest determined relative to GAPDH labeling intensity. Full length immunoblots of the anti-pro-AKAP4, AKAP4, and GAPDH antibodies used throughout this study are presented in **Supplementary Figure S3**.

Immunocytochemistry

Following 4HNE treatment, round spermatids, pachytene spermatocytes, and mature human and mouse spermatozoa, were fixed in 4% paraformaldehyde, washed 3× with 0.05 M glycine in phosphate-buffered saline (PBS). Each cell preparation was then carefully pipetted onto a poly-L-lysine-coated glass coverslip and the cells allowed to settle via overnight incubation at 4°C. Cells were permeabilized with 0.2% (v/v) Triton X-100, then placed in a humidified chamber and blocked with 3% (v/v) BSA/PBS for 1 h at RT. Each coverslip was then washed in PBS and incubated with either anti-proAKAP4, anti-AKAP4, anti-4HNE, anti-phospho-PKA substrate, or anti-phosphotyrosine primary antibodies as appropriate. All primary antibodies were diluted 1:100 in 1% (v/v) BSA/PBS before being applied to coverslips and incubated overnight at 4°C. Coverslips were next washed with three changes of PBS (5 min/wash) before applying the appropriate Alex Fluor-conjugated secondary antibodies (diluted 1:100 in 1% (v/v) BSA/PBS and incubating for 1 h at RT. Coverslips were washed with changes of PBS (3 × 5 min/wash) before mounting in a solution consisting of 10% (v/v) Mowiol 4-88 (Calbiochem) supplemented with 30% (v/v) glycerol in 0.2 M Tris (pH 8.5) and 2.5% (v/v) 1,4-diazabicyclo-(2.2.2)-octane (DABCO). Labeled cells were examined using a Zeiss LSM510 laser scanning confocal microscope (Carl Zeiss).

Proximity Ligation Assay

Duolink *in situ* primary ligation assays (PLAs) were conducted in accordance with the manufacturers' instructions (Sigma-Aldrich), on fixed cells adhered to poly-L-lysine-coated coverslips. Briefly, samples were blocked in Duolink blocking solution and then incubated with appropriate primary antibody pairings (anti-proAKAP4, anti-AKAP4, anti-4HNE or anti-amyloid fibrils OC antibodies) overnight at 4°C. Oligonucleotide-conjugated secondary antibodies (PLA probes; anti-rabbit plus, Duo92002; anti-mouse minus Duo82004; Duolink) were then applied for 1 h at 37°C and ligation of the PLA probes was performed. The fluorescent signal generated when molecules are in close association (<40 nm) was visualized using fluorescence microscopy and the number of cells deemed positive for PLA staining was recorded for untreated and 4HNE-treated populations. The specificity of the PLA reaction was ensured by performing proximity ligation with antibodies to the target antigens combined with anti-androgen receptor antibodies with which they should not interact.

Pharmacological Inhibition of proAKAP4 and AKAP4 Proteolysis

To prevent 4HNE-mediated proteolysis of proAKAP4 and AKAP4 in male germ cells and mature spermatozoa, the cells were treated with several broad-spectrum pharmacological suppressors of proteolytic activity (Complete Mini Protease Inhibitor Cocktail; Roche), or with a selective inhibitor of proteasomal activity (MG132). Alternatively, cells were treated with a selective inhibitor of arachidonate 15-lipoxygenase (PD146176; Tocris Bioscience, Bristol, United Kingdom), an enzyme involved in the propagation of oxidative stress via the metabolism of polyunsaturated fatty acids to 4HNE (Walters et al., 2018b). The concentrations of each inhibitor (Complete Mini Protease Inhibitor Cocktail at 1× working concentration; MG132, 10–25 μM; PD146176, 1 μM), were selected based on published IC_{50} values and from our previous use of these reagents to effectively block the loss of other 4HNE targeted proteins from the germ cell proteome (Bromfield et al., 2017b; Walters et al., 2018a). Germ cells and mature spermatozoa were pre-treated with each inhibitor for 15 min prior to exposure to 4HNE (protease inhibitor cocktail and MG132) or H_2O_2 (in the case of PD146176) and the inhibitor was retained for the duration of treatment thereafter to ensure adequate inhibition of each target. A DMSO vehicle control (1 μM) was also included in these experiments.

Functional Assessment of Human Spermatozoa

Computer Assisted Sperm Analysis (CASA): the movement characteristics of human spermatozoa were assessed using a Hamilton-Thorn motility analyzer (HTMA IVOS II; Hamilton-Thorn Research, Danvers, MA, United States). The settings for human spermatozoa were: 10× NH 160 mm objective, negative phase-contrast optics, recording rate 60 frames/s, minimum head brightness 171, minimum cell size 5 μm^2, maximum head size 50 μm^2 and measured in a chamber of 20 μm depth. The criteria of sperm movement assessed were average path velocity (VAP), curvilinear velocity (VCL), straight line velocity (VSL), progressive motility, characterized by a VAP of >25 μm/s and a STR (straightness) of >80%.

Acrosome reaction: Following the induction of capacitation as previously described (Zhou et al., 2017), spermatozoa were induced to acrosome react by supplementation of media with 2.5 μM A23187 for 30 min. The spontaneous rates of acrosome loss were assessed via the inclusion of a capacitated sperm control group, which were prepared under identical incubation conditions with the exception that they did not receive an A23187 stimulus. At the completion of this induction period, the cells were then incubated in pre-warmed hypo-osmotic swelling media (HOS; 0.07% w/v sodium citrate; 1.3% w/v fructose) for another 30 min at 37°C. After being fixed in 4% PFA, spermatozoa were aliquoted onto 12-well slides, air-dried and permeabilized with ice cold methanol for 10 min. Cells were then incubated with fluorescein isothiocyanate (FITC)-conjugated PSA (*Pisum sativum* agglutinin) (1 μg/μl) at 37°C for 15 min, and the acrosomal status of viable cells (possessing coiled tails as a result of incubation in HOS medium) were verified using fluorescence microscopy as previously described (Zhou et al., 2017).

Statistics

All experiments were replicated at least three times, with each biological replicate comprised of germ cells or mature spermatozoa from at least three mice, or in the case of human spermatozoa, three healthy normozoospermic individuals. Data are expressed as mean values ± SE. Experimental results were analyzed using two-tailed unpaired Student's *t*-tests (for two way comparison of 4HNE treatments to that of untreated controls) or by one-way analysis of variances (ANOVA) using Microsoft Excel (Version 14.0.0); *post hoc* comparison of group means was by

Fisher's PLSD (protected least significant difference). Differences were considered significant if a $p < 0.05$ was obtained.

RESULTS

ProAKAP4 and AKAP4 Are Targeted for 4HNE Adduction in Post-meiotic Male Germ Cells

Previous studies have established that several residues within the AKAP4 primary structure are vulnerable to 4HNE adduction in human spermatozoa. However, the implications of this form of chemical alkylation remain unknown. Here, we therefore, initially assessed the stability of both the AKAP4 and the precursor form, proAKAP4, in mouse germ cell populations treated with exogenous 4HNE (50 or 100 μM) for either 1 or 3 h at 37°C (**Figure 1**). Consistent with our previous findings (Bromfield et al., 2017a, 2019), the modest level of oxidative stress generated under these exposure regimens led to <20% loss of germ cell viability (**Supplementary Figure S1**). However, the 1 and 3 h 4HNE treatments did significantly reduce the abundance of both proAKAP4 (**Figures 1A,B**) and AKAP4 (**Figures 1C,D**) in post-meiotic round spermatids ($P < 0.05$). Further, the degree of reduction was similar for both the 50 or 100 μM 4HNE treatments (**Figures 1E,F**). As expected, based on its expression profile (Johnson et al., 1997), the proAKAP4 precursor was not detected in equivalent lysates of untreated pachytene spermatocytes (**Figures 1A,B**), a finding that confirmed germ cell preparation purity. To account for the possibility of 4HNE-mediated epitope masking, recombinant AKAP4 protein was treated under identical conditions to those imposed on germ cells (i.e., 50 μM 4HNE for 1 h at 37°C) prior to being prepared for immunoblotting. **Supplementary Figure S2** clearly demonstrates that 4HNE treated recombinant AKAP4 was detectable at an equivalent level of efficiency to the untreated control with both anti-proAKAP4 and anti-AKAP4 antibodies. Together, these data suggest that the demonstrable reduction in proAKAP4 and AKAP4 immunoreactivity in round spermatids challenged with 4HNE reflects a genuine reduction in the abundance of both precursor and mature forms of AKAP4. This result led us to next attempt to uncover the causative nature of the observed response.

Toward this goal, round spermatids were treated with 4HNE prior to assessing the cumulative levels of this aldehyde, and the extent of 4HNE co-localization with the proAKAP4 precursor; the isoform determined most affected by 4HNE treatment (**Figure 1E**). Consistent with the immunoblotting data, the accumulation of 4HNE throughout the cytosol of round spermatids was accompanied by a reciprocal reduction in the amount of immunoreactive proAKAP4 detected within these cells (**Figure 2A**). In addition, the residual proAKAP4 remaining in round spermatids appeared to co-localize with 4HNE labeling (**Figure 2A**). This co-localized accumulation profile for 4HNE and proAKAP4, was confirmed via use of the proximity ligation assay, which revealed intense labeling foci for the paired proAKAP4 and 4HNE antibodies throughout the round spermatid cytosol (**Figure 2B**). Notwithstanding the basal levels of 4HNE detected in untreated round spermatids via conventional immunolabeling (**Figure 2A**), this naïve cell population was characterized by very few PLA positive foci when assessed using the same antibody pairing (anti-proAKAP4 and anti-4HNE) (**Figure 2B**). The specificity of PLA labeling was confirmed via inclusion of two controls, namely; antibodies against the androgen receptor protein that is not known to interact with proAKAP4, as well as the use of a single antibody only (anti-proAKAP4) control. **Figure 2C** clearly shows that each control failed to generate a positive PLA signal (red fluorescence). This result confirms the close proximity of 4HNE to the proAKAP4 precursor in the cytosol of round spermatids.

The preceding data strongly suggests that elevated levels of intracellular 4HNE leads to proAKAP4 adduction, possibly destabilizing the structure of the precursor; a modification that would likely interfere with the formation of mature AKAP4. The ubiquitin-proteasome pathway has been previously implicated in the selective elimination of a variety of oxidatively damaged proteins (Davies, 2001; Shringarpure et al., 2001). We therefore, next assessed the contribution of the proteasomal pathway to the clearance of modified proAKAP4. For this purpose, round spermatids were co-incubated with 4HNE in tandem with MG132, a cell-permeable synthetic peptide that is widely used to repress proteasome activity. Unexpectedly however, MG132 co-incubation failed to rescue 4HNE-mediated loss of proAKAP4 in round spermatids (**Figures 3A,B**). Similarly, co-incubation with a broad-spectrum protease inhibitor cocktail also had minimal effect on the abundance of proAKAP4 in 4HNE-treated round spermatids, when used either alone, or in tandem with MG132 (data not shown). This result led to the conclusion that 4HNE-mediated loss of proAKAP4 in round spermatids is unlikely to involve conventional proteolytic degradation.

Acute 4HNE Exposure Reduces proAKAP4 and AKAP4 Abundance in Mouse and Human Spermatozoa

Given the pronounced 4HNE-mediated loss of proAKAP4 and AKAP4 in post-meiotic round spermatids, we next extended our analyses to assess the consequences of 4HNE treatment of mouse and human spermatozoa; terminally differentiated cells that have a reduced capacity to ameliorate the deleterious effects of oxidative insult compared to that of precursor germ cells. In mouse spermatozoa, 4HNE treatment reduced the abundance of both proAKAP4 and AKAP4 (**Figures 4A,D**). However, proAKAP4 appeared more sensitive in these cells, experiencing a highly significant ~40% reduction ($P < 0.01$), compared to the untreated controls (**Figures 4A,D**). Consistent with our data on the round spermatid (**Figure 2**), the application of PLA revealed intense co-labeling of 4HNE with proAKAP4 and AKAP4 within the expected domains of the sperm flagellum (**Figure 4B**). More specifically, PLA fluorescence was restricted to the proximal portion of the sperm flagellum for the 4HNE and proAKAP4 antibody pairing, whilst the 4HNE and AKAP4 pairing allowed for the visualization of fluorescent foci throughout the entire principal piece (**Figure 4B**). Together, these data indicate that

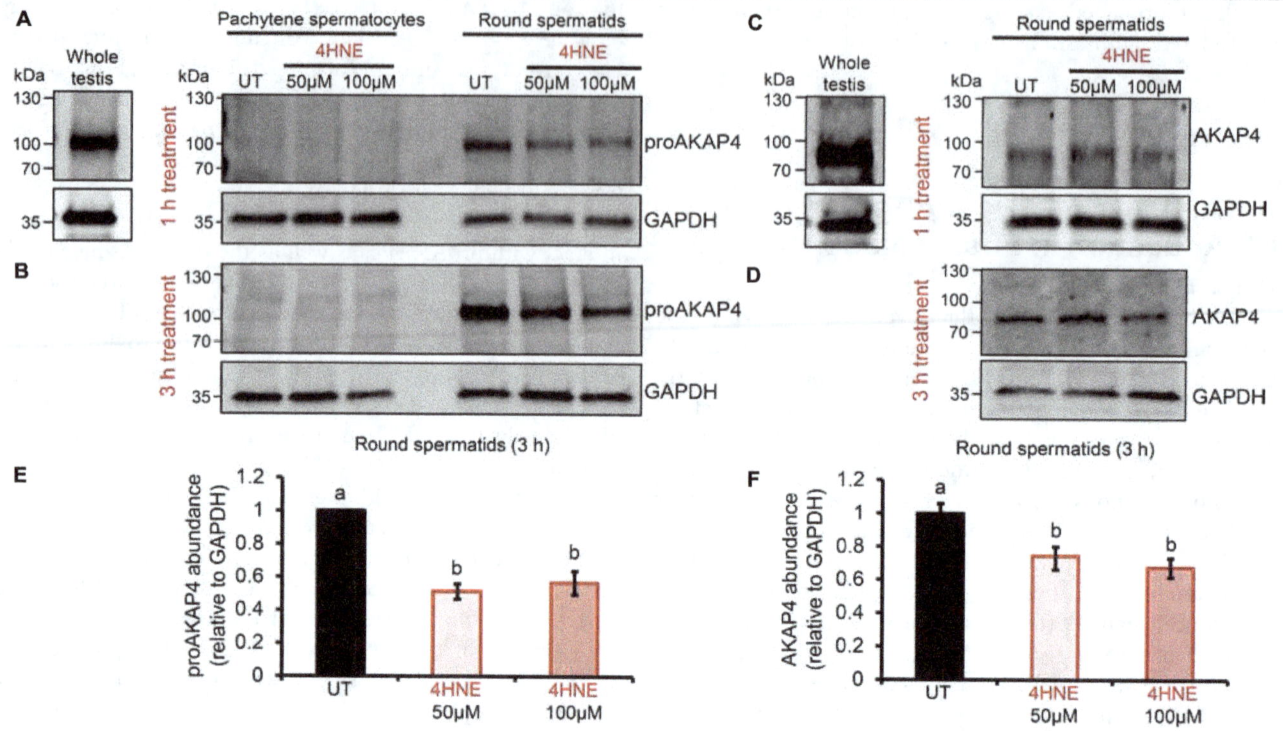

FIGURE 1 | Assessment of the impact of 4HNE treatment on both proAKAP4 and AKAP4 abundance in mouse male germ cells. **(A–D)** Mouse pachytene spermatocytes and round spermatids were exposed to 4-hydroxynonenal (4HNE) (50 or 100 μM) for intervals of either 1 or 3 h before being lysed and subjected to immunoblotting with either **(A,B)** anti-proAKAP4 or **(C,D)** anti-AKAP4 antibodies. Each blot was stripped and re-probed with anti-GAPDH antibodies to confirm equivalent protein loading. **(E,F)** Densitometric analysis of proAKAP4 and AKAP4 band intensity relative to that of GAPDH confirmed significant attenuation of both proteins in 4HNE treated comparted to untreated (UT) round spermatids. Data are expressed as mean ± SEM ($n = 3$). Differing lowercase letters denote statistical significance ($p < 0.05$) as determined by ANOVA.

residual proAKAP4 and AKAP4 proteins that remain within the flagellum of 4HNE treated mouse spermatozoa likely harbor substantial levels of aldehyde adducts. It is also important to note here that, as observed for 4HNE-treated round spermatids, co-incubation with the proteasome inhibitor, MG132, failed to rescue the loss of either proAKAP4 or AKAP4 in 4HNE-treated mature mouse spermatozoa (**Figures 4C,D**).

To determine if AKAP4 is similarly targeted for 4HNE-mediated adduction in human spermatozoa, these cells were treated as per their mouse counterparts. Initially, proAKAP4 and AKAP4 abundance was assessed in the spermatozoa of three healthy normozoospermic donors, with each sample subjected to acute 4HNE treatment (50 or 100 μM) for 1 h at 37°C. As shown in the representative immunoblots in **Figure 5A**, sperm from each donor responded to 4HNE challenge in an equivalent manner, that is; proAKAP4 and AKAP4 abundance was significantly reduced in a dose-dependent manner ($p < 0.01$). For the 100 μM 4HNE treatment, both the precursor and mature form of AKAP4 were reduced by as much as 70% compared to the untreated control samples (**Figure 5B**). Accordingly, immunocytochemistry revealed elevated levels of 4HNE and a concomitant reduction in proAKAP4 and AKAP4 abundance within the flagellum of each 4HNE-treated human sperm sample assessed (**Figures 6A,B**). Furthermore, PLA fluorescence was observed in the majority of these cells post-4HNE treatment when the 4HNE antibody was paired with either the proAKAP4 or AKAP4 antibody (**Figures 6C–F**). Although basal levels of PLA fluorescence were detected in untreated control spermatozoa, both the distribution and intensity of this labeling appeared equivalent to that detected in the irrelevant antibody control samples, suggesting that the detected signal was non-specific in nature (**Figures 6C,D**). Overall, these data are in general agreement with that generated for mouse spermatozoa (**Figure 4**), thus indicating cross-species conservation in terms of the vulnerability of both the precursor and mature form of AKAP4 to 4HNE insult as well as the fate of the alkylated proteins.

Consequences of 4HNE-Adduction of ProAKAP4 and AKAP4

To explore the causal nature of 4HNE-mediated attenuation of proAKAP4 and AKAP4 abundance, populations of round spermatids, mouse and human spermatozoa were treated with reduced glutathione (GSH) prior to, or after, implementing the 4HNE exposure. As anticipated based on the ability of GSH to directly alkylate and thereby reduce the bioavailability of 4HNE, pre-incubation of male gametes with this antioxidant conferred at least some degree of protection to proAKAP4 and AKAP4

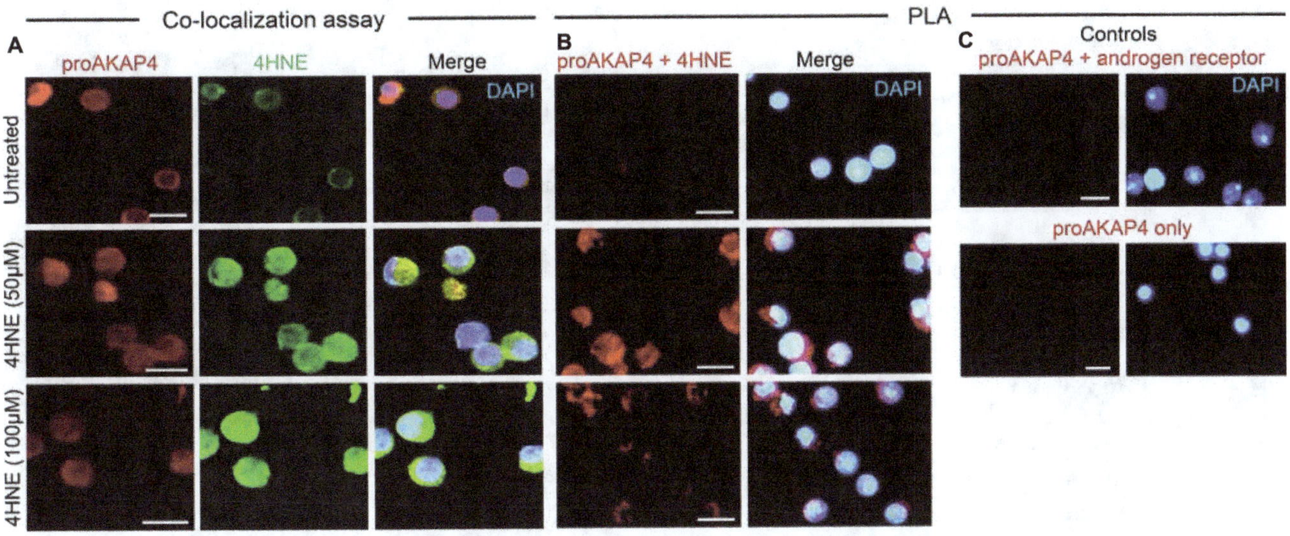

FIGURE 2 | Co-immunolocalization of 4HNE and proAKAP4 in mouse round spermatids. **(A)** Following exposure to 4HNE (50 or 100 μM for 1 h), round spermatids were fixed in paraformaldehyde and sequentially labeled with anti-proAKAP4 (red), anti-4HNE (green) and corresponding fluorescently labeled secondary antibodies. Cells were counterstained with the nuclear stain DAPI (blue). **(B)** Co-localization of target proAKAP4 and 4HNE antigens was confirmed through the application of a proximity ligation assay, whereby fixed round spermatids were incubated with target primary antibodies (anti-proAKAP4 and anti-4HNE) or **(C)** negative controls (anti-proAKAP4 and anti-androgen receptor; anti-proAKAP4 alone) and oligonucleotide-conjugated secondary antibodies (PLA probes). PLA probes were then ligated and the signal was amplified according to the manufacturer's instructions (Sigma-Aldrich). The red fluorescent signals generated when target antigens reside within <40 nm were visualized using fluorescence microscopy. Scale bars = 10 μm.

proteins. Indeed, the abundance of both proteins detected in pre-GSH treated round spermatids was statistically indistinguishable from that of the untreated control samples. An equivalent trend was observed in mouse and human spermatozoa, although in both instances the abundance of proAKAP4 and AKAP4 proteins was still reduced in pre-GSH treated cells versus that of their untreated counterparts. In terms of the response to the opposing post-GSH treatment, this again varied depending on the cell type analyzed. Thus, in the case of round spermatids, which retain some capacity for protein synthesis, proAKAP4 and AKAP4 levels were recovered to levels that proved statistically similar to that of untreated controls (**Figures 7A,B**). However, the retrospective application of GSH failed to rescue either proAKAP4 or AKAP4 levels in 4HNE treated mouse or human spermatozoa (**Figures 7C–F**). These results prompted us to explore whether alternative strategies could be used to prevent 4HNE-mediated reduction of proAKAP4 and AKAP4 in mature spermatozoa. With this goal in mind, we next investigated whether the abundance of the two AKAP4 isoforms could be maintained via the administration of a pharmacological inhibitor that acts upstream of 4HNE production. Specifically, spermatozoa were subjected to oxidative stress in the form of an H_2O_2 insult either alone, or in the presence of PD146176, a selective inhibitor of the lipoxygenase enzyme, arachidonate 15-lipoxygenase (ALOX15); an enzyme that drives a positive feedback loop of lipid peroxidation leading to amplification of 4HNE generation in male germ cells (Walters et al., 2018a). Accordingly, via the administration of H_2O_2 alone, we were able to reproduce the previously observed reduction in the abundance of both proAKAP4 and AKAP4 from mouse and human spermatozoa (**Figures 8A–D**). Further, in H_2O_2 alone treated samples, proAKAP4 and AKAP4 were reduced to levels similar to those elicited by the direct application of 4HNE. Unexpectedly however, co-incubation of PD146176 together with H_2O_2, led to only a partial recovery of proAKAP4 and AKAP4 levels in mouse spermatozoa (**Figures 8A,C**), and proved completely ineffective in the rescue of proAKAP4 and AKAP4 in human spermatozoa (**Figures 8B,D**).

In view of these data, we next attempted to determine if 4HNE adduction can act as a catalyst to destabilize either the precursor or mature form of AKAP4, in order to drive the protein toward aggregate formation. Thus, PLA was again employed to assess the dual labeling of either the proAKAP4 or AKAP4 antibody together with an amyloid fibrils OC-specific antibody (**Figure 8**). The amyloid fibril OC antibody was selected for inclusion in this analysis based on its recognition of generic epitopes common to many amyloid fibrils and fibrillary oligomers, but not prefibrillar oligomers or natively folded precursors. As shown in **Figure 9A**, PLA fluorescence was observed for both antibody pairings throughout the cytosol of 4HNE-treated round spermatids, with the labeling appearing more intense at the higher 4HNE concentration of 100 μM (**Figure 9A**). PLA fluorescence, albeit less intense, was also observed for both antibody pairings within the flagellum of 4HNE-treated mouse (**Figure 9B**) and human spermatozoa (**Figure 9C**). In all instances, PLA labeling was attenuated via prior incubation of the germ cells with GSH before they received 4HNE-exposure (**Figures 9A–C**). Taken together, these data suggest that in male germ cells, 4HNE adduction can result in the aggregation of both the precursor and mature forms of AKAP4.

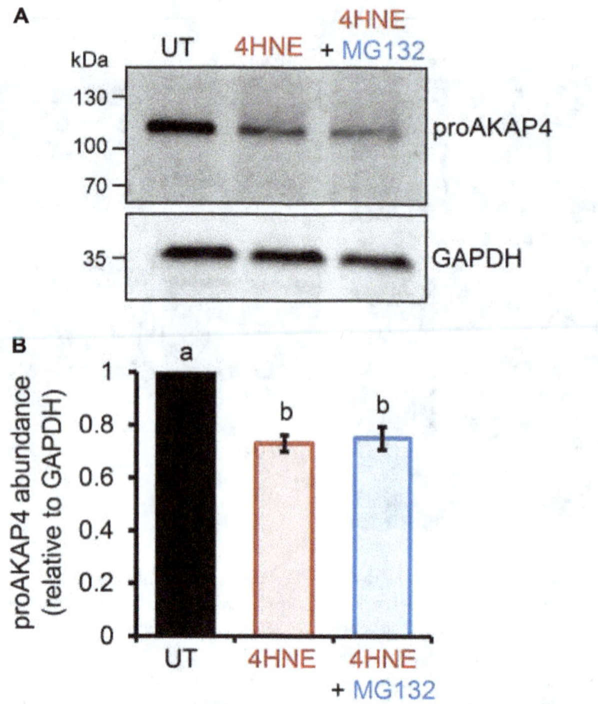

FIGURE 3 | Inhibition of proteasome activity does not rescue 4HNE mediated loss of proAKAP4 in round spermatids. **(A)** Round spermatids were pre-treated with MG132 (proteasome inhibitor) for 15 min prior to exposure to 4HNE (100 μM, 3 h at 37°C), with the inhibitor being retained for the duration of treatment. Cells were solubilized in an SDS based extraction buffer prior to being resolved by SDS-PAGE and prepared for immunoblotting with anti-proAKAP4 antibodies. Blots were subsequently stripped and reprobed with anti-GAPDH antibodies to ensure equivalent protein loading. **(B)** Labeled bands corresponding to proteins of interest were subjected to band densitometry analysis and mean values (±SEM) are presented relative to the corresponding GAPDH control (n = 3). Differing lowercase letters denote statistical significance ($p < 0.05$) as determined by ANOVA. UT = untreated control.

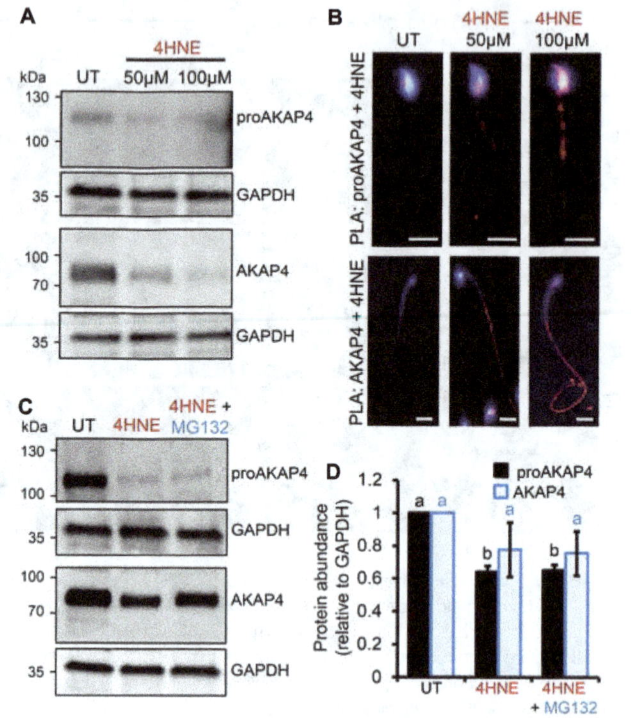

FIGURE 4 | Assessment of 4HNE adduction to proAKAP4 and AKAP4 in mature mouse spermatozoa. **(A,B)** Mouse spermatozoa were exposed to 4HNE (50 or 100 μM) alone or **(C,D)** in the presence of the proteasome inhibitor MG132 and incubated for 1 h at 37°C. **(A,C)** Spermatozoa were prepared for immunoblotting analysis with anti-proAKAP4 and anti-AKAP4 antibodies. Each blot was stripped and re-probed with anti-GAPDH antibodies to confirm equivalent protein loading. **(B)** The adduction of proAKAP4 and AKAP4 with 4HNE was assessed through the application of a proximity ligation assay, whereby fixed spermatozoa were incubated with target primary antibodies (anti-proAKAP4 or anti-AKAP4 and anti-4HNE) or **(C)** negative controls (anti-proAKAP4 and anti-AKAP4 and anti-androgen receptor; anti-proAKAP4 alone) and oligonucleotide-conjugated secondary antibodies (PLA probes). PLA probes were then ligated and the signal was amplified. The red fluorescent signals generated when target antigens reside within <40 nm were visualized using fluorescence microscopy and representative images of each treatment group are presented. **(D)** Protein abundance was quantified by band densitometry and mean values (±SEM) are presented relative to the corresponding GAPDH control (n = 3). Differing lowercase letters denote statistical significance ($p < 0.05$) as determined by ANOVA. Scale bars = 5 μm. UT = untreated control.

A potential consequence of 4HNE-mediated protein degradation and/or aggregation is dysregulation of the cAMP signaling framework assembled around the AKAP4 scaffold in mature spermatozoa. To address this possibility, human spermatozoa were subjected to 4HNE treatment before being driven to capacitate and assessed for the phosphorylation of PKA and tyrosine kinase substrates. Immunocytochemical analysis demonstrated that our 4HNE treatment regimen did not overtly impact the localization of proteins being phosphorylated during the capacitation of human spermatozoa, with prominent staining being evident throughout the sperm flagellum (**Figures 10A,B**). However, immunoblotting confirmed that 4HNE treatment did in fact lead to reduced levels of phosphorylation among a portion of the intermediary PKA targets, particularly the prominent bands resolving at ~35 and 100 kDa (**Figure 10C**). In addition, 4HNE elicited a more pronounced, global reduction in the phosphorylation levels of downstream tyrosine kinase substrates (**Figure 10D**). In both instances, these effects were reduced by prior incubation of the human spermatozoa with reduced GSH before the addition of 4HNE (**Figures 10A–D**).

Notably, the deleterious impact of 4HNE extended to alterations in the motility profile of capacitated human spermatozoa (**Figures 11A–D**), as well as the ability of these cells to undergo acrosomal exocytosis (**Figure 11E**). Interestingly in this regard, in addition to a subtle, albeit significant reduction in the proportion of human spermatozoa exhibiting some form of motility (i.e., total motile sperm count; **Supplementary Figure S1E**), the assessment of key parameters of sperm movement, including average path velocity, curvilinear velocity, straight line velocity, and progressive motility, were all significantly attenuated after incubation with 4HNE

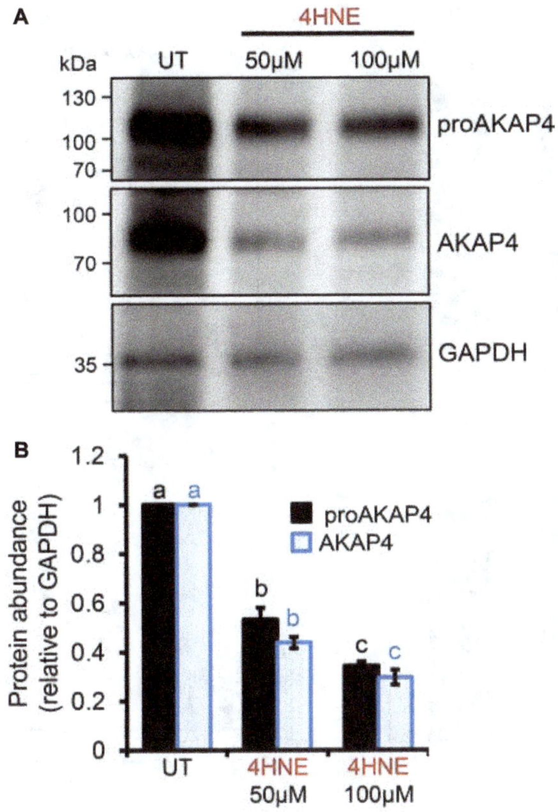

FIGURE 5 | Assessment of the impact of 4HNE adduction on proAKAP4/AKAP4 protein abundance in mature human spermatozoa. **(A)** Human spermatozoa were incubated with 4HNE (50 or 100 μM) for 1 h at 37°C to induce oxidative stress. Cells were subsequently prepared for immunoblotting analysis with anti-proAKAP4 and anti-AKAP4 antibodies. Each blot was stripped and re-probed with anti-GAPDH antibodies to confirm equivalent protein loading. This analysis was performed in triplicate using spermatozoa from three different donors and a representative blot is depicted. **(B)** Protein abundance was quantified by band densitometry and mean values (±SEM) are presented relative to the corresponding GAPDH control ($n = 3$). Differing lowercase letters denote statistical significance ($p < 0.05$) as determined by ANOVA. UT = untreated control.

(**Figures 11A–D**). Similarly, human spermatozoa experienced a significant, ~25% reduction in their ability to complete a calcium ionophore (A23187) induced acrosome reaction (**Figure 11E**). Once again, these damaging effects of 4HNE were ameliorated via pre-treatment of spermatozoa with GSH.

DISCUSSION

Driven by unprecedented rates of recourse to assisted reproductive technologies, there remains a pressing need to develop robust biomarkers capable of predicting fertilization success and discriminating the causative agents that can be targeted to prevent reproductive failure (Aitken et al., 2010). Consistent with these objectives, here, we examined the effects of sub-lethal doses of oxidative insult on the expression of proAKAP4 and of AKAP4; proteins that hold pivotal roles in the formation and structure of the sperm flagellar, in addition to coordination of capacitation-associated signaling (Luconi et al., 2011). We demonstrate that both proAKAP4 and AKAP4 are highly sensitive to oxidative challenge throughout the development of the male germ cell. Indeed, exposure to the lipid aldehyde, 4HNE, led to a substantive loss of both proAKAP4 and AKAP4 in round spermatids and mature spermatozoa. In addition, the residual proAKAP4 and AKAP4 that remained post-4HNE treatment were demonstrated to harbor the burden of 4HNE chemical alkylation; a modification that may perturb the stability of the protein native state, resulting in misfolding and nucleation of protein aggregates as has been shown in somatic cells (Maniti et al., 2015).

As the focus of this study, AKAP4 is a member of a large family of structurally diverse, but functionally conserved, anchoring proteins that coordinate the subcellular distribution of cAMP-mediated signaling networks (Colledge and Scott, 1999). Accordingly, a defining feature of the AKAP family is the presence of at least one PKA anchoring domain that serves to position the PKA holoenzyme at locations where it can rapidly respond to fluctuations in cAMP production. However, the multivalent nature of the AKAP scaffold has also implicated this protein in the physical tethering of several kinases, phosphatases, ion channels, and GTP binding proteins (Colledge and Scott, 1999). This property enables AKAPs to orchestrate the formation of macromolecular complexes compatible with the integration of cAMP and alternate intracellular signaling networks (Colledge and Scott, 1999). In the context of spermatozoa, the compartmentalization of cAMP signaling machinery coordinated by AKAP4 serves to regulate the specificity of signal transduction pathways responsible for the development, activation and maintenance of motility (Luconi et al., 2011; Sergeant et al., 2019). In accordance with this fundamental role, AKAP4 expression displays high evolutionary conservation, with *Akap4* transcripts and/or immunoreactive orthologs of AKAP4 having been characterized in the testes and spermatozoa of species as phylogenetically diverse as eutherian mammals (humans, rodents, bovine, equine, porcine) (Johnson et al., 1997; Turner et al., 1998; Moss et al., 1999; Teijeiro and Marini, 2012; Blommaert et al., 2019; Sergeant et al., 2019), marsupials (tammar wallaby, opossum) (Hu et al., 2009), monotremes (platypus) (Hu et al., 2009), and reptiles (crocodile) (Nixon et al., 2019).

In the mouse testes, AKAP4 is synthesized as a precursor of ~100 kDa (proAKAP4) during the post-meiotic phase of spermatogenesis, with transcripts first detected in early stage round spermatids (Johnson et al., 1997; Brown et al., 2003). Following synthesis, proAKAP4 is processed via the proteolytic cleavage of an N-terminal prodomain, yielding the mature AKAP4 protein (~82 kDa) (Carrera et al., 1994). AKAP4 is subsequently transported to the principal piece of developing flagellum to become the most abundant structural element of the nascent fibrous sheath; accounting for as much 50% of the protein within this specialized domain. The fate of proAKAP4 is somewhat less certain, with emerging evidence supporting interspecies differences in both the extent of its processing and distribution within the mature sperm flagellum. Thus,

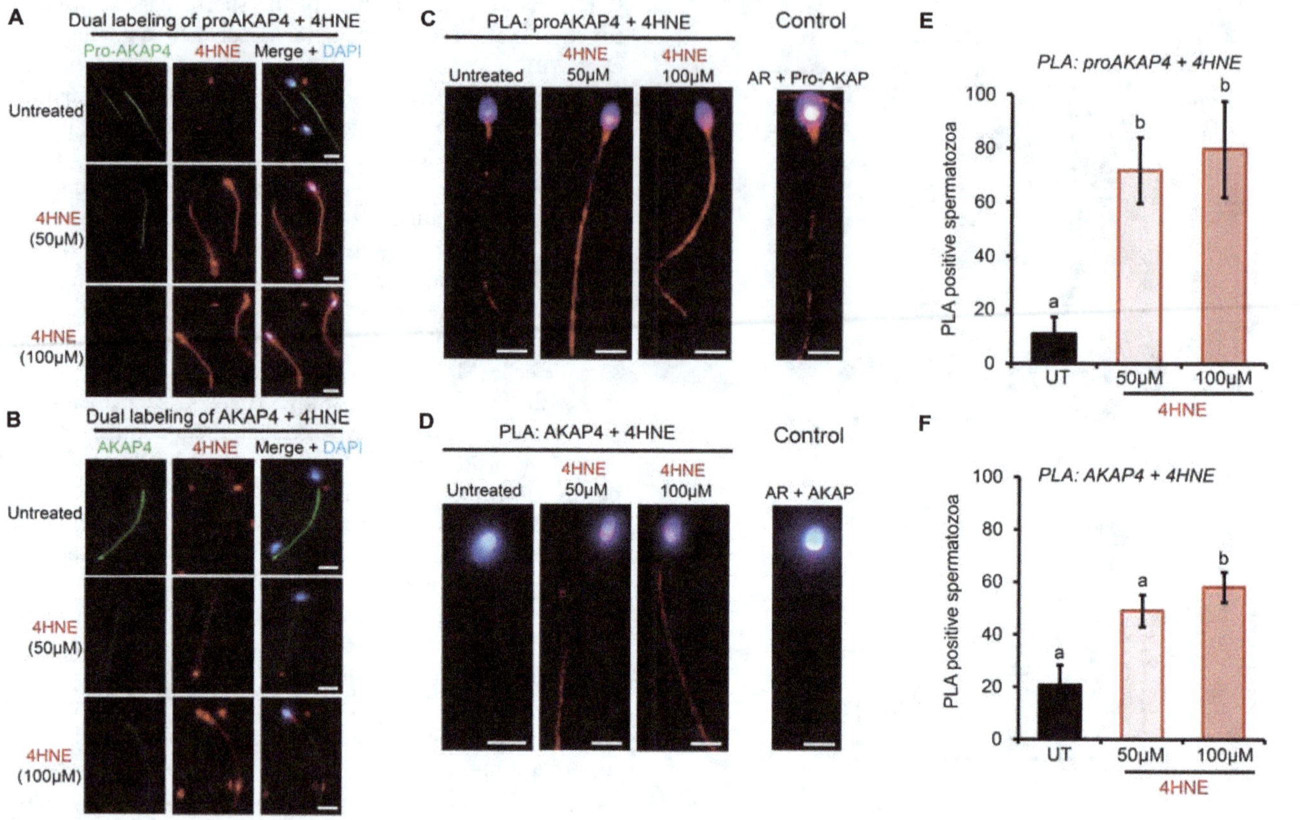

FIGURE 6 | Confirmation of 4HNE adduction to proAKAP4 and AKAP4 in mature human spermatozoa. Human spermatozoa were incubated with 4HNE (50 or 100 μM) for 1 h to induce oxidative stress before being fixed with paraformaldehyde. **(A,B)** Co-localization of proAKAP4 and AKAP4 with 4HNE was performed by dual labeling of spermatozoa with anti-proAKAP4, anti-AKAP4 and anti-4HNE primary antibodies, followed by incubation with corresponding Alexa Fluor conjugated secondary antibodies. This protocol was repeated in the absence of either primary antibody to generate a secondary antibody only control. Representative images were captured using fluorescence microscopy. **(C,D)** The adduction of proAKAP4 and AKAP4 with 4HNE was assessed through the application of a proximity ligation assay, whereby fixed spermatozoa were incubated with target primary antibodies (anti-proAKAP4 or anti-AKAP4 and anti-4HNE) or negative controls [anti-proAKAP4 or anti-AKAP4 and anti-androgen receptor (AR)] and oligonucleotide-conjugated secondary antibodies (PLA probes). PLA probes were then ligated and the signal was amplified. The red fluorescent PLA signals were visualized using fluorescence microscopy and representative images of each treatment group are presented. **(E,F)** Positive proAKAP4/AKAP4 and 4HNE interaction was assessed in a minimum of 100 cells per treatment group using fluorescence microscopy and the percentage of PLA positive cells is expressed as mean values ± SEM ($n = 3$). Differing lowercase letters denote statistical significance ($p < 0.05$) as determined by ANOVA. Scale bars = 5 μm. UT = untreated control.

proAKAP4 has been reported to localize along the entire length of the principal piece of mouse testicular spermatozoa before becoming restricted to the proximal portion of the flagellum in mature cauda epididymal spermatozoa (Johnson et al., 1997); suggestive of an additional wave of proAKAP4 processing during epididymal sperm maturation. By contrast, and in agreement with our own data, proAKAP4 is retained within the flagellum of mature human spermatozoa, where it co-localizes with AKAP4 throughout the fibrous sheath (Turner et al., 1998; Jumeau et al., 2018). Notably however, striking differences in proAKAP4 abundance have been documented in the semen of normozoospermic individuals, wherein the quantity of the protein is positively correlated with sperm motility; albeit in the high-quality cells recovered by density gradient centrifugation (Jumeau et al., 2018). Whilst these data invite speculation that the extent of proAKAP4 processing may reflect the integrity of post-testicular sperm maturation, and hence contribute to differences in the motility profile of human spermatozoa, there is currently no causal evidence to substantiate such an association. Rather, it has been postulated that proAKAP4 may serve as a "reservoir" that can be activated to generate mature AKAP4 and thus rescue sperm motility, if and when required (Jumeau et al., 2018; Sergeant et al., 2019).

Our collective findings confirm previous work in identifying AKAP4 as a primary target of 4HNE adduction in mature human spermatozoa. Indeed, studies by Baker et al. (2015) identified at least three AKAP4 peptides that harbor either one or two 4HNE modified residues after exogenous treatment of spermatozoa with the aldehyde. This study not only confirmed a significant 11-fold enrichment in modified AKAP4 peptides isolated after 4HNE treatment, but also revealed basal levels of endogenous 4HNE modification of AKAP4 in untreated spermatozoa (Baker et al., 2015); data that further reinforces the inherent sensitivity of AKAP4 to chemical alkylation

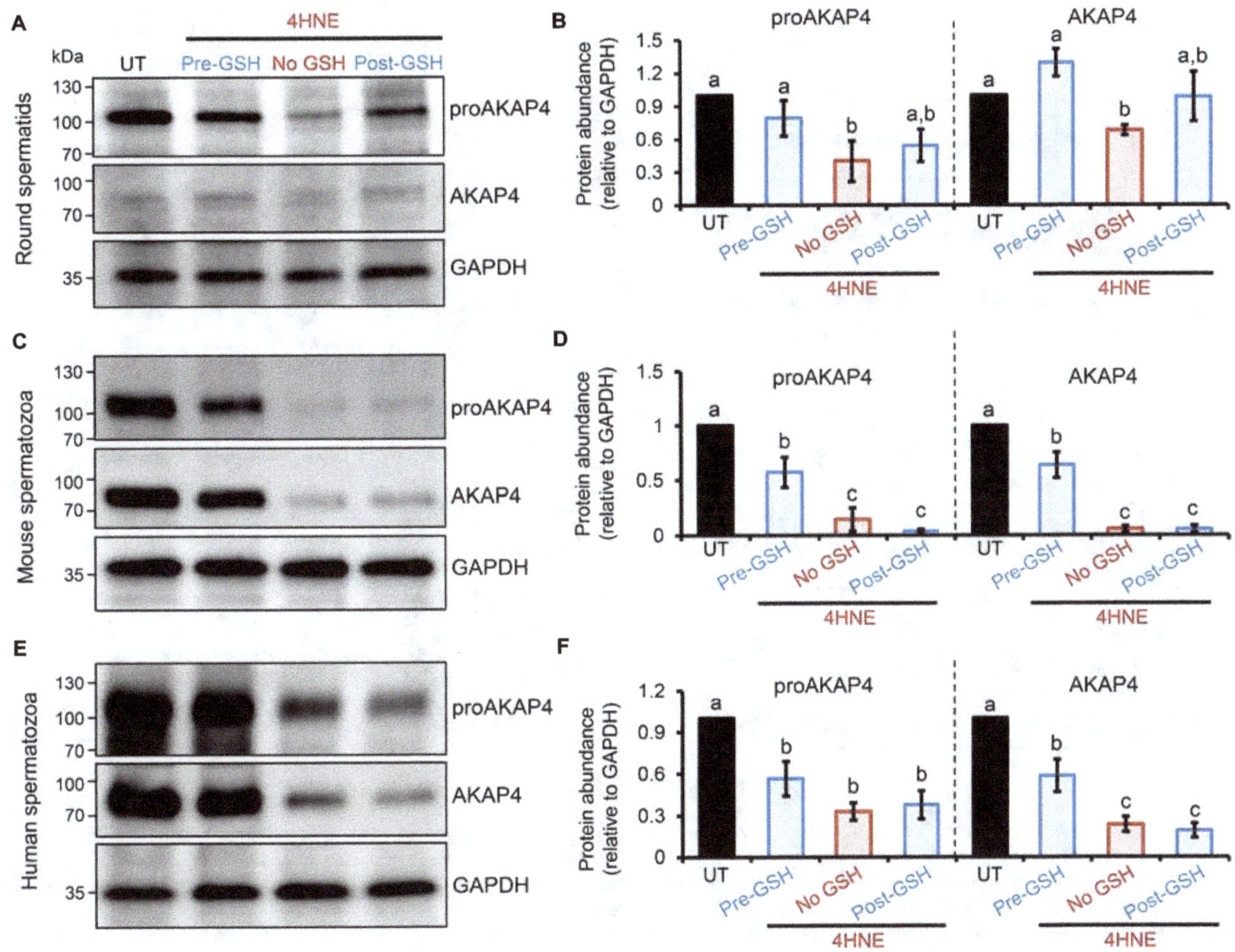

FIGURE 7 | Assessment of the impact of GSH on proAKAP4 and AKAP4 abundance in populations of 4HNE-treated round spermatids and mature spermatozoa. **(A,B)** Round spermatids, and mature **(C,D)** mouse and **(E,F)** human spermatozoa were pre-treated with reduced glutathione (GSH; 4 mM) for 10 min prior to the addition of 4HNE (100 μM). The cells were then co-incubated with both GSH and 4HNE throughout the exposure period (Pre-GSH). Alternatively, following the completion of 4HNE exposure, the cells were washed to remove residual 4HNE before resuspended in media supplemented with GSH (4 mM) and incubated for an additional 30 min (Post-GSH). At the completion of either treatment regimen, gametes were washed before being processed for immunoblotting with either anti-proAKAP4 or anti-AKAP4 antibodies. Each blot was stripped and re-probed with anti-GAPDH antibodies to confirm equivalent protein loading. This analysis was performed in triplicate and representative blots are depicted. **(B,D,F)** Protein abundance was quantified by band densitometry and mean values (±SEM) are presented relative to the corresponding GAPDH control (n = 3). Differing lowercase letters denote statistical significance ($p < 0.05$) as determined by ANOVA. UT = untreated control.

reactions. Though the full extent of AKAP4 damage elicited by insertion of bulky 4HNE (C-9) carbonyl adducts has yet to be investigated, our *in silico* modeling of 4HNE modified residues (K_{279}, K_{331}, C_{566} and C_{570}), indicates that these lie outside of the prodomain (M_1-N_{188}) and those regions implicated in the binding of PKA regulatory subunits (i.e., F_{219}–A_{232} and I_{336}–K_{345}) (Miki and Eddy, 1998, 1999). The 4HNE modified residues do however, reside close to several putative phosphorylation sites and include cysteine residues that may be involved in stabilization of AKAP4 tertiary structure. By analogy with other 4HNE targets, it is reasonable to suspect that these modifications could elicit protein mis-folding, poor substrate recognition, and/or degradation of the protein itself (Carbone et al., 2004a,b); lesions that likely contribute to the dysregulation of sperm motility witnessed in this study as well as that commonly reported in cells burdened by excessive ROS production (Aitken et al., 2010).

In extrapolating these data beyond motility, the importance of the signaling framework coordinated by AKAP4 (Luconi et al., 2011) raises the question of whether cAMP-responsive events associated with sperm capacitation are similarly affected by 4HNE adduction. In addition to the supporting data presented here on phosphorylation profiles and acrosome reaction rates, previous studies have also shown that exogenous 4HNE administration does compromise important correlates of the capacitation cascade including global increases in tyrosine phosphorylation (Baker et al., 2015) and downstream functional endpoints such as zona pellucida adhesion (Bromfield et al., 2015). However, as an important caveat in the interpretation of these data, we note that alternative elements of the

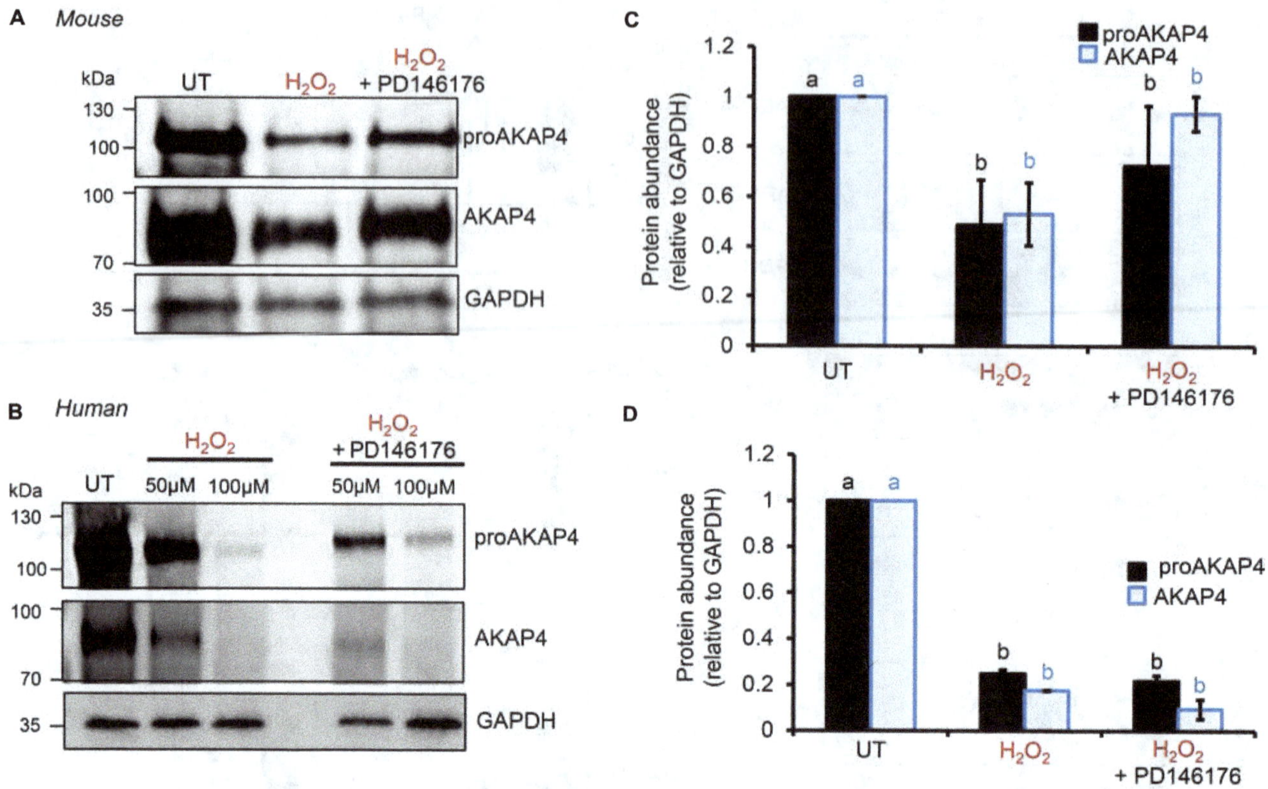

FIGURE 8 | Assessment of ALOX15 inhibition on proAKAP4 and AKAP4 in mouse and human spermatozoa. **(A,B)** Mouse and human sperm samples were pre-treated with PD146176 to inhibit ALOX15 (an enzyme implicated in driving a positive feedback loop of lipid peroxidation) for 15 min prior to exposure to H_2O_2 for 1 h at 37°C, with the inhibitor being retained for the duration of treatment. A DMSO vehicle control was also included in experiments. Sperm lysates were prepared for immunoblotting with anti-proAKAP4 and anti-AKAP4 antibodies. Blots were subsequently stripped and reprobed with anti-GAPDH antibodies to ensure equivalent protein loading. All **(A)** mouse and **(B)** human protein lysates were resolved on the same gels but have been cut and spliced for presentation purposes. **(C,D)** Labeled bands corresponding to proteins of interest were subjected to band densitometry analysis and mean values (±SEM) are presented expressed relative to the corresponding GAPDH control (n = 3). Differing lowercase letters denote statistical significance ($p < 0.05$) as determined by ANOVA. UT = untreated control.

motility apparatus (dynein, outer dense fiber protein 1) (Baker et al., 2015), capacitation signaling (PKA) (Baker et al., 2015), and membrane remodeling proteins (heat shock protein A2) (Bromfield et al., 2015) have been validated as primary targets of 4HNE-mediated modification. Such pervasive broad-spectrum effects make it extremely challenging to disentangle whether individual sperm proteins such as AKAP4 play a dominant role in the pathophysiological responses to 4HNE.

Of concern, these pleiotropic effects are elicited at concentrations of 4HNE that are well within the range attained under conditions of oxidative stress, which can reach as high as 5 mM (Uchida, 2003). They also proved refractory to a lipoxygenase inhibition strategy designed to disrupt the positive feedback loop of lipid peroxidation and hence prevent the induction of redox cycling cascades. In somatic and male germ cells alike, 4HNE adducted proteins are commonly targeted for proteolysis in order to mitigate the risk they pose to cellular homeostasis (Grune et al., 1995; Shang et al., 2001; Carbone et al., 2004b; Bromfield et al., 2017a). Here, we confirm that, despite differences in their solubility and putative interaction networks (Nipper et al., 2006), the innate stability of both proAKAP4 and AKAP4 is also significantly impacted by 4HNE adduction. Curiously however, our data do not support the mobilization of conventional proteolytic degradation pathways in the clearance of proAKAP4 and AKAP4, neither of which were rescued by pharmacological interventions intended to suppress proteasomal activity. Similarly, incubation of mature spermatozoa with GSH post-4HNE treatment also failed to rescue proAKAP4 and AKAP4 levels. A possible explanation for this response lies in the chemistry of 4HNE, which has the potential to form either Michael addition to thiol or amino compounds (via the C3 of the C2=C3 double bond) or Schiff bases (between the C1 carbonyl group and primary amines) (Dalleau et al., 2013). Notably, the kinetics of the Schiff base formation are inherently slow and reversible, whereas those of the Michael-adducts are more rapid and stable; hence Michael-adducts predominate (Dalleau et al., 2013). Although retro-Michael cleavage can occur, leading to resolution of 4HNE adducts, this is by no means a universal phenomenon and is instead heavily influenced by the context of the cellular environment in which this response is measured (Schaur et al., 2015). Irrespective, at present we remain uncertain what mechanism(s) may account for the loss of AKAP4 expression, however, we do not consider this an artifact caused by 4HNE adducts masking antibody recognition

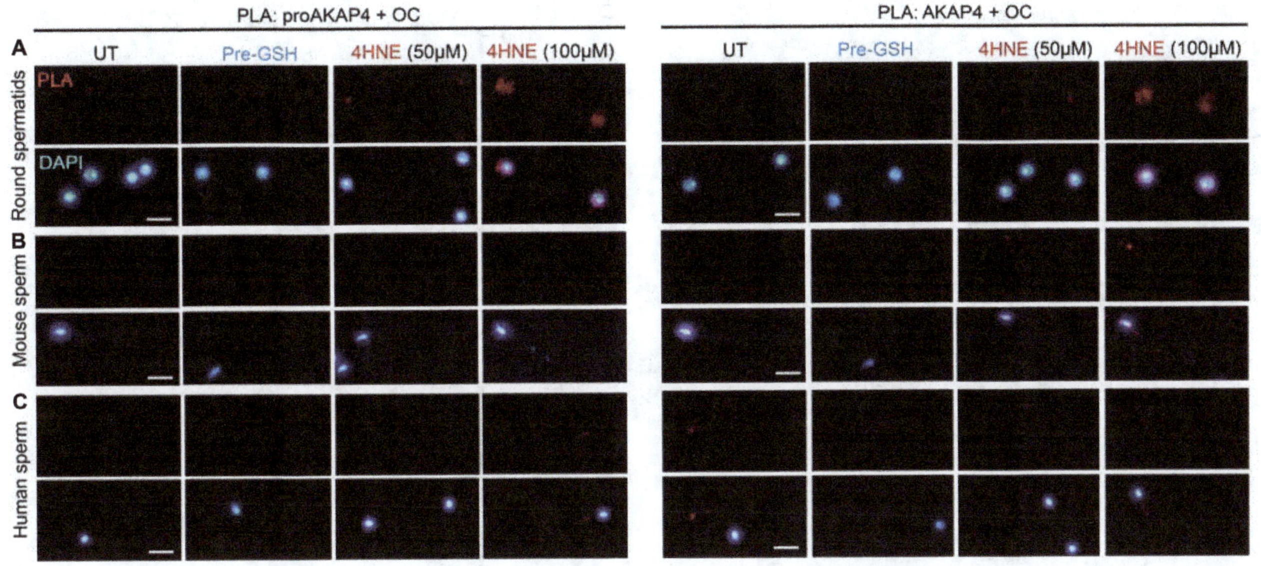

FIGURE 9 | Assessment of the aggregation potential of 4HNE modified proAKAP4 and AKAP4 in male germ cells. Populations of **(A)** round spermatids, **(B)** mouse spermatozoa, and **(C)** human spermatozoa were incubated with 4HNE (50 or 100 μM) for 1 h to induce oxidative stress before being fixed with paraformaldehyde. The propensity of 4HNE adducted proAKAP4 and AKAP4 to form aggregates was assessed through the application of PLA, whereby fixed spermatozoa were incubated with target primary antibodies (anti-proAKAP4 or anti-AKAP4 and anti-amyloid fibrils OC antibodies) and oligonucleotide-conjugated secondary antibodies (PLA probes). In addition to an untreated control (UT), gametes were also pre-treated with reduced glutathione (GSH; 4 mM) for 10 min prior to the addition of 4HNE (100 μM). The cells were then co-incubated with both GSH and 4HNE throughout the exposure period (Pre-GSH). PLA fluorescent signals were visualized using fluorescence microscopy and representative images of each treatment group are presented. This experiment was replicated three times and representative images are depicted. Scale bars = 10 μm.

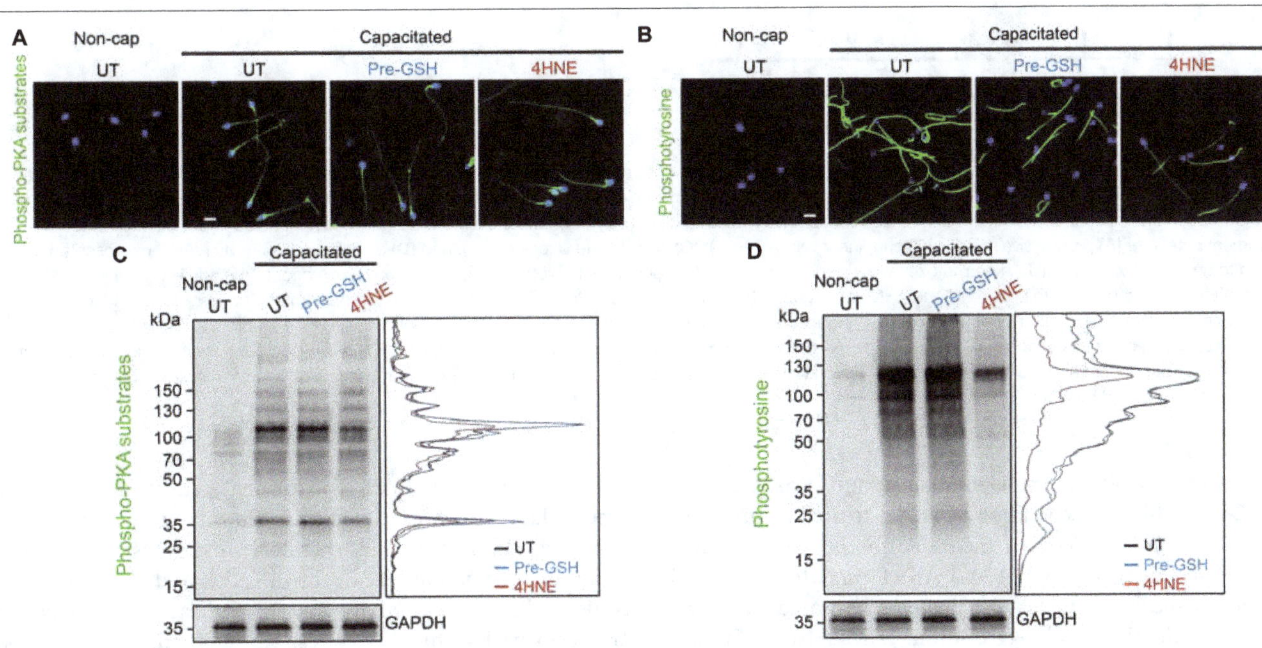

FIGURE 10 | 4HNE adduction of proAKAP4 and AKAP4 attenuates capacitation-associated signaling in human spermatozoa. Human spermatozoa treated with 4HNE (100 μM for 1 h at 37°C) were induced to capacitate (Capacitated) or held in a non-capacitated state (Non-cap) using standard protocols (Mitchell et al., 2007). Spermatozoa were subsequently prepared for either **(A,B)** immunocytochemistry or **(C,D)** immunoblotting with anti-phospho-PKA substrate or anti-phosphotyrosine antibodies. A densitometric trace of representative immunoblots is included to highlight changes in phospho-labeling in untreated (UT; black trace), GSH pre-treated (Pre-GSH; blue trace) and 4HNE treated (4HNE; red trace) spermatozoa. This experiment was replicated with samples from three separate donors and representative images are immunoblots are presented. Scale bars = 10 μm.

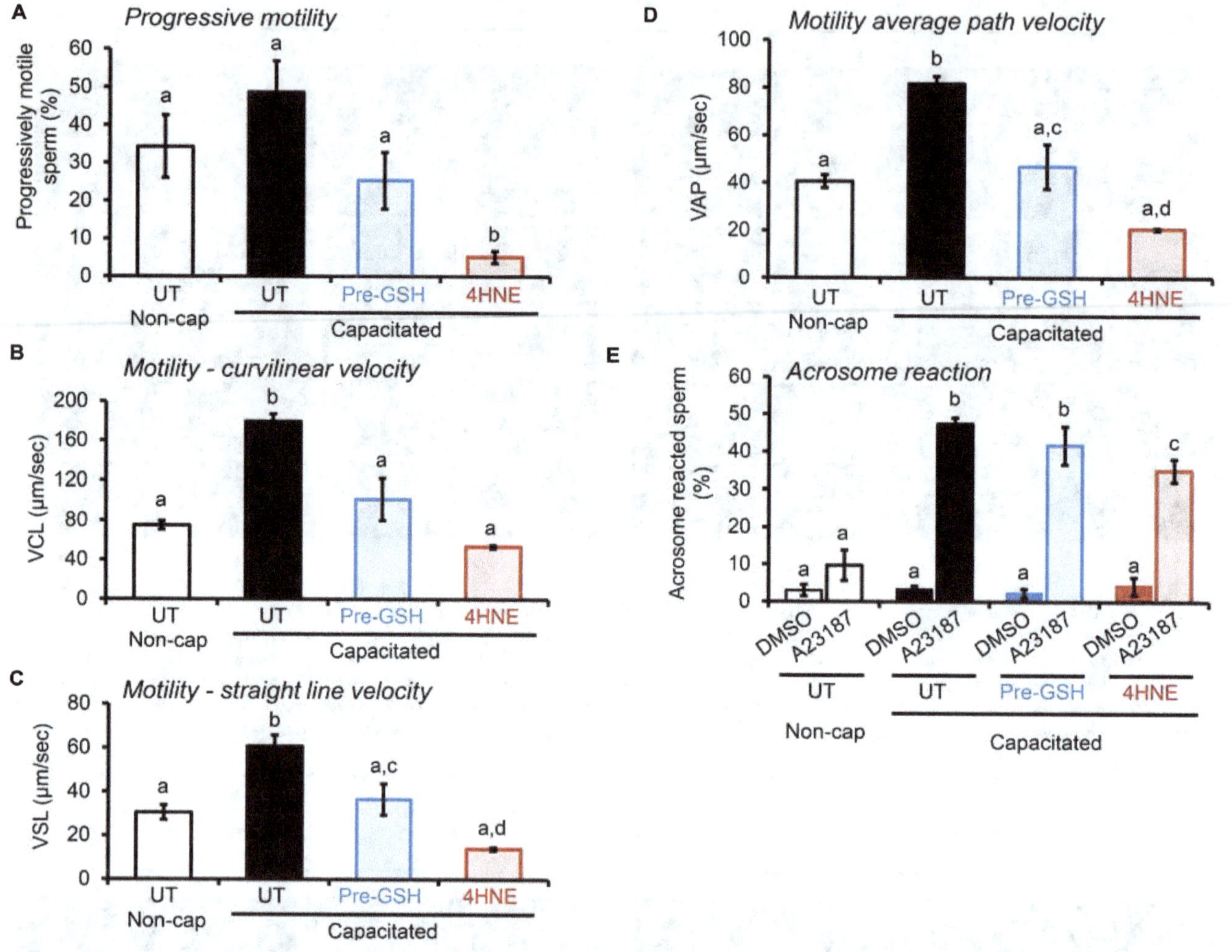

FIGURE 11 | 4HNE negatively impacts the motility profile and ability of human spermatozoa to complete an acrosome reaction. **(A–D)** Human spermatozoa treated with 4HNE (100 µM for 1 h at 37°C) were induced to capacitate (Capacitated) or held in a non-capacitated state (Non-cap) using standard protocols (Mitchell et al., 2007). Computer Assisted Sperm Analysis (CASA) was subsequently used to objectively track the movement characteristics of human spermatozoa and the assessment criteria of **(A)** progressive motility, **(B)** curvilinear velocity (VCL), **(C)** straight line velocity (VSL), and **(D)** average path velocity (VAP) are presented. In addition to an untreated control (UT), spermatozoa were also pre-treated with reduced glutathione (GSH; 4 mM) for 10 min prior to the addition of 4HNE and the cells were then co-incubated with both GSH and 4HNE throughout the exposure period (Pre-GSH). **(E)** Alternatively, the spermatozoa were assessed for their competence to complete a calcium ionophore (A23187) induced acrosome reaction, via staining with fluorescently labeled PSA as previously described (Zhou et al., 2017). The spontaneous rates of acrosome loss were assessed via the inclusion of a vehicle control group (DMSO). These experiments were replicated with samples from three separate donors and representative images are and mean values (±SEM) are presented. Differing lowercase letters denote statistical significance ($p < 0.05$) as determined by ANOVA.

motifs. Indeed, we were able to demonstrate anti-proAKAP4 and anti-AKAP4 antibody recognition of 4HNE-treated recombinant AKAP4 protein. Moreover, these antibodies also readily labeled the residual proAKAP4 and AKAP4 *in situ* post-4HNE treatment, a setting in which the proteins harbored signatures of 4HNE adduction and aggregation. These latter findings are supported by independent evidence that heavily oxidized proteins resisting degradation have a propensity to crosslink and aggregate (Castro et al., 2017). Indeed, evidence from the somatic cell literature, has established that 4HNE oxidative modifications can inactivate target proteins by rendering them prone to formation of oligomers; both in solution and in the intracellular environment (Maniti et al., 2015). Accordingly, we have also shown that 4HNE treatment can result in significant accumulation of cytosolic protein deposits in the male germline (Cafe et al., 2019). We therefore, hypothesize that 4HNE induced aggregation of the proAKAP4 and AKAP4 proteins could reduce their activity and the efficacy with which they are recovered from cell lysates; although this prospect awaits further investigation.

CONCLUSION

Here, we have confirmed the vulnerability of both proAKAP4 and AKAP4 to 4HNE modification throughout male germ cell development. Such modification leads to a range of adverse sequela that not only affect proAKAP4 and AKAP4 stability, but also compromises their functions in mature spermatozoa. These findings provide a physiological explanation for the loss of sperm motility and capacitation competence commonly encountered in response to oxidative stress and raise the prospect that such defects may help reduce the likelihood of sperm harboring oxidative DNA lesions from participating in fertilization. In this sense, oxidative damage of both proAKAP4 and AKAP4 may be considered a protective mechanism that limits the transmission of an altered male genome to the next generation. In any event, these data add to a growing body of literature emphasizing the need for novel therapeutic interventions to alleviate the burden of oxidative-stress mediated dysfunction in the male germline.

ETHICS STATEMENT

The studies involving human participants were reviewed and approved by The University of Newcastle Human Ethics Committee. All donors provided their written informed consent to participate in this study. The animal study was reviewed and approved by The University of Newcastle Animal Care and Ethics Committee.

AUTHOR CONTRIBUTIONS

BN conceived the study and wrote the first draft of the manuscript. IB, SC, AA, and NT were responsible for the study execution and data analysis. MD, NS, AE, TL, GD, MDD, and EB contributed to the conception and design of the study, and participated in the data analysis. All authors contributed to the manuscript revision, read, and approved the submitted version.

FUNDING

This project was supported by a National Health and Medical Research Council of Australia (NHMRC) Project Grant (APP1163319) awarded to BN and EB. SC and NT are the recipients of University of Newcastle Postgraduate Research Scholarships. EB is the recipient of a NHMRC CJ Martin Early Career Fellowship. BN is the recipient of a NHMRC Senior Research Fellowship. MDD is the recipient of a Cancer Institute NSW Early Career Fellowship.

ACKNOWLEDGMENTS

The authors gratefully acknowledge the support of the University of Newcastle, Priority Research Centre for Reproductive Science.

REFERENCES

Aitken, R. J. (2018). Not every sperm is sacred; a perspective on male infertility. *Mol. Hum. Reprod.* 24, 287–298. doi: 10.1093/molehr/gay010

Aitken, R. J., Baker, M. A., De Iuliis, G. N., and Nixon, B. (2010). New insights into sperm physiology and pathology. *Handb. Exp. Pharmacol.* 198, 99–115. doi: 10.1007/978-3-642-02062-9_7

Aitken, R. J., Gibb, Z., Baker, M. A., Drevet, J., and Gharagozloo, P. (2016). Causes and consequences of oxidative stress in spermatozoa. *Reprod. Fertil. Dev.* 28, 1–10. doi: 10.1071/RD15325

Aitken, R. J., and Nixon, B. (2013). Sperm capacitation: a distant landscape glimpsed but unexplored. *Mol. Hum. Reprod.* 19, 785–793. doi: 10.1093/molehr/gat067

Aitken, R. J., Whiting, S., De Iuliis, G. N., McClymont, S., Mitchell, L. A., and Baker, M. A. (2012). Electrophilic aldehydes generated by sperm metabolism activate mitochondrial reactive oxygen species generation and apoptosis by targeting succinate dehydrogenase. *J. Biol. Chem.* 287, 33048–33060. doi: 10.1074/jbc.m112.366690

Baker, M. A., Weinberg, A., Hetherington, L., Villaverde, A. I., Velkov, T., Baell, J., et al. (2015). Defining the mechanisms by which the reactive oxygen species by-product, 4-hydroxynonenal, affects human sperm cell function. *Biol. Reprod.* 92, 108. doi: 10.1095/biolreprod.114.126680

Bjorndahl, L., Barratt, C. L., Mortimer, D., and Jouannet, P. (2016). 'How to count sperm properly': checklist for acceptability of studies based on human semen analysis. *Hum. Reprod.* 31, 227–232. doi: 10.1093/humrep/dev305

Blommaert, D., Sergeant, N., Delehedde, M., Jouy, N., Mitchell, V., Franck, T., et al. (2019). Expression, localization, and concentration of A-kinase anchor protein 4 (AKAP4) and its precursor (proAKAP4) in equine semen: promising marker correlated to the total and progressive motility in thawed spermatozoa. *Theriogenology* 131, 52–60. doi: 10.1016/j.theriogenology.2019.03.011

Bromfield, E. G., Aitken, R. J., Anderson, A. L., McLaughlin, E. A., and Nixon, B. (2015). The impact of oxidative stress on chaperone-mediated human sperm-egg interaction. *Hum. Reprod.* 30, 2597–2613. doi: 10.1093/humrep/dev214

Bromfield, E. G., Aitken, R. J., McLaughlin, E. A., and Nixon, B. (2017a). Proteolytic degradation of heat shock protein A2 occurs in response to oxidative stress in male germ cells of the mouse. *Mol. Hum. Reprod.* 23, 91–105. doi: 10.1093/molehr/gaw074

Bromfield, E. G., Mihalas, B. P., Dun, M. D., Aitken, R. J., McLaughlin, E. A., Walters, J. L., et al. (2017b). Inhibition of arachidonate 15-lipoxygenase prevents 4-hydroxynonenal-induced protein damage in male germ cells. *Biol. Reprod.* 96, 598–609. doi: 10.1093/biolre/iox005

Bromfield, E. G., Walters, J. L. H., Cafe, S. L., Bernstein, I. R., Stanger, S. J., Anderson, A. L., et al. (2019). Differential cell death decisions in the testis: evidence for an exclusive window of ferroptosis in round spermatids. *Mol. Hum. Reprod.* 25, 241–256. doi: 10.1093/molehr/gaz015

Brown, P. R., Miki, K., Harper, D. B., and Eddy, E. M. (2003). A-kinase anchoring protein 4 binding proteins in the fibrous sheath of the sperm flagellum. *Biol. Reprod.* 68, 2241–2248. doi: 10.1095/biolreprod.102.013466

Cafe, S. L., Nixon, B., Roman, S. D., Bernstein, I. R. and Bromfield, E. G. (2019). Oxidative stress dysregulates protein homeostasis within the male germ line. *Antioxid. Redox Signal.* doi: 10.1089/ars.2019.7832 [Epub ahead of print].

Carbone, D. L., Doorn, J. A., Kiebler, Z., Sampey, B. P., and Petersen, D. R. (2004a). Inhibition of Hsp72-mediated protein refolding by 4-hydroxy-2-nonenal. *Chem. Res. Toxicol.* 17, 1459–1467. doi: 10.1021/tx049838g

Carbone, D. L., Doorn, J. A., and Petersen, D. R. (2004b). 4-Hydroxynonenal regulates 26S proteasomal degradation of alcohol dehydrogenase. *Free Radic. Biol. Med.* 37, 1430–1439. doi: 10.1016/j.freeradbiomed.2004.07.016

Carrera, A., Gerton, G. L., and Moss, S. B. (1994). The major fibrous sheath polypeptide of mouse sperm: structural and functional similarities to the A-kinase anchoring proteins. *Dev. Biol.* 165, 272–284. doi: 10.1006/dbio.1994.1252

Carrera, A., Moos, J., Ning, X. P., Gerton, G. L., Tesarik, J., Kopf, G. S., et al. (1996). Regulation of protein tyrosine phosphorylation in human sperm by a calcium/calmodulin-dependent mechanism: identification of A kinase anchor proteins as major substrates for tyrosine phosphorylation. *Dev. Biol.* 180, 284–296. doi: 10.1006/dbio.1996.0301

Castro, J. P., Jung, T., Grune, T., and Siems, W. (2017). 4-Hydroxynonenal (HNE) modified proteins in metabolic diseases. *Free Radic. Biol. Med.* 111, 309–315. doi: 10.1016/j.freeradbiomed.2016.10.497

Chen, Z. H., and Niki, E. (2006). 4-hydroxynonenal (4-HNE) has been widely accepted as an inducer of oxidative stress. *Is this the whole truth about it or can* 4-HNE also exert protective effects? *IUBMB Life* 58, 372–373. doi: 10.1080/15216540600686896

Colledge, M., and Scott, J. D. (1999). AKAPs: from structure to function. *Trends Cell Biol.* 9, 216–221. doi: 10.1016/s0962-8924(99)01558-5

Dalleau, S., Baradat, M., Gueraud, F., and Huc, L. (2013). Cell death and diseases related to oxidative stress: 4-hydroxynonenal (HNE) in the balance. *Cell Death. Differ* 20, 1615–1630. doi: 10.1038/cdd.2013.138

Davies, K. J. (2001). Degradation of oxidized proteins by the 20S proteasome. *Biochimie* 83, 301–310. doi: 10.1016/s0300-9084(01)01250-0

Dohle, G. R., Colpi, G. M., Hargreave, T. B., Papp, G. K., Jungwirth, A., Weidner, W., et al. (2005). EAU guidelines on male infertility. *Eur. Urol.* 48, 703–711.

Dun, M. D., Anderson, A. L., Bromfield, E. G., Asquith, K. L., Emmett, B., McLaughlin, E. A., et al. (2012). Investigation of the expression and functional significance of the novel mouse sperm protein, a disintegrin and metalloprotease with thrombospondin type 1 motifs number 10 (ADAMTS10). *Int. J. Androl.* 35, 572–589. doi: 10.1111/j.1365-2605.2011.01235.x

Eddy, E. M. (2007). The scaffold role of the fibrous sheath. *Soc. Reprod. Fertil. Suppl.* 65, 45–62.

Eddy, E. M., Toshimori, K., and O'Brien, D. A. (2003). Fibrous sheath of mammalian spermatozoa. *Microsc. Res. Tech.* 61, 103–115. doi: 10.1002/jemt.10320

Fang, X., Huang, L. L., Xu, J., Ma, C. Q., Chen, Z. H., Zhang, Z., et al. (2019). Proteomics and single-cell RNA analysis of Akap4-knockout mice model confirm indispensable role of Akap4 in spermatogenesis. *Dev. Biol.* 454, 118–127. doi: 10.1016/j.ydbio.2019.06.017

Frapsauce, C., Pionneau, C., Bouley, J., Delarouziere, V., Berthaut, I., Ravel, C., et al. (2014). Proteomic identification of target proteins in normal but nonfertilizing sperm. *Fertil. Steril.* 102, 372–380. doi: 10.1016/j.fertnstert.2014.04.039

Grune, T., Reinheckel, T., Joshi, M., and Davies, K. J. (1995). Proteolysis in cultured liver epithelial cells during oxidative stress. Role of the multicatalytic proteinase complex, proteasome. *J. Biol. Chem.* 270, 2344–2351. doi: 10.1074/jbc.270.5.2344

Hauck, A. K., and Bernlohr, D. A. (2016). Oxidative stress and lipotoxicity. *J. Lipid Res.* 57, 1976–1986. doi: 10.1194/jlr.r066597

Hu, Y., Yu, H., Pask, A. J., O'Brien, D. A., Shaw, G., and Renfree, M. B. (2009). A-kinase anchoring protein 4 has a conserved role in mammalian spermatogenesis. *Reproduction* 137, 645–653. doi: 10.1530/REP-08-0337

Johnson, L. R., Foster, J. A., Haig-Ladewig, L., VanScoy, H., Rubin, C. S., Moss, S. B., et al. (1997). Assembly of AKAP82, a protein kinase A anchor protein, into the fibrous sheath of mouse sperm. *Dev. Biol.* 192, 340–350. doi: 10.1006/dbio.1997.8767

Jumeau, F., Sigala, J., Dossou-Gbete, F., Frimat, K., Barbotin, A. L., Buee, L., et al. (2018). A-kinase anchor protein 4 precursor (pro-AKAP4) in human spermatozoa. *Andrology* 6, 854–859. doi: 10.1111/andr.12524

LoPachin, R. M., Gavin, T., Petersen, D. R., and Barber, D. S. (2009). Molecular mechanisms of 4-hydroxy-2-nonenal and acrolein toxicity: nucleophilic targets and adduct formation. *Chem. Res. Toxicol* 22, 1499–1508. doi: 10.1021/tx900147g

Lord, T., Martin, J. H., and Aitken, R. J. (2015). Accumulation of electrophilic aldehydes during postovulatory aging of mouse oocytes causes reduced fertility, oxidative stress, and apoptosis. *Biol. Reprod.* 92:33. doi: 10.1095/biolreprod.114.122820

Luconi, M., Cantini, G., Baldi, E., and Forti, G. (2011). Role of a-kinase anchoring proteins (AKAPs) in reproduction. *Front. Biosci.* 16, 1315–1330. doi: 10.2741/3791

Maniti, O., Francois-Moutal, L., Lecompte, M. F., Vial, C., Lagarde, M., Guichardant, M., et al. (2015). Protein "amyloid-like" networks at the phospholipid membrane formed by 4-hydroxy-2-nonenal-modified mitochondrial creatine kinase. *Mol. Membr. Biol.* 32, 1–10. doi: 10.3109/09687688.2015.1023376

Mihalas, B. P., Bromfield, E. G., Sutherland, J. M., De Iuliis, G. N., McLaughlin, E. A., Aitken, R. J., et al. (2018). Oxidative damage in naturally aged mouse oocytes is exacerbated by dysregulation of proteasomal activity. *J. Biol. Chem.* 293, 18944–18964. doi: 10.1074/jbc.RA118.005751

Mihalas, B. P., De Iuliis, G. N., Redgrove, K. A., McLaughlin, E. A., and Nixon, B. (2017). The lipid peroxidation product 4-hydroxynonenal contributes to oxidative stress-mediated deterioration of the ageing oocyte. *Sci. Rep.* 7:6247. doi: 10.1038/s41598-017-06372-z

Miki, K., and Eddy, E. M. (1998). Identification of tethering domains for protein kinase A type Ialpha regulatory subunits on sperm fibrous sheath protein FSC1. *J. Biol. Chem.* 273, 34384–34390. doi: 10.1074/jbc.273.51.34384

Miki, K., and Eddy, E. M. (1999). Single amino acids determine specificity of binding of protein kinase A regulatory subunits by protein kinase A anchoring proteins. *J. Biol. Chem.* 274, 29057–29062. doi: 10.1074/jbc.274.41.29057

Miki, K., Willis, W. D., Brown, P. R., Goulding, E. H., Fulcher, K. D., and Eddy, E. M. (2002). Targeted disruption of the Akap4 gene causes defects in sperm flagellum and motility. *Dev. Biol.* 248, 331–342. doi: 10.1006/dbio.2002.0728

Mitchell, L. A., Nixon, B., and Aitken, R. J. (2007). Analysis of chaperone proteins associated with human spermatozoa during capacitation. *Mol. Hum. Reprod.* 13, 605–613. doi: 10.1093/molehr/gam043

Moretti, E., Scapigliati, G., Pascarelli, N. A., Baccetti, B., and Collodel, G. (2007). Localization of AKAP4 and tubulin proteins in sperm with reduced motility. *Asian J. Androl.* 9, 641–649. doi: 10.1111/j.1745-7262.2007.00267.x

Moss, S. B., Turner, R. M., Burkert, K. L., VanScoy Butt, H., and Gerton, G. L. (1999). Conservation and function of a bovine sperm A-kinase anchor protein homologous to mouse AKAP82. *Biol. Reprod.* 61, 335–342. doi: 10.1095/biolreprod61.2.335

Nipper, R. W., Jones, B. H., Gerton, G. L., and Moss, S. B. (2006). Protein domains govern the intracellular distribution of mouse sperm AKAP4. *Biol. Reprod.* 75, 189–196. doi: 10.1095/biolreprod.106.050963

Nixon, B., Johnston, S. D., Skerrett-Byrne, D. A., Anderson, A. L., Stanger, S. J., Bromfield, E. G., et al. (2019). Modification of crocodile spermatozoa refutes the tenet that post-testicular sperm maturation is restricted to mammals. *Mol. Cell. Proteomics* 18, S59–S76. doi: 10.1074/mcp.RA118.000904

Nixon, B. J., Katen, A. L., Stanger, S. J., Schjenken, J. E., Nixon, B., and Roman, S. D. (2014). Mouse spermatocytes express CYP2E1 and respond to acrylamide exposure. *PLoS One* 9:e94904. doi: 10.1371/journal.pone.0094904

Peddinti, D., Nanduri, B., Kaya, A., Feugang, J. M., Burgess, S. C., and Memili, E. (2008). Comprehensive proteomic analysis of bovine spermatozoa of varying fertility rates and identification of biomarkers associated with fertility. *BMC Syst. Biol.* 2:19. doi: 10.1186/1752-0509-2-19

Petersen, D. R., and Doorn, J. A. (2004). Reactions of 4-hydroxynonenal with proteins and cellular targets. *Free Radic. Biol. Med.* 37, 937–945. doi: 10.1016/j.freeradbiomed.2004.06.012

Redgrove, K. A., Anderson, A. L., Dun, M. D., McLaughlin, E. A., O'Bryan, M. K., Aitken, R. J., et al. (2011). Involvement of multimeric protein complexes in mediating the capacitation-dependent binding of human spermatozoa to homologous zonae pellucidae. *Dev. Biol.* 356, 460–474. doi: 10.1016/j.ydbio.2011.05.674

Redgrove, K. A., Nixon, B., Baker, M. A., Hetherington, L., Baker, G., Liu, D. Y., et al. (2012). The molecular chaperone HSPA2 plays a key role in regulating the expression of sperm surface receptors that mediate sperm-egg recognition. *PLoS One* 7:e50851. doi: 10.1371/journal.pone.0050851

Reid, A. T., Lord, T., Stanger, S. J., Roman, S. D., McCluskey, A., Robinson, P. J., et al. (2012). Dynamin regulates specific membrane fusion events necessary for acrosomal exocytosis in mouse spermatozoa. *J. Biol. Chem.* 287, 37659–37672. doi: 10.1074/jbc.M112.392803

Schaur, R. J., Siems, W., Bresgen, N., and Eckl, P. M. (2015). 4-Hydroxy-nonenal-A Bioactive Lipid Peroxidation Product. *Biomolecules* 5, 2247–2337. doi: 10.3390/biom5042247

Sergeant, N., Briand-Amirat, L., Bencharif, D., and Delehedde, M. (2019). The sperm specific protein proAKAP4 as an innovative marker to evalulate sperm quaility and fertility. *Dairy Vet. Sci. J.* 11:555803.

Shang, F., Nowell, T. R. Jr., and Taylor, A. (2001). Removal of oxidatively damaged proteins from lens cells by the ubiquitin-proteasome pathway. *Exp. Eye Res.* 73, 229–238. doi: 10.1006/exer.2001.1029

Shringarpure, R., Grune, T., and Davies, K. J. (2001). Protein oxidation and 20S proteasome-dependent proteolysis in mammalian cells. *Cell Mol. Life Sci.* 58, 1442–1450. doi: 10.1007/pl00000787

Teijeiro, J. M., and Marini, P. E. (2012). The effect of oviductal deleted in malignant brain tumor 1 over porcine sperm is mediated by a signal transduction pathway that involves pro-AKAP4 phosphorylation. *Reproduction* 143, 773–785. doi: 10.1530/REP-11-0314

Towbin, H., Staehelin, T., and Gordon, J. (1979). Electrophoretic transfer of proteins from polyacrylamide gels to nitrocellulose sheets: procedure and some applications. *Proc. Natl. Acad. Sci. U.S.A.* 76, 4350–4354. doi: 10.1073/pnas.76.9.4350

Tremellen, K. (2008). Oxidative stress and male infertility–a clinical perspective. *Hum. Reprod. Update* 14, 243–258. doi: 10.1093/humupd/dmn004

Turner, R. M., Johnson, L. R., Haig-Ladewig, L., Gerton, G. L., and Moss, S. B. (1998). An X-linked gene encodes a major human sperm fibrous sheath protein, hAKAP82. Genomic organization, protein kinase A-RII binding, and distribution of the precursor in the sperm tail. *J. Biol. Chem.* 273, 32135–32141. doi: 10.1074/jbc.273.48.32135

Uchida, K. (2003). 4-Hydroxy-2-nonenal: a product and mediator of oxidative stress. *Prog. Lipid Res.* 42, 318–343. doi: 10.1016/s0163-7827(03)00014-6

Walsh, A., Whelan, D., Bielanowicz, A., Skinner, B., Aitken, R. J., O'Bryan, M. K., et al. (2008). Identification of the molecular chaperone, heat shock protein 1 (chaperonin 10), in the reproductive tract and in capacitating spermatozoa in the male mouse. *Biol. Reprod.* 78, 983–993. doi: 10.1095/biolreprod.107.066860

Walters, J. L. H., De Iuliis, G. N., Dun, M. D., Aitken, R. J., McLaughlin, E. A., Nixon, B., et al. (2018a). Pharmacological inhibition of arachidonate 15-lipoxygenase protects human spermatozoa against oxidative stress. *Biol. Reprod.* 98, 784–794. doi: 10.1093/biolre/ioy058

Walters, J. L. H., De Iuliis, G. N., Nixon, B., and Bromfield, E. G. (2018b). oxidative stress in the male germline: a review of novel strategies to reduce 4-hydroxynonenal production. *Antioxidants* 7:E132. doi: 10.3390/antiox7100132

Zhou, W., Anderson, A. L., Turner, A. P., De Iuliis, G. N., McCluskey, A., McLaughlin, E. A., et al. (2017). Characterization of a novel role for the dynamin mechanoenzymes in the regulation of human sperm acrosomal exocytosis. *Mol. Hum. Reprod.* 23, 657–673. doi: 10.1093/molehr/gax044

Zhou, W., Sipila, P., De Iuliis, G. N., Dun, M. D., and Nixon, B. (2018). Analysis of epididymal protein synthesis and secretion. *J. Vis. Exp.* 138:e58308. doi: 10.3791/58308

15

Quantitative Intracellular pH Determinations in Single Live Mammalian Spermatozoa Using the Ratiometric Dye SNARF-5F

*Julio C. Chávez, Alberto Darszon, Claudia L. Treviño and Takuya Nishigaki**

Departamento de Genética del Desarrollo y Fisiología Molecular, Instituto de Biotecnología, Universidad Nacional Autónoma de México, Cuernavaca, Mexico

***Correspondence:**
Takuya Nishigaki
takuya@ibt.unam.mx

Intracellular pH (pH_i) plays a crucial role in mammalian sperm physiology. However, it is a challenging task to acquire quantitative single sperm pH_i images due to their small size and beating flagella. In this study, we established a robust pH_i imaging system using the dual-emission ratiometric pH indicator, SNARF-5F. Simultaneous good signal/noise ratio fluorescence signals were obtained exciting with a green high-power LED (532 nm) and acquiring with an EM-CCD camera through an image splitter with two band-pass filters (550–600 nm, channel 1; 630–650 nm, channel 2). After *in vivo* calibration, we established an imaging system that allows determination of absolute pH_i values in spermatozoa, minimizing cell movement artifacts. Using this system, we determined that bicarbonate increases non-capacitated human pH_i with slower kinetics than in mouse spermatozoa. This difference suggests that distinct ionic transporters might be involved in the bicarbonate influx into human and mouse spermatozoa. Alternatively, pH_i regulation downstream bicarbonate influx into spermatozoa could be different between the two species.

Keywords: intracellular pH, alkalization, spermatozoa, dual emission, image splitter, ratiometric

INTRODUCTION

The pH is fundamental for most proteins to ensure their proper function, as it influences the electrostatic status of their side chains that, in turn, affect protein structure (folding and conformation) and their interaction with other molecules (Zhou and Pang, 2018). Therefore, intracellular pH (pH_i) changes serve as crucial signals in many cell types.

In spermatozoa, pH_i critically regulates motility (Ho et al., 2002; Nishigaki et al., 2014). In mammals, spermatozoa remain quiescent in the epididymis due to the acidic environment created by vacuolar-type H^+-ATPase (V-ATPase) found in the apical plasma membrane of epithelial cells (Acott and Carr, 1984; Brown et al., 1997). Flagellar beating is suppressed in acidic environments as dynein ATPases, the motor molecules that propel the flagellum, are highly pH_i dependent (Crhisten et al., 1983). Upon ejaculation and contact with the seminal fluid sperm pH_i increases, and the flagellum starts beating. The initial flagellar beat is symmetric with low amplitude and high frequency. Subsequently in the oviduct, the flagellar beat pattern becomes vigorous (asymmetric with high amplitude and low frequency), a process called hyperactivation (Ho and Suarez, 2001). Hyperactivated motility is essential for mammalian spermatozoa since it is required to approach the oocyte and to penetrate its investments (Stauss et al., 1995; Suarez and Pacey, 2006). In order to induce and maintain hyperactivation, an increase in intracellular Ca^{2+} concentration ($[Ca^{2+}]_i$)

is required (Ho et al., 2002), which is mediated through a sperm-specific Ca^{2+} channel, named CatSper (Ren et al., 2001). Although there are species-specific activation mechanisms of CatSper (Lishko et al., 2011), this channel is moderately voltage dependent and highly up regulated by intracellular alkalization (Kirichok et al., 2006). In mouse, the sperm-specific Na^+/H^+ exchanger (sNHE) is essential for the regulation of sperm motility and has been proposed as an activator of CatSper by elevating pH_i (Wang et al., 2003; Navarro et al., 2008). On the other hand, in human spermatozoa, a voltage-gated H^+ channel (Hv1) has been documented to be the main H^+ transporter that activates CatSper rather than sNHE (Lishko et al., 2010). In sea urchin sperm, CatSper is a predominant player in chemotaxis toward sperm-attracting peptides (Seifert et al., 2015; Espinal-Enríquez et al., 2017) and sNHE has been shown to be critical for modulating CatSper activity (González-Cota et al., 2015; Windler et al., 2018).

External bicarbonate (HCO_3^-) is fundamental for capacitation in mammalian spermatozoa (Lee and Storey, 1986; Visconti et al., 1995). Both the pH and the HCO_3^- concentration of the oviductal fluid are higher in uterine and tubal fluids compared to plasma (Vishwakarma, 1962). Moreover, pH in the rhesus monkey female tract elevates dramatically, concomitantly with ovulation (Maas et al., 1977), which might promote sperm capacitation *in vivo*. In mammalian spermatozoa, several HCO_3^- transporters were reported as candidates to mediate HCO_3^- influx across the plasma membrane such as Na^+/HCO_3^- cotransporter (NBC) (Demarco et al., 2003), Cl^-/HCO_3^- exchangers (Chavez et al., 2012), and CFTR (Hernández-González et al., 2007; Xu et al., 2007), as well as its indirect entrance via CO_2 diffusion with subsequent hydration by intracellular carbonic anhydrases (CA) (Wandernoth et al., 2010; José et al., 2015). Besides an increase in the pH_i, a cytosolic HCO_3^- elevation is crucial for activation of the sperm soluble adenylyl cyclase (Okamura et al., 1985; Buck et al., 1999).

To understand how sperm pH_i is regulated, it is indispensable to determine where and when it changes in individual cells. Although sperm pH_i measurements in suspension have been performed using fluorescence indicators for more than three decades (Schackmann and Boon Chock, 1986; Darszon et al., 2004; Hamzeh et al., 2019), there are few reports of imaging single sperm pH_i (Zeng et al., 1996; Chávez et al., 2014, 2018; González-Cota et al., 2015). All these experiments were performed with BCECF (Rink et al., 1982), the most popular fluorescent pH_i indicator in cell physiology. This fluorescence probe is ratiometric but requires dual-excitation (Rink et al., 1982). Consequently, there is a time lag between two subsequent images excited by two different wavelengths and therefore, cell movement artifacts can be significant. Furthermore, BCECF is highly phototoxic to cells (Nishigaki et al., 2006), which was also confirmed in this study.

To overcome the BCECF disadvantages stated above we employed SNARF-5F acetoxymethyl ester (AM) (Liu et al., 2001) whose fluorescence spectra changes (shift of the peak wavelength) depending on pH (pKa: 7.2). This dye allowed us to perform dual-emission ratiometric pH_i imaging using an image splitter with a single EMCCD camera. In this report, we detail our pH_i imaging setup and conditions. Furthermore, we found kinetic differences in the pH_i changes induced by HCO_3^- in human and mouse spermatozoa which could suggest that HCO_3^- influx pathways are distinct in human and mouse spermatozoa.

MATERIALS AND METHODS

Materials

Dimethyl sulfoxide (DMSO, cat. D2650), ammonium chloride (NH_4Cl, cat. A9434), nigericin (cat. N7143), progesterone (cat. P8783), and concanavalin A (cat. C2010) were purchased from Sigma–Aldrich. Pluronic F-127 (cat. P6867), SNARF-5F AM (5-(and-6)-carboxylic acid, acetoxymethyl ester) (cat. S23923), and 2′, 7′-Bis-(2-carboxyethyl)-5-(and-6)-carboxyfluorescein, acetoxymethyl ester (BCECF AM) (cat. B1170) were obtained from ThermoFisher Scientific.

Biological Sample Collection

Human Spermatozoa

Human spermatozoa samples were obtained from healthy donors under written informed consent and with the approval of the Bioethics Committee of the Instituto de Biotecnología, Universidad Nacional Autónoma de México (IBt-UNAM). Only ejaculates that fulfilled the World Health Organization guidelines were used in all the experiments (Cao et al., 2010). Motile cells were recovered using the swim-up technique in HTF medium (in mM: 90 NaCl, 4.7 KCl, 1.6 $CaCl_2$, 0.3 KH_2PO_4, 1.2 $MgSO_4$, 2.8 glucose, 0.3 pyruvic acid, 23.8 HEPES, and 21.4 lactic acid, 25 $NaHCO_3$) pH 7.4 (Mata-Martínez et al., 2013). Briefly, 400 μl of liquefied semen was placed in glass test tubes and 1 ml HTF medium was carefully added on the top of the semen without mixing the phases. Samples were incubated for 1 h at 37°C under 5% CO_2. The upper layer (700 μl) with motile spermatozoa was then collected. Cell density was determined using a Makler chamber and adjusted to 10×10^6 spermatozoa/ml.

Mouse Spermatozoa

All experimental protocols were approved by the Bioethics Committee of the IBt-UNAM). Motile spermatozoa were obtained from epididymal cauda of 3-month-old CD-1 mouse by placing incised epididymis in an Eppendorf tube containing 1 ml of in TYH medium (in mM: 119 NaCl, 4.7 KCl, 1.7 $CaCl_2$, 1.2 KH_2PO_4, 1.2 $MgSO_4$, 5.6 dextrose, 0.5 pyruvic acid, and 20 HEPES) pH 7.4. Spermatozoa were allowed to swim-out during 15 min at 37°C. The upper layer (800 μl) with motile spermatozoa was collected and the cell density was adjusted to 10×10^6 spermatozoa/ml using a Makler counting chamber (Irvine Scientific, Santa Ana, CA, United States).

In vitro Fluorescence Spectra of SNARF-5F

Fluorescence spectra of SNARF-5F were determined with a Perkin-Elmer LS 55 (Perkin-Elmer, Waltham, MA, United States) fluorescence spectrometer using the software FL WinLab version 4.00.03 for data acquisition (**Figure 1**). SNARF-5F non-permeable and AM versions were used at 20 μM final

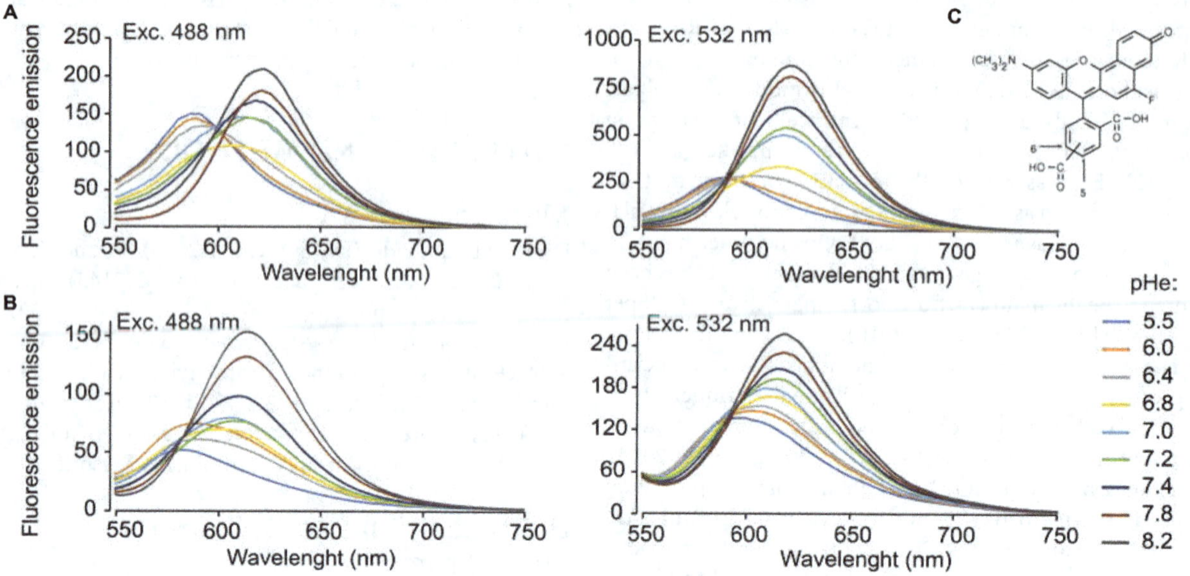

FIGURE 1 | SNARF-5F emission spectra at 488 and 532 nm excitation wavelengths, in 50 mM potassium phosphate buffers at various pH values. Emission spectra of non-permeable SNARF-5F **(A)** using a fixed excitation wavelength of 488 nm (**A**,left) and 532 nm (**A**,right). Emission spectra of SNARF-5F-AM **(B)** with 10 × 10^6 sperm/ml treated with 0.1% Triton X-100, using a fixed excitation wavelength of 488 nm (**B**,left) and 532 nm (**B**,right). The lines are representative fluorescence spectra at different pH_e (5.5, 6.0, 6.4, 6.8, 7.0, 7.2, 7.4, 7.8, and 8.2), indicated by color lines. **(C)** SNARF-5F chemical structure. Typically, SNARF-5F possess two emission wavelengths, at 575 and 640 nm; *n* = 4.

concentration in 50 mM potassium phosphate buffer (see table in **Supplementary Figure S1**). Multiple spectra were acquired using various excitation wavelengths (405, 440, 465, 488, 510, 532, and 543 nm) and different pH_e (5.5, 6.0, 6.4, 6.8, 7.0, 7.2, 7.4, 7.8, and 8.2) (**Supplementary Figure S1**).

SNARF-5F and BCECF Incorporation Into Spermatozoa

Motile mouse/human spermatozoa (10 × 10^6/ml) were incubated with 20 μM SNARF-5F AM in the presence of 0.1% pluronic F-127 during 90 min at 37°C with 5% CO_2 in the dark. The cells were washed once by centrifugation at 200 × *g* for 5 min and resuspended with fresh medium. To obtain fluorescence spectra of SNARF-5F incorporated into spermatozoa, human spermatozoa loaded with SNARF-5F AM were diluted in the media of different pH_e as described above and treated with 0.1% Triton-X 100 detergent. Fluorescence spectra of the lysed spermatozoa were acquired at excitation wavelengths 488 and 532 nm. For single cell recordings, spermatozoa were attached to Concanavalin A-treated coverslips for 2–3 min and mounted in recording chambers.

For BCECF experiments, motile mouse/human spermatozoa (10 × 10^6/ml) were incubated with 1 μM BCECF AM without pluronic acid during 15 min at 37°C with 5% CO_2 in the dark and the unincorporated dye was removed by centrifugation as the case of SNARF-5F.

Imaging Setup

Single cell images were acquired using two different setups: (1) Olympus iX71 LED-light source epifluorescence microscope and (2) Olympus iX81 laser widefield/total internal reflection fluorescence (TIRF) microscope (Olympus, Japan). The LED setup was equipped with a PlanApo N 60X/1.42 oil objective and a 3A 532 nm LED coupled to Opto-LED light controller (Cairn Research, United Kingdom). The laser setup was equipped with an Apo N (TIRF) 60X/1.49 oil objective and a 488 nm laser with high speed imaging shutter. To acquire dual emission images of SNARF-5F, an image splitter OptoSplit II (Cairn Research, United Kingdom) was used for both setups, LED (with band-pass filter ET 530/30X) and laser. To acquire the images with SNARF-5F, a wide band-pass filter ET 575/50 M (channel 1) and a band-pass filter ET 640/20 M (channel 2) were employed as dual emission filters combined with a dichroic mirror DC 610lp (Chroma Technology, United States) (**Figure 2**). For BCECF experiments, a 3.15 A 465 nm LED (Luminus Devices, Woburn, MA, United States) with bandpass filter HQ 480/40X was used for excitation light, combined with a dichroic mirror (Q505lp) and an emission filter (HQ 535/50M) (Chroma Technology, United States). Each setup has a 512 × 512 Andor iXon 3 EMCCD camera (model X3 DU897E-CS0) (Oxford Instruments, United Kingdom).

Images were acquired with the software Andor iQ version 2.9.1 (LED set-up) (Oxford Instruments, United Kingdom) and Xcellence version 1.2 (laser set-up) (Olympus, Japan). Fluorescence images of both SNARF-5F and BCECF were taken with 1 × 1 binning, 5 images/s (5 ips), with an exposure time of 10 ms for the LED setup and 30 ms (laser potency 35%) for the laser setup. Images were analyzed with ImageJ version 1.52n (NIH, United States), obtaining mean fluorescence intensities, selecting heads and flagellum as regions of interest.

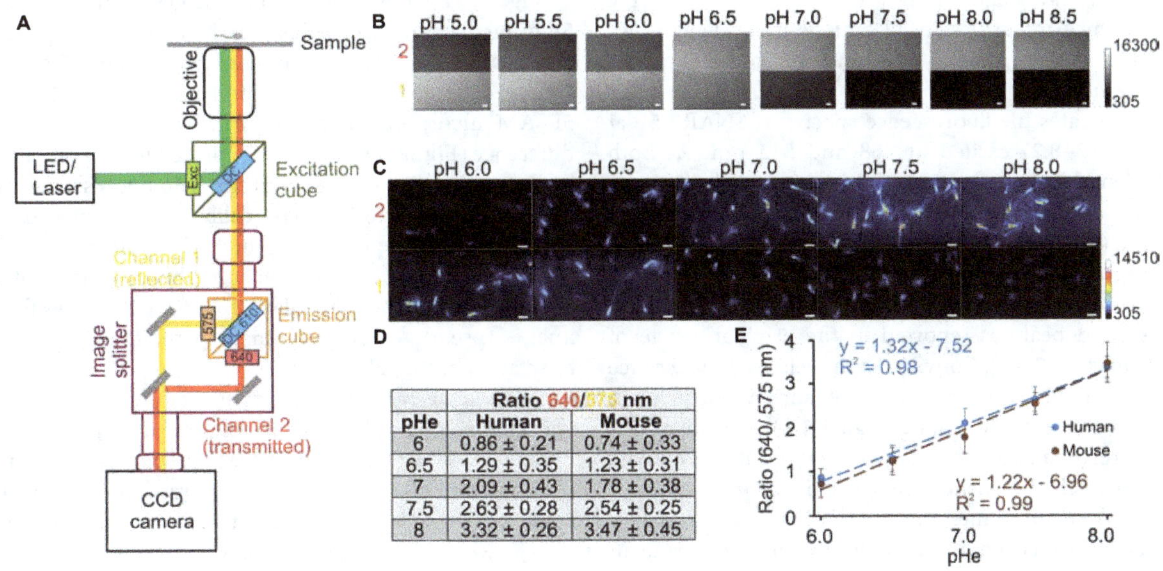

FIGURE 2 | Imaging set-up configuration to visualize the dual emission wavelengths of SNARF-5F. Diagram of imaging set-up **(A)**, indicating LED (532 nm) or laser (488 nm) as an illumination source. A different excitation cube (green square) was used for the LED set-up (ET 530/30X, dichroic mirror DC 550 LP) and the laser set-up (D485/25X, dichroic DC510 LP). To visualize at the same time the two emission wavelengths of SNARF-5F, we used an image splitter (in purple), which has an emission cube (orange square) (ET575/50M, ET640/20M, and dichroic mirror DC610 LP), that divides the emission in reflected (channel 1, corresponding to emission wavelength 575 nm) or transmitted (channel 2, corresponding to emission wavelength 640 nm) images. The image splitter is coupled to the microscope on one side, and to the detector (CCD camera) on the other. Fluorescence images obtained from epifluorescence (laser set-up) microscope with 60× (Plan Apo N, 1.49 numerical aperture) objective, using 20 μM non-permeable SNARF-5F **(B)** or 20 μM SNARF-5F-AM loaded in human and mouse (not shown) spermatozoa in the presence of nigericin 10 μM **(C)** in 50 mM potassium phosphate buffers at indicated pH. **(D)** Ratio values were obtained (referred from panel **C**) at each pH_e (6.0, 6.5, 7.0, 7.5, and 8.0) in human and mouse spermatozoa, using channel 1 (575 nm) and channel 2 (640 nm) fluorescence values. **(E)** Lineal correlation between pH_e and fluorescence ratio in human and mouse spermatozoa, obtaining R^2 = 0.99 and 0.98, respectively. Numbers 1 (yellow) and 2 (red) to the left in panels **B** and **C** refer to channel 1 (emission 575 nm) and channel 2 (emission 640 nm). Scale bar in panels **B** and **C** is equal to 10 μm; n = 3.

In vivo pH_i Calibration

To convert fluorescence data to pH values *in vitro*, the following equation is commonly used:

$$pH = pK_a - \log\left[\frac{R - R_B}{R_A - R} \times \frac{F_{B(\lambda_2)}}{F_{A(\lambda_2)}}\right]$$

where R is the ratio $F\lambda_1/F\lambda_2$ of fluorescence intensities (F) measured at two wavelengths λ_1 and λ_2 and the subscripts A and B represent the values at the acidic and basic conditions, respectively (Whitaker et al., 1991). However, it is difficult to maintain live spermatozoa in highly acidic and alkaline condition to obtain $F_{B(\lambda_2)}/F_{A(\lambda_2)}$ values from the same cells. Therefore, we performed *in vivo* pH_i calibration by fixing external pH (pH_e) between 6.0 and 8.0 as reported previously (Grillo-Hill et al., 2014). Briefly, spermatozoa suspensions were incubated for 15 min with calibration medium (in mM: 120 KCl, 25 HEPES, 1 $MgCl_2$, and 0.01 nigericin, at different pH_e: 6.0, 6.5, 7.0, 7.5, and 8.0, adjusted with KOH). We measured the fluorescence intensity at two emissions, 575 (channel 1) and 640 nm (channel 2), always subtracting the fluorescence background value in each channel. As fluorescence ratio values ($R_{F640/F575}$) have a lineal relation with pH_i values (between 6.0 and 8.0) (**Figures 2D,E**), we used the following equations to estimate pH_i from the fluorescence ratio values, for human: $pH_i = (R_{F640/F575} + 6.96)/1.22$ and for mouse: $pH_i = (R_{F640/F575} + 7.52)/1.32$.

Statistical Analysis

The results are expressed as the mean ± SEM of at least three independent experiments (three different donors or mice), with a minimum of 200 cells per condition. The data were analyzed by a comparison test between the groups, using the non-parametric Mann–Whitney U-test with 95% statistical significance. The paired tests were carried out comparing the head and the flagellum of the same cell. Additionally, the Bonferroni correction was used when multiple comparisons were made.

RESULTS

Emission Spectra of SNARF-5F With Distinct Excitation Wavelengths

To perform ratiometric fluorescence measurements with a good signal to noise ratio (S/N ratio), it is important to acquire bright fluorescence images in both channels. In other words, if we detect dim fluorescence signals in one channel, the S/N ratio of the dual-emission ratio values become undesirably low even when we detect bright signals in the other channel. As spermatozoa possess a quite reduced cytoplasm, it is crucial to use an appropriate excitation wavelength and emission filters. Therefore, we first determined the fluorescence spectra of SNARF-5F at several pH_e values (5.5–8.2), exciting with various wavelengths (405–543 nm). As shown in **Supplementary Figure S1**, the longer excitation wavelength (longer than 465 nm) gives the higher fluorescence intensities in all emission wavelengths we explored (550–750 nm). Namely, 543 nm produced the highest fluorescence values.

Figure 1 illustrates the fluorescence spectra of SNARF-5F at different pH_e (5.5–8.2) excited at 488 and 532 nm. At both exciting wavelengths, the fluorescence intensities around 575 nm (the first peak) decrease when the pH increases, while those of around 640 nm (the second peak) increase at the same conditions. When exciting at 532 nm, the relative fluorescence intensities within the first peak at different pH_e are much smaller than those within the second peak, as reported in the original article of SNARF-5F (Liu et al., 2001). Conversely, the relative fluorescence intensities within the two peaks became almost equal when 488 nm was used as excitation light (**Figure 1A**). In spite of this favorable feature, their absolute fluorescence intensities are small. Considering these characteristics, we selected 532 nm as the best compromise between brightness and peak balance for this study.

To evaluate the incorporation of the membrane permeant dye SNARF-5F AM into the spermatozoa, we incubated human spermatozoa with 20 μM of this dye for 90 min. After the excess dye was washed out by centrifugation, the cells were lysed with 0.1% Triton X-100 and the fluorescence spectra were acquired (**Figure 1B**). The spectra of the dye incorporated into human spermatozoa were not identical to SNARF-5F *in vitro*, suggesting that SNARF-5F AM was not completely hydrolyzed in the cell and/or some of the dye was bound to certain molecules of the cell. Nevertheless, SNARF-5F AM incorporated into the cell responded to pH_e changes similarly to SNARF-5F AM.

Dual-Emission pH_i Imaging System and *in vivo* Calibration of pH_i

A conventional dual-emission fluorescence imaging setup usually is composed of an epi-fluorescence microscope, a CCD camera, and a filter wheel, which exchanges two emission filters alternatively. In this type of setup, there is always a time lag between the image in one channel and the image in the other channel. Since spermatozoa are small and motile cells, the presence of a time lag between two images of each channel is undesirable. Therefore, we used an image splitter (Kinosita et al., 1991) that allows the simultaneous capture of the images from the two channels with a single camera (**Figure 2A**). In a common configuration of dual-emission ratiometric imaging, emission lights are divided into two components (two channels) at the isosbestic point, around 595 nm in the case of SNARF-5F AM excited by 532 nm. However, because the fluorescence intensity of the first peak (575 nm) is lower than the second peak (640 nm) as described previously (**Figure 1**), we separated the emission light at 610 nm (about 15 nm longer than the isosbestic point) by a dichroic mirror. Consequently, we collected a wide range of wavelengths, 550–600 nm, as the fluorescence signals in the first channel (channel 1). Then, we collected 630–650 nm wavelengths as the longer wavelength fluorescence (channel 2). This configuration gives us comparable fluorescence intensities from the two channels without the insertion of a neutral density filter (**Figure 2A**).

Figure 2B shows fluorescence images (gray scale) of SNARF-5F in media at different pHs, clearly demonstrating the opposite changes of fluorescence intensity between Channel 1 and Channel 2. Since fluorescence spectra of SNARF-5F and SNARF-5F AM incorporated into human spermatozoa show a slight difference (**Figures 1A,B**), we performed *in vivo* calibration using human spermatozoa to convert the ratio fluorescence values into pH_i values. To perform *in vivo* calibration, spermatozoa pH_i was equilibrated to the pH_e using high K^+ (120 mM) media in the presence of 10 μM nigericin (an ionophore that facilitates K^+/H^+ exchange across the lipid bilayer). **Figure 2C** shows fluorescence images (pseudo color) of human spermatozoa, whose pH_i was fixed at different pH_e (6.0–8.0).

The mean ratio values of fluorescence intensities of the two channels (F640/F575) in distinct pH_i are summarized in **Figure 3C** and these ratio values are plotted as a function of pH_i (**Figure 2D**). The ratio values increase proportionally to pH_i between 6.0 and 8.0 with excellent linearity (human spermatozoa: $R_{F640/F575} = 1.22 \times pH_i - 6.96$, $R^2 = 0.99$; mouse spermatozoa: $R_{F640/F575} = 1.32 \times pH_i - 7.52$, $R^2 = 0.98$) (**Figure 2E**).

Phototoxicity of SNARF-5F to Spermatozoa

BCECF is known to be quite phototoxic to spermatozoa and this effect can be easily detected as flagellar beat attenuation and as a decrease in the fluorescence intensity (photo-bleaching) during the intense exposure of excitation light (Nishigaki et al., 2006; González-Cota et al., 2015). In this study, we confirmed the phototoxic effect of BCECF on sperm using the same setup utilized for SNARF-5F (**Supplementary Figure S2**). Particularly, the 488 nm laser excitation attenuated the flagellar beat of human and mouse spermatozoa after around 60 and 20 s illuminations, respectively. Subsequently, notable photobleaching of BCECF was observed in both human and mouse spermatozoa (**Supplementary Figures S2A,C**). On the other hand, LED illumination caused less photobleaching in human spermatozoa (**Supplementary Figure S2B**), but certain level of photobleaching was still observed in 40% of mouse spermatozoa (**Supplementary Figure S2D**). This result suggests that mouse sperm are more susceptible to oxidative stress than human spermatozoa.

In contrast, SNARF-5F incorporated into spermatozoa is much less toxic to the cells than BCECF (**Figure 3**). The fluorescence intensities excited by LED and 488 nm laser (epi-fluorescence mode) did not cause photo-bleaching of the dye during our experimental periods (5 ips for 250 s) (**Figures 3A,B**). However, we observed a slight photobleaching of SNARF-5F when excited by the 488 nm laser in the TIRF configuration (**Figure 3C**). This photobleaching was negligible when we reduced the frequency of image acquisition from 5 to 2.5 ips (data not shown).

Comparison of Epi-Fluorescence and TIRF Images

In our previous study of pH_i imaging (epi-fluorescence mode) of sea urchin spermatozoa using BCECF, fluorescence intensities of

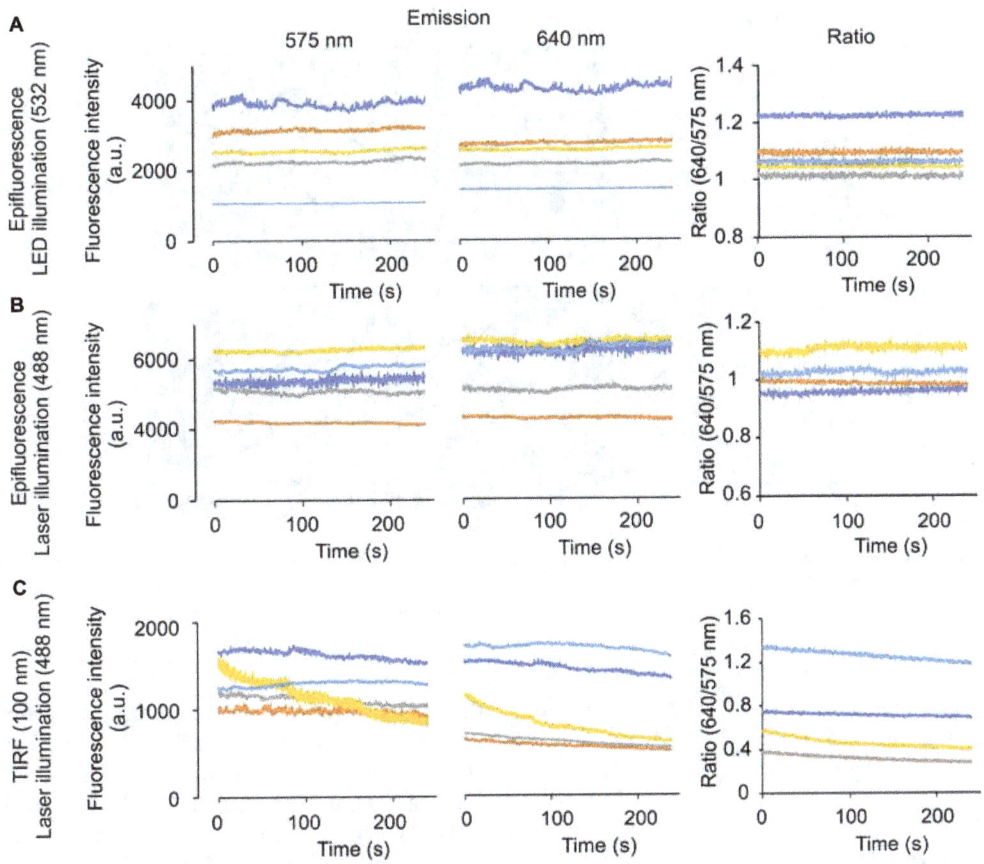

FIGURE 3 | Time-lapse experiments in the microscope set-up did not cause significant photobleaching in mammal spermatozoa, using LED or laser as an illumination source. Representative recordings from emission wavelength time lapse experiments, using 20 μM SNARF-5F-AM in human spermatozoa. Images were taken every 200 ms, exposure time 4 ms with 60× objective. An image splitter was used for the experiments, allowing us to measure emission fluorescence at 575 (left) and 640 (center) nm, and obtaining the ratio from both wavelengths (right). The illumination source was LED 532 **(A)** or laser 488 nm **(B,C)**, in the epifluorescence **(A,B)** or TIRF 100 nm **(C)** configuration. Traces in each panel show representative single cell pH_i. Same color at both emission wavelengths indicates the same cell; $n = 3$.

the flagellum were much lower than those of the heads and their fluorescence signals were noisy with a poor S/N ratio (González-Cota et al., 2015). We thought that the use of TIRF would improve this aspect, avoiding the saturation of fluorescence signal in the head. However, the difference of SNARF-5F images between the two configurations (epi-fluorescence and TIRF) was relatively small in both human (**Figure 4A**) and mouse spermatozoa (**Figure 4B**). Particularly, in mouse spermatozoa, the TIRF fluorescence signals in the head and the flagellum (primarily mid piece) are very similar to the epi-fluorescence images. This result is probably due to the thin hook-like shape of the mouse sperm head. As a consequence, an important difference between the two systems (epi-fluorescence and TIRF) is not significant for mouse spermatozoa.

Spermatozoa Responses to pH_i Manipulation

Using the epi-fluorescence configuration with the LED as a light source, we acquired fluorescence images upon pH_i manipulations. During image acquisition, we added HTF or TYH medium as control in human and mouse spermatozoa, respectively. As additional control, 10 mM NH_4Cl and 5 mM HCl were added to increase and reduce the pH_i, respectively. The upper panels of **Figures 5A,B** show human sperm fluorescence signals from the two channels in the head and the flagellum, respectively. Changes of fluorescence intensities were observed during the additions even in control conditions (indicated with arrows). Also, fluorescence signals from some cells are noisy probably due to the continuous movement associated to the flagellar beat. Once the dual emission signals were converted into the ratio and pH_i values (**Figures 5A,B**, lower panels), the problems of addition artifacts and movement were eliminated in the both regions, demonstrating the advantage of the dual-emission ratiometric imaging. Additionally, the effects of NH_4Cl and HCl can be clearly observed as an increase and a decrease of the ratio and the pH_i, respectively. **Figure 6** basically demonstrates the same results as **Figure 5** but using mouse spermatozoa. In this experiment, the fluorescence signal of the flagellum arises mainly from the mid piece since mouse spermatozoa flagellum is much longer than that of human spermatozoa and therefore it is difficult to capture the

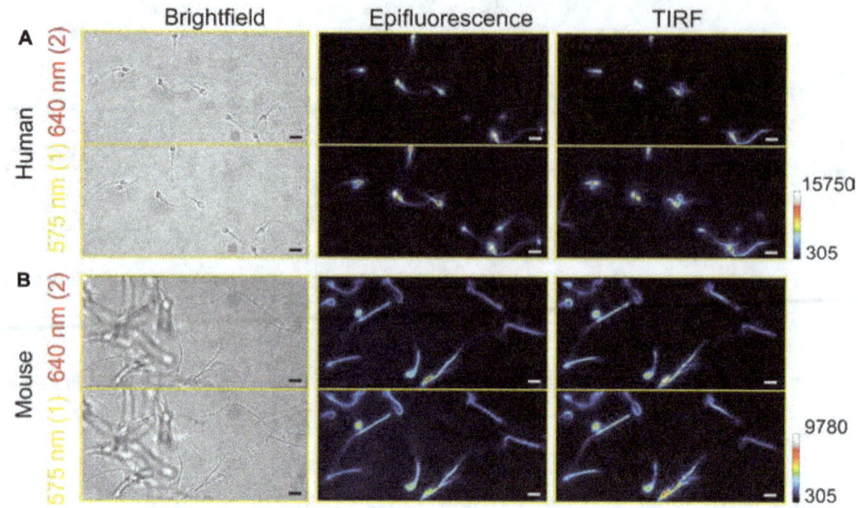

FIGURE 4 | Comparison between epifluorescence and total internal reflection fluorescence (TIRF) images. Representative images from human **(A)** and mouse **(B)** spermatozoa in the two emission channels for SNARF-5F dye, 640 (red) and 575 nm (yellow). Images were taken using the epifluorescence (center) or TIRF (right) configuration. For reference, brightfield images (left) are shown. Scale bar is equal to 10 μm. Reference bar for fluorescence intensity is also depicted. Scale bar is equal to 10 μm; $n = 3$.

image of the entire flagellum of mouse spermatozoa. In these experiments, the average pH_i of non-capacitated human and mouse spermatozoa was 6.72 ± 0.19 (SEM) and 6.63 ± 0.23 (SEM), respectively; $n = 3$.

Response to HCO_3^-

To obtain new insights of mammalian spermatozoa pH_i regulation, we determined the effect of HCO_3^- (10 and 25 mM) on pH_i in non-capacitated human and mouse spermatozoa using our dual-emission imaging system (**Figure 7**). In these experiments, we confirmed that HCO_3^- increases the pH_i of human (**Figure 7A**) and mouse (**Figure 7B**) spermatozoa, in a concentration-dependent manner. We did not observe statistical differences in the pH_i increase induced by HCO_3^- between human and mouse spermatozoa (**Figure 7C**). However, we found a significant difference in the kinetics of the pH_i increase between the two species. Namely, HCO_3^- rapidly increases the pH_i of mouse spermatozoa, and the time to reach 50% of the maximum pH_i increase (t_{50}) was around 10 s. In contrast, HCO_3^- increases human sperm pH_i gradually with a longer t_{50} (40 s) in our experimental conditions (**Figure 7D**). Moreover, the pH_i increase in human spermatozoa was slightly, but significantly, slower in the flagellum compared to the head with 10 and 25 mM HCO_3^- additions.

Response to Progesterone in Human Spermatozoa

In the literature, there is some controversy about the effect of progesterone on human sperm pH_i. A decrease (Garcia and Meizel, 1996; Cross and Razy-Faulkner, 1997), no change (Fraire-Zamora and González-Martínez, 2004) or a slow increase (Hamamah et al., 1996) in pH_i have been reported by different groups in response to this hormone. Therefore, we determined the effect of different progesterone concentrations on pH_i in human spermatozoa. **Figure 8** shows that progesterone at 500 nM (I), 1 μM (II), and 10 μM (III) did not change pH_i neither in the head (**Figure 8A**) nor in the flagellum (**Figure 8B**) of these cells. As a control we tested 1 μM monensin, a Na^+ ionophore that exchanges Na^+/H^+ (Babcock, 1983). As anticipated, this ionophore alkalized pH_i in these cells in both head (**Figure 8A**, IV) and flagellum (**Figure 8B**, IV).

DISCUSSION

Advantages of the New System to Determine Spermatozoa pH_i

In this study we established a dual-emission ratiometric imaging system using SNARF-5F AM, which has negligible photo-toxicity compared to BCECF (**Figure 3** and **Supplementary Figure S2**). Our system allows determining mammalian spermatozoa (head and flagellum) pH_i with minimum artifacts associated to cell movements and focus alteration upon addition or exchange of bath solutions (**Figures 5–7**). Commonly, the ratio of dual fluorescence signals utilizes the dye isosbestic point (595 nm in our condition). However, the first peak fluorescence intensity (575 nm) of SNARF-5F excited at 532 nm is much smaller than the second peak (640 nm). Therefore, we divided the fluorescence at 610 nm, 15 nm longer than the isosbestic point, and employed a wide band-pass filter (550–600 nm) for Channel 1. In this configuration, fluorescence signals of the two channels are comparable (**Figure 2**), which is a critical point to obtain the ratio values with a good S/N ratio. This type of optical filter configuration (division of fluorescence signals not at the isosbestic point) could be applied to other dual-emission indicators such as GEM-GECO (Zhao et al., 2011) and Asante

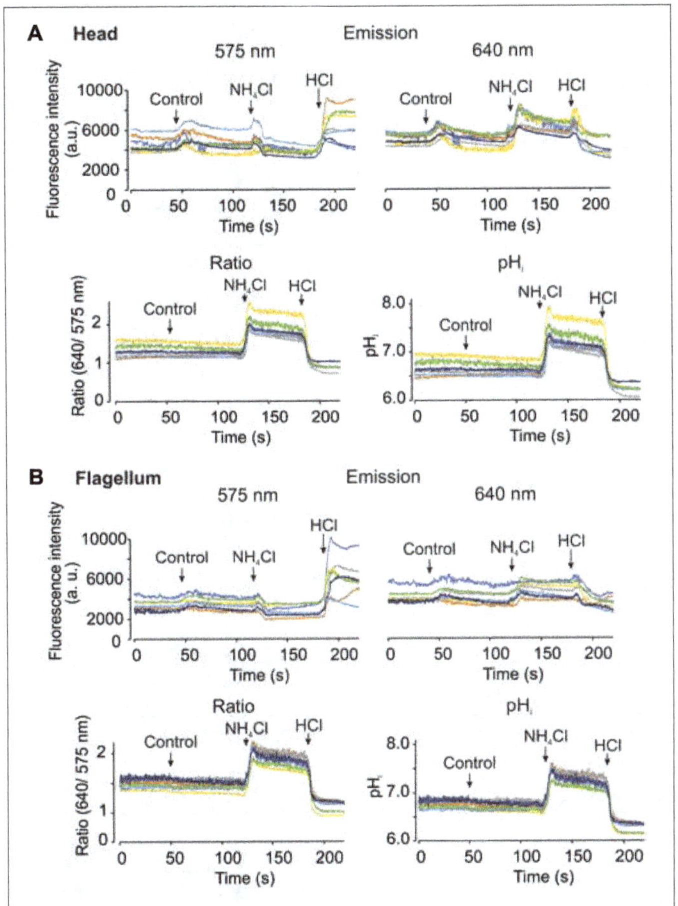

FIGURE 5 | It is possible to measure pH_i using SNARF-5F in human spermatozoa, in the head and flagellum regions. Representative recordings from head **(A)** and flagellum **(B)** regions, measuring fluorescence changes at the two emission wavelengths of SNARF-5F, 575 (Top left) and 640 nm (Top right). Ratio recordings (Bottom left) are obtained from both emission fluorescence values, and converted to pHi (Bottom right) utilizing the calibration curve as shown in **Figure 2**. The micropipette manual addition of HTF medium (control), 10 mM NH_4Cl, and 5 mM HCl is indicated by arrows in each panel. Traces in each panel show representative single cell pH_i responses. Same color at both emission wavelengths and in both regions (head and flagellum) correspond to the same cell; $n = 3$.

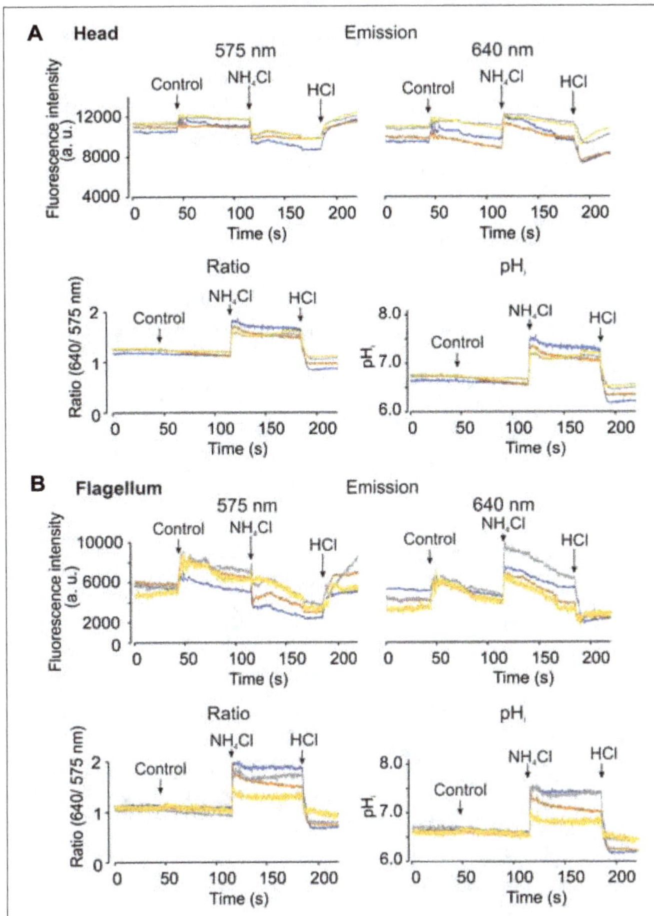

FIGURE 6 | It is possible to measure pH_i using SNARF-5F in mouse spermatozoa, in the head and flagellum regions. Representative fluorescence recordings from head **(A)** and flagellum **(B)** regions, measuring changes at the dual emission wavelengths of SNARF-5F, 575 (Top left) and 640 nm (Top right). Ratio recordings (Bottom left) are obtained from both emission fluorescence values, and converted to pH_i (Bottom right) using the calibration curve shown before. The micropipette manual addition of TYH medium (control), 10 mM NH_4Cl, and 5 mM HCl are indicated by arrows in each panel. Traces in each panel show representative single cell pH_i. The same color at both emission wavelengths and in both regions (head and flagellum) correspond to the same cell; $n = 3$.

Calcium Red (Hyrc et al., 2013) because their dual-emission signals are quite asymmetric.

pH_i Calibration

We observed a slight difference between the fluorescence spectra of SNARF-5F *in vitro* and inside human spermatozoa. Therefore, in order to convert the fluorescence emission values into the pH_i, we performed an *in vivo* pH_i calibration with human and mouse spermatozoa using a high K^+ solution combined with nigericin in order to equal pH_i to the pH_e. This protocol is based on the assumption that the cytoplasmic K^+ concentration is 120 mM in human and mouse spermatozoa, as determined in bovine spermatozoa (Babcock, 1983). Therefore, depending on the real cytoplasmic K^+ concentration in human and mouse spermatozoa, the absolute pH_i values could be different. In our conditions, we determined that the pH_i value in non-capacitated human and mouse spermatozoa is 6.72 ± 0.19 and 6.63 ± 0.23, respectively. These values were measured in the head, but no significant differences were observed in the flagellum (see below). There are several reports of pH_i determinations (most of them in cell population experiments and a few using single cell determination) of non-capacitated spermatozoa from distinct mammalian species: 6.24 (Parrish et al., 1989a) and 6.7 (Vredenburgh-Wilberg and Parrish, 1995) in bovine spermatozoa, 6.55 (Balderas et al., 2013), 6.54 (Zeng et al., 1996), and 6.8 (Carlson et al., 2007) in mouse sperm, and 6.7 (Hamamah et al., 1996; Fraire-Zamora and González-Martínez, 2004) and 6.94 (Cross and Razy-Faulkner, 1997) in human spermatozoa. Our findings that pH_i values of non-capacitated mammalian spermatozoa are >6.5 are consistent with the

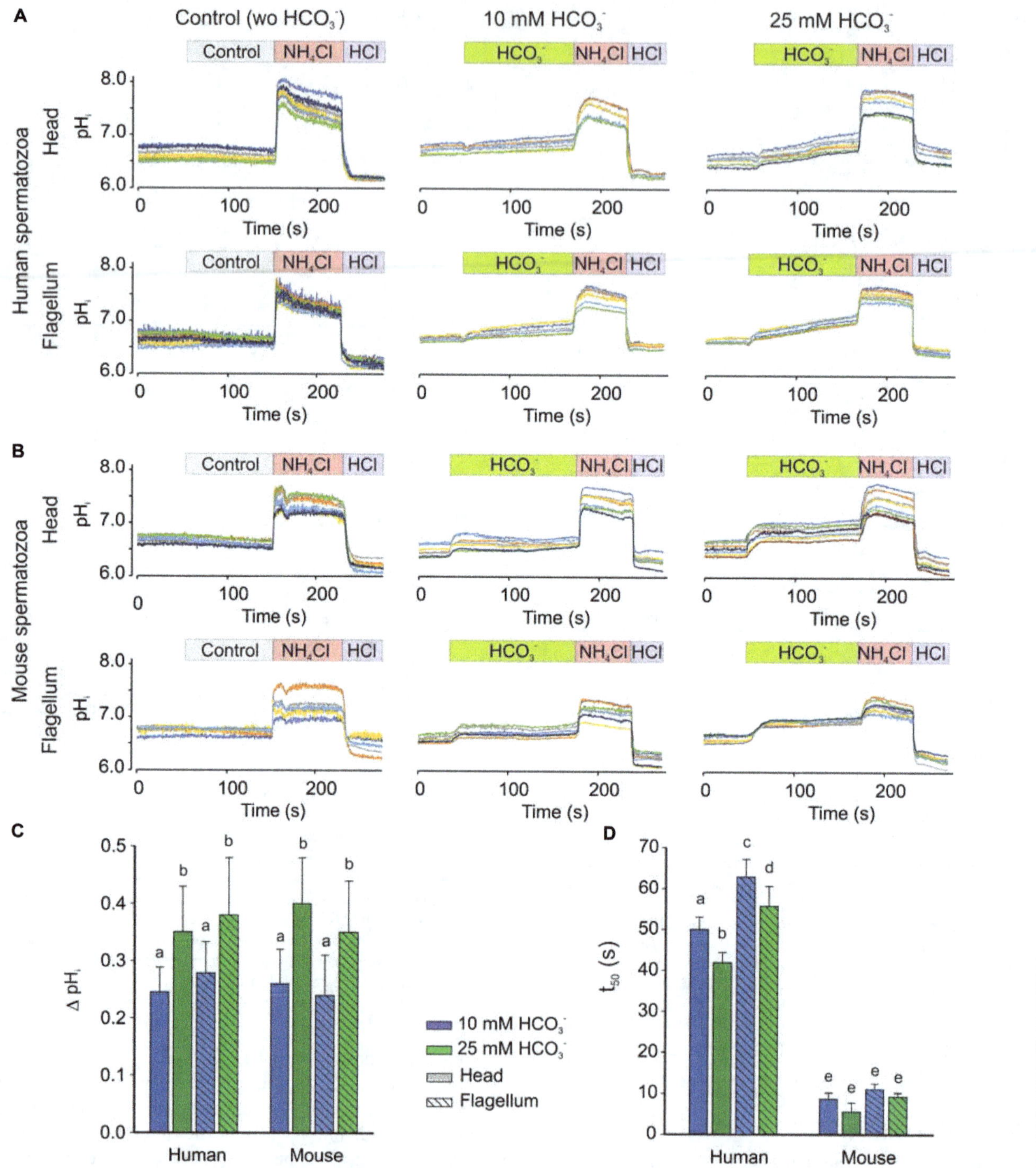

FIGURE 7 | HCO$_3^-$ increased pH$_i$ in a concentration-dependent manner in both, head and flagellum, regions using human and mouse spermatozoa. Representative recordings from human **(A)** and mouse **(B)** spermatozoa, measuring pH$_i$ using 20 μM SNARF-5F in head (Top) and flagellum (Bottom) regions. The perfused addition of medium (HTF and TYH for human and mouse, respectively) (left, control in gray rectangle), 10 (center in green rectangle) or 25 mM (right in green rectangle) HCO$_3^-$ are showed. As positive controls, perfused addition of 10 mM NH$_4$Cl (red rectangle) and 5 mM HCl (purple rectangle) are showed in each panel. Traces in each panel show representative single cell pH$_i$. Same color in both, head and flagellum, indicate to the same cell. Maximum change in pH$_i$ (ΔpH$_i$) **(C)** and average of t_{50} **(D)**, time to reach 50% of the maximum fluorescent intensity, before and after 10 (blue bars), 25 (green bars) mM HCO$_3^-$ addition, in head (shaded) or flagellum (diagonal lines) regions. The bars in **C,D** indicated means ± SEM. Different letters indicate significant differences at the $p \leq 0.05$ level, according to Mann–Whitney *U*-test; $n = 5$.

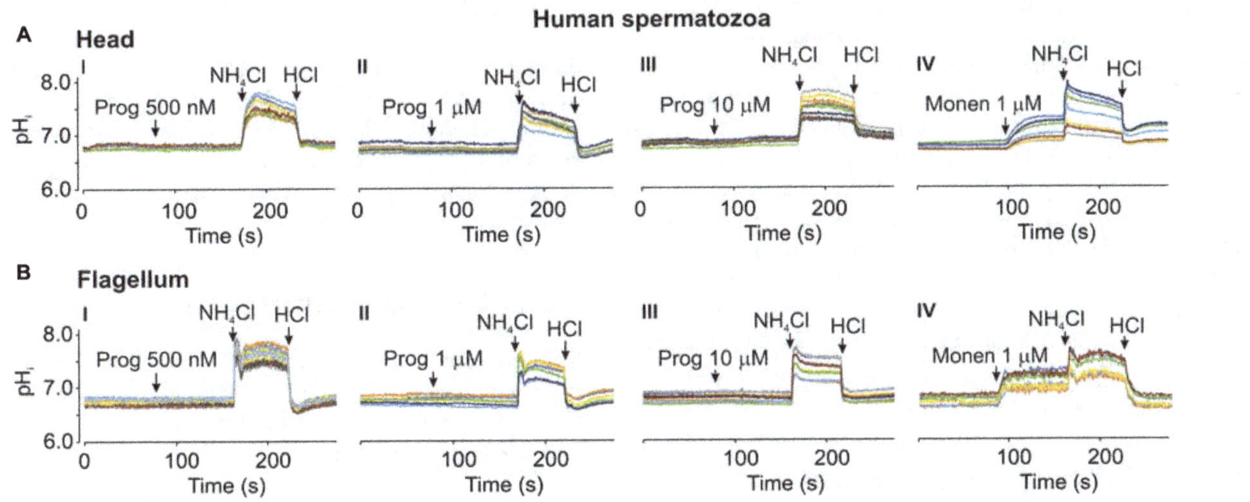

FIGURE 8 | Progesterone did not changed pH_i in human spermatozoa. Representative recordings using 20 μM SNARF-5F in human spermatozoa in the head **(A)** and flagellum **(B)** regions. Micropipette manual progesterone (Prog) additions of 500 nM (I), 1 μM (II), and 10 μM (III), as well as 1 μM of monensin (Monen) (IV) are indicated by arrows in each panel. As controls, 10 mM NH_4Cl and 5 mM HCl additions were performed (see arrows). Traces in each panel show representative single cell pH_i. The same color at both emission wavelengths and in both regions (head and flagellum) corresponds to the same cell; $n = 3$.

report that detergent-demembranated bovine spermatozoa do not exhibit motility at pH 6.5, although they are highly motile at pH 7.0 (Ho et al., 2002).

Regional pH_i Difference in the Head and the Flagellum

We did not observe significant differences between the head and the flagellum in the basal pH_i in non-capacitated spermatozoa, although the head pH_i tends to be slightly higher than the flagellar pH_i both in human (6.72 ± 0.19 and 6.69 ± 0.24, respectively) and mouse spermatozoa (6.63 ± 0.23 and 6.60 ± 0.26, respectively). Our results are similar to those reported in bovine spermatozoa (Vredenburgh-Wilberg and Parrish, 1995). In general, the epifluorescent signal from an indicator incorporated into the sperm head is generally much higher than in the flagellum, independently of the species. Therefore, we examined if TIRF microscopy would reduce the fluorescence difference between the head and the flagellum. However, we did not observe significant differences nor advantages of TIRF microscopy compared to epifluorescence microscopy (**Figure 4**) either in mouse or human spermatozoa for measuring pH_i. With these data, we can conclude that epifluorescence microscopy with SNARF-5F AM allows performing reliable single spermatozoa pH_i imaging with a good S/N ratio in both spermatozoa head and flagellum (mid piece of flagellum in the case of mouse).

Difference of pH_i Responses to HCO_3^- Between Human and Mouse Spermatozoa

HCO_3^- is an essential ion for mammalian sperm to acquire the ability to fertilize the oocyte (Lee and Storey, 1986). In fact, the HCO_3^- concentrations in rabbit uterine and tubal fluids are approximately twice as high as in the blood plasma, which results in pH values of 7.4 and 8.1–8.3, respectively (Vishwakarma, 1962). In rhesus monkeys, the pH and HCO_3^- concentration in the oviduct lumen change during the menstrual cycle. Namely, these values are similar to those of the blood plasma during the follicular phase, but they suddenly increase concomitantly with ovulation (Maas et al., 1977). This observation supports the importance of HCO_3^- for fertilization in mammals. The principal role of cytoplasmic HCO_3^- in mammalian spermatozoa is considered to be the activation of the soluble adenylyl cyclase, which increases cAMP (Okamura et al., 1985; Buck et al., 1999; Chen et al., 2000), leading to protein kinase A (PKA) stimulation. The enhanced PKA activity increases flagellar beat frequency (Wennemuth, 2003) and elevates CatSper activity (Carlson et al., 2003; Orta et al., 2018), among many other things.

In this work, we observed that HCO_3^- elevates the pH_i in both human and mouse spermatozoa (**Figure 7D**). In contrast, Carlson et al. (2007) reported that HCO_3^- did not induce a pH_i increase in mouse spermatozoa. Interestingly, we found a difference in the kinetics of HCO_3^--induced pH_i increase between the two species (**Figure 7D**), namely a faster increase in mouse compared to human spermatozoa, but of similar magnitude (**Figure 7C**). So far, several mechanisms have been reported for HCO_3^- influx, such as the NBC (Demarco et al., 2003), Cl^-/HCO_3^- exchangers (Chavez et al., 2012), and the CFTR channel (Hernández-González et al., 2007; Xu et al., 2007). However, the physiological relevance of each transporter is unclear as well as differences between the two species. In addition to HCO_3^- transporters, CO_2 diffusion with subsequent hydration by intracellular CA contributes to an increase in cytoplasmic HCO_3^- concentration (Carlson et al., 2007; Wandernoth et al., 2010; José et al., 2015). Curiously, a general CA inhibitor, ethoxyzolamide, potently affects human but not mouse sperm motility (José et al., 2015), suggesting a difference in the involvement of CAs in the motility of the two species. Another explanation is that human spermatozoa may have higher pH buffering capacity than mouse spermatozoa. This might be correlated to the time required for capacitation (>6 h in human compared to 1–2 h in mouse spermatozoa). Indeed, the pH_i of mammalian spermatozoa studied so far increases around 0.14–0.4 units during capacitation (Parrish et al., 1989b; Vredenburgh-Wilberg and Parrish, 1995; Hamamah et al., 1996; Zeng et al., 1996; Cross and Razy-Faulkner, 1997; Fraire-Zamora and González-Martínez, 2004; Balderas et al., 2013). A significant part of this pH_i change can be attributed to the HCO_3^- influx into the cell. Therefore, further studies are required for a better understanding of the mechanism of HCO_3^--induced pH_i increase during capacitation. The pH_i imaging system established in this study should contribute to this issue.

Effect of Progesterone in Human Spermatozoa

Progesterone increases $[Ca^{2+}]_i$ in human spermatozoa at concentrations as low as 300 nM, through CatSper activation (Tesarik et al., 1992; Harper et al., 2003; Achikanu et al., 2018). Recently it was described that the progesterone receptor in these cells is a α/β hydrolase domain-containing protein (ABHD2), which depletes the endocannabinoid 2-arachinoylglycerol (2AG) from membrane and removes CatSper inactivation (Miller et al., 2016; Mannowetz et al., 2017). In contrast, there is inconsistency regarding how progesterone affects pH_i. Some groups suggest that this hormone acidifies, others that it alkalizes or does not induce pH_i changes (Garcia and Meizel, 1996; Hamamah et al., 1996; Cross and Razy-Faulkner, 1997; Fraire-Zamora and González-Martínez, 2004). In the present work, progesterone did change pH_i in human spermatozoa even at concentrations as high as 10 μM (**Figure 8**). Our result supports that progesterone activates CatSper in a pH-independent manner, possibly exclusively via ABHD2-2AG.

Progesterone-induced Ca^{2+} influx through CatSper may affect the activity of transporters and enzymes that can affect pH_i such as PMCA (Wennemuth et al., 2003; Okunade et al., 2004) and NOX5 (Baker and Aitken, 2004; Musset et al., 2012). Both PMCA and NOX5 may acidify pH_i when they are activated, namely when the $[Ca^{2+}]_i$ is high. However, the pH_i acidification together with the membrane potential depolarization caused by Ca^{2+} influx through CatSper and electron efflux through NOX5 could activate Hv1 channel (Lishko et al., 2010; Berger et al., 2017) and may rapidly neutralize the acidification (alkalize the pH_i). Depending on the experimental conditions, one activity (acidifying or alkalizing) may exceed the other when progesterone stimulates human CatSper. This may account for part of the discrepancies regarding human sperm pH_i responses to progesterone. Further studies are required to confirm this hypothesis.

ETHICS STATEMENT

The studies involving human participants/donors were reviewed and approved by the Bioethics Committee of the Instituto de Biotecnología. The donors provided their written informed consent to participate in this study. The animal study was reviewed and approved by the Bioethics Committee of the Instituto de Biotecnología.

AUTHOR CONTRIBUTIONS

TN conceived the project. JC performed most of the experiments and prepared the figures. All authors proposed the experiments, discussed the results, and wrote, revised, and approved the manuscript.

FUNDING

This work was supported by the PAPIIT DGAPA (Grant Numbers IA200419 to JC, IN200919 to AD, IN202519 to CT, and IN205719 to TN) and CONACyT (Fronteras 71).

ACKNOWLEDGMENTS

We thank Gastón Contreras from the National Laboratory in Advanced Microscopy Facilities, in addition to José L. De la Vega-Beltrán, Yoloxóchitl Sánchez-Guevara, and Paulina Torres for technical assistance. Also, we would like to thank Shirley Ainsworth for library services, and the people of the animal facilities Elizabeth Mata, Graciela Cabeza, and Sergio González. We acknowledge Juan Manuel Hurtado, Roberto Rodríguez, Omar Arriaga, and Arturo Ocádiz for computer services.

SUPPLEMENTARY MATERIAL

FIGURE S1 | Spectral characterization of the pH sensitive dye SNARF-5F. Representative emission spectra in 405, 440, 465, 488, 510, 532, and 543 nm excitation wavelengths, in 50 mM potassium phosphate buffers at the proportions indicated in Table 1, obtaining pH_e: 5.5, 6.0, 6.4, 6.8, 7.0, 7.2, 7.4, 7.8, and 8.2. The lines are representative fluorescence spectra at indicated excitation wavelength in each pH_e; $n = 3$.

FIGURE S2 | Single cell pH_i measurements with BCECF using laser of led excitation causes significant photobleaching and a reduced response to alkalization and acidification. Representative normalized recordings using BCECF-loaded spermatozoa in human **(A,B)** and mouse **(C,D)**. Laser **(A,C)** and LED **(B,D)** were used as the excitation light source. Arrows indicate the manual addition of 10 mM NH_4Cl and 5 mM HCl in each panel. Each trace represents the response of a single cell; $n = 3$.

REFERENCES

Achikanu, C., Pendekanti, V., Teague, R., and Publicover, S. (2018). Effects of pH manipulation, CatSper stimulation and Ca2+-store mobilization on [Ca2+]i and behaviour of human sperm. *Hum. Reprod.* 33, 1802–1811. doi: 10.1093/humrep/dey280

Acott, T. S., and Carr, D. W. (1984). Inhibition of bovine spermatozoa by caudal epididymal fluid: ii. interaction of pH and a quiescence factor. *Biol. Reprod.* 30, 926–935. doi: 10.1095/biolreprod30.4.926

Babcock, D. F. (1983). Examination of the intracellular ionic environment and of ionophore action by null point measurements employing the fluorescein chromophore. *J. Biol. Chem.* 258, 6380–6389.

Baker, M. A., and Aitken, R. J. (2004). The importance of redox regulated pathways in sperm cell biology. *Mol. Cell. Endocrinol.* 216, 47–54. doi: 10.1016/j.mce.2003.10.068

Balderas, E., Sánchez-Cárdenas, C., Chávez, J. C., De La Vega Beltrán, J. L., Gómez-Lagunas, F., Treviño, C. L., et al. (2013). The anti-inflammatory drug celecoxib inhibits t-type Ca2+ currents in spermatogenic cells yet it elicits the acrosome reaction in mature sperm. *FEBS Lett.* 587, 2412–2419. doi: 10.1016/j.febslet.2013.05.068

Berger, T. K., Fußhöller, D. M., Goodwin, N., Bönigk, W., Khesroshahi, N. D., Brenker, C., et al. (2017). Posttranslational cleavage of Hv1 in human sperm tunes pH- and voltage-dependent gating. *J. Physiol.* 595, 1533–1546. doi: 10.1113/JP273189

Brown, D., Smith, P. J., and Breton, S. (1997). Role of V-ATPase-rich cells in acidification of the male reproductive tract. *J. Exp. Biol.* 200, 257–262.

Buck, J., Sinclair, M. L., Schapal, L., Cann, M. J., and Levin, L. R. (1999). Cytosolic adenylyl cyclase defines a unique signaling molecule in mammals. *Proc. Natl. Acad. Sci. U.S.A.* 96, 79–84. doi: 10.1073/pnas.96.1.79

Cao, X. W., Lin, K., Li, C. Y., and Yuan, C. W. (2010). *A Review of WHO Laboratory Manual for the Examination and Processing of Human Semen*, 5th Edn, Vol. 17. Geneva: World Health Organization, 287.

Carlson, A. E., Hille, B., and Babcock, D. F. (2007). External Ca2+ acts upstream of adenylyl cyclase SACY in the bicarbonate signaled activation of sperm motility. *Dev. Biol.* 312, 183–192. doi: 10.1016/j.ydbio.2007.09.017

Carlson, A. E., Westenbroek, R. E., Quill, T., Ren, D., Clapham, D. E., Hille, B., et al. (2003). CatSper1 required for evoked Ca2+ entry and control of flagellar function in sperm. *Proc. Natl. Acad. Sci. U.S.A.* 100, 14864–14868. doi: 10.1073/pnas.2536658100

Chávez, J. C., De la Vega-Beltrán, J. L., José, O., Torres, P., Nishigaki, T., Treviño, C. L., et al. (2018). Acrosomal alkalization triggers Ca2+ release and acrosome reaction in mammalian spermatozoa. *J. Cell. Physiol.* 233, 4735–4747. doi: 10.1002/jcp.26262

Chávez, J. C., Ferreira, J. J., Butler, A., De La Vega Beltrán, J. L., Treviño, C. L., Darszon, A., et al. (2014). SLO3 K+ channels control calcium entry through CATSPER channels in sperm. *J. Biol. Chem.* 289, 32266–32275. doi: 10.1074/jbc.M114.607556

Chavez, J. C., Hernandez-Gonzalez, E. O., Wertheimer, E., Visconti, P. E., Darszon, A., and Trevino, C. L. (2012). Participation of the Cl-/HCO3- exchangers SLC26A3 and SLC26A6, the Cl- channel CFTR, and the regulatory factor SLC9A3R1 in mouse sperm capacitation. *Biol. Reprod.* 86, 1–14. doi: 10.1095/biolreprod.111.094037

Chen, Y., Cann, M. J., Litvin, T. N., Iourgenko, V., Sinclair, M. L., Levin, L. R., et al. (2000). Soluble adenylyl cyclase as an evolutionarily conserved bicarbonate sensor. *Science* 289, 625–628. doi: 10.1126/science.289.5479.625

Crhisten, R., Schackmann, R. W., and Shapiro, B. M. (1983). Metabolism of Sea Urchin Sperm Interrelationships between intracellular pH, ATPase activity, and mitochondrial respiration. *J. Biol. Chem.* 258, 5392–5399. doi: 10.1086/281606

Cross, N. L., and Razy-Faulkner, P. (1997). Control of human sperm intracellular pH by cholesterol and its relationship to the response of the acrosome to progesterone. *Biol. Reprod.* 56, 1169–1174. doi: 10.1095/biolreprod56.5.1169

Darszon, A., Wood, C. D., Beltrán, C., Sánchez, D., Rodríguez-Miranda, E., Gorelik, J., et al. (2004). Measuring ion fluxes in sperm. *Methods Cell Biol.* 74, 545–576. doi: 10.1016/s0091-679x(04)74022-4

Demarco, I. A., Espinosa, F., Edwards, J., Sosnik, J., De la Vega-Beltrán, J. L., Hockensmith, J. W., et al. (2003). Involvement of a Na+/HCO3- cotransporter in mouse sperm capacitation. *J. Biol. Chem.* 278, 7001–7009. doi: 10.1074/jbc.M206284200

Espinal-Enríquez, J., Priego-Espinosa, D. A., Darszon, A., Beltrán, C., and Martínez-Mekler, G. (2017). Network model predicts that CatSper is the main Ca2+ channel in the regulation of sea urchin sperm motility. *Sci. Rep.* 7:4236. doi: 10.1038/s41598-017-03857-9

Fraire-Zamora, J. J., and González-Martínez, M. T. (2004). Effect of intracellular pH on depolarization-evoked calcium influx in human sperm. *Am. J. Physiol. Cell Physiol.* 287, C1688–C1696. doi: 10.1152/ajpcell.00141.2004

Garcia, M. A., and Meizel, S. (1996). Importance of sodium ion to the progesterone-initiated acrosome reaction in human sperm. *Mol. Reprod. Dev.* 45, 513–520. doi: 10.1002/(sici)1098-2795(199612)45:4<513::aid-mrd14>3.0.co;2-x

González-Cota, A. L., Silva, P. Â, Carneiro, J., and Darszon, A. (2015). Single cell imaging reveals that the motility regulator speract induces a flagellar alkalinization that precedes and is independent of Ca2+ influx in sea urchin spermatozoa. *FEBS Lett.* 589, 2146–2154. doi: 10.1016/j.febslet.2015.06.024

Grillo-Hill, B. K., Webb, B. A., and Barber, D. L. (2014). Ratiometric imaging of pH probes. *Methods Cell Biol.* 123, 429–448. doi: 10.1016/B978-0-12-420138-5.00023-9

Hamamah, S., Magnoux, E., Royere, D., Barthelemy, C., Dacheux, J. L., and Gatti, J. L. (1996). Internal pH of human spermatozoa: effect of ions, human follicular fluid and progesterone. *Mol. Hum. Reprod.* 2, 219–224.

Hamzeh, H., Alvarez, L., Strünker, T., Kierzek, M., Brenker, C., Deal, P. E., et al. (2019). Kinetic and photonic techniques to study chemotactic signaling in sea urchin sperm. *Methods Cell Biol.* 151, 487–517. doi: 10.1016/bs.mcb.2018.12.001

Harper, C. V., Kirkman-Brown, J. C., Barratt, C. L. R., and Publicover, S. J. (2003). Encoding of progesterone stimulus intensity by intracellular [Ca2+] ([Ca2+]i) in human spermatozoa. *Biochem. J.* 372, 407–417. doi: 10.1042/BJ20021560

Hernández-González, E. O., Treviño, C. L., Castellano, L. E., De La Vega-Beltrán, J. L., Ocampo, A. Y., Wertheimer, E., et al. (2007). Involvement of cystic fibrosis transmembrane conductance regulator in mouse sperm capacitation. *J. Biol. Chem.* 282, 24397–24406. doi: 10.1074/jbc.M701603200

Ho, H.-C., Granish, K. A., and Suarez, S. S. (2002). Hyperactivated motility of bull sperm is triggered at the axoneme by Ca2+ and not cAMP. *Dev. Biol.* 250, 208–217. doi: 10.1006/dbio.2002.0797

Ho, H. C., and Suarez, S. S. (2001). Hyperactivation of mammalian spermatozoa: function and regulation. *Reproduction* 122, 519–526. doi: 10.1530/rep.0.1220519

Hyrc, K. L., Minta, A., Escamilla, P. R., Chan, P. P. L., Meshik, X. A., and Goldberg, M. P. (2013). Synthesis and properties of Asante Calcium Red-A novel family of long excitation wavelength calcium indicators. *Cell Calcium* 54, 320–333. doi: 10.1016/j.ceca.2013.08.001

José, O., Torres-Rodríguez, P., Forero-Quintero, L. S., Chávez, J. C., De La Vega-Beltrán, J. L., Carta, F., et al. (2015). Carbonic anhydrases and their functional differences in human and mouse sperm physiology. *Biochem. Biophys. Res. Commun.* 468, 713–718. doi: 10.1016/j.bbrc.2015.11.021

Kinosita, K., Itoh, H., Ishiwata, S., Hirano, K., Nishizaka, T., and Hayakawa, T. (1991). Dual-view microscopy with a single camera: real-time imaging of molecular orientations and calcium. *J. Cell Biol.* 115, 67–73. doi: 10.1083/jcb.115.1.67

Kirichok, Y., Navarro, B., and Clapham, D. E. (2006). Whole-cell patch-clamp measurements of spermatozoa reveal an alkaline-activated Ca2+ channel. *Nature* 439, 737–740. doi: 10.1038/nature04417

Lee, M. A., and Storey, B. T. (1986). Bicarbonate mouse sperm is essential for fertilization of mouse eggs: mouse sperm require it to undergo the acrosome reaction. *Biol. Reprod.* 56, 349–356. doi: 10.1095/biolreprod34.2.349

Lishko, P. V., Botchkina, I. L., Fedorenko, A., and Kirichok, Y. (2010). Acid extrusion from human spermatozoa is mediated by flagellar voltage-gated proton channel. *Cell* 140, 327–337. doi: 10.1016/j.cell.2009.12.053

Lishko, P. V., Botchkina, I. L., and Kirichok, Y. (2011). Progesterone activates the principal Ca2+ channel of human sperm. *Nature* 471, 387–391. doi: 10.1038/nature09767

Liu, J., Diwu, Z., and Leung, W. Y. (2001). Synthesis and photophysical properties of new fluorinated benzo[c]xanthene dyes as intracellular pH indicators. *Bioorg. Med. Chem. Lett.* 11, 2903–2905. doi: 10.1016/S0960-894X(01)00595-9

Maas, D. H., Storey, B. T., and Mastroianni, L. (1977). Hydrogen ion and carbon dioxide content of the oviductal fluid of the rhesus monkey (*Macaca mulatta*). *Fertil. Steril.* 28, 981–985. doi: 10.1016/S0015-0282(16)42801-3

Mannowetz, N., Miller, M. R., and Lishko, P. V. (2017). Regulation of the sperm calcium channel CatSper by endogenous steroids and plant triterpenoids. *Proc. Natl. Acad. Sci. U.S.A.* 114, 5743–5748. doi: 10.1073/pnas.1700367114

Mata-Martínez, E., José, O., Torres-Rodríguez, P., Solís-López, A., Sánchez-Tusie, A. A., Sánchez-Guevara, Y., et al. (2013). Measuring intracellular Ca^{2+} changes in human sperm using four techniques: conventional fluorometry, stopped flow fluorometry, flow cytometry and single cell imaging. *J. Vis. Exp.* 75:50344. doi: 10.3791/50344

Miller, M. R., Mannowetz, N., Iavarone, A. T., Safavi, R., Gracheva, E. O., Smith, J. F., et al. (2016). Unconventional endocannabinoid signaling governs sperm activation via the sex hormone progesterone. *Science* 352, 555–559. doi: 10. 1126/science.aad6887

Musset, B., Clark, R. A., DeCoursey, T. E., Petheo, G. L., Geiszt, M., Chen, Y., et al. (2012). NOX5 in human spermatozoa: expression, function, and regulation. *J. Biol. Chem.* 287, 9376–9388. doi: 10.1074/jbc.M111.314955

Navarro, B., Kirichok, Y., Chung, J. J., and Clapham, D. E. (2008). Ion channels that control fertility in mammalian spermatozoa. *Int. J. Dev. Biol.* 52, 607–613. doi: 10.1387/ijdb.072554bn

Nishigaki, T., José, O., González-Cota, A. L., Romero, F., Treviño, C. L., and Darszon, A. (2014). Intracellular pH in sperm physiology. *Biochem. Biophys. Res. Commun.* 450, 1149–1158. doi: 10.1016/j.bbrc.2014.05.100

Nishigaki, T., Wood, C. D., Shiba, K., Baba, S. A., and Darszon, A. (2006). Stroboscopic illumination usine light-emitting diodes reduces phototoxicity in fluorescence cell imaging. *Biotechniques* 41, 191–197. doi: 10.2144/000112220

Okamura, N., Tajima, Y., Soejima, A., Masuda, H., and Sugita, Y. (1985). Sodium bicarbonate in seminal plasma stimulates the motility of mammalian spermatozoa through direct activation of adenylate cyclase. *J. Biol. Chem.* 260, 9699–9705.

Okunade, G. W., Miller, M. L., Pyne, G. J., Sutliff, R. L., O'Connor, K. T., Neumann, J. C., et al. (2004). Targeted ablation of plasma membrane Ca2+-ATPase (PMCA) 1 and 4 indicates a major housekeeping function for PMCA1 and a critical role in hyperactivated sperm motility and male fertility for PMCA4. *J. Biol. Chem.* 279, 33742–33750. doi: 10.1074/jbc.M404628200

Orta, G., Vega-Beltran, J. L., Hidalgo, D., Santi, C. M., Visconti, P., and Darszon, A. (2018). CatSper channels are regulated by protein kinase A. *J. Biol. Chem.* 293, 16830–16841. doi: 10.1074/jbc.RA117.001566

Parrish, J. J., Susko-Parrish, J. L., and Furst, N. L. (1989a). Capacitation of Bovine Sperm by Heparin: inhibitory Effect of Glucose and Role of Intracellular pH. *Biol. Reprod.* 41, 683–699. doi: 10.1095/biolreprod41.4.683

Parrish, J. J., Susko-Parrish, J. L., Handrow, R. R., Sims, M. M., and First, N. L. (1989b). Capacitation of bovine spermatozoa by oviduct fluid. *Biol. Reprod.* 40, 1020–1025. doi: 10.1095/biolreprod40.5.1020

Ren, D., Navarro, B., Perez, G., Jackson, A. C., Hsu, S., Shi, Q., et al. (2001). A sperm ion channel required for sperm motility and male fertility. *Nature* 413, 603–609. doi: 10.1038/35098027

Rink, T. I., Tsien, R. Y., and Pozzan, T. (1982). Cytoplasmic pH and free Mg2+ in lymphocytes. *J. Cell Biol.* 95, 189–196. doi: 10.1083/jcb.95.1.189

Schackmann, R. W., and Boon Chock, P. (1986). Alteration of intracellular [Ca2+] in sea urchin sperm by the egg peptide speract. Evidence that increased intracellular Ca2+ is coupled to Na+ entry and increased intracellular pH. *J. Biol. Chem.* 261, 8719–8728.

Seifert, R., Flick, M., Bönigk, W., Alvarez, L., Trötschel, C., Poetsch, A., et al. (2015). The CatSper channel controls chemosensation in sea urchin sperm. *EMBO J.* 34, 379–392. doi: 10.15252/embj.201489376

Stauss, C. R., Votta, T. J., and Suarez, S. S. (1995). Sperm motility hyperactivation facilitates penetration of the hamster Zona Pellucida'. *Biol. Reprod.* 53, 1280–1285. doi: 10.1095/biolreprod53.6.1280

Suarez, S. S., and Pacey, A. A. (2006). Sperm transport in the female reproductive tract. *Hum. Reprod. Update* 12, 23–37. doi: 10.1093/humupd/dmi047

Tesarik, J., Mendoza, C., Moos, J., Fénichel, P., and Fehlmann, M. (1992). Progesterone action through aggregation of a receptor on the sperm plasma membrane. *FEBS Lett.* 308, 116–120. doi: 10.1016/0014-5793(92)81256-l

Visconti, P. E., Moore, G. D., Bailey, J. L., Leclerc, P., Connors, S. A., Pan, D., et al. (1995). Capacitation of mouse spermatozoa. II. Protein tyrosine phosphorylation and capacitation are regulated by a cAMP-dependent pathway. *Development* 121, 1139–1150.

Vishwakarma, P. (1962). The pH and bicarbonate-ion content of the oviduct and uterine fluids. *Fertil. Sterl.* 13, 481–485. doi: 10.1016/S0015-0282(16)34633-7

Vredenburgh-Wilberg, W. L., and Parrish, J. J. (1995). Intracellular pH of bovine sperm increases during capacitation. *Mol. Reprod. Dev.* 40, 490–502. doi: 10. 1002/mrd.1080400413

Wandernoth, P. M., Raubuch, M., Mannowetz, N., Becker, H. M., Deitmer, J. W., Sly, W. S., et al. (2010). Role of carbonic anhydrase IV in the bicarbonate-mediated activation of murine and human sperm. *PLoS One* 5:e15061. doi: 10.1371/journal.pone.0015061

Wang, D., King, S. M., Quill, T. A., Doolittle, L. K., and Garbers, D. L. (2003). A new sperm-specific Na+/H+ Exchanger required for sperm motility and fertility. *Nat. Cell Biol.* 5, 1117–1122. doi: 10.1038/ncb1072

Wennemuth, G. (2003). Bicarbonate actions on flagellar and Ca2+-channel responses: initial events in sperm activation. *Development* 130, 1317–1326. doi: 10.1242/dev.00353

Wennemuth, G., Babcock, D. F., and Hille, B. (2003). Calcium clearance mechanisms of mouse sperm. *J. Gen. Physiol.* 122, 115–128. doi: 10.1085/jgp. 200308839

Whitaker, J. E., Haugland, R. P., and Prendergast, F. G. (1991). Spectral and photophysical studies of benzo[c]xanthene dyes: dual emission pH sensors. *Anal. Biochem.* 194, 330–344. doi: 10.1016/0003-2697(91) 90237-N

Windler, F., Bönigk, W., Körschen, H. G., Grahn, E., Strünker, T., Seifert, R., et al. (2018). The solute carrier SLC9C1 is a Na+/H+-exchanger gated by an S4-type voltage-sensor and cyclic-nucleotide binding. *Nat. Commun.* 9:2809. doi: 10.1038/s41467-018-05253-x

Xu, W. M., Shi, Q. X., Chen, W. Y., Zhou, C. X., Ni, Y., Rowlands, D. K., et al. (2007). Cystic fibrosis transmembrane conductance regulator is vital to sperm fertilizing capacity and male fertility. *Proc. Natl. Acad. Sci. U.S.A.* 104, 9816–9821. doi: 10.1073/pnas.0609253104

Zeng, Y., Oberdorf, J. A., and Florman, H. M. (1996). pH regulation in mouse sperm: identification of Na+-, Cl–, and[formula]dependent and arylaminobenzoate-dependent regulatory mechanisms and characterization of their roles in sperm capacitation. *Dev. Biol.* 173, 510–520. doi: 10.1006/dbio. 1996.0044

Zhao, Y., Araki, S., Wu, J., Teramoto, T., Chang, Y.-F., Nakano, M., et al. (2011). An expanded palette of genetically encoded Ca2+ indicators. *Science* 333, 1888–1891. doi: 10.1126/science.1208592

Zhou, H. X., and Pang, X. (2018). Electrostatic interactions in protein structure, folding, binding, and condensation. *Chem. Rev.* 118, 1691–1741. doi: 10.1021/ acs.chemrev.7b00305

16

Successful ICSI in Mice Using Caput Epididymal Spermatozoa

Raúl Fernández-González**, Ricardo Laguna, Priscila Ramos-Ibeas, Eva Pericuesta, Víctor Alcalde-Lopez, Serafín Perez-Cerezales and Alfonso Gutierrez-Adan

Departamento de Reproducción Animal, INIA, Madrid, Spain

***Correspondence:**
Raúl Fernández-González
raulfg@inia.es;
agutierr@inia.es

Spermatozoa undergo their last phase of spermiogenesis, known as maturation, as they pass through the epididymis. A recent report indicates that mouse immature spermatozoa retrieved from the caput epididymis for intracytoplasmic sperm injection (ICSI) give rise to embryos with multiple developmental defects. Further, these embryos were unable to develop to term after their transfer to surrogate mothers. Herein, we examined the potential of mouse caput spermatozoa to produce normal embryos by comparing the use of caput vs. cauda epididymal spermatozoa for *in vitro* fertilization (IVF) or ICSI. Two methods for the separation of sperm heads prior to ICSI were also compared: freezing/thawing or drawing through a syringe. We found that in contrast to caudal spermatozoa, caput spermatozoa failed to produce embryos via IVF, confirming their immature state. However, regardless of the method employed for the separation of sperm heads, similar efficiencies of blastocyst production *in vitro* and development to term after transfer to surrogate mothers were observed following ICSI using both caput and cauda epididymal spermatozoa. It therefore seems that mice spermatozoa recovered from the caput epididymis are as valid as caudal spermatozoa for the production of embryos and offspring by ICSI.

Keywords: ICSI, caput, epididymis, mice, sperm

INTRODUCTION

Spermatozoa acquire their final mature state during passage through the epididymis. Mammalian immature sperm produced in the testis move from the ducts of the testis into the caput epididymis, where they are completely immobile and unable to fertilize an egg cell; then they are transported through the epididymis to the cauda region as a result of rhythmic contractions of this organ, where they undergo complex modifications, acquire motility and become fertilization-competent, denominating then mature sperm (Gervasi and Visconti, 2017). Thus, in theory, ejaculated sperm should have a better fertilizing capacity than sperm recovered from the testis as they have transited through the epididymis, where the final steps of maturation take place. These steps include compaction of sperm chromatin, formation of disulfide bridges between protamines and epigenetic remodeling (Ariel et al., 1994; Haidl et al., 1994; Perez-Cerezales et al., 2012). Chromatin maturation is required to fully stabilize and protect DNA from damage induced by endogenous nucleases or reactive oxygen species during sperm passage through the epididymis (Irvine et al., 2000; Perez-Cerezales et al., 2012). The importance of sperm maturation in the epididymis has also been confirmed by *in vitro* fertilization (IVF) assays performed with spermatozoa collected from different sites of the epididymis. In these assays, sperm retrieved from the distal part acquire a higher motility and ability to fertilize the oocyte (Sullivan and Mieusset, 2016). The epididymis is also able to eliminate defective or immature germ cells (Ramos-Ibeas et al., 2013).

Recently, it has been reported that small RNAs are trafficked to mammalian sperm during the process of post-testicular maturation in the epididymis (Sharma et al., 2018). It has been also described that 2-cell embryos generated via intracytoplasmic sperm injection (ICSI) using sperm obtained from the proximal (caput) versus distal (cauda) epididymis show similar RNA expression, but as development progresses, their gene expression profiles diverge (Conine et al., 2018). Further, embryos arising from caput spermatozoa (caput embryos) have been shown to have multiple developmental defects, and when transferred to surrogate mothers were unable to reach term (Conine et al., 2018). However, the injection of cauda- specific microRNAs (miRNAs) into caput zygotes was observed to suppress the specific gene expression profile of caput embryos and rescue their potential for development. These results indicate that dynamic small RNAs are essential for sperm maturation and also necessary for successful development and were taken as evidence that sperm-borne small RNAs derived from near the cauda region are critical for fetal development (Conine et al., 2018; Sharma et al., 2018). However, both testis spermatids and sperm support full-term development when injected into oocytes (Kimura and Yanagimachi, 1995; Moreira et al., 2016). In this context, the findings of Conine et al. (2018) suggest that the ability of sperm to support full-term embryo development after ICSI is acquired in the testis, then lost in the caput epididymis, and re-acquired during epididymal transit prior to arriving at the cauda. However, this hypothesis contradicts the results reported by others showing that ICSI produces normal offspring using caput sperm (Suganuma et al., 2005; Zhou et al., 2019).

Our hypothesis is that the developmental potential of caput and cauda fertilized embryo is similar and that the discrepancies of the results reported by Conine et al. (2018) respect to the literature could be due to differences in ICSI protocols, mainly in the technique used to separate the head from the tail of the sperm, since the different techniques can produce different degrees of alterations in the sperm (Tateno, 2008). Mouse spermatozoa are particularly sensitive to mechanical damage (Mazur et al., 2000), and these damages can be more decisive for the sperm of the caput, since it has been shown that there are more DNA fragmentation and less chromatin compaction in the caput than in the cauda epididymal spermatozoa (Perez-Cerezales et al., 2012), and that sperm obtained from the caput are more susceptible to nuclease-dependent DNA damage than sperm obtained from other epididymal regions (Yamauchi et al., 2007). Moreover, it has been reported that ICSI in mice using DNA-fragmented sperm has been linked to altered gene expression at the preimplantation stage, reduction of fetal development, an increased risk of genetic and epigenetic abnormalities both in embryos and offspring (Ramos-Ibeas et al., 2014). Separation of the sperm heads from the tail prior to ICSI is commonly conducted by sonication, by fine needle shearing, by unprotected freezing, by piezo pulses, or by detergent treatment, and all these protocols may produce different level of chromosome aberrations in mouse (Martin et al., 1988; Tateno, 2008).

Our study addresses the reproductive potential of caput spermatozoa used for IVF or ICSI. As a positive control, we used caudal spermatozoa, regularly used for these procedures in mice. Our objective was to test the reported inability of caput spermatozoa to produce viable ICSI-derived mice by injecting into oocytes caput or cauda epididymal sperm recovered from standard B6D2F1 hybrid and inbred B6 mouse strains using similar protocols to previously described (Conine et al., 2018).

MATERIALS AND METHODS

Handling of Mice and Sperm Samples

Experiments in mice were carried out in strict accordance with recommendations of the guidelines of the European Community Council Directive 86/609/EEC. The study protocol was approved by the Committee on the Ethics of Animal Experiments of the INIA (2016 permit number CEEA 2014/025). Spermatozoa were collected from the caput and caudal epididymis of 20-week-old B6D2F1 males (C57/BL/6JxDBA/2J) and B6 (C57BL/6NHsd) mice (**Figure 1**). Sperm were released by making an incision in the epididymal tissue and then squeezing to release its contents. The sperm were then suspended in M2 medium (Sigma–Aldrich, Madrid, Spain) for the ICSI experiments, or in human tubal fluid medium (HTF) supplemented with 1% BSA for IVF tests. To capacitate the sperm for the IVF experiments, samples were incubated for 30 min under an atmosphere of 5% CO_2 at 37°C.

Intracytoplasmic Sperm Injection (ICSI) and *in vitro* Fertilization (IVF)

For our ICSI experiments, the caput and caudal epididymis of the same animal were dissected separately, and sperm collected in M2 medium (6 adult individuals) as described previously (Perez-Cerezales et al., 2012). The sperm was mixed with five volumes of a 10% solution of polyvinyl-pyrrolidone in M2. ICSI was performed in M2 medium at room temperature (Ramos-Ibeas et al., 2014). Sperm heads were decapitated by the freezing-thawing method (Moreira et al., 2003) or by drawing the sperm repeatedly through a fine-gauge needle (25G) into a 1 mL syringe 20–30 times (Conine et al., 2018). In parallel, oocytes were collected at metaphase II from B6D2F1 8-week-old females, which were superovulated by standard intraperitoneal injection (Moreira et al., 2005), and incubated with hyaluronidase (300 μg/mL) to remove cumulus cells. After allowing their recovery for 15 min, sperm were injected into the oocytes in M2 at room temperature. Surviving zygotes were cultured until the blastocyst stage to check their development or until the 2-cell stage for the embryo transfer experiments.

For the IVF experiments, oocytes were obtained from superovulated female mice as described above. The method used has been described elsewhere (Hourcade et al., 2010). Briefly, 2.5–10.0 μL of fresh caput or cauda epididymal sperm were added to each fertilization drop to achieve a final concentration of ~1–2 × 10^6 spermatozoa/mL. Four hours after oocyte and sperm co-incubation at 37°C in a humidified atmosphere of 5% CO_2 in air, putative zygotes were washed and cultured in KSOM.

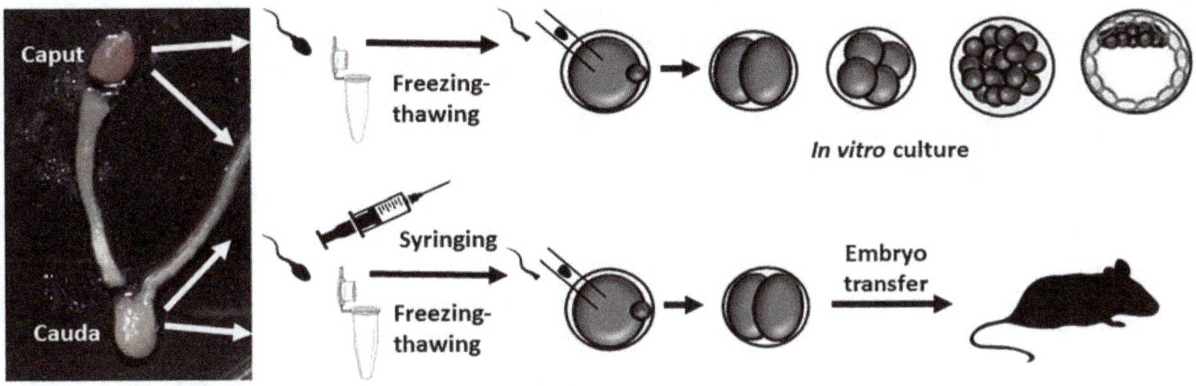

FIGURE 1 | Outline of the experiments carried out. Epididymis dissections showing the caput and cauda regions used. Paired caput and cauda sperm samples (from the same animal) were injected into control oocytes, and 2-cell embryos were *in vitro* cultured or transferred to pseudo-pregnant females.

Statistical differences between caput- and cauda- derived embryos and offspring were assessed using an unpaired *t*-test and ANOVA (SigmaStat package), respectively. Significance was set at $p < 0.05$.

RESULTS

Sperm from the cauda and caput epididymis were collected from six 20-week-old sexually mature B6D2F1 and four inbred B6 male mice (Perez-Cerezales et al., 2012) and prepared according to requirements for IVF or ICSI (**Figure 1**). For IVF, the sperm were capacitated for 30 min and for ICSI the sperm were frozen without a cryoprotectant (Moreira et al., 2003) or drawn repeatedly through a fine-gauge needle into a 1 mL syringe 20–30 times (Conine et al., 2018) to obtain tail-free sperm heads. Our IVF experiments revealed that only caudal sperm had the capacity to fertilize oocytes. Thus, using caudal sperm, 96.29 ± 3.70% of fertilized oocytes (n = 48) underwent 2-cell cleavage and all of these embryos developed to blastocysts. In contrast, no fertilization was produced with sperm obtained from the caput epididymis: only 4 out of 128 (3.25 ± 3.25%) fertilized oocytes developed to the 2-cell stage, and none developed into blastocysts. This result could be explained by a lack of motility of caput sperm.

We next microinjected caput and caudal sperm (heads decapitated by freezing-thawing) of B6D2 mice into oocytes and found that embryos produced with both sperm types developed *in vitro* to the blastocyst stage at similar efficiencies (**Figure 2**). Given that caput-derived embryos were perfectly capable of developing to the blastocyst stage *in vitro* (57% of blastocysts produced by caput sperm vs. 63% by caudal sperm, four replicates and more than 100 embryos produced in each group), we then generated both caput- and cauda-derived embryos by ICSI using paired sperm samples from the same animal, and surgically transferred 15–20 2-cell embryos into pseudopregnant surrogate mothers to analyze their *in vivo* developmental capacity. First, we used our classic method of fast freezing/thawing to separate sperm heads. As we show in **Table 1**, we found similar percentages of cleaved embryos and live offspring using caput or caudal sperm. We then used the drawing through a syringe method to decapitate sperm (Conine et al., 2018), and using both B6D2 and B6 mice, we also observed similar percentages of 2-cell embryos and live offspring derived from caput or caudal sperm. Interestingly, we noted a small but non-significant reduction in the number of live offspring when sperm were treated with the syringe, and also a non-significant reduction in the percentage of live offspring generated from caput sperm. In total, 20 and 30 pups were obtained by both procedures from caput and cauda sperm, respectively. Birth weights and blastocyst development were similar between the caput and cauda groups and both males and females were fertile (n = 8 per group).

DISCUSSION

A recent report describes that embryos generated via ICSI using immature sperm derived from the caput epididymis show multiple defects during the peri-implantation period and quickly fail to undergo implantation (Conine et al., 2018). The authors

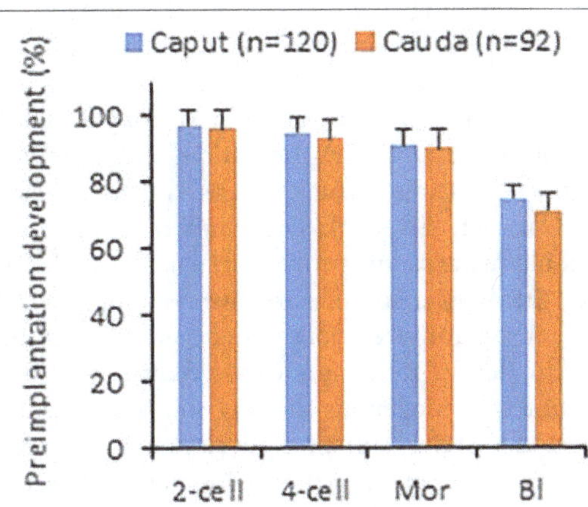

FIGURE 2 | *In vitro* development of embryos produced by injecting sperm from caput or cauda epididymis into oocytes. Percentages shown are calculated with respect to oocytes surviving injection. Mor, morulae; Bl, blastocyst. Values are mean ± SEM. No significant differences between groups were detected (unpaired *t*-test, $p \leq 0.05$).

TABLE 1 | Development of oocytes injected with sperm from caput vs. caudal epididymis.

Sperm source	Mouse strain	Sperm treatment	Oocytes surviving injection (%)	2-cell embryos at 24 h (% surviving)	No. embryos transferred (no. recipients)[a]	No. live offspring (% implantations)
Caput	B6D2	Freezing/thawing	167/192 (86.9)	134 (80.2)	134 (5)	15 (11.2)
Cauda	B6D2	Freezing/thawing	90/116 (77.6)	78 (86.7)	78 (4)	19 (24.4)
Caput	B6D2	DWG T syringe	46/53 (86.8)	35 (76.1)	35 (2)	3 (8.6)
Cauda	B6D2	DWG T syringe	44/60 (73.3)	36 (81.8)	36 (3)	6 (16.7)
Caput	B6	DWG T syringe	39/50 (78)	32 (76.9)	32 (2)	2 (6.3)
Cauda	B6	DWG T syringe	38/50 (76)	31 (81.6)	31 (2)	5 (16.7)

Four independent experiments were conducted. B6D2 = C57/BL/6 JxDBA/2 J; B6 = C57BL/6NHsd; DWG T syringe = Drawing through syringe. [a]All recipients were pregnant. P > 0.05 Chi-square analysis.

of this paper also observed that these defects could be rescued by the injection of small RNAs derived from extracellular vesicles (epididymosomes), which deliver their small RNA repertoire to mature sperm, suggesting that small RNAs in mature sperm play major roles during early mouse embryogenesis. Here, we report that similar embryo development and offspring production results for ICSI using immature sperm from the caput epididymis or mature sperm from the caudal epididymis.

In mice, ICSI is performed with isolated sperm heads. However, sperm heads can be obtained by different protocols and this could have an appreciable impact on the sperm. In our hands, both protocols used to generate individual sperm heads (freezing/thawing, the standard method used in our laboratory, and drawing through a syringe, the method employed by Conine et al. (2018) produced healthy offspring from immature caput sperm. However, the number of live offspring generated with caput sperm was slightly lower than that generated with caudal sperm. In effect, this could be due to differences in maturation and sperm chromatin status between caput and caudal sperm. We earlier reported that the immaturity of mouse spermatozoa in the caput epididymis was revealed by a higher permeability of membranes to propidium iodide (PI) (Perez-Cerezales et al., 2012). Sperm chromatin undergoes the formation of disulfide bridges between protamines during the transit through the epididymis, increasing compaction of the genetic material (Golan et al., 1996). Also, using the comet assay and sperm chromatin structure assay (SCSA), we previously described different maturation stages of spermatozoa along the epididymis consisting of more DNA fragmentation and less chromatin compaction in the caput- than cauda epididymal spermatozoa (Perez-Cerezales et al., 2012). These differences in chromatin structure could make caput sperm more sensitive to decapitation procedures. Perhaps, a more aggressive technique will lead to more severe chromatin alterations in spermatozoa from the caput epididymis, or leave DNA more exposed and thus susceptible to degradation by endogenous or exogenous nucleases. Oocytes can support the preimplantation development of sperm with damaged chromatin, but major developmental defects appear later, after implantation (Fernandez-Gonzalez et al., 2008). This is in line with clinical observations that ejaculated sperm with damaged DNA go through normal preimplantation embryonic stages but fail to develop beyond this stage (Tesarik et al., 2004). Further, another two procedures designed to separate the sperm head from tail have been used to produce normal offspring from caput sperm (Suganuma et al., 2005; Zhou et al., 2019). The sperm head can be separated from the midpiece and tail by applying one or a few piezo pulses (Suganuma et al., 2005) or through sonication or the use of detergents like Triton X-100 or 3-[(3-cholamidopropyl) dimethylammonio]-1-propanesulfonate (Zhou et al., 2019).

There are several methodological differences between Conine et al. (2018) and previous studies (Suganuma et al., 2005; Zhou et al., 2019) which could potentially account for the discrepancy about the ability of caput-derived embryos to implant. In our experiments we used similar protocols to Conine et al. (2018) with the exception of the mouse strain background (we use B6D2 hybrids and inbred B6, and Conine et al. (2018) use inbred FVB). Further, other inbred mice have been also used, like 129Sc (Suganuma et al., 2005), showing to produce normal caput-derived mice. Although we cannot eliminate the possibility that the ability of caput-derived embryos to implant could be affected by strain background our results rule out the general character of the findings reported by Conine et al. (2018) for the mouse species.

In summary, sperm from the caput region of the epididymis are incapable of IVF but, contrary to recent findings (Conine et al., 2018), we here confirm that healthy fertile mice can be produced by ICSI from caput sperm.

ETHICS STATEMENT

The animal study was reviewed and approved by the Committee on the Ethics of Animal Experiments of the INIA (2016 permit number CEEA 2014/025).

AUTHOR CONTRIBUTIONS

RF-G and RL produced the ICSI mice and collaborated in the phenotyping. PR-I, EP, VA-L, and SP-C performed all the experiments and co-wrote the manuscript. AG-A conceived the experiments and co-wrote the manuscript.

FUNDING

This work was supported by Grant RTI2018-093548-B-I00 from the Spanish Ministry of Science, Innovation and Universities. PR-I was funded by a Talent Attraction Fellowship from the Madrid Community (2017-T2/BIO-5182). SP-C was supported by the Ramón y Cajal Programme (RYC-2016-20147).

REFERENCES

Ariel, M., Cedar, H., and Mccarrey, J. (1994). Developmental changes in methylation of spermatogenesis-specific genes include reprogramming in the epididymis. *Nat. Genet.* 7, 59–63. doi: 10.1038/ng0594-59

Conine, C. C., Sun, F., Song, L., Rivera-Perez, J. A., and Rando, O. J. (2018). Small RNAs gained during epididymal transit of sperm are essential for embryonic development in mice. *Dev. Cell* 46, 470.e3–480.e3. doi: 10.1016/j.devcel.2018.06.024

Fernandez-Gonzalez, R., Moreira, P. N., Perez-Crespo, M., Sanchez-Martin, M., Ramirez, M. A., Pericuesta, E., et al. (2008). Long-term effects of mouse intracytoplasmic sperm injection with DNA-fragmented sperm on health and behavior of adult offspring. *Biol. Reprod.* 78, 761–772. doi: 10.1095/biolreprod.107.065623

Gervasi, M. G., and Visconti, P. E. (2017). Molecular changes and signaling events occurring in spermatozoa during epididymal maturation. *Andrology* 5, 204–218. doi: 10.1111/andr.12320

Golan, R., Cooper, T. G., Oschry, Y., Oberpenning, F., Schulze, H., Shochat, L., et al. (1996). Changes in chromatin condensation of human spermatozoa during epididymal transit as determined by flow cytometry. *Hum. Reprod.* 11, 1457–1462. doi: 10.1093/oxfordjournals.humrep.a019419

Haidl, G., Badura, B., and Schill, W. B. (1994). Function of human epididymal spermatozoa. *J. Androl.* 15(Suppl.), 23S–27S.

Hourcade, J. D., Perez-Crespo, M., Fernandez-Gonzalez, R., Pintado, B., and Gutierrez-Adan, A. (2010). Selection against spermatozoa with fragmented DNA after postovulatory mating depends on the type of damage. *Reprod. Biol. Endocrinol.* 8:9. doi: 10.1186/1477-7827-8-9

Irvine, D. S., Twigg, J. P., Gordon, E. L., Fulton, N., Milne, P. A., and Aitken, R. J. (2000). DNA integrity in human spermatozoa: relationships with semen quality. *J. Androl.* 21, 33–44.

Kimura, Y., and Yanagimachi, R. (1995). Mouse oocytes injected with testicular spermatozoa or round spermatids can develop into normal offspring. *Development* 121, 2397–2405.

Martin, R. H., Ko, E., and Rademaker, A. (1988). Human sperm chromosome complements after microinjection of hamster eggs. *J. Reprod. Fertil.* 84, 179–186. doi: 10.1530/jrf.0.0840179

Mazur, P., Katkov, I. I., Katkova, N., and Critser, J. K. (2000). The enhancement of the ability of mouse sperm to survive freezing and thawing by the use of high concentrations of glycerol and the presence of an *Escherichia coli* membrane preparation (Oxyrase) to lower the oxygen concentration. *Cryobiology* 40, 187–209. doi: 10.1006/cryo.2000.2238

Moreira, P., Perez-Cerezales, S., Laguna, R., Fernandez-Gonzalez, R., Sanjuanbenito, B. P., and Gutierrez-Adan, A. (2016). Transgenic mouse offspring generated by ROSI. *J. Reprod. Dev.* 62, 37–42. doi: 10.1262/jrd.2015-105

Moreira, P. N., Fernandez-Gonzalez, R., Rizos, D., Ramirez, M., Perez-Crespo, M., and Gutierrez-Adan, A. (2005). Inadvertent transgenesis by conventional ICSI in mice. *Hum. Reprod.* 20, 3313–3317. doi: 10.1093/humrep/dei237

Moreira, P. N., Jimenez, A., Fernandez, R., Bury-Madrid, N., De La Fuente, J., Pintado, B., et al. (2003). Mouse ICSI with frozen-thawed sperm: the impact of sperm freezing procedure and sperm donor strain. *Mol. Reprod. Dev.* 66, 98–103. doi: 10.1002/mrd.10335

Perez-Cerezales, S., Miranda, A., and Gutierrez-Adan, A. (2012). Comparison of four methods to evaluate sperm DNA integrity between mouse caput and cauda epididymidis. *Asian J. Androl.* 14, 335–337. doi: 10.1038/aja.2011.119

Ramos-Ibeas, P., Calle, A., Fernandez-Gonzalez, R., Laguna-Barraza, R., Pericuesta, E., Calero, A., et al. (2014). Intracytoplasmic sperm injection using DNA-fragmented sperm in mice negatively affects embryo-derived embryonic stem cells, reduces the fertility of male offspring and induces heritable changes in epialleles. *PLoS One* 9:e95625. doi: 10.1371/journal.pone.0095625

Ramos-Ibeas, P., Pericuesta, E., Fernandez-Gonzalez, R., Ramirez, M. A., and Gutierrez-Adan, A. (2013). Most regions of mouse epididymis are able to phagocytose immature germ cells. *Reproduction* 146, 481–489. doi: 10.1530/REP-13-0145

Sharma, U., Sun, F., Conine, C. C., Reichholf, B., Kukreja, S., Herzog, V. A., et al. (2018). Small RNAs are trafficked from the epididymis to developing mammalian sperm. *Dev. Cell* 46:e486. doi: 10.1016/j.devcel.2018.06.023

Suganuma, R., Yanagimachi, R., and Meistrich, M. L. (2005). Decline in fertility of mouse sperm with abnormal chromatin during epididymal passage as revealed by ICSI. *Hum. Reprod.* 20, 3101–3108. doi: 10.1093/humrep/dei169

Sullivan, R., and Mieusset, R. (2016). The human epididymis: its function in sperm maturation. *Hum. Reprod. Update* 22, 574–587. doi: 10.1093/humupd/dmw015

Tateno, H. (2008). Chromosome aberrations in mouse embryos and fetuses produced by assisted reproductive technology. *Mutat. Res.* 657, 26–31. doi: 10.1016/j.mrgentox.2008.09.002

Tesarik, J., Greco, E., and Mendoza, C. (2004). Late, but not early, paternal effect on human embryo development is related to sperm DNA fragmentation. *Hum. Reprod.* 19, 611–615. doi: 10.1093/humrep/deh127

Yamauchi, Y., Ajduk, A., Riel, J. M., and Ward, M. A. (2007). Ejaculated and epididymal mouse spermatozoa are different in their susceptibility to nuclease-dependent DNA damage and in their nuclease activity. *Biol. Reprod.* 77, 636–647. doi: 10.1095/biolreprod.107.062406

Zhou, D., Suzuki, T., Asami, M., and Perry, A. C. F. (2019). Caput epididymidal mouse sperm support full development. *Dev. Cell* 50, 5–6. doi: 10.1016/j.devcel.2019.05.012

17

Transient Sperm Starvation Improves the Outcome of Assisted Reproductive Technologies

Felipe A. Navarrete[1], Luis Aguila[1], David Martin-Hidalgo[1,2], Darya A. Tourzani[1], Guillermina M. Luque[3], Goli Ardestani[1], Francisco A. Garcia-Vazquez[4,5], Lonny R. Levin[6], Jochen Buck[6], Alberto Darszon[7], Mariano G. Buffone[3], Jesse Mager[1], Rafael A. Fissore[1], Ana M. Salicioni[1], María G. Gervasi[1] and Pablo E. Visconti[1]**

[1] *Department of Veterinary and Animal Sciences, Integrated Sciences Building, University of Massachusetts Amherst, Amherst, MA, United States,* [2] *Research Group of Intracellular Signaling and Technology of Reproduction, Institute of Biotechnology in Agriculture and Livestock (INBIO G + C), University of Extremadura, Cáceres, Spain,* [3] *Instituto de Biología y Medicina Experimental, Consejo Nacional de Investigaciones Científicas y Técnicas, Buenos Aires, Argentina,* [4] *Department of Physiology, Veterinary School, International Excellence Campus for Higher Education and Research, University of Murcia, Murcia, Spain,* [5] *Institute for Biomedical Research of Murcia, IMIB-Arrixaca, Murcia, Spain,* [6] *Department of Pharmacology, Weill Cornell Medical College, Cornell University, New York, NY, United States,* [7] *Departamento de Genética del Desarrollo y Fisiología Molecular, Instituto de Biotecnología, Universidad Nacional Autónoma de México, Cuernavaca, Mexico*

***Correspondence:**
María G. Gervasi
mariagracia@vasci.umass.edu
Pablo E. Visconti
pvisconti@vasci.umass.edu

To become fertile, mammalian sperm must undergo a series of biochemical and physiological changes known as capacitation. These changes involve crosstalk between metabolic and signaling pathways and can be recapitulated *in vitro*. In this work, sperm were incubated in the absence of exogenous nutrients (starved) until they were no longer able to move. Once immotile, energy substrates were added back to the media and sperm motility was rescued. Following rescue, a significantly higher percentage of starved sperm attained hyperactivated motility and displayed increased ability to fertilize *in vitro* when compared with sperm persistently incubated in standard capacitation media. Remarkably, the effects of this treatment continue beyond fertilization as starved and rescued sperm promoted higher rates of embryo development, and once transferred to pseudo-pregnant females, blastocysts derived from treated sperm produced significantly more pups. In addition, the starvation and rescue protocol increased fertilization and embryo development rates in sperm from a severely sub-fertile mouse model, and when combined with temporal increase in Ca^{2+} ion levels, this methodology significantly improved fertilization and embryo development rates in sperm of sterile CatSper1 KO mice model. Intracytoplasmic sperm injection (ICSI) does not work in the agriculturally relevant bovine system. Here, we show that transient nutrient starvation of bovine sperm significantly enhanced ICSI success in this species. These data reveal that the conditions under which sperm are treated impact post-fertilization development and suggest that this "starvation and rescue method" can be used to improve assisted reproductive technologies (ARTs) in other mammalian species, including humans.

Keywords: sperm, blastocyst, embryo transfer, IVF, ICSI, capacitation

INTRODUCTION

Sperm capacitation is defined as all the biochemical and physiological events occurring after epididymal maturation that are necessary for the sperm to acquire fertilizing capacity (Yanagimachi, 1994; Gervasi and Visconti, 2016). Following this definition, capacitation ends once the sperm fuses with a metaphase II (MII)-arrested egg to become a zygote. The zygote follows a series of complex cell biological processes leading to the first cleavage, continuing with pre-implantation development and differentiation, implantation, and finally, birth of an offspring (White et al., 2018). Among these processes, capacitation, fertilization, and early embryo development can be mimicked *in vitro* in defined media (Ventura-Junca et al., 2015). Fertilization can also be achieved by intracytoplasmic sperm injection (ICSI) effectively bypassing many physiological events preceding gamete fusion (Palermo et al., 2017). These techniques are well established in many mammalian species including humans. However, the efficiency of these methods is species-specific, and success depends on other factors including the age of male and female gametes, environmental factors, and genetic background (Meldrum et al., 2016). Although many problems in capacitation can be overcome using ICSI, obtaining good quality preimplantation embryos at the blastocyst stage is a major limiting factor of successful pregnancies (Sadeghi, 2017).

Sperm capacitation depends upon crosstalk between metabolic and signaling pathways (Goodson et al., 2012). In mouse sperm, changes in motility pattern associated with capacitation (i.e., hyperactivation) are based on ATP produced by glycolysis (Miki et al., 2004). However, it is also clear that the Krebs cycle and oxidative phosphorylation are active in these cells (Goodson et al., 2012) and mammalian sperm capacitation media contain fuels for both glycolysis (i.e., glucose) and oxidative phosphorylation (i.e., pyruvate). To explore the specific role of these fuels for capacitation, initially, we incubated mouse sperm in media devoid of all nutrients (starvation step). Once sperm became motionless, defined energy molecules (e.g., glucose and pyruvate) were added back (rescue step). We hypothesized that after energy depletion, adding back nutrients to the sperm incubation media would induce recovery of sperm functionality. Indeed, the recovery was observed; however, the starvation and rescue protocol significantly increased the percentage of sperm achieving hyperactivated motility and also enhanced *in vitro* fertilization (IVF) rates when compared with sperm persistently incubated in standard capacitation media containing glucose and pyruvate. Also unexpectedly, the embryos fertilized with previously starved and recovered sperm were more efficient in reaching the blastocyst stage; and these blastocysts produced approximately three times more pups when transferred to pseudo-pregnant females.

The need for capacitation is often overcome by the use of ICSI. Although this procedure is highly successful in mice, ICSI with bovine sperm presents severe challenges and only succeeds when the egg is artificially activated (Catt and Rhodes, 1995; Malcuit et al., 2006). We now show that the starvation and rescue protocol improves ICSI success rates in the bovine system. Together, these results indicate that sperm incubation conditions can improve the outcome of embryo development and that capacitation-associated changes occurring in sperm before fertilization are still relevant for post-fertilization events. The molecular basis of these changes is still not known and warrants future investigation. Some of the hypotheses regarding these mechanisms will be briefly mentioned in the section "Discussion."

RESULTS

Sperm from CD1 mice incubated in TYH media lacking glucose and pyruvate stopped moving after ~40 min (**Supplementary Video S1**). We reasoned that these sperm had ceased swimming because they had consumed all available stored nutrients, and we refer to them as "starved." Once immotile, glucose and pyruvate were added back to reach standard concentrations in TYH media (5.56 mM glucose and 0.5 mM pyruvate, **Supplementary Video S1**). For the purpose of comparison, parallel control incubations were done resuspending sperm in standard TYH capacitating conditions persistently incubated in the presence of nutrients. Counter-intuitively, a higher percentage of starved and capacitated sperm were motile (**Figure 1A**) and became hyperactivated (**Figure 1B**) after addition of nutrients compared to control sperm persistently incubated in the presence of nutrients in standard TYH capacitating conditions. Hereafter, we refer to this procedure, in which sperm energy is recovered after starvation, using the acronym SER.

Considering that SER produced a higher percentage of hyperactivated sperm, we hypothesized that SER-treated sperm would also improve fertilization rates. IVF using sperm from CD1 mice is highly efficient (over 90%). Therefore, to test the effectiveness of SER in IVF and other assisted reproductive technologies (ARTs), we switched to using sperm from inbred C57BL/6J which have lower IVF and embryo development rates (Liu et al., 2009). C57BL/6J sperm were capacitated in standard TYH media with BSA and HCO_3^- (CAP) containing nutrients or incubated in nutrient-free CAP TYH media until becoming immotile and then rescued by addition of glucose and pyruvate (SER). Similar to sperm from CD1 mice, SER increased motility (**Figure 1C**) and hyperactivation rates (**Figure 1D**) of C57BL/6J sperm. In addition, SER-treated C57BL/6J sperm yielded more eggs reaching the two-cell stage when incubated with heterologous CD1 MII-arrested eggs (**Figure 2A**; $n = 38$) as well as when incubated with homologous MII-arrested eggs from C57BL/6J females (**Figure 2D**; $n = 15$). Representative images of two-cell stage embryos are displayed in **Figure 2G**.

More surprising than the improvement observed in fertilization rates, in both homologous and heterologous conditions, a significantly higher percentage of two-cell embryos reached blastocyst stage (**Figures 2B,E** blastocyst % from two-cell). Representative images of blastocyst development are shown in **Figure 2H**. To compare the efficiency of the treatments, these results were also presented as the percentage of the initial number of eggs reaching blastocyst stage (**Figures 2C,F**, blastocyst % from initial number of eggs). For more information, these data are also presented in **Supplementary Figure S1** and tabulated

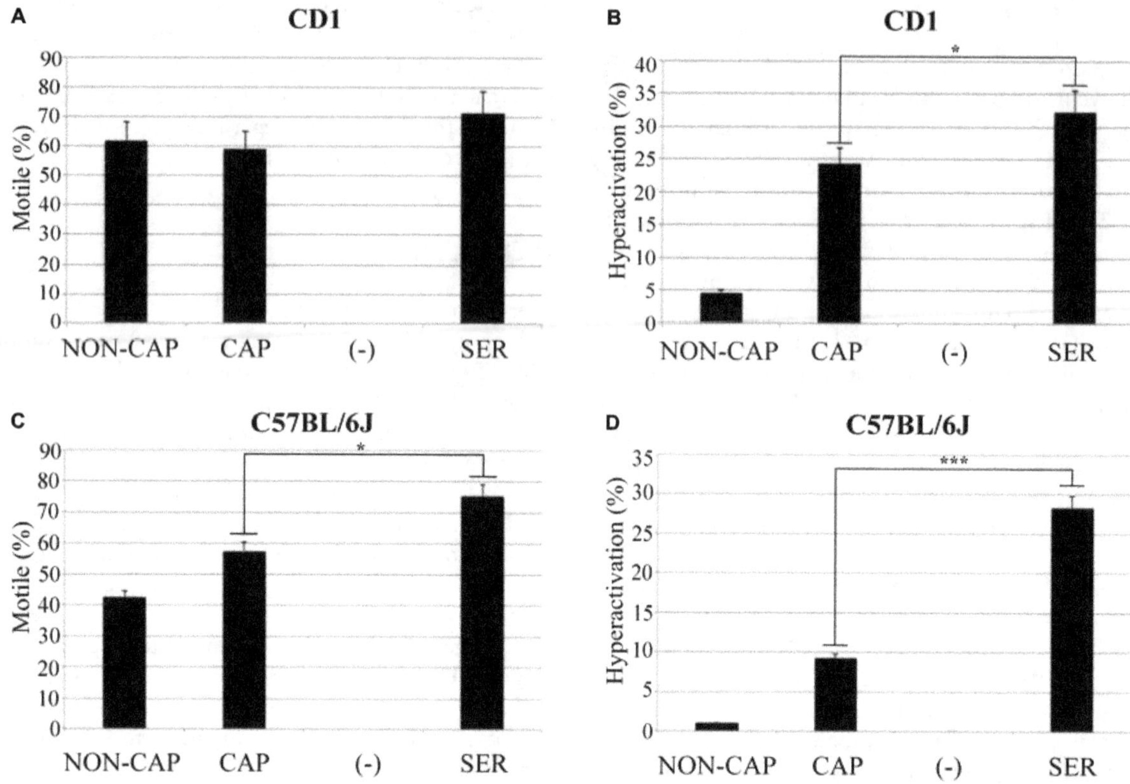

FIGURE 1 | Sperm energy restriction and recovery (SER) treatment improves sperm motility. Experimental conditions non-capacitated (NON-CAP), capacitated (CAP), sperm energy restriction without recovery (-) or sperm energy restriction and recovery (SER) were established by the incubation in different media as indicated in the section "Materials and Methods." After treatment under the different conditions, sperm motility was analyzed by computer-assisted sperm analysis (CASA). Two different strains of mice were analyzed, as follows: **(A)** Percentage of total motility for sperm of the outbred mice strain CD1. **(B)** Percentage of hyperactivated motility (out of total motile) for sperm of the outbred mice strain CD1. **(C)** Percentage of total motility for sperm of the inbred mouse strain C57BL/6J. **(D)** Percentage of hyperactivated motility (out of total motile) for sperm of the inbred mouse strain C57BL/6J. In each panel, significant differences are indicated as: $^{*}p < 0.05$ and $^{***}p < 0.001$, $n = 5$.

in **Supplementary Table S1** according to male mice age. To evaluate blastocyst developmental potential, in a fraction of the experiments described above ($n = 19$, $n = 15$ for heterologous CD1 female x C57BL/6J male IVF and $n = 4$ for homologous C57BL/6J female x C57BL/6J male), an equal number of blastocysts derived from CAP or SER-treated sperm were non-surgically transferred to pseudo-pregnant females. Unexpectedly, the number of pups born from SER-treated sperm derived blastocysts was over three times higher than the number of pups born from control blastocysts (**Figure 3A** for heterologous IVF and **Supplementary Table S1** for heterologous and homologous IVF). The improvement in embryo development is reflected in the increased ratio of transferred blastocysts producing offspring (**Figure 3B** and **Supplementary Table S1**). In addition, blastocyst quality was also assessed by counting the total cell number present at the blastocyst stage (**Figure 3C**) as well as by blastocyst outgrowth (**Figure 3D**). These analyses revealed a higher number of cells and percentage of outgrowth of blastocysts derived from SER-treated sperm. Thus, these data indicate that transient nutrient withdrawal provides a qualitative improvement in the ability of sperm to produce embryos, and this effect is not simply due to increased ability to fertilize oocytes.

The aforementioned experiments indicate an overall better success in fertilization, embryo development, and pregnancy rates when SER-treated sperm are used. We next sought to determine if this methodology enhances IVF and embryo development rates in sub-fertile and sterile mouse models. Recently, we showed that sperm derived from $FER^{DR/DR}$ mice, in which the FER tyrosine kinase is replaced by a non-active mutant, are severely sub-fertile *in vitro* (Alvau et al., 2016). When compared to sperm incubated in standard capacitation media, SER-treated $FER^{DR/DR}$ sperm significantly increased fertilization rates (**Figure 4A**) and embryo development (**Figures 4B,C**). When these embryos were transferred to pseudo-pregnant females, live pups were born (**Figure 4D**). We next tested the SER treatment on sperm from CatSper1 KO mice, which are sterile (Ren et al., 2001). We recently found that a short incubation of CatSper1 KO sperm with Ca^{2+} ionophore A_{23187} induced fertilizing capacity in these normally infertile sperm (Navarrete et al., 2016). SER treatment alone did not rescue the fertilizing capacity of CatSper1 KO sperm. However, the two treatments proved to be synergistic; sequential treatment of CatSper1 KO sperm with SER and A_{23187} significantly increased fertilization (**Figure 5A**) and embryo development (**Figure 5B**) rates when

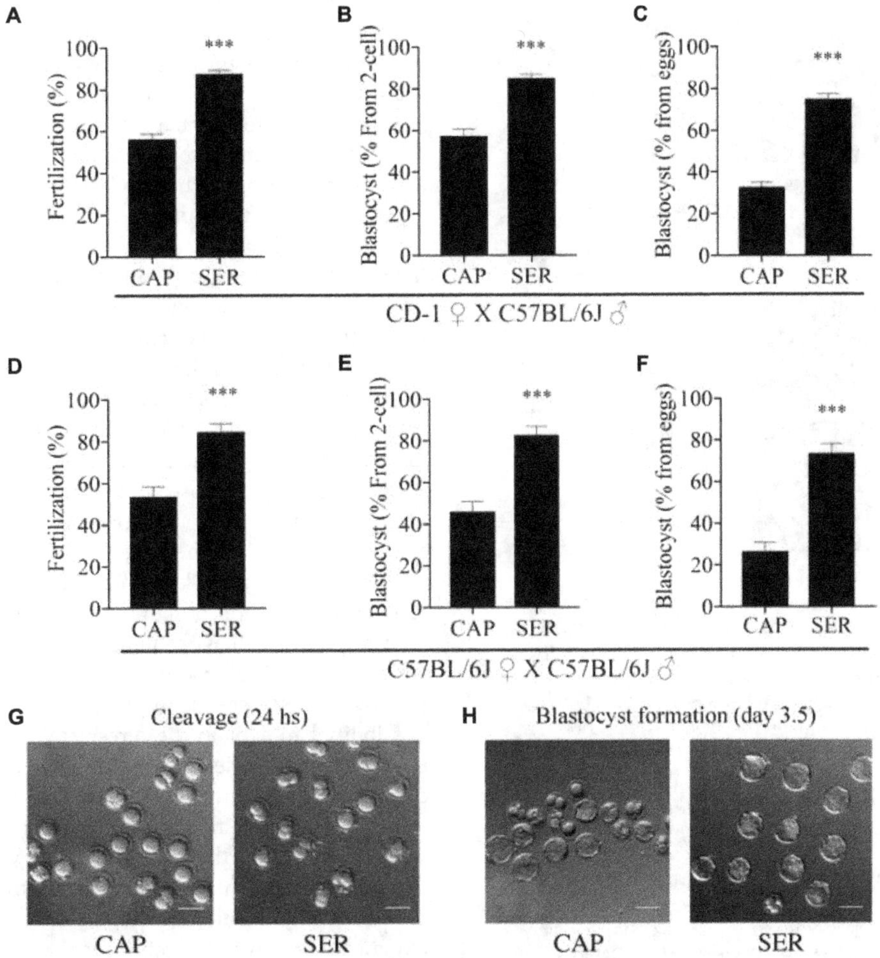

FIGURE 2 | Sperm energy restriction and recovery (SER) treatment improves fertilization and embryo development rates in C57BL/6J male mice. Sperm obtained from C57BL/6J mice were incubated in C-TYH, containing glucose and pyruvate (CAP) or in F-TYH media, not containing nutrients; sperm in this medium will then be rescued by energy sources replenishment as explained in the section "Materials and Methods," and the treatment abbreviated (SER). After treatment (CAP or SER) sperm from each condition were added to the insemination drops containing cumulus-enclosed female oocytes (COCs). **(A)** Percentage of fertilization calculated as percentage of oocytes that reached a two-cell embryo stage after heterologous fertilization between CD-1 female oocytes and C57BL/6J sperm (n = 38, total number of oocytes CAP = 2030, total number of oocytes SER = 2024). **(B)** Percentage of blastocyst development calculated as percentage of two-cell embryos that reached 3.5-day blastocyst stage corresponding to embryo cultures after heterologous CD-1 female oocytes and C57BL/6J sperm IVF (n = 38). **(C)** Percentage of total blastocyst development calculated as the percentage of 3.5-day blastocyst stage embryos out of the total number of inseminated eggs corresponding to embryo cultures after heterologous CD-1 female oocytes and C57BL/6J sperm IVF (n = 38). **(D)** Percentage of fertilization calculated as percentage of oocytes that reached two-cell embryo stage after homologous fertilization between C57BL/6J female oocytes and C57BL/6J sperm (n = 15, total number of oocytes CAP = 608, total number of oocytes SER = 685). **(E)** Percentage of blastocyst development calculated as percentage of the two-cell embryos that reached 3.5-day blastocyst stage from embryo cultures after homologous C57BL/6J female oocytes and C57BL/6J sperm IVF (n = 15). **(F)** Percentage of total blastocyst development calculated as the percentage of 3.5-day blastocyst stage embryos out of the total number of inseminated eggs from embryo cultures after homologous C57BL/6J female oocytes and C57BL/6J sperm IVF (n = 15). In each panel, significant differences are indicated as $^{***}p < 0.001$. **(G)** Representative images of two-cell embryos obtained after heterologous, CD-1 female oocytes and C57BL/6J sperm, SER, or control IVF. Scale bar = 100 μm. **(H)** Representative images of heterologous IVF-derived blastocyst development at 3.5 days. Scale bar = 100 μm.

compared with A_{23187} alone. When blastocysts (**Figure 5C**) from these experiments were transferred to pseudo-pregnant females, live pups were born (Table in **Figure 5D**).

While ICSI in the mouse is quite successful, the efficiency of this technique in bovines is very poor when compared to other species (Salamone et al., 2017). Therefore, we used frozen bovine sperm and *in vitro* matured bovine oocytes to test if SER can also improve ICSI success rates. Contrary to mouse sperm, bovine sperm motility was reduced but did not completely stop during incubation in the absence of exogenous energy sources. Bovine capacitation media normally contain pyruvate and lactate but do not contain glucose; therefore, after 3 h in the absence (starvation step) of nutrients, pyruvate and lactate were added back, and normal motility was restored. Individual bovine sperm were injected into oocytes (ICSI) and the number of zygotes undergoing cleavage divisions was evaluated. The percentage of two-cell embryos was increased over threefold in SER-treated bovine sperm relative to controls persistently

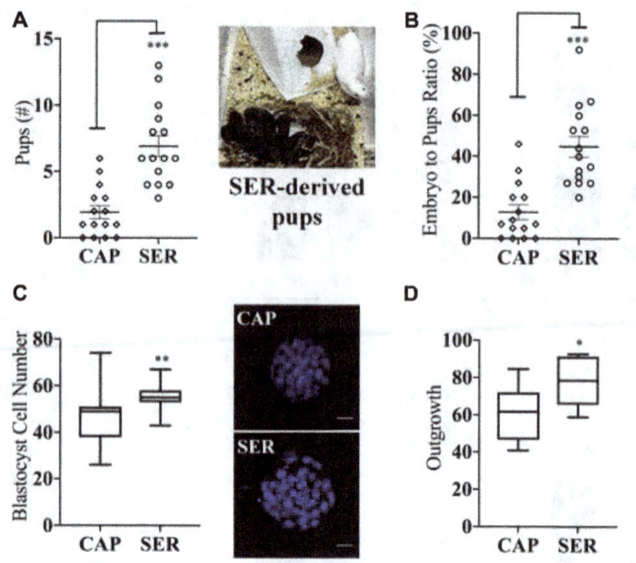

FIGURE 3 | Sperm energy restriction and recovery (SER) treatment impacts on embryonic parameters and implantation potential after non-surgical embryo transfer. A fraction of the blastocysts derived from CAP or SER treatments as described in **Figure 2** were used to evaluate the impact of these treatments in blastocyst potential. **(A)** Blastocysts derived from CAP- or SER-treated sperm were transferred to pseudo-pregnant recipient female mice. The total number of pups obtained from either CAP or SER treatment (n = 15) is indicated. Image shown is representative of a litter obtained after transfer of SER-derived embryos. **(B)** Percentage of pups born per number of embryos transferred is indicated. **(C)** Blastocysts derived from CAP- or SER-treated sperm were stained with Hoechst as indicated in the section "Materials and Methods." The number of stained nuclei that represents the number of cells in each blastocyst was counted (n = 3, 35 blastocysts/treatment counted). Representative images of stained embryos are shown. Scale bar = 25 μm. **(D)** Blastocyst derived from CAP or SER-treated sperm were assayed for outgrowth *in vitro* as explained in the section "Materials and Methods" (n = 10, 205 and 210 blastocysts counted for CAP and SER-derived blastocysts, respectively). In each panel, significant differences are indicated as: $^*p < 0.05$; $^{**}p < 0.01$, and $^{***}p < 0.001$. Experiments represented in this figure were done using blastocysts obtained by heterologous fertilization.

incubated in the presence of nutrients. Importantly, almost 17% of these two-cell embryos developed into blastocysts compared to zero blastocysts obtained from sperm incubated in standard capacitation conditions (**Table 1**).

DISCUSSION

Infertility and sub-fertility are critical health problems with social and economic consequences. About 9% of couples worldwide present signs of infertility. Since the first successful "Test-Tube" baby in 1978, over 5 million babies were born using ARTs. ARTs include IVF, artificial insemination (AI), ICSI, *in vitro* maturation of oocytes, superovulation, cryopreservation, and embryo transfer techniques. In addition to their use in human clinical application, ARTs are also used for agricultural domestic species and for production and maintenance of valuable laboratory animals which often present reproductive problems (Behringer et al., 2014). Despite their frequent use, ART methods are usually expensive, time consuming, and can be plagued by limited successful pregnancy rates (de Mouzon et al., 2010; Mantikou et al., 2013). At the basic research level, our group has recently shown that we can induce *in vitro* fertilizing capacity in sperm from sterile knock-out genetic models using a short incubation with the Ca^{2+} ionophore A_{23187} (Navarrete et al., 2016). Interestingly, short treatment with A_{23187} also increased fertilization and embryo development rates of control inbred C57BL/6J mice sperm (Navarrete et al., 2016) suggesting that embryo development can be affected by differential sperm incubation conditions during capacitation.

Capacitation can be achieved *in vitro* in defined media containing ions, a cholesterol binding source, and energy substrates (reviewed in Gervasi and Visconti (2016)). In the mouse, capacitation and IVF can be achieved with TYH medium containing only glucose and pyruvate as energy compounds (Toyoda and Yokoyama, 2016). Here, we observed that mouse sperm incubated in the absence of these exogenous nutrients become immotile in less than 40 min and motility can be rescued with the addition of glucose and pyruvate. Once rescued, starved sperm achieved higher percentages of hyperactivation and IVF rates. We do not yet know the molecular basis for this improvement in sperm functional parameters. Two alternative possibilities to explain these results are that due to the need for energy sources molecules limiting capacitation competence are consumed during the starvation stage; or that during rescue, molecules supporting capacitation are upregulated. Another possibility is that the starvation followed by rescue protocol induces changes in metabolites, supporting an increase of certain metabolites that could be beneficial for the development of sperm hyperactivated motility and fertilization. Finally, we cannot discard changes in the production of radical oxygen species (ROS) which have been associated with deleterious effects on sperm motility as well as with beneficial effects on capacitation (de Lamirande and Gagnon, 1995; Aitken, 2017). Further investigations are being performed to test these hypotheses.

Unexpectedly, eggs fertilized with SER-treated sperm showed significantly greater percentage of two-cell embryos reaching the blastocyst stage. Moreover, at 3.5 days post-fertilization, blastocysts derived from SER-treated sperm had a higher percentage of outgrowth and higher number of total cells, parameters that are indicative of good implantation potential (Binder et al., 2015). Furthermore, when transferred to pseudo-pregnant females, blastocysts derived from SER-treated sperm gave rise to a higher number of pups than those obtained with sperm incubated in standard capacitation conditions. These experiments indicate that blastocysts derived from SER-treated sperm have advantages over those obtained from sperm incubated in standard capacitation media. In concordance with our findings, it has been proposed that sperm incubation conditions for IVF can affect embryonic development (Jaakma et al., 1997; Matas et al., 2003; Zheng et al., 2018). However, the molecular basis of sperm-derived post-fertilization effects remains unknown. We hypothesize that the post-fertilization effects observed after sperm SER treatment are related to epigenetic changes in the male gamete. Environmental factors can

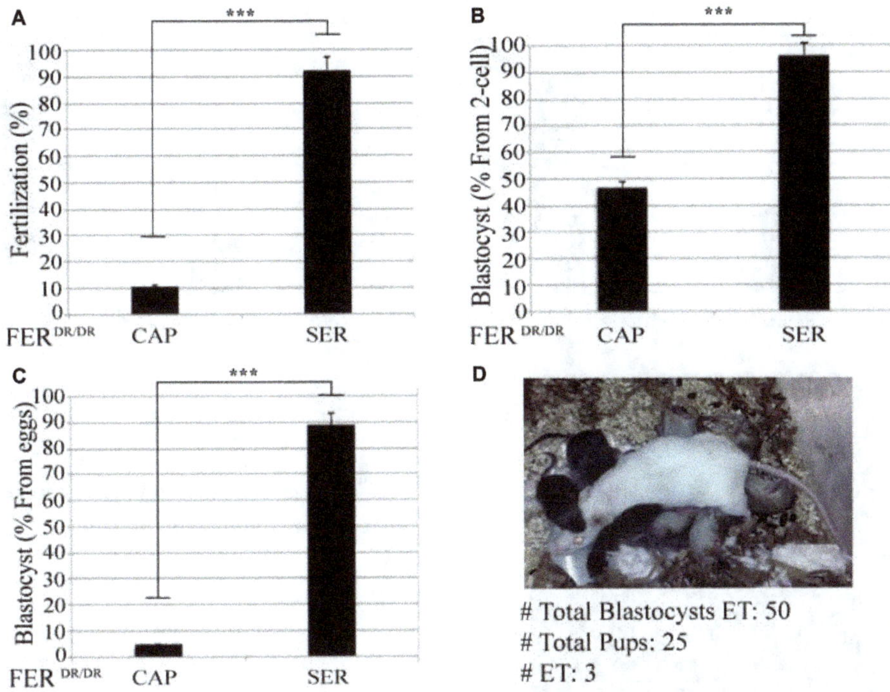

FIGURE 4 | Sperm energy restriction and recovery (SER) treatment rescues sperm fertilization capacity and embryo development of a sub-fertile mouse strain. Sperm obtained from $Fer^{DR/DR}$ mice were treated under CAP or SER conditions and used for insemination as described in the section "Materials and Methods." **(A)** Percentage of fertilization of $Fer^{DR/DR}$ sperm calculated as percentage of oocytes that reached two-cell embryo stage. **(B)** Percentage of blastocyst development calculated as percentage of the two-cell embryos that reached 3.5-day blastocyst stage. **(C)** Percentage of total blastocyst formation calculated as the percentage of 3.5-day blastocyst stage embryos out of the total number of inseminated eggs. **(D)** Representative image of a recipient female with its embryo-transferred pups. A total of three embryo transfers (ET) were performed as indicated in **Supplementary Table S1**. In each panel, significant differences are indicated as ***$p < 0.001$.

influence epigenetic processes, change gene expression, and have a great impact on development. Epigenetic marks such as, DNA methylation, and histone tail modifications, show asymmetrical distribution between male and female gamete and play critical roles in embryo development (Marcho et al., 2015; Canovas et al., 2017). Recent evidence suggests that small non-coding RNAs in sperm have a role in non-genomic inheritance of paternal traits (Chen et al., 2016; Sharma et al., 2016; Conine et al., 2018). One intriguing possibility is that SER treatment can affect RNA levels including the pool of non-coding RNAs, which could impact post-fertilization development. On the other hand, it has been shown that the state of the sperm chromatin contains critical information for the regulation of gene expression after fertilization (Jung et al., 2017, 2019). One possibility is that SER treatment is inducing changes in the sperm chromatin prior fertilization, and that those changes have a direct impact in the development of the embryo. We are currently studying these possibilities.

Intracytoplasmic sperm injection is a technique by which sperm are directly introduced into the egg, bypassing the need for capacitation. In mice, ICSI is very successful, effectively rescuing several sperm sterile phenotypes (Kuretake et al., 1996; Yanagimachi et al., 2004; Ihara et al., 2005). In contrast, embryo development after ICSI is compromised in bovines, and successful development requires additional treatments with reagents that induce egg activation (Catt and Rhodes, 1995; Malcuit et al., 2006; Salamone et al., 2017). ICSI has also been achieved by pre-treating bovine sperm or eggs with diverse reagents (Rho et al., 1998; Aguila et al., 2017; Canel et al., 2017). At present, it is not clear why bovine sperm do not induce egg activation, but our data suggest that SER treatment of bovine sperm stimulates their ability to activate oocytes. One of the best characterized sperm contributions to early embryo development is the phospholipase C zeta (PLCζ)-mediated induction of Ca^{2+} oscillations (Saunders et al., 2002). We hypothesized that in bovine sperm, the PLCζ protein and its activity are closely guarded such that its release requires active nuclear remodeling. Consistently, our group has recently shown that injected bovine sperm are resistant to nuclear remodeling and decondensation by *in vitro* matured bovine oocytes and that treating these oocytes with ionomycin plus cycloheximide (CHX) to chemically induce acute activation and sperm head decondensation can partially overcome the poor success of this technique in this species (Aguila et al., 2017). In addition, it has been recently shown that the sperm-borne protein glutathione-S-transferase omega 2 facilitates nuclear decondensation after fertilization (Hamilton et al., 2019). These results suggest that during penetration through the cumulus and zona pellucida layers, bovine sperm undergo changes that induce or support nuclear remodeling, which facilitate the subsequent exposure and/or activation of PLCζ. Our data indicate that SER treatment of bovine sperm stimulates their ability to activate oocytes

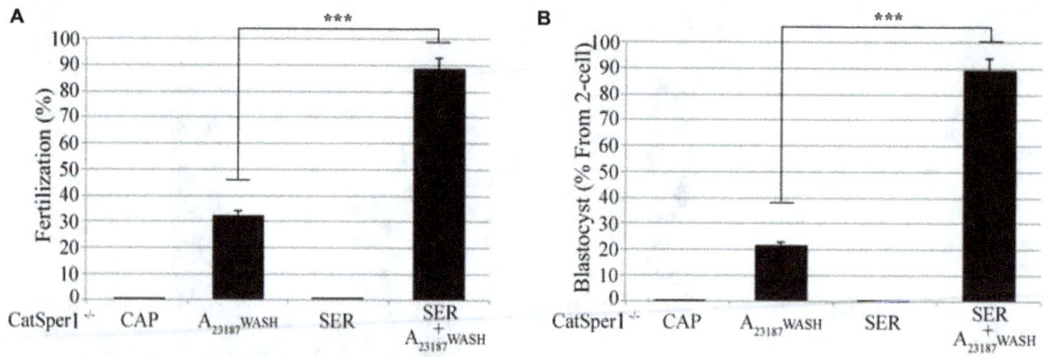

C

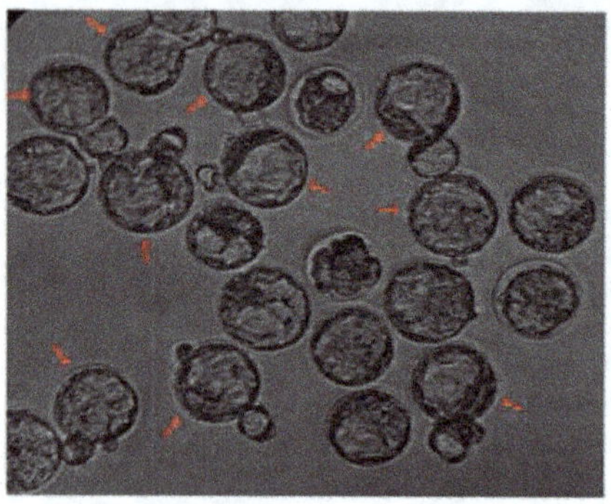

D

Treatment	Number of embryos transferred	Number of pups (% out of transferred)
A_{23187} WASH	27	6 (22 %)
SER + A_{23187} WASH	45	16 (36 %)

FIGURE 5 | Combination of sperm energy restriction and recovery (SER) treatment and A23187 (transient treatment) rescues sperm fertilization capacity and embryo development of infertile CatSper1 KO mice. Sperm from CatSper1 KO mice were incubated in four conditions as detailed in the section "Materials and Methods." Briefly, the experimental conditions applied were: (1) capacitating conditions in the presence of glucose and pyruvate (CAP); (2) A23187 transient treatment (A23187 WASH); (3) capacitating conditions in the absence of glucose and pyruvate followed by replenishment of energy substrates (SER); and (4) SER treatment followed by A23187 transient treatment (SER + A23187 WASH). Sperm were used for IVF of cumulus-enclosed CD1 female oocytes. After 18 h, two-cell embryos were transferred to KSOM media and further incubated for a total of 3.5 days until blastocyst stage. **(A)** Percentage of fertilization calculated as percentage of oocytes that reached two-cell embryo stage. **(B)** Percentage of blastocyst development calculated as percentage of the two-cell embryos that reached 3.5-day blastocyst stage. **(C)** Representative image of 3.5-day blastocysts formation from combined SER treatment followed by A23187 transient treatment. Arrows indicate blastocysts hatching. **(D)** Results showing total 3.5-day blastocysts obtained from either SER-treated alone, or SER + A23187-treated sperm, that were NSET-transferred to pseudo-pregnant female recipients (n = 3), and the number of pups born after 21 days of gestation. In each panel, significant differences are indicated as ***$p < 0.001$.

following fertilization by ICSI. We hypothesize that in bovine sperm, SER conditions induce remodeling of the sperm head facilitating nuclear decondensation and PLCζ release, just as it occurs during the process of natural sperm entry and fertilization. It will be interesting to determine whether the mechanism increasing sperm functional parameters and improving embryo development success rates in mice are related to the molecular changes which increase egg activation rates in bovines.

In all ARTs, the limiting step for a successful pregnancy is the attainment of embryos competent for implantation that can develop into viable fetuses (Geary and Moon, 2006; Patrizio et al., 2007). Poor quality of embryos results in higher rates of implantation failure (Takeuchi et al., 2017). Not surprisingly, most clinical research in humans and species of economic relevance has focused on improving embryo culture techniques (Summers, 2013) and selecting the best embryos to be transferred to the female (Castello et al., 2016; Vaiarelli et al., 2016). In particular, embryos can be selected by monitoring embryo development in real time using imaging technology or by preimplantation genetic diagnostic (PGD; Castello et al., 2016; Vaiarelli et al., 2016). In comparison, less research has been conducted to investigate sperm contributions to embryo quality. For ICSI, recent efforts focused on selecting high quality sperm using high microscopy magnification (Goswami et al., 2018), a method, known as morphologically selected sperm injection (IMSI). IMSI has been used by different clinics with a variety of outcomes (De Vos et al., 2013; Luna et al., 2015). More recently, thermotaxis was used to select sperm for ICSI using temperature gradients (Perez-Cerezales et al., 2018). After ICSI, thermotaxis-selected sperm resulted in higher percentage of blastocyst development and better implantation rates than non-selected sperm (Perez-Cerezales et al., 2018). These investigations

TABLE 1 | Effect of SER treatment on the *in vitro* development of bovine embryos generated by ICSI, piezoelectric-aided.

Treatment	*n* (total)	Day 3 cleaved embryos (%)	Day 8 Blastocyst/cleaved embryos (%)
ICSI control	5 (80)	13 (16)[b]	0 (0)[b]
ICSI + SER	5 (84)	42 (50)[a]	7 (17)[a]

Data followed by different superscripts (a,b) are significantly different ($p < 0.05$).

suggest that the condition of the sperm prior to fertilization contributes to embryo development and that sperm selection prior to ICSI has the potential to be used in the clinic to improve pregnancy rates. Similarly, SER-treated sperm increased embryo development and pregnancy rates; however, instead of selecting the best sperm, SER appears to improve the overall sperm quality increasing their chances to produce high-quality embryos.

Translationally, SER treatment can be used for more efficient transgenic mouse production. SER treatment increased fertilization and embryo development rates of $Fer^{DR/DR}$ mice which have a severely *in vitro* sub-fertile phenotype (Alvau et al., 2016). As another model, CatSper1 KO mice are infertile (Ren et al., 2001). In previous work, we showed that a short exposure of Ca^{2+} ionophore A_{23187} to sperm induced IVF rates of 30% in CatSper1 KO mice (Navarrete et al., 2016). SER treatment alone was not able to induce fertilizing capacity in sperm from sterile CatSper1 KO mice. One important difference between these two models is that while $FER^{DR/DR}$ mouse model is fertile *in vivo*, CatSper1 KO is completely sterile. We hypothesize that SER treatment is able to bypass lack of tyrosine phosphorylation in $FER^{DR/DR}$ because sperm from these mice are still able to fertilize. In this case, SER is only improving their ability to fertilize. On the other hand, CatSper1 KO mice are completely sterile *in vivo* and *in vitro*. When we combined both treatments, we found a synergistic increase of fertilization and embryo development rates in CatSper1 KO mice. These experiments suggest that an increase in sperm $[Ca^{2+}]_i$ is still required for SER to work.

Overall, the sperm energy restriction treatment is a novel method that improves both sperm fertilization rates and embryo development after IVF. The molecular mechanisms triggered by the sperm SER treatment prior IVF or ICSI are still not understood. Our data raise a series of very important still unanswered questions that call for new investigations in the field of reproductive biology and early embryo development. Importantly, our results indicate that sperm capacitation conditions continue to be relevant after fertilization has occurred, opening new avenues to study the relationship between sperm capacitation and early embryo development. The overall SER improvements in sperm function before and after fertilization have the potential to be applied to other mammalian species including humans and to impact ART practices worldwide.

MATERIALS AND METHODS

Materials

Chemicals and other lab reagents were purchased as follows: 4-Bromo-Ca^{2+} Ionophore A_{23187} (B7272), bovine serum albumin (BSA, fatty acid-free, A0281) for media, pregnant mare serum gonadotropin (PMSG) (G4877), and human chorionic gonadotropin (hCG) (CG5) from Sigma (St. Louis, MO, United States). Non-surgical embryo transfer (NSET) device was acquired from Paratechs (Billerica, MA, United States). Light mineral oil (ES-005-C) and EmbryoMax® KSOM Medium (1X) with 1/2 Amino Acids (MR-106-D) were obtained from Millipore (Billerica, MA, United States). Paraformaldehyde was purchased from Electron Microscopy Sciences (Hatfield, PA, United States). Hoechst 33342 was obtained from ThermoFisher Scientific (Agawam, MA, United States).

Animals

All procedures involving experimental animals were performed in accordance with Protocol 2016-0026 approved by the University of Massachusetts Amherst Institutional Animal Care and Use Committee (IACUC). Male CD-1 (ICR) retired breeders, female CD1 (ICR) 8–12 weeks of age, and male CD-1 (ICR) vasectomized mice were obtained from Charles River Laboratories (Wilmington, MA, United States). Male C57BL/6J (different ages) and female C57BL/6J 8-weeks of age mice were obtained from The Jackson Laboratory (Farmington, CT, United States). Male Fer $^{DR/DR}$ mice (Craig et al., 2001) were obtained from Dr. Greer from Queen's University, Kingston (ON, Canada). Infertile CatSper1 KO (Ren et al., 2001) mice were obtained from Dr. Clapham and Dr. Chung from Harvard University, Boston (MA, United States).

Computer-Assisted Sperm Analysis (CASA)

Sperm incubation for analysis of motility was performed in a HEPES modified Toyoda–Yokoyama–Hosi (HEPES-TYH) medium (Toyoda et al., 1971) containing 119.37 mM NaCl, 4.7 mM KCl, 1.71 mM $CaCl_2.2H_2O$, 1.2 mM KH_2PO_4, 1.2 mM $MgSO_4.7H_2O$, 0.51 mM Na-pyruvate, 5.56 mM glucose, and 20 mM HEPES (pH 7.4). This medium does not contain HCO_3^- or BSA and does not support capacitation; it was named (NON-CAP-HEPES-TYH) and abbreviated as NON-CAP in **Figure 1**. The same medium supplemented with 15 mM HCO_3^- and 5 mg/mL BSA support capacitation, it was named CAP-HEPES-TYH and abbreviated as CAP in **Figure 1**. Starvation was done in CAP medium in which glucose and pyruvate were omitted; this medium was named Free-CAP-HEPES-TYH and notated with the symbol (-) in **Figure 1**. Finally, rescue was performed by incubating sperm first in FREE-HEPES-TYH until motility stopped and then recovered in CAP-HEPES-TYH medium. Following the same abbreviation used throughout this manuscript, this procedure was abbreviated as SER in **Figure 1**.

To conduct computer-assisted sperm analyses (CASA), for each replicate, cauda epididymides from two mice were dissected, cut in half, and distributed in specific media as follows: (1) for non-capacitating conditions (NON-CAP), two half epididymis from each mouse were collected in NON-CAP-HEPES-TYH containing energy substrates but lacking $NaHCO_3$ and BSA; (2) for capacitating conditions (CAP), two half epididymis from each mouse were collected in CAP-HEPES-TYH containing energy substrates and supplemented with 15 mM $NaHCO_3$ and 5 mg/mL of BSA; (3 and 4) the remaining half epididymides were collected in FREE-CAP-HEPES-TYH medium devoid of glucose and pyruvate supplemented with 15 mM $NaHCO_3$ and 5 mg/mL of BSA. In all these cases, after 10 min of sperm swim-out, epididymides were removed and samples were washed by two sequential centrifugations, using the respective incubation media. Sperm were then counted for each condition; equal number of sperm ($\sim$2 million sperm) were then divided in four aliquots (notice that starved sperm in FREE-CAP-HEPES-TYH are divided in two different aliquots) and incubated at 37°C in 500 μL of their respective medium. After ~40 min (when sperm in starvation conditions stop moving), to facilitate washing, additional 1.5 mL of the appropriate media (as defined in the next sentence) was added to each aliquot. Appropriate media mean: for condition 1 (NON-CAP), NON-CAP-HEPES-TYH; for condition 2 (CAP), CAP-HEPES-TYH, for condition 3 (-), FREE-CAP-HEPES-TYH; and for condition 4 (SER), same as for condition 2, CAP-HEPES-TYH. Sperm suspensions were then centrifuged for 5 min at 150 × *g* at room temperature, 1.7 mL of supernatants was removed leaving the bottom 300 μL in the tubes to avoid losing sperm cells. Additional 200 μL of the respective media was added and each aliquot incubated for 60 additional minutes. After this period, sperm suspensions (25 μL) were loaded into pre-warmed chamber slide (depth, 100 μm) (Leja slide, Spectrum Technologies) and placed on a microscope stage at 37°C. Sperm motility was examined using the CEROS computer-assisted semen analysis (CASA) system (Hamilton Thorne Research, Beverly, MA, United States) as previously described (Sanchez-Cardenas et al., 2018). The default settings include the following: frames acquired: 90; frame rate: 60 Hz; minimum cell size: 4 pixels; static head size: 0.13–2.43; static head intensity: 0.10–1.52; and static head elongation: 5–100. Sperm with hyperactivated motility, defined as motility with high amplitude thrashing patterns and short distance of travel, were sorted and analyzed using the CASAnova software (Goodson et al., 2011). At least five microscopy fields corresponding to a minimum of 200 sperm were analyzed for each treatment in each experiment.

Sperm Preparation for *in vitro* Fertilization (IVF)

Media used for IVF assay did not contain HEPES; instead pH 7.4 was maintained using HCO_3^-/CO_2 buffer system. For these assays, we used Toyoda–Yokoyama–Hosi Complete TYH (C-TYH) medium (Toyoda et al., 1971) containing 119.37 mM NaCl, 4.7 mM KCl, 1.71 mM $CaCl_2.2H_2O$, 1.2 mM KH_2PO_4, 1.2 mM $MgSO_4$. $7H_2O$, 25.1 mM $NaHCO_3$, 0.51 mM Na-pyruvate, 5.56 mM glucose, and 4 mg/mL BSA, 10 μg/mL gentamicin and phenol red 0.0006% equilibrated at 5% CO_2 to reach pH 7.4. For media used for starvation, glucose and pyruvate were omitted from the medium described above and was called F-TYH.

For IVF, spermatozoa were collected from the cauda epididymis. In each case, the two epididymides from the same mouse were separated and incubated in different conditions. One of the cauda was placed in 2 mL of C-TYH, containing glucose and pyruvate and abbreviated as CAP in **Figures 2–5**. The other one was placed in 2 mL of F-TYH media, not containing nutrients; sperm in this medium will then be rescued and the treatment abbreviated SER in **Figures 2–5**. After 10 min of sperm swim-out, each cauda epididymis was removed from the tubes, and sperm were washed by two sequential centrifugations using the respective incubation medium as follows. First, sperm suspensions were centrifuged for 5 min at 300 × *g* at room temperature. After that, supernatants were removed, and sperm were re-suspended in 2 mL of C-TYH for the control, and 2 mL of F-TYH for the SER treatment. Samples were centrifuged for additional 5 min at 150 × *g* at room temperature, supernatants were removed, and sperm re-suspended in 500 μL of C-TYH for the CAP control and 500 μL of F-TYH for the SER treatment. Both sperm suspensions were incubated at 5% CO_2 at 37°C until sperm from F-TYH stopped moving (~40 min). Then, 1.5 mL of C-TYH was added to both CAP- and SER-treated sperm. Sperm suspensions were then centrifuged for 5 min at 150 × *g* at room temperature and 1.7 mL of supernatants was removed leaving the bottom 300 μL in the tubes. To maintain the initial sperm concentration, additional 200 μL of C-TYH was added to both samples.

Ca^{2+} Ionophore Treatment for IVF

Ca^{2+} ionophore 4Br-A_{23187} was used at a final concentration of 20 μM in C-TYH as previously described (Navarrete et al., 2016). Briefly, sperm were incubated with Ca^{2+} ionophore 4Br-A_{23187} for 10 min in 5% CO_2 at 37°C, and subsequently washed twice by mild 5 min centrifugations (150 × *g*) in C-TYH media. For SER and Ca^{2+} ionophore A_{23187} combination, SER treatment was done as explained above with minor modifications. At 35 min of incubation in F-TYH, just before sperm stopped their movement, Ca^{2+} ionophore 4Br-A_{23187} was added for 5 min. Next, 1.5 mL of C-TYH was added and the sperm suspension was centrifuged for 5 min at 150 × *g* at room temperature. Supernatant was removed, and 2 mL of C-TYH was added. Then, the sperm sample was centrifuged once more for 5 min at 150 × *g* and the supernatant removed leaving the bottom 300 μL in the tube. Additional 200 μL of C-TYH was added to reach a final volume of 500 μL.

Sperm Motility Video Recordings

Sperm were incubated in F-TYH or C-TYH as described above. The respective sperm suspensions (25 μL) were loaded into glass-bottom culture dishes (MatTek Corp., Ashland, MA, United States). Videos were captured using NIS-Elements software on a Nikon TE300 inverted microscope (Chiyoda, Tokyo, Japan) fitted with 20X objective lenses (Plan Apo, NA 0.75) and equipped with a cMOS camera (Andor Zyla, Belfast, Northern Ireland). Temperature of the samples was maintained at 37°C using a stage warmer (Frank E. Fryer scientific instruments, Carpentersville, IL, United States).

In vitro Fertilization

Metaphase II-arrested mouse oocytes were collected from 6–8-week-old super ovulated CD-1 (ICR) or C57BL/6J female mice (Charles River Laboratories, Wilmington, MA, United States) as previously described (Navarrete et al., 2015). Each female was injected with 7.5–10 IU PMSG and hCG 48 h apart. Super-ovulated females were then sacrificed 13 h post-hCG injection, oviducts were dissected, and cumulus-oocyte complexes (COCs) were collected in TL-HEPES medium [containing 114 mM NaCl, 3.22 mM KCl, 2.04 mM $CaCl_2.2H_2O$, 0.35 mM $NaH_2PO_4.2H_2O$, 0.49 mM $MgCl_2.6H_2O$, 2.02 mM $NaHCO_3$, 10 mM Lactic acid (sodium salt), and 10.1 mM Hepes]. Then, COCs were washed in C-TYH medium, and subsequently placed into a 90 μL drop of C-TYH covered with mineral oil previously equilibrated in an incubator with 5% CO_2 at 37°C. Fertilization drops containing two to three COCs (~40–60 eggs) were inseminated with 100,000 sperm incubated in different conditions as described above. Fertilization dishes were kept in an incubator with 5% CO_2 at 37°C. After 4 h of insemination, eggs were washed, put in fresh C-TYH media, and incubated overnight in 5% CO_2 at 37°C. Fertilization rates (in percentage) were evaluated 24 h post-insemination and were calculated as the total number of two-cell embryos divided by the total number of inseminated oocytes multiplied by 100.

Embryo Culture and Embryo Transfer

Twenty-four hours post-fertilization, two-cell embryos were transferred to drops containing KSOM media and further incubated for 3.5 days in 5% CO_2 at 37°C. At this stage, the percentage of blastocyst formation was evaluated. In some cases, 12–18 blastocysts were transferred to 2.5 days post-coitum (dpc) pseudo-pregnant CD-1 recipient females using the non-surgical uterine embryo transfer device NSET (Bin Ali et al., 2014). The number of blastocysts for transfer was selected considering the minimum number of blastocysts available which in all cases corresponded to those obtained from sperm incubated in standard capacitation media. The pseudo-pregnant CD-1 recipient females were obtained by mating with vasectomized males (obtained from Charles River) 2.5 days before the embryo transfers were performed. Only female mice with a visible plug were chosen as embryo recipients.

Blastocyst Nuclear Staining

A total cell count of 35 individual 3.5-day blastocysts for each condition (control or SER treatment) was performed. Embryos were removed from culture and washed two times in 100 μL drops of PBS containing 1 mg/mL BSA. Then, embryos were fixed in a 100-μL drop of paraformaldehyde solution [4% (w/v) in PBS, pH 7.4] for 20 min at room temperature and washed three times in 100 μL PBS-BSA. After that, embryos were transferred to a 100-μL drop of 1 μg/mL Hoechst 33342 (ThermoFisher Scientific, Agawam, MA, United States) in PBS-BSA and incubated for 10 min at room temperature. Then, embryos were washed two times in 100-μL drops of PBS-BSA and mounted on slides.

Images were taken using an A1 HD25 resonant scanning confocal microscope (Nikon) equipped with an sCMOS camera using a 40X (Plan Fluor, NA 1.3) objective. For each embryo, 10–12 z-stacks of 0.9 μm were taken, and cell number was calculated as the total number of nuclei stained per embryo.

Blastocysts Outgrowth Assay

Blastocysts were collected and transferred gently into a culture plate coated with 0.1% gelatin (Sigma–Aldrich, St. Louis, MO, United States) and cultured in DMEM (Lonza, Allendale, NJ, United States) containing 10% fetal calf serum (Atlanta Biologicals, Flowery Branch, GA, United States) and 1X GlutaMAX (Thermo Fisher Scientific, Agawam, MA, United States). Outgrowth assays were conducted at 37°C in a humidified atmosphere of 5% CO_2 for 3 days and were observed daily. Blastocysts outgrowth was considered positive when: (1) they were able to hatch out of the zona pellucida by 24 h, (2) they had attached to the culture plate by 48 h, and (3) they had formed inner cell mass (ICM) colonies with surrounding trophoblast cells at 72 h.

Bovine Sperm Preparation and SER Treatment

Bovine sperm were obtained from frozen semen samples kindly donated by American Breeder Services (DeForest, WI, United States). Sperm containing straws were thawed at 38°C for 1 min. After that, sperm were separated using a Percoll gradient (45%/90%) by centrifugation 600 × g for 15 min.

After Percoll centrifugation, sperm (5 × 10^6 spermatozoa/mL) were washed in 3 mL of either Sp-TALP [containing 100 mM NaCl, 3.1 mM KCl, 2.04 mM $CaCl_2.2H_2O$, 0.35 mM $NaH_2PO_4.2H_2O$, 0.4 mM $MgCl_2.6H_2O$, 25 mM $NaHCO_3$, 21.6 mM lactic acid (sodium salt), and 1 mM pyruvate] (Parrish et al., 1988) or pyruvate-lactate-free Sp-TALP (free-Sp-TALP) medium, and centrifuged at 150 × g for 5 min at room temperature. After that, supernatants were removed, and sperm were re-suspended in 0.5 mL of Sp-TALP for the control, and 0.5 mL of free-Sp-TALP for the SER treatment. Both sperm suspensions were incubated at 5% CO_2 at 38°C until sperm from free-Sp-TALP showed a considerable reduction in their motility (~3 h). Then, 1.5 mL of Sp-TALP was added to both control and SER-treated sperm. The samples were then centrifuged for 5 min at 150 × g at room temperature, 1.7 mL of supernatants was removed leaving the bottom 300 μL. Sperm were used for ICSI as explained below.

Bovine Intracytoplasmic Sperm Injection

Intracytoplasmic sperm injection was carried out as previously described (Kurokawa and Fissore, 2003), according to standard protocols, using Narishige manipulators (Medical System Corp., Great Neck, NY, United States) mounted on a Nikon diaphot microscope (Nikon Inc., Garden City, NY, United States). Before ICSI, oocytes were denuded of granulosa cells by gently pipetting in the presence of 1 mg/mL of hyaluronidase and selected by the presence of the first polar body. All matured oocytes were randomly allocated to groups. One part of the sperm suspension was mixed with one part of PBS containing 10% polyvinylpyrrolidone (PVP, M.W. 360 kDa; Sigma). Bovine sperm were immobilized by applying a few piezo pulses to the sperm tail, and the whole sperm was injected. Sperm were delivered into the oocyte's cytosol using a piezo micropipette-driving unit (Piezodrill; Burleigh Instruments Inc., Rochester, NY, United States).

Statistical Analysis

Data from all experiments were analyzed using SIGMA plot software[1]. Data are expressed as the means ± SEM. The difference

[1] www.sigmaplot.com

between groups mean values was analyzed by one-way analysis of variance (ANOVA) followed by Tukey's test. P-values < 0.05 were considered significant, and statistical significances were indicated in the figure legends.

ETHICS STATEMENT

The animal study was reviewed and approved by the University of Massachusetts, Amherst Institutional Animal Care and Use Committee (IACUC), protocol 2016-0026.

AUTHOR CONTRIBUTIONS

FN, MG, and PV were responsible for the organization and design of the whole work, data analysis, and preparation of manuscript. FN, LA, DM-H, DT, GL, GA, FG-V, and MG performed the experiments. AS, LL, JB, MB, AD, JM, MG, RF, and PV contributed with experimental design, animal protocols, discussion of findings, and correction of the manuscript.

FUNDING

This study was supported by NIH grants HD-038082 (to PV), HD-088571 (to JB, LL, and PV), and HD-92499 (to RF). FG-V was supported by Jiménez de la Espada Mobility Program-Fundación Séneca 2015 (19935/EE/15). DM-H was a recipient of a postdoctoral fellowship from the Government of Extremadura (Spain) and the Fondo Social Europeo (PO14005).

ACKNOWLEDGMENTS

The authors would like to thank Dr. Peter Greer for the donation of $Fer^{DR/DR}$ mice. Confocal images were taken at the Light Microscopy Facility and Nikon Center of Excellence at the Institute for Applied Life Sciences, University of Massachusetts Amherst, which is supported by the Massachusetts Life Sciences Center.

SUPPLEMENTARY MATERIAL

FIGURE S1 | Sperm energy restriction and recovery (SER) treatment improves fertilization and embryo development rates in C57BL/6J male mice of different ages. Sperm obtained from C57BL/6J mice of different ages were incubated in C-TYH, containing glucose and pyruvate (CAP) or in F-TYH media, not containing nutrients; sperm in this medium will then be rescued by energy sources replenishment as explained in Methods, and the treatment abbreviated (SER). After treatment (CAP or SER) sperm from each condition were added to the insemination drops containing cumulus-enclosed female oocytes (COCs). In all cases, left panels represent percentages of fertilization calculated as the percentage of oocytes that reached 2-cell embryo stage. Middle panels represent percentages of blastocyst formation calculated as percentage of the 2-cell embryos that reached a 3.5-day blastocyst stage. Right panels represent percentages of total blastocysts calculated as the percentage of 3.5-day blastocyst stage embryos out of the total number of inseminated eggs. **(A–C)** Results from IVF and embryo cultures after heterologous fertilization between CD1 female oocytes and 2–6 months old C57BL/6J sperm (**A**, $n = 18$); 7–12 months old C57BL/6J sperm (**B**, $n = 10$); or 13–24 months old C57BL/6J sperm (**C**, $n = 10$). **(D–F)** Results from IVF and embryo culture after homologous fertilization between C57BL/6J female oocytes and 2–6 months old C57BL/6J sperm (**D**, $n = 5$); 7–12 months old C57BL/6J sperm (**E**, $n = 5$); or 13–24 months old C57BL/6J sperm (**F**, $n = 5$). In each panel, statistically significant differences are indicated as: $^{*}p < 0.05$; $^{**}p < 0.01$, and $^{***}p < 0.001$.

TABLE S1 | Compilation of IVF, embryo development, and pups born after embryo transfer.

VIDEO S1 | Sperm energy restriction and recovery (SER) treatment. Sperm were incubated in F-TYH at 5% CO_2 at 37°C until stopped moving (~40 min). Then, an aliquot was loaded into glass-bottom culture dishes and filmed in an inverted microscope as explained in Methods. C-TYH was added after 10 sec of recording and sperm regained motility.

REFERENCES

Aguila, L., Felmer, R., Arias, M. E., Navarrete, F., Martin-Hidalgo, D., Lee, H. C., et al. (2017). Defective sperm head decondensation undermines the success of ICSI in the bovine. *Reproduction* 154, 307–318. doi: 10.1530/REP-17-0270

Aitken, R. J. (2017). Reactive oxygen species as mediators of sperm capacitation and pathological damage. *Mol. Reprod. Dev.* 84, 1039–1052. doi: 10.1002/mrd.22871

Alvau, A., Battistone, M. A., Gervasi, M. G., Navarrete, F. A., Xu, X., Sanchez-Cardenas, C., et al. (2016). The tyrosine kinase FER is responsible for the capacitation-associated increase in tyrosine phosphorylation in murine sperm. *Development* 143, 2325–2333. doi: 10.1242/dev.136499

Behringer, R., Gertsenstein, M., Vintersten Nagy, K., and Nagy, A. (2014). "Assisted Reproduction: Ovary transplantation, *in vitro* fertilization, artificial insemination, and intracytoplasmic sperm injection," in *Manipulating the Mouse Embryo: A Laboratory Manual*, Fourth Edn, eds J. Cuddihy, R. Behringer, M. Gertsenstein, K. Vintersten Nagy, and A. Nagy, (Cold Spring Harbor, NY: Cold Spring Harbor Laboratory Press), 593–600.

Bin Ali, R., van der Ahe, F., Braumuller, T. M., Pritchard, C., Krimpenfort, P., Berns, A., et al. (2014). Improved pregnancy and birth rates with routine application of nonsurgical embryo transfer. *Transgenic Res.* 23, 691–695. doi: 10.1007/s11248-014-9802-3

Binder, N. K., Hannan, N. J., and Gardner, D. K. (2015). *In vitro* embryo outgrowth is a bioassay of *in vivo* embryo implantation and development. *Asian Pac. J. Reprod.* 4, 240–241. doi: 10.1016/j.apjr.2015.06.009

Canel, N. G., Bevacqua, R. J., Hiriart, M. I., Rabelo, N. C., de Almeida Camargo, L. S., Romanato, M., et al. (2017). Sperm pretreatment with heparin and l-glutathione, sex-sorting, and double cryopreservation to improve intracytoplasmic sperm injection in bovine. *Theriogenology* 93, 62–70. doi: 10.1016/j.theriogenology.2016.12.018

Canovas, S., Ross, P. J., Kelsey, G., and Coy, P. (2017). DNA methylation in embryo development: epigenetic impact of ART (Assisted Reproductive Technologies). *Bioessays* 39:1700106. doi: 10.1002/bies.201700106

Castello, D., Motato, Y., Basile, N., Remohi, J., Espejo-Catena, M., and Meseguer, M. (2016). How much have we learned from time-lapse in clinical IVF? *Mol. Hum. Reprod.* 22, 719–727. doi: 10.1093/molehr/gaw056

Catt, J. W., and Rhodes, S. L. (1995). Comparative intracytoplasmic sperm injection (ICSI) in human and domestic species. *Reprod. Fertil. Dev.* 7, 161–166.

Chen, Q., Yan, M., Cao, Z., Li, X., Zhang, Y., Shi, J., et al. (2016). Sperm tsRNAs contribute to intergenerational inheritance of an acquired metabolic disorder. *Science* 351, 397–400. doi: 10.1126/science.aad7977

Conine, C. C., Sun, F., Song, L., Rivera-Perez, J. A., and Rando, O. J. (2018). Small RNAs gained during epididymal transit of sperm are essential for embryonic development in mice. *Dev. Cell* 46, 470–480.e3. doi: 10.1016/j.devcel.2018.06.024

Craig, A. W., Zirngibl, R., Williams, K., Cole, L. A., and Greer, P. A. (2001). Mice devoid of fer protein-tyrosine kinase activity are viable and fertile but display reduced cortactin phosphorylation. *Mol. Cell. Biol.* 21, 603–613. doi: 10.1128/mcb.21.2.603-613.2001

de Lamirande, E., and Gagnon, C. (1995). Impact of reactive oxygen species on spermatozoa: a balancing act between beneficial and detrimental effects. *Hum. Reprod.* 10(Suppl. 1), 15–21. doi: 10.1093/humrep/10.suppl_1.15

de Mouzon, J., Goossens, V., Bhattacharya, S., Castilla, J. A., Ferraretti, A. P., Korsak, V., et al. (2010). Assisted reproductive technology in Europe, 2006: results generated from European registers by ESHRE. *Hum. Reprod.* 25, 1851–1862. doi: 10.1093/humrep/deq124

De Vos, A., Polyzos, N. P., Verheyen, G., and Tournaye, H. (2013). Intracytoplasmic morphologically selected sperm injection (IMSI): a critical and evidence-based review. *Basic Clin. Androl.* 23:10. doi: 10.1186/2051-4190-23-10

Geary, S., and Moon, Y. S. (2006). The human embryo *in vitro*: recent progress. *J. Reprod. Med.* 51, 293–302.

Gervasi, M. G., and Visconti, P. E. (2016). Chang's meaning of capacitation: a molecular perspective. *Mol. Reprod. Dev.* 83, 860–874. doi: 10.1002/mrd.22663

Goodson, S. G., Qiu, Y., Sutton, K. A., Xie, G., Jia, W., and O'Brien, D. A. (2012). Metabolic substrates exhibit differential effects on functional parameters of mouse sperm capacitation. *Biol. Reprod.* 87:75.

Goodson, S. G., Zhang, Z., Tsuruta, J. K., Wang, W., and O'Brien, D. A. (2011). Classification of mouse sperm motility patterns using an automated multiclass support vector machines model. *Biol. Reprod.* 84, 1207–1215. doi: 10.1095/biolreprod.110.088989

Goswami, G., Sharma, M., Jugga, D., and Gouri, D. M. (2018). Can intracytoplasmic morphologically selected spermatozoa injection be used as first choice of treatment for severe male factor infertility patients? *J. Hum. Reprod. Sci.* 11, 40–44. doi: 10.4103/jhrs.JHRS_74_17

Hamilton, L. E., Suzuki, J., Aguila, L., Meinsohn, M. C., Smith, O. E., Protopapas, N., et al. (2019). Sperm-borne glutathione-S-transferase omega 2 accelerates the nuclear decondensation of spermatozoa during fertilization in mice. *Biol. Reprod.* 101, 368–376. doi: 10.1093/biolre/ioz082

Ihara, M., Kinoshita, A., Yamada, S., Tanaka, H., Tanigaki, A., Kitano, A., et al. (2005). Cortical organization by the septin cytoskeleton is essential for structural and mechanical integrity of mammalian spermatozoa. *Dev. Cell* 8, 343–352. doi: 10.1016/j.devcel.2004.12.005

Jaakma, U., Zhang, B. R., Larsson, B., Niwa, K., and Rodriguez-Martinez, H. (1997). Effects of sperm treatments on the *in vitro* development of bovine oocytes in semidefined and defined media. *Theriogenology* 48, 711–720. doi: 10.1016/s0093-691x(97)00295-1

Jung, Y. H., Kremsky, I., Gold, H. B., Rowley, M. J., Punyawai, K., Buonanotte, A., et al. (2019). Maintenance of CTCF- and transcription factor-mediated interactions from the gametes to the early mouse embryo. *Mol. Cell* 75, 154.e5–171.e5. doi: 10.1016/j.molcel.2019.04.014

Jung, Y. H., Sauria, M. E. G., Lyu, X., Cheema, M. S., Ausio, J., Taylor, J., et al. (2017). Chromatin states in mouse sperm correlate with embryonic and adult regulatory landscapes. *Cell Rep.* 18, 1366–1382. doi: 10.1016/j.celrep.2017.01.034

Kuretake, S., Maleszewski, M., Tokumasu, A., Fujimoto, H., and Yanagimachi, R. (1996). Inadequate function of sterile tw5/tw32 spermatozoa overcome by intracytoplasmic sperm injection. *Mol. Reprod. Dev.* 44, 230–233. doi: 10.1002/(sici)1098-2795(199606)44:2<230::aid-mrd12>3.3.co;2-j

Kurokawa, M., and Fissore, R. A. (2003). ICSI-generated mouse zygotes exhibit altered calcium oscillations, inositol 1,4,5-trisphosphate receptor-1 down-regulation, and embryo development. *Mol. Hum. Reprod.* 9, 523–533. doi: 10.1093/molehr/gag072

Liu, L., Nutter, L. M., Law, N., and McKerlie, C. (2009). Sperm freezing and *in vitro* fertilization in three substrains of C57BL/6 mice. *J. Am. Assoc. Lab. Anim. Sci.* 48, 39–43.

Luna, D., Hilario, R., Duenas-Chacon, J., Romero, R., Zavala, P., Villegas, L., et al. (2015). The IMSI procedure improves laboratory and clinical outcomes without compromising the aneuploidy rate when compared to the classical ICSI procedure. *Clin. Med. Insights Reprod. Health* 9, 29–37. doi: 10.4137/CMRH.S33032

Malcuit, C., Maserati, M., Takahashi, Y., Page, R., and Fissore, R. A. (2006). Intracytoplasmic sperm injection in the bovine induces abnormal [Ca2+]i responses and oocyte activation. *Reprod. Fertil. Dev.* 18, 39–51.

Mantikou, E., Youssef, M. A., van Wely, M., van der Veen, F., Al-Inany, H. G., Repping, S., et al. (2013). Embryo culture media and IVF/ICSI success rates: a systematic review. *Hum. Reprod. Update* 19, 210–220. doi: 10.1093/humupd/dms061

Marcho, C., Cui, W., and Mager, J. (2015). Epigenetic dynamics during preimplantation development. *Reproduction* 150, R109–R120. doi: 10.1530/REP-15-0180

Matas, C., Coy, P., Romar, R., Marco, M., Gadea, J., and Ruiz, S. (2003). Effect of sperm preparation method on *in vitro* fertilization in pigs. *Reproduction* 125, 133–141. doi: 10.1530/reprod/125.1.133

Meldrum, D. R., Casper, R. F., Diez-Juan, A., Simon, C., Domar, A. D., and Frydman, R. (2016). Aging and the environment affect gamete and embryo potential: can we intervene? *Fertil. Steril.* 105, 548–559. doi: 10.1016/j.fertnstert.2016.01.013

Miki, K., Qu, W., Goulding, E. H., Willis, W. D., Bunch, D. O., Strader, L. F., et al. (2004). Glyceraldehyde 3-phosphate dehydrogenase-S, a sperm-specific glycolytic enzyme, is required for sperm motility and male fertility. *Proc. Natl. Acad. Sci. U.S.A.* 101, 16501–16506. doi: 10.1073/pnas.0407708101

Navarrete, F. A., Alvau, A., Lee, H. C., Levin, L. R., Buck, J., Leon, P. M., et al. (2016). Transient exposure to calcium ionophore enables *in vitro* fertilization in sterile mouse models. *Sci. Rep.* 6:33589. doi: 10.1038/srep33589

Navarrete, F. A., Garcia-Vazquez, F. A., Alvau, A., Escoffier, J., Krapf, D., Sanchez-Cardenas, C., et al. (2015). Biphasic role of calcium in mouse sperm capacitation signaling pathways. *J. Cell. Physiol.* 230, 1758–1769. doi: 10.1002/jcp.24873

Palermo, G. D., O'Neill, C. L., Chow, S., Cheung, S., Parrella, A., Pereira, N., et al. (2017). Intracytoplasmic sperm injection: state of the art in humans. *Reproduction* 154, F93–F110. doi: 10.1530/REP-17-0374

Parrish, J. J., Susko-Parrish, J., Winer, M. A., and First, N. L. (1988). Capacitation of bovine sperm by heparin. *Biol. Reprod.* 38, 1171–1180.

Patrizio, P., Bianchi, V., Lalioti, M. D., Gerasimova, T., and Sakkas, D. (2007). High rate of biological loss in assisted reproduction: it is in the seed, not in the soil. *Reprod. Biomed. Online* 14, 92–95. doi: 10.1016/s1472-6483(10)60769-9

Perez-Cerezales, S., Laguna-Barraza, R., de Castro, A. C., Sanchez-Calabuig, M. J., Cano-Oliva, E., de Castro-Pita, F. J., et al. (2018). Sperm selection by thermotaxis improves ICSI outcome in mice. *Sci. Rep.* 8:2902. doi: 10.1038/s41598-018-21335-8

Ren, D., Navarro, B., Perez, G., Jackson, A. C., Hsu, S., Shi, Q., et al. (2001). A sperm ion channel required for sperm motility and male fertility. *Nature* 413, 603–609. doi: 10.1038/35098027

Rho, G. J., Kawarsky, S., Johnson, W. H., Kochhar, K., and Betteridge, K. J. (1998). Sperm and oocyte treatments to improve the formation of male and female pronuclei and subsequent development following intracytoplasmic sperm injection into bovine oocytes. *Biol. Reprod.* 59, 918–924. doi: 10.1095/biolreprod59.4.918

Sadeghi, M. R. (2017). Poor quality embryos hamper the development of high quality ones. *J. Reprod. Infertil.* 18, 211–212.

Salamone, D. F., Canel, N. G., and Rodriguez, M. B. (2017). Intracytoplasmic sperm injection in domestic and wild mammals. *Reproduction* 154, F111–F124. doi: 10.1530/REP-17-0357

Sanchez-Cardenas, C., Montoya, F., Navarrete, F. A., Hernandez-Cruz, A., Corkidi, G., Visconti, P. E., et al. (2018). Intracellular Ca2+ threshold reversibly switches flagellar beat off and on. *Biol. Reprod.* 99, 1010–1021. doi: 10.1093/biolre/ioy132

Saunders, C. M., Larman, M. G., Parrington, J., Cox, L. J., Royse, J., Blayney, L. M., et al. (2002). PLC zeta: a sperm-specific trigger of Ca(2+) oscillations in eggs and embryo development. *Development* 129, 3533–3544.

Sharma, U., Conine, C. C., Shea, J. M., Boskovic, A., Derr, A. G., Bing, X. Y., et al. (2016). Biogenesis and function of tRNA fragments during sperm maturation and fertilization in mammals. *Science* 351, 391–396. doi: 10.1126/science.aad6780

Summers, M. C. (2013). A brief history of the development of the KSOM family of media. *J. Assist. Reprod. Genet.* 30, 995–999. doi: 10.1007/s10815-013-0097-8

Takeuchi, M., Seki, M., Furukawa, E., Takahashi, A., Saito, K., Kobayashi, M., et al. (2017). Improvement of implantation potential in mouse blastocysts derived from IVF by combined treatment with prolactin, epidermal growth factor and 4-hydroxyestradiol. *Mol. Hum. Reprod.* 23, 557–570. doi: 10.1093/molehr/gax035

Toyoda, Y., and Yokoyama, M. (2016). The early history of the TYH medium for *in vitro* fertilization of mouse ova. *J. Mamm. Ova Res.* 33, 3–10. doi: 10.1274/032.033.0103

Toyoda, Y., Yokoyama, M., and Hosi, T. (1971). Studies on the fertilization of mouse eggs *in vitro*. I. *In vitro* fertilization of eggs by fresh epididymal sperm. *Jpn. J. Anim. Reprod.* 16, 147–151.

Vaiarelli, A., Cimadomo, D., Capalbo, A., Orlando, G., Sapienza, F., Colamaria, S., et al. (2016). Pre-implantation genetic testing in ART: who will benefit and what is the evidence? *J. Assist. Reprod. Genet.* 33, 1273–1278. doi: 10.1007/s10815-016-0785-2

Ventura-Junca, P., Irarrazaval, I., Rolle, A. J., Gutierrez, J. I., Moreno, R. D., and Santos, M. J. (2015). *In vitro* fertilization (IVF) in mammals: epigenetic and developmental alterations. Scientific and bioethical implications for IVF in humans. *Biol. Res.* 48:68. doi: 10.1186/s40659-015-0059-y

White, M. D., Zenker, J., Bissiere, S., and Plachta, N. (2018). Instructions for assembling the early mammalian embryo. *Dev. Cell* 45, 667–679. doi: 10.1016/j.devcel.2018.05.013

Yanagimachi, R. (1994). "Mammalian fertilization," in *The Phyisiology of Reproduction*, eds E. Knobil, and J. D. Neill, (New York, NY: Raven Press), 189–317.

Yanagimachi, R., Wakayama, T., Kishikawa, H., Fimia, G. M., Monaco, L., and Sassone-Corsi, P. (2004). Production of fertile offspring from genetically infertile male mice. *Proc. Natl. Acad. Sci. U.S.A.* 101, 1691–1695. doi: 10.1073/pnas.0307832100

Zheng, W. W., Song, G., Wang, Q. L., Liu, S. W., Zhu, X. L., Deng, S. M., et al. (2018). Sperm DNA damage has a negative effect on early embryonic development following *in vitro* fertilization. *Asian J. Androl.* 20, 75–79. doi: 10.4103/aja.aja_19_17

Permissions

All chapters in this book were first published by Frontiers; hereby published with permission under the Creative Commons Attribution License or equivalent. Every chapter published in this book has been scrutinized by our experts. Their significance has been extensively debated. The topics covered herein carry significant findings which will fuel the growth of the discipline. They may even be implemented as practical applications or may be referred to as a beginning point for another development.

The contributors of this book come from diverse backgrounds, making this book a truly international effort. This book will bring forth new frontiers with its revolutionizing research information and detailed analysis of the nascent developments around the world.

We would like to thank all the contributing authors for lending their expertise to make the book truly unique. They have played a crucial role in the development of this book. Without their invaluable contributions this book wouldn't have been possible. They have made vital efforts to compile up to date information on the varied aspects of this subject to make this book a valuable addition to the collection of many professionals and students.

This book was conceptualized with the vision of imparting up-to-date information and advanced data in this field. To ensure the same, a matchless editorial board was set up. Every individual on the board went through rigorous rounds of assessment to prove their worth. After which they invested a large part of their time researching and compiling the most relevant data for our readers.

The editorial board has been involved in producing this book since its inception. They have spent rigorous hours researching and exploring the diverse topics which have resulted in the successful publishing of this book. They have passed on their knowledge of decades through this book. To expedite this challenging task, the publisher supported the team at every step. A small team of assistant editors was also appointed to further simplify the editing procedure and attain best results for the readers.

Apart from the editorial board, the designing team has also invested a significant amount of their time in understanding the subject and creating the most relevant covers. They scrutinized every image to scout for the most suitable representation of the subject and create an appropriate cover for the book.

The publishing team has been an ardent support to the editorial, designing and production team. Their endless efforts to recruit the best for this project, has resulted in the accomplishment of this book. They are a veteran in the field of academics and their pool of knowledge is as vast as their experience in printing. Their expertise and guidance has proved useful at every step. Their uncompromising quality standards have made this book an exceptional effort. Their encouragement from time to time has been an inspiration for everyone.

The publisher and the editorial board hope that this book will prove to be a valuable piece of knowledge for researchers, students, practitioners and scholars across the globe.

List of Contributors

Upasna Sharma
Department of Molecular, Cell and Developmental Biology, University of California, Santa Cruz, CA, United States

Souvik Dey, Cameron Brothag and Srinivasan Vijayaraghavan
Department of Biological Sciences, Kent State University, Kent, OH, United States

Gerhard van der Horst and Liana Maree
Department of Medical Biosciences, University of the Western Cape, Bellville, South Africa

Sanet H. Kotzé
Division of Clinical Anatomy, Department of Biomedical Sciences, Stellenbosch University, Stellenbosch, South Africa

M. Justin O'Riain
Institute for Communities and Wildlife in Africa, Department of Biological Sciences, University of Cape Town, Cape Town, South Africa

Alaaeldin Saleh, Angelos Thanassoulas, Bared Safieh-Garabedian and Michail Nomikos
Member of QU Health, College of Medicine, Qatar University, Doha, Qatar

Junaid Kashir
College of Medicine, Alfaisal University, Riyadh, Saudi Arabia
Department of Comparative Medicine, King Faisal Specialist Hospital and Research Center, Riyadh, Saudi Arabia
School of Biosciences, Cardiff University, Cardiff, United Kingdom

F. Anthony Lai
Member of QU Health, College of Medicine, Qatar University, Doha, Qatar
Biomedical Research Center, Qatar University, Doha, Qatar

Carla Ritagliati, Cintia Stival, Darío Krapf and Carolina Baro Graf
CONICET-UNR, Laboratoty of Cell Signal Transduction Networks, Instituto de Biología Molecular y Celular de Rosario, Rosario, Argentina
UNR, Laboratorio de Medicina Reproductiva, Facultad de Ciencias Bioquímicas y Farmacéuticas, Rosario, Argentina

Paula A. Balestrini and Mariano G. Buffone
Consejo Nacional de Investigaciones Científicas y Tecnológicas, Instituto de Biología y Medicina Experimental, Buenos Aires, Argentina

Hui Gao
State Key Laboratory of Stem Cell and Reproductive Biology, Institute of Zoology, Chinese Academy of Sciences, Beijing, China

Muhammad Babar Khawar and Wei Li
State Key Laboratory of Stem Cell and Reproductive Biology, Institute of Zoology, Chinese Academy of Sciences, Beijing, China
University of Chinese Academy of Sciences, Beijing, China

Emily L. Fishman
Department of Biological Sciences, College of Natural Sciences and Mathematics, The University of Toledo, Toledo, OH, United States

Tomer Avidor-Reiss, Matthew Mazur and Puneet Sindhwani
Department of Biological Sciences, College of Natural Sciences and Mathematics, The University of Toledo, Toledo, OH, United States
Department of Urology, College of Medicine and Life Sciences, The University of Toledo, Toledo, OH, United States

Katarzyna Kent and Thomas X. Garcia
Department of Pathology & Immunology, Baylor College of Medicine, Houston, TX, United States
Department of Biology and Biotechnology, University of Houston–Clear Lake, Houston, TX, United States
Center for Drug Discovery, Baylor College of Medicine, Houston, TX, United States

Madelaine Johnston and Natasha Strump
Department of Pathology & Immunology, Baylor College of Medicine, Houston, TX, United States
Center for Drug Discovery, Baylor College of Medicine, Houston, TX, United States

Carolina Baro Graf and Dario Krapf
Laboratory of Cell Signal Transduction Networks, Instituto de Biología Molecular y Celular de Rosario (IBR), CONICET-UNR, Rosario, Argentina
Laboratorio de Medicina Reproductiva, Facultad de Ciencias Bioquímicas y Farmacéuticas, Universidad Nacional de Rosario, Rosario, Argentina

Valentina Torres-Monserrat and Carlos Carizza
Fertya, Medicina Reproductiva, Rosario, Argentina

Mariano G. Buffone
Instituto de Biología y Medicina Experimental (IBYME), CONICET, Buenos Aires, Argentina

Iván Oseguera-López
Unidad Iztapalapa, Universidad Autónoma Metropolitana, Mexico City, Mexico

Priscila Ramos-Ibeas and Serafín Pérez-Cerezales
Department of Animal Reproduction, Instituto Nacional de Investigación y Tecnología Agraria y Alimentaria, Madrid, Spain

Sara Ruiz-Díaz
Mistral Fertility Clinics S.L., Clínica Tambre, Madrid, Spain
Department of Animal Reproduction, Instituto Nacional de Investigación y Tecnología Agraria y Alimentaria, Madrid, Spain

Lis C. Puga Molina, Stephanie Gunderson, Joan Riley, Aluet Borrego-Alvarez, Emily S. Jungheim and Celia M. Santi
Department of Obstetrics & Gynecology, Washington University School of Medicine, St Louis, MO, United States

Pascal Lybaert
Laboratory of Experimental Hormonology, School of Medicine, Université Libre de Bruxelles, Brussels, Belgium

Judit Castillo, Orleigh Adeleccia Bogle, Meritxell Jodar and David Delgado-Dueñas
Molecular Biology of Reproduction and Development Research Group, Institut d'Investigacions Biomèdiques August Pi I Sunyer (IDIBAPS), Fundació Clínic per a la Recerca Biomèdica, Department of Biomedical Sciences, Faculty of Medicine and Health Sciences, Universitat de Barcelona, Barcelona, Spain

Forough Torabi and David Miller
LIGHT Laboratories, Leeds Institute of Cardiovascular and Metabolic Medicine, University of Leeds, Leeds, United Kingdom

Josep Maria Estanyol
Proteomics Unit, Scientific and Technical Services, Universitat de Barcelona, Barcelona, Spain

Josep Lluís Ballescà
Clinic Institute of Gynaecology, Obstetrics and Neonatology, Hospital Clínic, Barcelona, Spain

Rafael Oliva
Biochemistry and Molecular Genetics Service, Hospital Clínic, Barcelona, Spain

Muhammet Rasit Ugur Thu Dinh and Erdogan Memili
Department of Animal and Dairy Sciences, Mississippi State University, Starkville, MS, United States

Mustafa Hitit
Department of Animal and Dairy Sciences, Mississippi State University, Starkville, MS, United State
Department of Animal Genetics, Kastamonu University, Kastamonu, Turkey

Abdullah Kaya
Department of Reproduction and Artificial Insemination, Selçuk University, Konya, Turkey

Einko Topper and Bradley Didion
Alta Genetics, Inc., Watertown, WI, United States

Brett Nixon, Ilana R. Bernstein, Shenae L. Cafe, Amanda L. Anderson, Natalie A. Trigg, Andrew L. Eamens, Tessa Lord and Geoffry N. De Iuliis
Priority Research Centre for Reproductive Science, School of Environmental and Life Sciences, Discipline of Biological Sciences, The University of Newcastle, Callaghan, NSW, Australia
Pregnancy and Reproduction Program, Hunter Medical Research Institute, New Lambton Heights, NSW, Australia

Maryse Delehedde
SPQI - 4BioDx-Breeding Section, Lille, France

Nicolas Sergeant
SPQI - 4BioDx-Breeding Section, Lille, France
University of Lille, INSERM UMRS, Lille, France

Matthew D. Dun
Cancer Signalling Research Group, School of Biomedical Sciences and Pharmacy, Faculty of Health and Medicine, University of Newcastle, Callaghan, NSW, Australia
Priority Research Centre for Cancer Research Innovation and Translation, Hunter Medical Research Institute, New Lambton Heights, NSW, Australia

Elizabeth G. Bromfield
Priority Research Centre for Reproductive Science, School of Environmental and Life Sciences, Discipline of Biological Sciences, The University of Newcastle, Callaghan, NSW, Australia
Pregnancy and Reproduction Program, Hunter Medical Research Institute, New Lambton Heights, NSW, Australia
Department of Biochemistry and Cell Biology, Faculty of Veterinary Medicine, Utrecht University, Utrecht, Netherlands

Julio C. Chávez, Alberto Darszon, Claudia L. Treviño and Takuya Nishigaki
Departamento de Genética del Desarrollo y Fisiología Molecular, Instituto de Biotecnología, Universidad Nacional Autónoma de México, Cuernavaca, Mexico

Raúl Fernández-González, Ricardo Laguna, Priscila Ramos-Ibeas, Eva Pericuesta, Víctor Alcalde-Lopez, Serafín Perez-Cerezales and Alfonso Gutierrez-Adan
Departamento de Reproducción Animal, INIA, Madrid, Spain

Felipe A. Navarrete, Luis Aguila, Darya A. Tourzani, Goli Ardestani, Jesse Mager, Rafael A. Fissore, Ana M. Salicioni, María G. Gervasi and Pablo E. Visconti
Department of Veterinary and Animal Sciences, Integrated Sciences Building, University of Massachusetts Amherst, Amherst, MA, United States

David Martin-Hidalgo
Department of Veterinary and Animal Sciences, Integrated Sciences Building, University of Massachusetts Amherst, Amherst, MA, United States
Research Group of Intracellular Signaling and Technology of Reproduction, Institute of Biotechnology in Agriculture and Livestock (INBIO G C C), University of Extremadura, Cáceres, Spain

Guillermina M. Luque and Mariano G. Buffone
Instituto de Biología y Medicina Experimental, Consejo Nacional de Investigaciones Científicas y Técnicas, Buenos Aires, Argentina

Francisco A. Garcia-Vazquez
Department of Physiology, Veterinary School, International Excellence Campus for Higher Education and Research, University of Murcia, Murcia, Spain
Institute for Biomedical Research of Murcia, IMIB-Arrixaca, Murcia, Spain

Lonny R. Levin and Jochen Buck
Department of Pharmacology, Weill Cornell Medical College, Cornell University, New York, NY, United States

Index

www.ingramcontent.com/pod-product-compliance
Lightning Source LLC
LaVergne TN
LVHW060058220926
848484LV00008BA/2188